Atlas of NUCLEAR MEDICINE

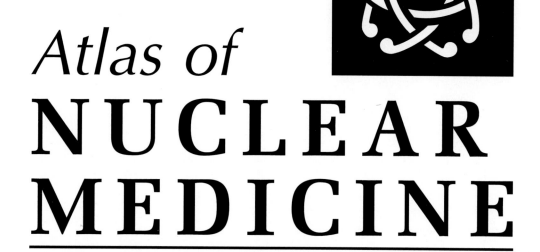

Marc Coel, M.D.
Director, Nuclear Medicine
The Queen's Medical Center
Professor of Radiology
John A. Burns School of Medicine
University of Hawaii
Honolulu, Hawaii

Jimmy Leung, M.D.
University of Hawaii
Honolulu, Hawaii
currently at
Hospital of the University of Pennsylvania
Resident, Department of Radiology
Philadelphia, Pennsylvania

W.B. SAUNDERS COMPANY
A Division of Harcourt Brace & Company
Philadelphia   London   Toronto   Montreal   Sydney   Tokyo

W.B. SAUNDERS COMPANY
A Division of Harcourt Brace & Company

The Curtis Center
Independence Square West
Philadelphia, Pennsylvania 19106

Library of Congress Cataloging-in-Publication Data

Coel, Marc.
 Atlas of nuclear medicine / Marc Coel, Jimmy Leung.

   p.   cm.

 ISBN 0–7216–3578–4

  1. Radioisotope scanning—Atlases.   I. Leung, Jimmy.   II. Title.
  [DNLM: 1. Radionuclide Imaging—atlases.   2. Nuclear Medicine—
atlases.   WN 17 C672a 1996]

 RC78.7.R4C64 1996   616.07′575′0222—dc20

 DNLM/DLC   96–16717

Atlas of Nuclear Medicine   ISBN 0–7216–3578–4

Printed in the United States of America

Last digit is the print number: 9   8   7   6   5   4   3   2   1

Dedicated to our parents,
who gave us the desire to learn,
and our wives, who helped us learn.

Foreword

The initial interpretation of a nuclear medicine procedure is made without any prior information that might introduce bias. At this stage, the results are considered "working diagnoses," expressed as the names of diseases and the probability that each is present.

It is essential that the nuclear medicine physician know the conditional probability of observing specific results of the nuclear medicine procedure as they are observed in different diseases. The probability that a finding is present is referred to as the sensitivity of the finding for the specific disease. The probability that the same finding will be observed in all other diseases or in normal persons is called the specificity of the finding. Knowledge of both is essential.

As the diagnostic process goes forward, the physician forms a dichotomy consisting of the set of diseases that the patient may have and a set of diseases that he or she probably does not have. Working diagnoses are reached at several stages: after the taking of the medical history; after the physical examination; after discussion with the patient's other physicians; after other diagnostic tests, including nuclear medicine procedures, are obtained; and during further observations of the course of the patient's illness. The physician can wait in making decisions until a sufficient amount of information is available.

This book is organized according to the international classification of diseases, which begins by classifying a disease according to its anatomic location, and then according to its etiology (such as congenital, metabolic, and so forth). This is called the gamut approach. The authors begin by describing findings in the nuclear medicine images, such as solitary skeletal lesions, as distinct from multiple lesions, and then relate these to different diseases.

The great value of the atlas is that it is based on the extensive personal experience of the authors, supplemented by cases provided by others. There are examples of most manifestations of disease found in nuclear medicine, with several variations of individual entities. This is of greatest value to the practicing nuclear medicine physician, who can use this book to help with unusual presentations of disease or to reconfirm a diagnosis.

This new atlas will help educate medical students and residents in nuclear medicine and other specialties in the objective interpretation of the findings in nuclear medicine procedures. It will aid the practicing nuclear medicine physician in building a differential diagnosis.

The atlas should be kept close at hand in all nuclear medicine departments and should be used in conjunction with textbooks that can provide details of the theory, techniques, and usefulness of the procedures.

Because of the ever-increasing number of valuable nuclear medicine procedures, this new atlas can be recommended with great enthusiasm to all practitioners of nuclear medicine and students. They should find the cases, techniques, tips, algorithms, and gamut lists informative and easy to use.

HENRY N. WAGNER, JR., M.D.

Preface

When this nuclear medicine atlas was first conceived, we had two groups of people in mind—the practicing nuclear medicine physician and trainees. This focus was especially appropriate, as the authors are an experienced practicing nuclear medicine physician and a resident in radiology. For the clinical practitioner we hope that this book will serve as a quick reference to examples of disease entities, both classic and variant. We felt that including variant cases was particularly important, as these represent many of the "problem cases" in clinical practice. As much as possible, multiple relevant examples of disease entities are included to pictorially describe a spectrum of clinical presentations.

On the other side of the coin, different disease entities can present similarly on nuclear imaging. Hence, we designed a book of "image gamuts," combining the gamuts format with a clinical atlas. The chapters are organized by organ systems, with the notable exception of the infection and tumor chapters. Each chapter is divided into sections based on broad categories of scan findings (e.g., solitary bony abnormalities, multiple bony abnormalities, and so on). The individual clinical cases in each section are presented in the order of normal to disease in various pathologic categories. Wherever relevant, the cases are presented in the following order:

1. Normal/Normal Variant
2. Congenital Conditions
3. Autoimmune Disorders/ Arthritides
4. Metabolic Disorders
5. Infectious/Inflammatory Diseases
6. Trauma and Postsurgical Abnormalities
7. Vascular Disorders
8. Neoplastic Diseases
9. Miscellaneous

Two major exceptions are the infection chapter and the tumor chapter, which for obvious reasons, could not be divided in this manner. Furthermore, there are numerous cases that, for various reasons, could have fit into more than one chapter or section. For this reason, we have included redundancy (e.g., lung tumor cases in both the lung chapter and the tumor chapter). There are many cross references to guide the reader to similar or related cases in other parts of the book. As much as possible, we attempted to arrange the cases in an order that would entice the reader to continue on.

A number of differential diagnoses are also included among the images. As this was not intended to be a written text, lists and prose are kept brief. We have refrained from using references but would like to acknowledge the innumerable authors who have contributed to our body of knowledge. We thank all those who shared their research experiences. We suggest using this atlas in conjunction with a full-scale reference work, such as the text written by Dr. F. Datz[1] and the one by Dr. Henry Wagner Jr.[2] Algorithms and some points on technique are also included in this atlas. The algorithms are intended as suggestions to the clinical practitioner to aid in clinical decision-making. They are not intended to describe the standard

---

1. Frederick L. Datz, Gamuts in Nuclear Medicine, 3rd ed. St. Louis, CV Mosby, 1995.
2. Wagner HN, Szabo Z, Buchanan JW: Principles of Nuclear Medicine, 2nd ed. Philadelphia, WB Saunders, 1995.

of care. Several technical points are described in the context of the clinical cases Medical Center.

For the resident, we hope that this atlas will provide a comprehensive teaching file in nuclear medicine. The clinical cases chosen will afford the resident or student a broad exposure to a spectrum of clinical problems. Classic examples of disease entities are presented along with variations on the theme. An important aspect of this atlas for the trainee is the inclusion of "teaching points." These teaching points are also used to comment on the correlation between nuclear imaging and clinical or radiologic presentation. The atlas is best used as a visual, or image teaching file. We suggest that the resident use this atlas in conjunction with a standard textbook of nuclear medicine to provide the details of theory, technique, and utility of the images presented here.

Finally, it should be noted that this atlas cannot be all-inclusive. Many interesting cases and teaching points could not be incorporated. New scan findings and new applications for nuclear imaging are constantly being described, as evidenced by the many excellent papers in the literature. PET scanning and tumor imaging are particularly dynamic areas. We suspect that by the publication date many new discoveries will have been made in these fields. However, it is exactly this aspect of nuclear medicine that makes it an exciting, interesting field and a challenging endeavor. It is our ultimate and sincere hope that this atlas will encourage and sustain enthusiasm for nuclear medicine in practitioners, residents, and students alike.

An effort such as this, several years in the preparation, requires the help and support of many people and organizations. First and foremost, our efforts would have gone nowhere without the excellent and untiring secretarial efforts of Ms. Susan Block. We would like to thank the nuclear medicine technologists at The Queen's Medical Center for the excellence of their work and their patience when asked to do "one more view." The quality photography of Teresa Hanifin is evident throughout this book. The administration at Queen's has been supportive. We hope that this text will reflect positively on this facility, which has been dedicated to the care of the Hawaiian people for 140 years. And last, but by no means least: our families, Elaine, Deborah, Rachel, and Rebecca Coel and Susan Leung, who saw little of us on the many weekends and evenings as we strived to complete a project that we had thought so easy and that took four years instead of the expected one.

MARC COEL, M.D.
JIMMY LEUNG, M.D.

Contents

SECTION I

BONE

Chapter 1

Solitary Bony Abnormalities

NORMAL WHOLE BODY BONE SCAN

Patient 1: Adult

FIGURE 1–1   A.

Anterior and Posterior Blood Pool Scintigraphy: The relatively homogeneous and symmetric blood pool was acquired over 20 minutes.

FIGURE 1–1   B.

Anterior and Posterior Delayed Bone Scan: There are no areas of increased activity except for the normal sacroiliac (SI) joints and the anterior iliac crests.

Illustration continued on following page

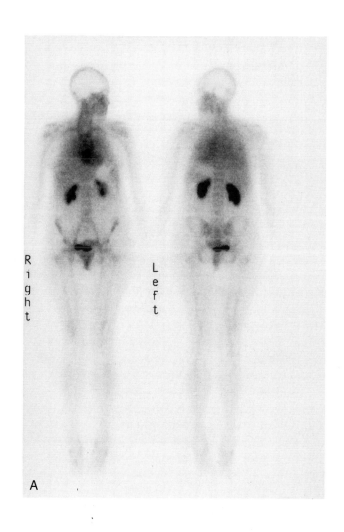

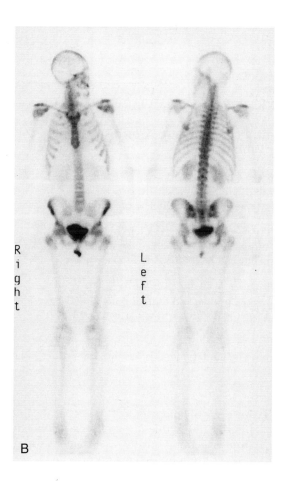

Patient 2: Adolescent

FIGURE 1–1   C.

Anterior and Posterior Bone Scan: The growth plates have intense, linear activity.

NOTE. The growth plates should be symmetric and have the same shape on both blood pool and delayed images.

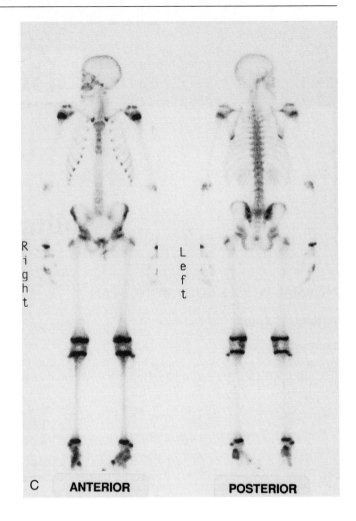

CERVICAL FACET OSTEOARTHRITIS

Patient: Post-traumatic Arthritis 4 Months After Whiplash Injury

FIGURE 1–2   A.

Posterior Bone Scan: There is a focal area of increased osteogenesis involving the left side of C3–C4.

FIGURE 1–2   B.

Left Anterior Oblique Bone Scintigraphy: From this angle, the abnormality can be localized to the facet joint.

FIGURE 1–2   C to E.

Transverse, Coronal, and Sagittal Bone SPECT Scans: The left C3–C4 facet joint has increased activity *(arrows)*.

FIGURE 1–2   F.

CT Scan: The left facet joint is narrowed, sclerotic, and hypertrophic.

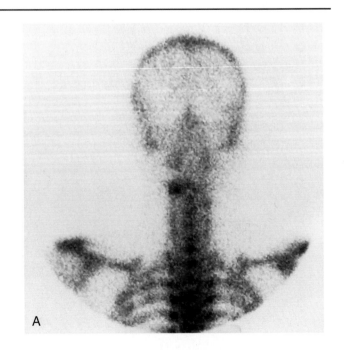

NOTE. Anterior oblique views of the cervical spine can help in differentiating apophyseal joint disease from vertebral body disease, which is where metastases are more likely to occur.

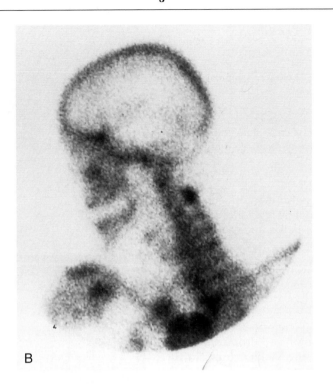

B

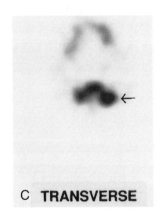

C **TRANSVERSE**

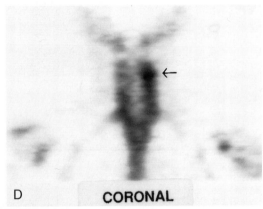

D **CORONAL**

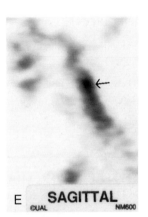

E **SAGITTAL**

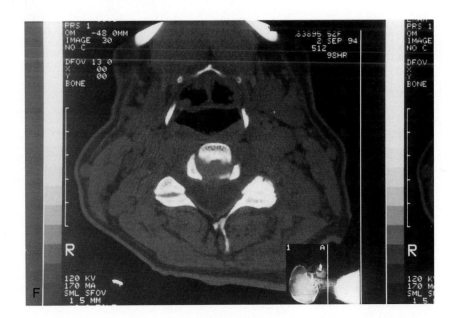

F

EARLY PAGET'S DISEASE OF PELVIS

FIGURE 1–3   A.

Posterior Pelvis Delayed Bone Scan: There is an irregular abnormality of the left iliac crest *(arrowhead)*.

FIGURE 1–3   B.

Plain Film X-ray: There are coarse trabeculae along the superior ilium *(arrowheads)*, along with increased sacral ala density.

NOTE 1. Paget's disease of the pelvis most often involves the iliopubic and ilioischial lines, although any or all portions of the pelvis and sacrum may be involved.

NOTE 2. Paget's disease can involve any bone and may be difficult to differentiate from blastic metastases or fibrous dysplasia.

NOTE 3. Paget's disease (osteitis deformans) is rare in Asia and Africa, common in Europe and Australia, and of decreasing incidence in North America.

Cross References

Chapter 2: Multiple Bony Abnormalities—Varying Patterns of Paget's Disease

Chapter 4: Pelvic Abnormalities—Pelvic Metastases vs. Paget's Disease

Chapter 5: Skull Abnormalities—Benign Focal Abnormalities of the Skull

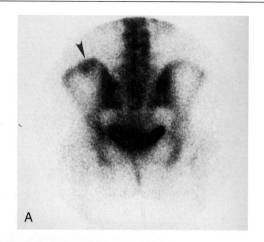

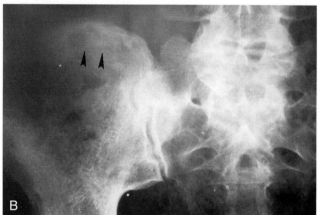

METAPHYSEAL HYPEREMIA AND OSTEOMYELITIS

Patient 1

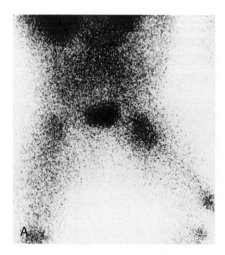

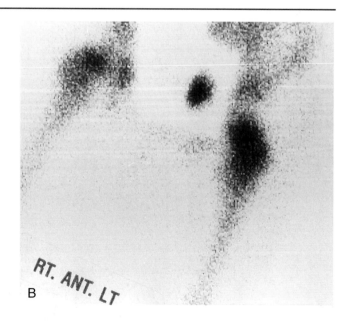

FIGURE 1–4   A.

Blood Pool Scintigraphy: There is marked hyperemia of the left proximal femur in this 6 month old child.

FIGURE 1–4   B.

Delayed Bone Scintigraphy: The marked increased osteogenesis involves the left femoral neck and intertrochanteric ridge as well as the metaphysis.

Patient 2

FIGURE 1–4   C.

Blood Pool Scintigraphy: There is loss of definition of the proximal left tibial growth plate, with hyperemia extending into the metaphysis.

FIGURE 1–4   D and E.

Delayed Bone Scintigraphy: There is increased activity in the left proximal tibial metaphysis *(arrow)* as compared with the normal.

NOTE 1. Hyperemia is almost always present with osteomyelitis, although it may not be seen in the first 24 hours. The hyperemia involves the soft tissues in virtually all cases.

NOTE 2. The growth plate in a child should be well defined.

Cross References

Chapter 8: Hyperemia—Hyperemia vs. Extent of Bone Activity in Osteogenesis

Chapter 9: ''Cold'' Abnormalities—''Cold'' to ''Hot'' Osteomyelitis on Bone Scan

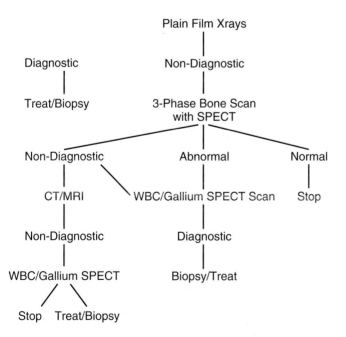

SUSPECT ACUTE OSTEOMYELITIS

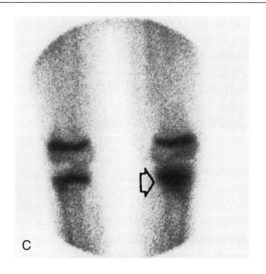

C

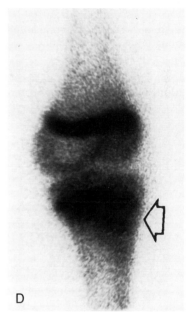

D

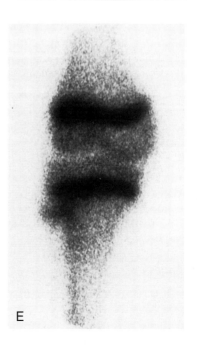

E

EPIPHYSEAL OSTEOMYELITIS

FIGURE 1–5.
Delayed Bone Scintigraphy: There is subtle increased activity involving the proximal right medial tibial epiphysis *(arrow).*

NOTE. In young children, magnification views of the affected joints should be obtained.

Cross Reference

Chapter 71: Infectious Diseases—WBC Scanning

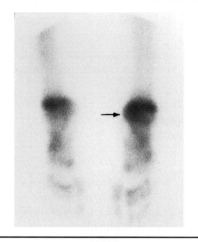

OSTEOMYELITIS AND CELLULITIS

FIGURE 1–6   A.
Blood Pool Scintigraphy: There is hyperemia along the dorsum of the right foot and the medial malleolus.

FIGURE 1–6   B.
Delayed Bone Scintigraphy: There is marked increased osteogenesis of the medial malleolus from osteomyelitis. The rest of the foot has generalized mild increased activity due to the hyperemia.

FIGURE 1–6   C.
Indium-111 White Blood Cell Scan: The diffuse activity over the dorsum of the foot is due to cellulitis. The medial malleolar activity proved to be osteomyelitis.

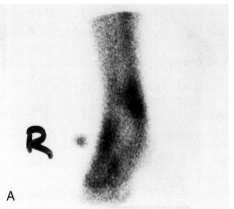

A

ABNORMAL WBC ACCUMULATION IN BONE	
Osteomyelitis	Neoplasms, including osteochondromas and primary malignant, often necrotic, tumors
Periostitis	
Active arthritides	
Healing fracture	Large osteophytes or sesamoid bones with marrow
Heterotopic ossification	
Compacted bone marrow from prostheses	Areas of expanded marrow, e.g., anemias
Paget's disease	

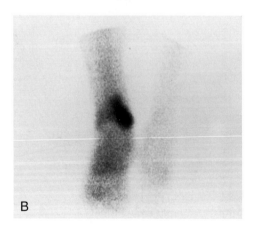

B

NOTE 1. A negative bone scan virtually rules out osteomyelitis.

NOTE 2. A WBC or gallium scan may be necessary in questionable cases, e.g., after trauma, with loose prostheses, or to see the extent of soft tissue involvement.

Cross References

Chapter 8: Hyperemia—Hyperemia vs. Extent of Bone Activity in Osteogenesis

Chapter 71: Infectious Diseases—Paraspinal Abscess

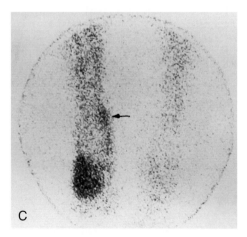

C

STUMP INFECTION

Patient 1: Stump Osteomyelitis

FIGURE 1–7 A.

Bone Scan: There is marked increased activity in the stump end of an above-the-knee amputation, beyond what one might expect from prosthetic and weight-bearing pressure. Note the soft tissue activity from the cellulitis surrounding the bone.

Patient 2: Normal Stump

FIGURE 1–7 B.

Bone Scan: There is normal osteogenesis at the stump tip and slightly greater activity along the shaft.

NOTE. The healthy stump has normal to mildly increased activity due to the stress of direct pressure from a prosthesis.

Cross Reference

Chapter 11: Soft Tissue Abnormalities—Cellulitis on Bone Scan

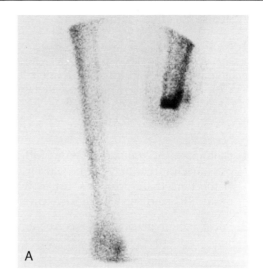

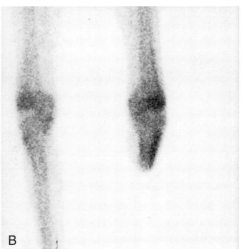

CHRONIC OSTEOMYELITIS

Patient 1: Bone Abscess

FIGURE 1–8 A.

Delayed Bone Scintigraphy: There is diffuse increased osteogenesis of virtually the entire right femur.

FIGURE 1–8 B and C.

Gallium Scans: There is focal involvement of the distal femoral diaphysis and metaphysis. The round accumulation of the gallium suggests a bone abscess, a process that requires surgical intervention.

Illustration continued on following page

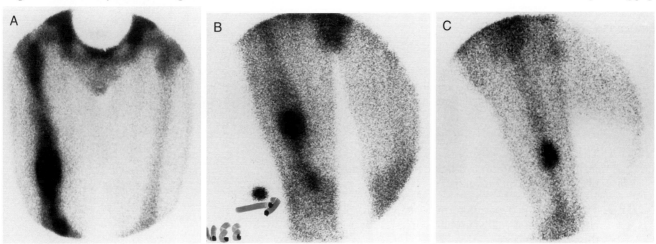

Patient 2: False Positive Gallium Scan

FIGURE 1–8 D and E.
Lateral Gallium Scintigraphy: There is diffuse increased gallium accumulation in the right tibia with cellulitis in the lower half of the lower leg, surrounding the skin ulcer. Results of bone biopsy were negative.

NOTE 1. Gallium can accumulate in a bone with chronic osteomyelitis that may not be actively infected at the time (false positive scan). A WBC scan or an MRI study may be more accurate.

NOTE 2. Focal gallium activity suggests osteomyelitis.

Cross Reference

Chapter 2: Multiple Bony Abnormalities—Progression of Acute Osteomyelitis to Chronic Osteomyelitis

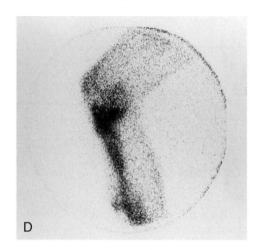

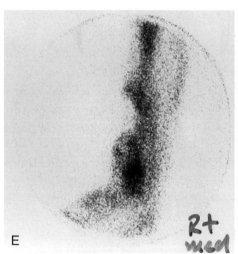

REACTIVATION OF CHRONIC OSTEOMYELITIS: GALLIUM VS. WBC

FIGURE 1–9 A.
Blood Pool Scan: There is hyperemia of the left mandibular ramus and coronoid process.

FIGURE 1–9 B and C.
Delayed Bone Scan: The entire left side of the mandible, including the mentum, has marked increased osteogenesis.

FIGURE 1–9 D.
Gallium Scan: The left side of the mandible is abnormal.

FIGURE 1–9 E.
WBC Scan: There is abnormal WBC accumulation in the angle of the mandible, the ramus, and the coronoid process.

NOTE 1. The WBC scan is positive only in actively infected areas. Gallium can be positive in "inactive" chronic osteomyelitis.

NOTE 2. The area of hyperemia in reactivation of chronic osteomyelitis usually corresponds to the active process.

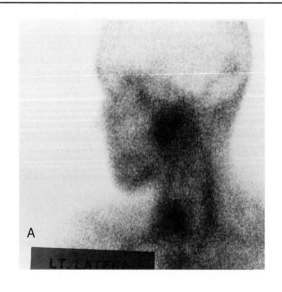

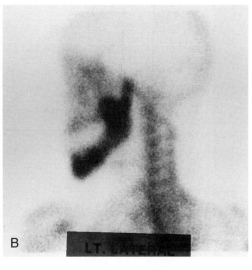

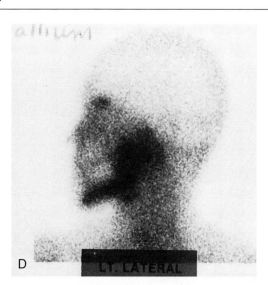

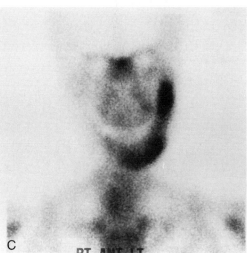

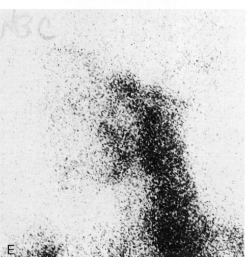

BRODIE'S ABSCESS OF ILIUM

FIGURE 1–10   A.

CT Scan: There is a small lucency with sclerotic borders within the right ilium *(arrow)*.

FIGURE 1–10   B.

Posterior Blood Pool Scan: There is no hyperemia of the right SI joint.

FIGURE 1–10   C and D.

Axial and Coronal SPECT Scans: The right SI joint region has increased activity.

FIGURE 1–10   E.

Axial STIR MRI: The abscess *(arrow)* can be seen as an area of increased signal intensity.

NOTE. Brodie's abscesses are well-demarcated fluid collections in bone that may be "sterile" or grow organisms of low virulence.

Cross Reference

Chapter 4: Pelvic Abnormalities—Sacroiliac Joint Infection

Illustration continued on following page

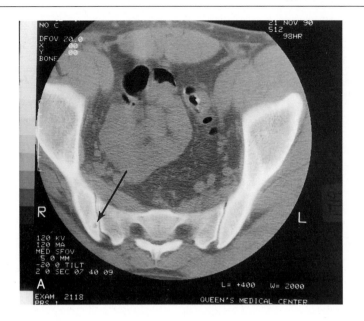

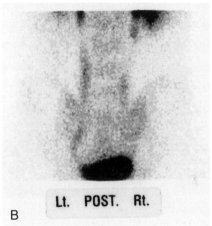

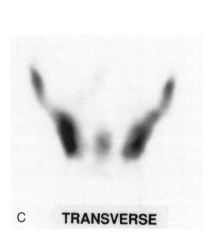

C **TRANSVERSE**

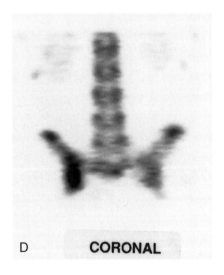

D **CORONAL**

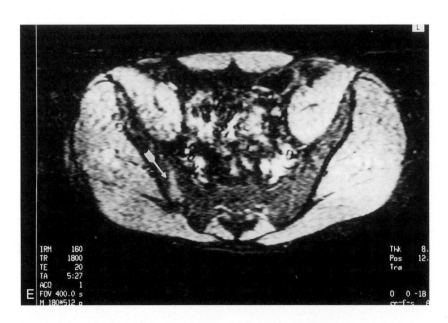

WBC ACCUMULATION IN A FRACTURE FRAGMENT

FIGURE 1–11 A.
Anterior Femoral WBC Scan: The left femoral fracture site has "abnormal" WBC accumulation.

FIGURE 1–11 B.
Anterior Femoral Colloid Marrow Scan: There is also colloid accumulation in a fracture fragment that contains living marrow.

NOTE. Infected bone marrow will accumulate WBCs but not radiocolloid. The two radiopharmaceuticals are best used for infections of fractures, metallic fixation devices (e.g., intramedullary rods), and prostheses.

Cross References

Chapter 10: Prostheses—Marrow Compression with Normal Hip Prosthesis

Chapter 71: Infectious Diseases—Gallium Uptake in Benign Fractures

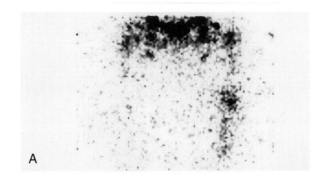

A

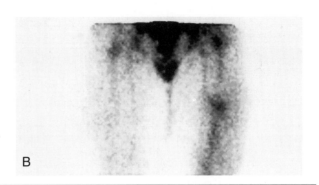

B

SEPTIC ARTHRITIS

Patient 1

FIGURE 1–12 A.
Anterior Knee Blood Flow Scan: There is markedly increased blood flow to the left knee.

FIGURE 1–12 B and C.
Anterior and Left Lateral Blood Pool Scintigraphy: There is marked hyperemia of the knee joint, bursa, and lateral femoral condyle.

FIGURE 1–12 D and E.
Anterior and Left Lateral Delayed Bone Scans: The intense osteogenesis involves the bones along the joint.

FIGURE 1–12 F to H.
Anterior and Both Lateral ^{111}In-WBC Scans: The WBC accumulation surrounds the bones, especially the lateral femoral condyle.

Illustration continued on following page

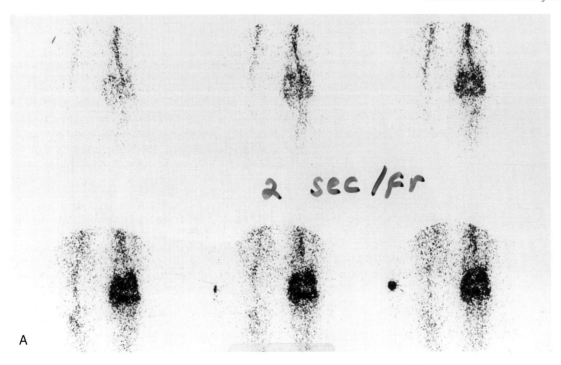

A

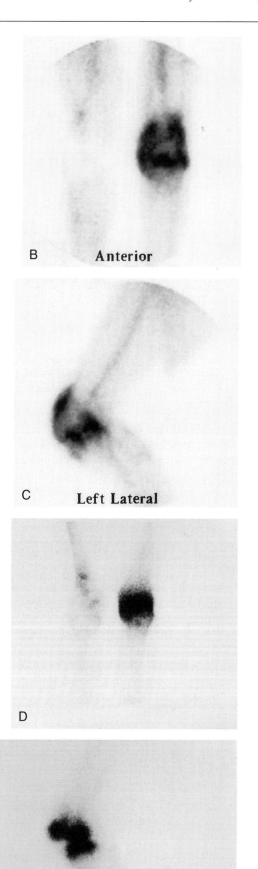

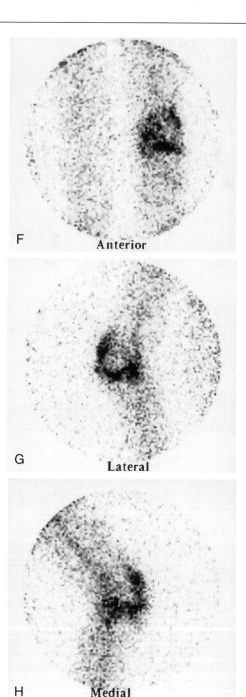

NOTE 1. Any soft tissue hyperemia will increase osteogenesis locally, creating increased activity in cortical bone. A periostitis cannot always be excluded.

NOTE 2. A WBC scan may be necessary to rule out osteomyelitis when the degree of bone reaction to the surrounding infection is intense.

Cross References

Chapter 1: Multiple Bony Abnormalities—Meniscal Disease and Osseous Changes of the Knee

Chapter 8: Hyperemia—Hyperemia in Septic Arthritis

TROCHANTERIC BURSITIS

Patient 1

FIGURE 1–13   A.

Blood Pool Scintigraphy: There is minimal hyperemia in the region of the left greater trochanter.

FIGURE 1–13   B.

Delayed Bone Scintigraphy: The linear increased osteogenesis is virtually pathognomonic for trochanteric bursitis.

FIGURE 1–13   C.

Plain Film X-ray: There is irregularity of the cortex of the greater trochanter *(arrows)*.

Patient 2

FIGURE 1–13   D.

Anterior Hip Gallium Scan: There is increased gallium accumulating along the right greater trochanter (the scan was done for lymphoma).

NOTE 1. There is increased osteogenesis of the greater trochanter in bursitis because of local periosteal reaction.

NOTE 2. Gallium will accumulate in any active inflammatory process.

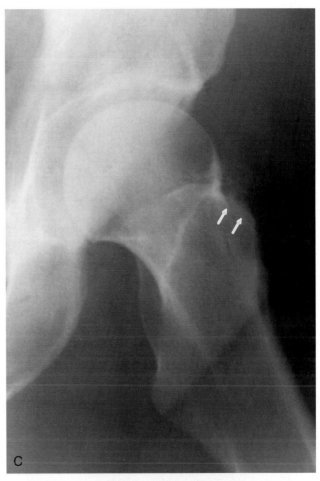

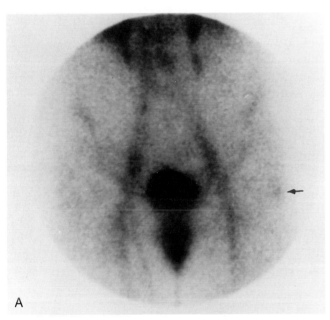

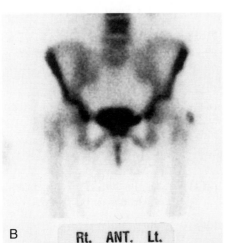

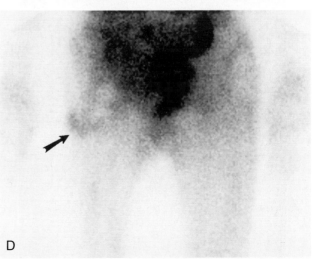

HIP FRACTURE IN THE ELDERLY

SUSPECT FRACTURE

Plain Film Xray

Diagnostic — Non-Diagnostic

Treat

In Elderly, Wait 48 Hr

3-Phase Bone Scan
with SPECT

Non-Diagnostic — Diagnostic

CT/MRI — Treat

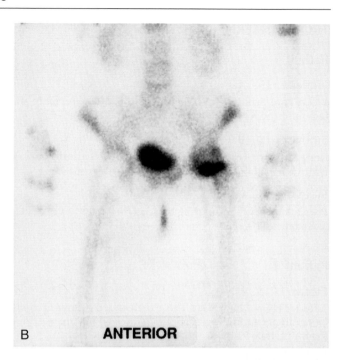

B   **ANTERIOR**

Patient 1: 75 Year Old Female

FIGURE 1–14 A.
Plain Film X-ray of the Left Hip: There is a questionable cortical break *(arrowheads)* in this severely arthritic and osteoporotic hip.

FIGURE 1–14 B.
Anterior Bone Scan: A definite linear abnormality traverses the femoral neck.

FIGURE 1–14 C.
T2-weighted Coronal MRI of the Hips: There is high signal in the femoral neck, indicative of a fracture *(arrow)*.

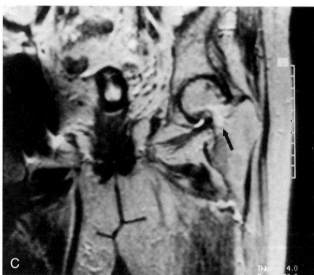

C

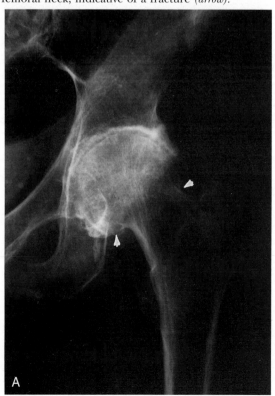

A

Patient 2: 82 Year Old Female

FIGURE 1–14 D.
Hip Blood Pool Scan: There is marked hyperemia in the right hip region.

FIGURE 1–14 E.
Delayed Bone Scan: The fracture involves the greater trochanter and the interchanteric ridge, with bony reaction extending into the femoral neck.

NOTE 1. In the elderly, a hip fracture may take up to 72 hours to be positive on bone scan.

NOTE 2. Hyperemia is usually less evident in elderly patients with acute fractures.

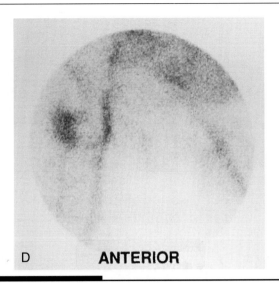

D   **ANTERIOR**

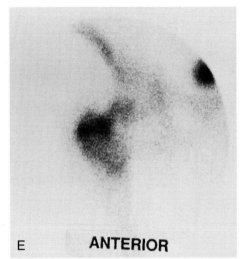

E   **ANTERIOR**

OSTEOCHONDRITIS DISSECANS

Patient 1: 60 Year Old Male with Knee Pain

FIGURE 1–15   A.

Blood Pool Scintigraphy: There is hyperemia of a focal area within the medial compartment of the left knee *(arrowhead)*.

FIGURE 1–15   B.

Delayed Bone Scintigraphy: There is focal, marked increased osteogenesis of the left medial femoral condyle along the articular surface. These findings are virtually diagnostic of subchondral bony injury.

Patient 2: 14 Year Old Female Dancer

FIGURE 1–15   C.

Blood Pool Scintigraphy: There is focal hyperemia involving the left ankle.

FIGURE 1–15   D.

Delayed Bone Scintigraphy: There is a focal area of increased osteogenesis at the posterior left ankle joint.

FIGURE 1–15   E.

Plain Film Tomography: There is a defect in the cortex extending into the subchondral bone of the tibia, indicative of osteochondritis dissecans.

Patient 3: 50 Year Old Male with Tibial Plateau Fracture and Unsuspected Femoral Osteochondritis Dissecans

FIGURE 1–15   F and G.

Blood Pool Scintigraphy: There is marked increased blood flow and hyperemia of the right knee involving both the medial femoral condyle and the medial tibial plateau.

FIGURE 1–15   H and I.

Anterior and Posterior Delayed Bone Scans: There is increased osteogenesis of the medial tibial plateau as well as a more focal abnormality of the medial femoral condyle.

FIGURE 1–15   J.

Plain Film X-ray: There is a fracture of the medial tibial plateau. The femoral fracture is hard to see *(arrow)*.

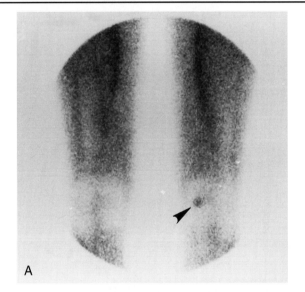

A

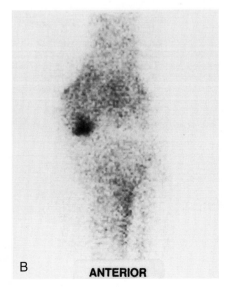

B   **ANTERIOR**

Illustration continued on following page

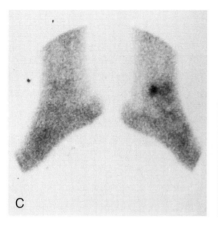

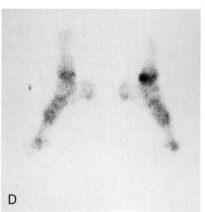

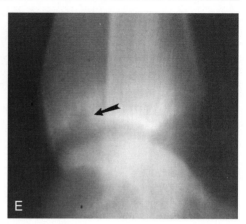

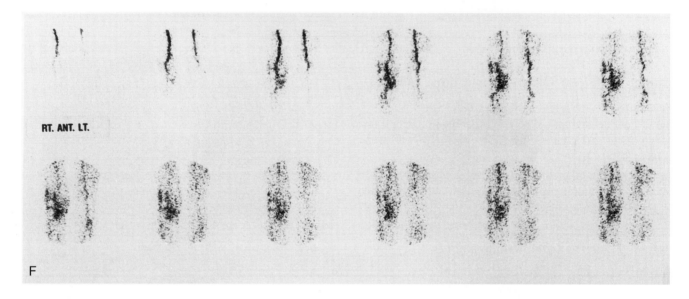

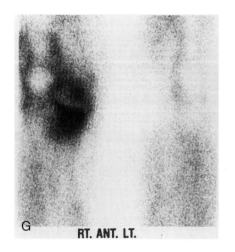

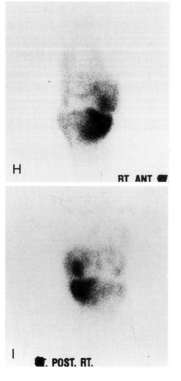

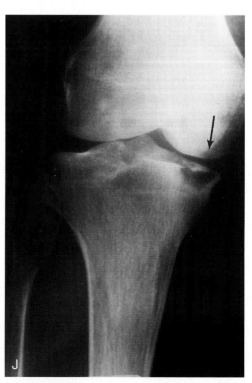

Patient 4: 47 Year Old Tennis Player

FIGURE 1–15   K.

Blood Pool Scan: There is hyperemia surrounding the right medial femoral condyle and the medial tibial plateau.

FIGURE 1–15   L.

Anterior Planar Delayed Bone Scan: There is a focal abnormality in the subchondral bone of the left medial femoral condyle.

FIGURE 1–15   M to O.

SPECT Bone Scan: The abnormality is better localized to the posterior aspect of the condyle.

NOTE 1. MRI or arthroscopy is necessary to see if there is any communication of the joint space across the cartilage into the subchondral bone.

NOTE 2. A bone scan can be useful to identify additional fractures, which might be missed on plain film x-ray.

NOTE 3. A hemarthrosis or an associated synovitis will have hyperemia in trauma cases.

Cross Reference

Chapter 8: Hyperemia—Osteochondritis Dissecans

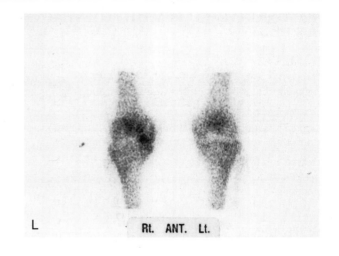

L   Rt. ANT. Lt.

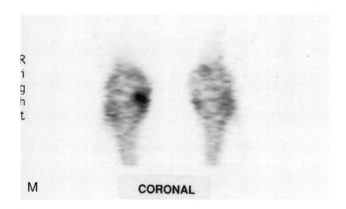

M   CORONAL

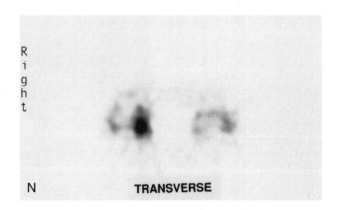

N   TRANSVERSE

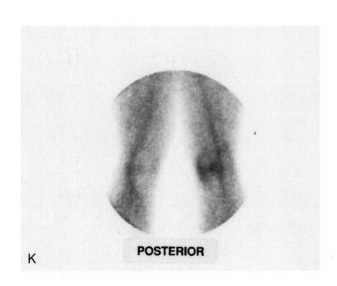

K   POSTERIOR

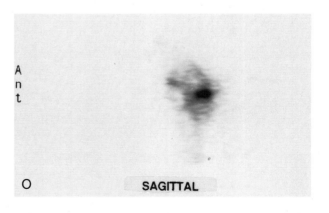

O   SAGITTAL

NONUNION FRACTURE WITH POTENTIAL FOR HEALING

FIGURE 1–16   A.
Plain Film X-ray: There is a tibial fracture with some callus formation but a persistent fracture line lucency.

FIGURE 1–16   B and C.
Blood Flow and Blood Pool Scintigraphy: There is increased blood flow and hyperemia at the fracture site *(arrow)*.

FIGURE 1–16   D.
Delayed Bone Scintigraphy: The fracture has increased osteogenesis.

NOTE. If there is no hyperemia associated with an un-united fracture, the potential for healing is small, and some intervention is warranted.

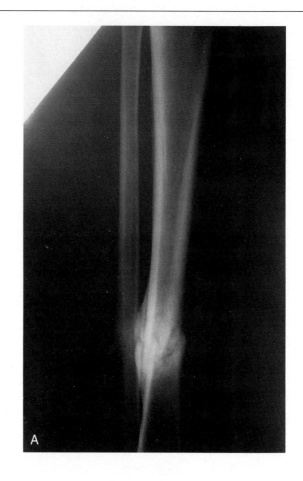

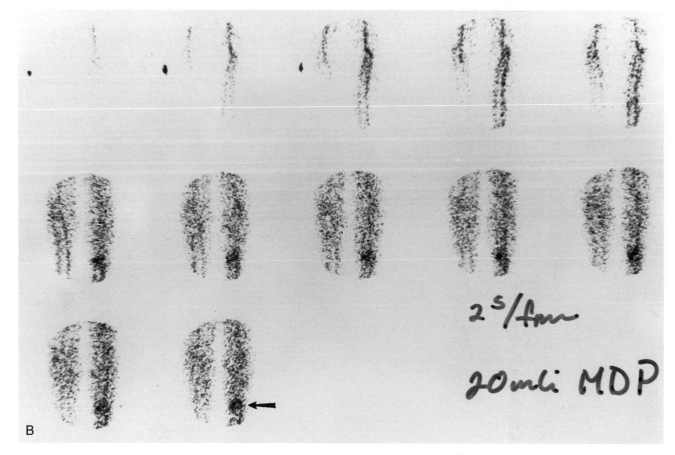

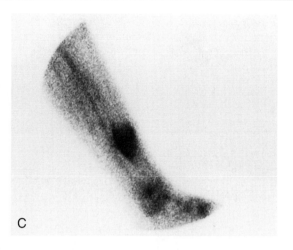

C

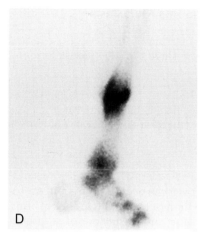

D

PATHOLOGIC FRACTURES

Patient 1: Aneurysmal Bone Cyst

FIGURE 1–17 A.

Plain Film X-ray: There is a fracture through the proximal right humerus in an area of permeative destruction of bone.

FIGURE 1–17 B and C.

Delayed Planar Bone Scan: There is a focal abnormality in the region of the fracture but also more diffuse activity proximal to the fracture.

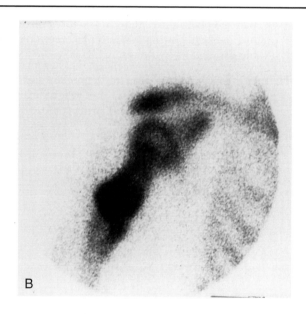

B

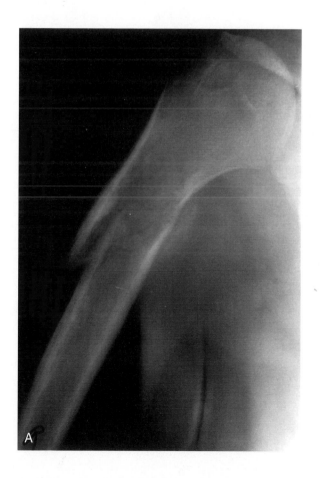

A

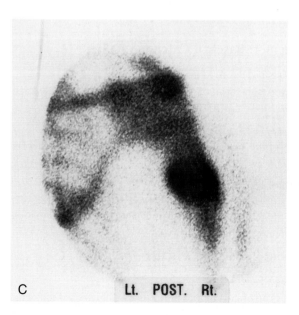

C   Lt. POST. Rt.

Illustration continued on following page

Patient 2: Lung Carcinoma Metastasis

FIGURE 1–17 D.

Delayed Bone Scintigraphy: There is a large metastasis to the right femoral diaphysis.

FIGURE 1–17 E.

Four Months Later: Delayed Bone Scintigraphy: There is linear photopenia in the middle of the metastasis, indicative of a widely separated pathologic fracture.

NOTE 1. Elongated activity can occur with fractures associated with benign or malignant lesions of bone but should raise the suspicion of a pathologic fracture.

NOTE 2. "Cold" areas are much more common in acute pathologic fractures than in fractures through normal bone, owing to the replacement of viable osteoblasts by tumor.

NOTE 3. It is important to warn the clinician and the patient of metastases to the weight-bearing bones, the shoulders and arms, before they break.

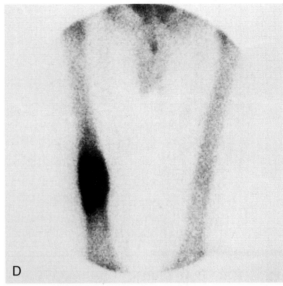

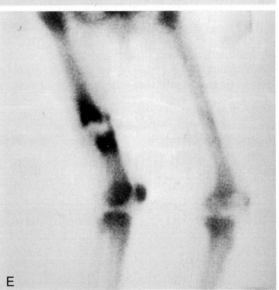

SOLITARY STRESS FRACTURES

Patient 1: Baseball Catcher

FIGURE 1–18 A.

Delayed Bone Scan of the Hip: There is focal increased activity in the inferior femoral neck.

FIGURE 1–18 B.

X-ray of the Right Hip: At the time of the bone scan there were no abnormalities.

FIGURE 1–18 C.

X-ray of the Right Hip at 48 Days: There is an area of new periosteal reaction along the medial femoral neck *(arrowheads)*.

Patient 2: Baseball Pitcher

FIGURE 1–18 D.

Bone Scan of the Elbow: There is marked increased osteogenesis of the olecranon. There is also a medial epicondyle abnormality, "pitcher's elbow" *(arrowhead)*.

Patient 3: Runner

FIGURE 1–18 E and F.

Blood Pool and Right Medial Delayed Bone Scan of the Feet: There is abnormal cuboid activity *(arrow)*. Older injuries of the navicular and first cuneiform bones are evident on the delayed scans only.

Patient 4: Ballet Dancer

FIGURE 1–18 G.

Delayed Bone Scan: There is increased activity in the posterior ankle in the region of the os trigonum or posterior talus.

FIGURE 1–18 H.

Planar X-ray: The talus is elongated posteriorly, but a fracture cannot be seen. There is no os trigonum.

Illustration continued on page 22

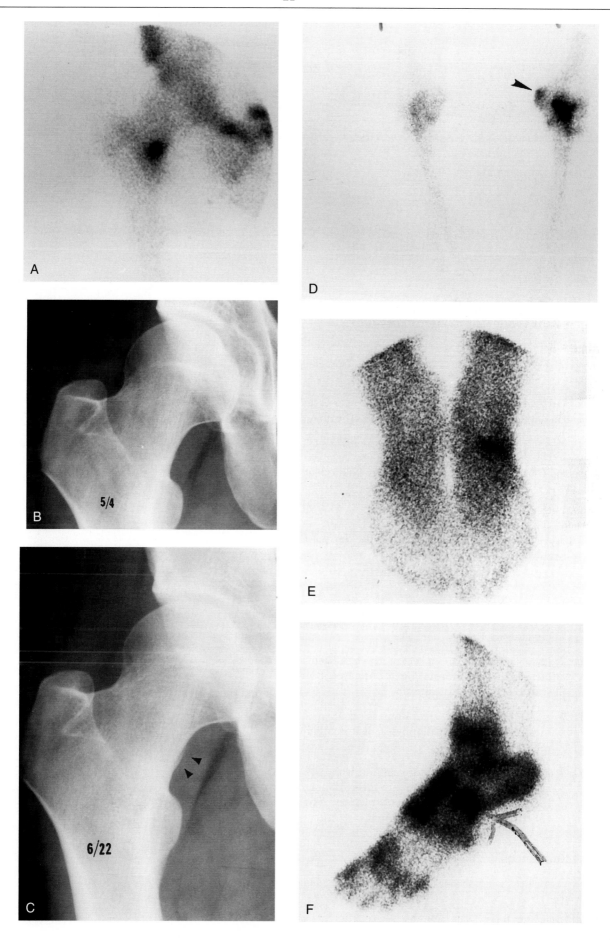

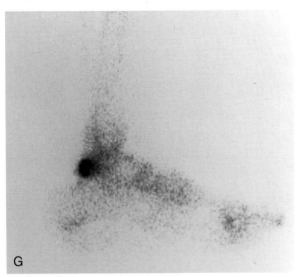

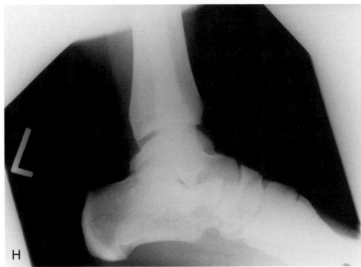

Patient 5: 16 Year Old Third Baseman with Sudden Pain While Throwing to First Base

FIGURE 1–18   I.

Anterior Planar Bone Scan: There is a small focus of increased osteogenesis behind the right clavicle.

FIGURE 1–18   J.

RAO Maximum Pixel Array Projection Bone Scan: The first rib abnormality is clearly separate from other bones.

FIGURE 1–18   K.

Coronal SPECT Bone Scan: The first rib fracture is quite prominent.

FIGURE 1–18   L.

Plain Film Rib X-Ray: The fracture can be seen to traverse the entire first rib. There is no evidence for an underlying pathologic process to predispose the rib to fracture.

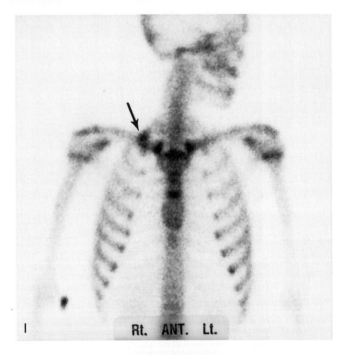

NOTE 1. In stress fractures, bone scans are often positive 2 weeks before any radiographic changes are present.

NOTE 2. Hyperemia indicates a recent injury. Older injuries will be abnormal on the delayed bone scan but have no hyperemia.

NOTE 3. The most frequent stress injuries occur in the metatarsals and tibial diaphyses, in athletes and military recruits.

NOTE 4. First rib fractures are unusual and when seen after trauma are associated with severe damage, including ruptured bronchi or tracheas. A first rib stress fracture is also unusual.

Cross References

Chapter 2: Multiple Bony Abnormalities—Bony Stress Reactions; Shin Splints

Chapter 7: Hands and Feet—Talar Fracture Simulating an Os Trigonum

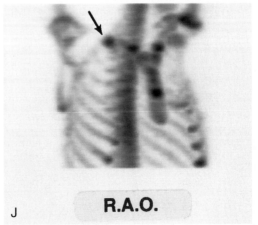

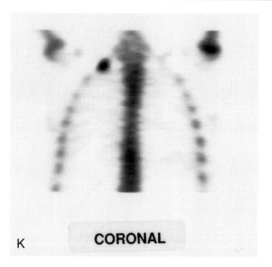

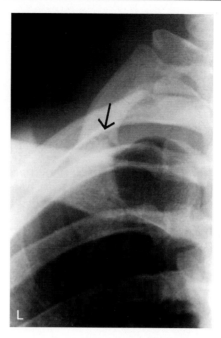

FALSE NEGATIVE BONE SCAN
FOR FRACTURE

Patient: 52 Year Old Male Patient with Pelvic Trauma 48 Hours Prior to Scan

FIGURE 1–19   A.

Plain Film X-ray: The left superior pubic ramus fracture overlaps the acetabulum *(arrow)*, while there is a step-off of the left ischiopubic junction *(arrowheads)*. The SI joint did not appear abnormal on x-ray or CT.

FIGURE 1–19   B and C.

Anterior and Posterior Blood Pool Scans: There is hyperemia of the left SI joint, which was separated, but the left superior pubic ramus and the left ischiopubic junction have less conspicuous increased blood pools.

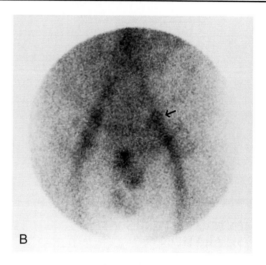

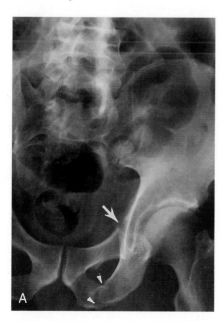

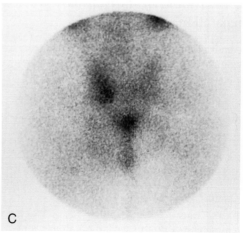

Illustration continued on following page

FIGURE 1–19 D and E.

Planar Bone Scan of the Pelvis: The left ischiopubic junction fracture is not evident (nor was it on SPECT scan). The left superior ramus fracture at the acetabulum and the left SI joint have increased activity.

NOTE 1. On bone scan, the left superior ramus fracture may be confused with acetabular osteoarthritis.

NOTE 2. Old fractures, un-united fractures, acute fractures in elderly patients, and, rarely, acute fractures in younger patients may not be evident on bone scan.

NOTE 3. Repeat bone scans 48 to 72 hours after the injury should demonstrate virtually all acute fractures.

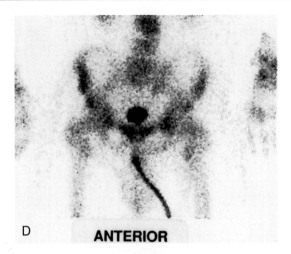

D   **ANTERIOR**

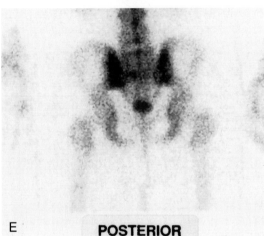

E   **POSTERIOR**

LIGAMENTOUS INJURIES WITH JOINT SEPARATION

Patient 1: Acute Acromioclavicular Joint Separation

FIGURE 1–20 A.

Right Shoulder Bone Scan: The acromioclavicular (AC) joint has a focal area of increased activity.

FIGURE 1–20 B.

Left Shoulder Bone Scan: The activity of the AC joint is homogeneous.

Patient 2: Sacroiliac Joint Separation

FIGURE 1–20 C and D.

Coronal and Transverse SPECT Bone Scan: The left SI joint has increased activity due to separation after trauma.

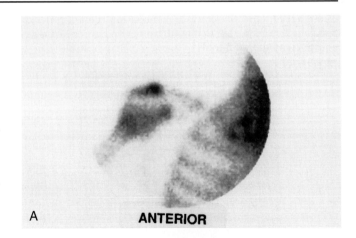

A   **ANTERIOR**

NOTE. Ligamentous injuries cause pulling on Sharpey's fibers with subsequent increased bony response.

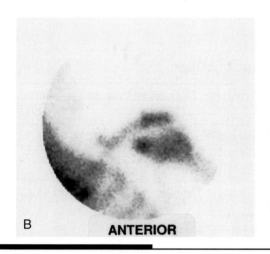

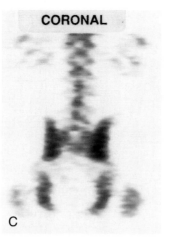

CORONAL

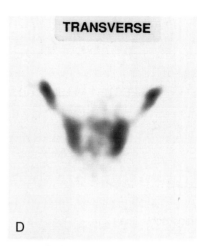

TRANSVERSE

B ANTERIOR

C

D

ISCHIAL ENTHESOPATHY

Patient: Tri-athlete

FIGURE 1–21 A.
Posterior Blood Pool: There is hyperemia in the left ischial region *(arrow)*.

FIGURE 1–21 B.
Posterior Pelvic Bone Scan: The left ischium has increased activity due to adductor muscle attachment injury.

NOTE. An enthesopathy is an abnormality due to abnormal stress or injury at the attachment of a muscle to a bone. In tendinitis, the abnormality on bone scan is in the tendon itself.

Cross Reference

Chapter 11: Soft Tissue Abnormalities—Tendinitis on Bone Scan

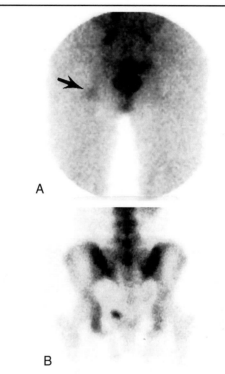

A

B

MENISCAL DISEASE AND OSSEOUS CHANGES OF THE KNEE

FIGURE 1–22.
Anterior Bone Scan: The medial compartment disease is associated with a varus deformity, not present on the left side.

NOTE 1. Unilateral, single compartment disease is probably related to meniscal or articular cartilage disease, usually lumped together as "degenerative changes" on scan reports.

NOTE 2. Meniscal tears often have abnormal bone scans even before there is joint space narrowing or degenerative arthritis evident on x-ray.

NOTE 3. A SPECT scan may be best to demonstrate these changes early.

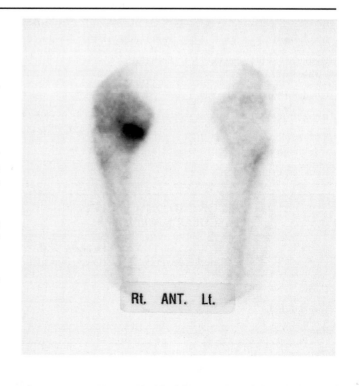

Rt. ANT. Lt.

SUSPECTED AVASCULAR NECROSIS

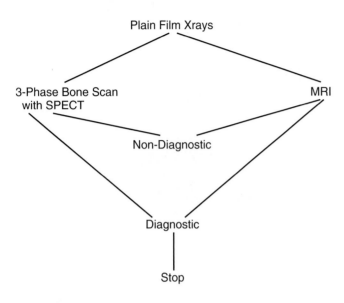

Plain Film Xrays

3-Phase Bone Scan with SPECT

MRI

Non-Diagnostic

Diagnostic

Stop

CAUSES OF OSTEONECROSIS

Common	Less Common
Femoral neck fractures (must be intracapsular)	Cushing's disease
Femoral head dislocation	Increased intracapsular pressure (e.g., septic arthritis)
Slipped capital femoral epiphysis	Gout
Steroid therapy	Gaucher's disease
Alcoholism	Pancreatitis
Dysbaric insults (caisson disease)	Radiation
Collagen vascular diseases	
Idiopathic or spontaneous	
Sickle cell and other hemoglobinopathies	
Renal transplantation	

STAGES OF OSTEONECROSIS (AVASCULAR NECROSIS)

	Blood Flow/Pool	Delayed Scan (Osteogenesis)
Early	↓	↓
Intermediate	↔	↓ ↔ ↑
Late	↑	↑

DIFFERENTIAL DIAGNOSIS OF DECREASED BLOOD POOL

Avascular necrosis (osteonecrosis)	Vascular insufficiency
Joint fluid	Stomach with food or liquid
Transient synovitis	Recent treatment with ice packs
Reflex sympathetic dystrophy	Methylmethacrylate
Prostheses	Radiation change
Artifacts	Fluid collections, e.g., pleural or peritoneal fluid
Metallic fixation devices	
Cysts	
Hematoma	

DIFFERENTIAL DIAGNOSIS OF A "HOT" EPIPHYSIS

Osteonecrosis (avascular necrosis, aseptic necrosis)	Fracture
	Osteomyelitis
Severe degenerative osteoarthritis	Septic arthritis
Rheumatoid and other inflammatory arthritides	Transient or aseptic synovitis (late phase)
Transient or migratory osteoporosis	Slipped capital femoral epiphysis

EARLY OSTEONECROSIS

Patient: Legg-Perthes Disease

FIGURE 1–23   A and B.

Blood Pool and Delayed Planar Scintigrams: The right femoral head has both decreased blood flow and osteogenesis *(thin arrow)*. There is activity within the left femoral head, indicating an intact blood supply *(thick arrow)*.

NOTE 1. Decreased activity on blood pool and bone scans is seen in the earliest stage of osteonecrosis.

NOTE 2. The re-establishment of the blood supply allows for attempts at bony repair, resorption of dead bone, and ultimately collapse and fragmentation.

NOTE 3. Decreased activity can also be seen with joint effusions, i.e., transient synovitis, hemarthrosis, and septic arthritis.

Cross References

Chapter 2: Multiple Bony Abnormalities—Multifocal Osteonecrosis

Chapter 9: "Cold" Abnormalities—"Cold" Abnormality in Early Osteonecrosis of the Hip

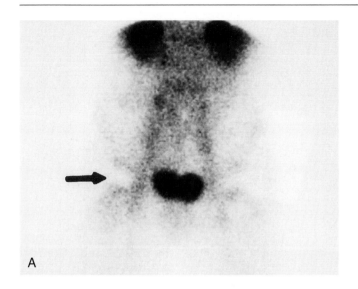

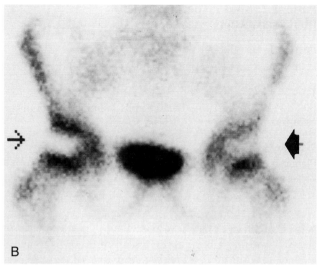

INTERMEDIATE PHASE OF OSTEONECROSIS

Patient 1: Normal Blood Pool with "Cold" Femoral Head

FIGURE 1–24   A and B.

Anterior and Posterior Blood Pool Scintigraphy: There is hyperemia of the right femoral neck but normal activity of the femoral head.

FIGURE 1–24   C.

Planar Bone Scan: The right femoral head has a central area of decreased activity surrounded by increased osteogenesis.

FIGURE 1–24   D.

Coronal SPECT Bone Scan: There is no apparent osteogenesis in the central right femoral head. It was necrotic at surgery.

Illustration continued on following page

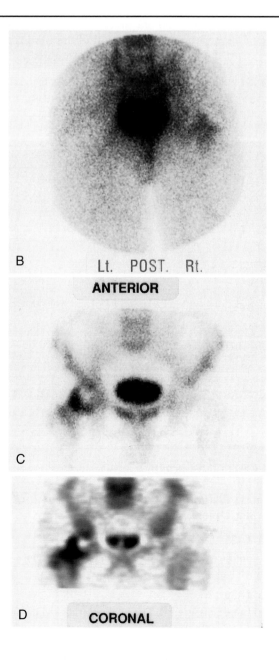

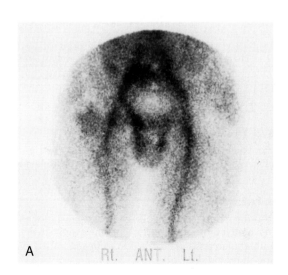

Patient 2: Mild Hyperemia with Increased Osteogenesis

FIGURE 1–24 E.

Plain Film X-ray: The appearance of the hips is normal.

FIGURE 1–24 F.

Blood Pool Scintigraphy: There is only mild hyperemia of the right hip.

FIGURE 1–24 G.

Planar Bone Scan: The subarticular weight-bearing bone has marked increased activity.

NOTE 1. Always place a urinary bladder catheter when doing a bone SPECT scan of the hips to avoid computer overshoot and loss of data across the hips.

NOTE 2. The intermediate phase of osteonecrosis occurs with re-establishment of the blood supply to the bone, prior to microfractures.

NOTE 3. Negative or equivocal bone scans for osteonecrosis may occur at this stage, requiring an MRI for further assessment.

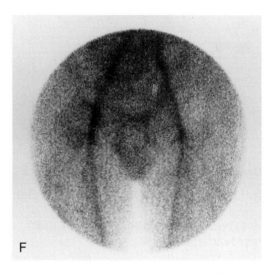

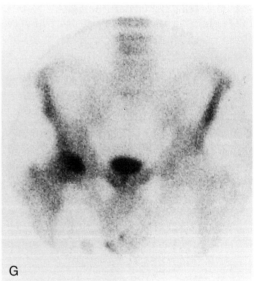

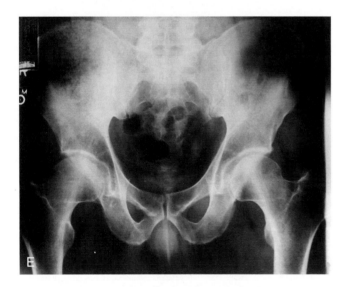

LATE OSTEONECROSIS

Patient 1: Osteonecrosis of the Humerus in a Deep Sea Diver

FIGURE 1–25 A.

Blood Pool Scintigraphy: There is marked hyperemia of the left humeral head.

FIGURE 1–25 B.

Delayed Bone Scintigraphy: The left humeral head has marked increased osteogenesis.

Patient 2: Osteonecrosis of the Knee

FIGURE 1–25 C and D.

Blood Pool Scintigraphy: There is hyperemia of the right knee, especially in the medial femoral condyle. The diffuse hyperemia may be due to an associated synovitis.

FIGURE 1–25 E and F.

Delayed Bone Scintigraphy: There is increased osteogenesis of the right medial femoral condyle. The increased activity of the medial tibial plateau is probably due to degenerative changes, including meniscal damage.

NOTE 1. Late osteonecrosis has hyperemia and increased osteogenesis as the bone develops microfractures and eventually fragments, followed by collapse.

NOTE 2. Osteonecrosis of the knee is indistinguishable from trabecular fractures (''bone bruise'') or even cortical fractures.

NOTE 3. Severe osteoarthritis can simulate osteonecrosis.

Cross Reference

Chapter 2: Multiple Bony Abnormalities—Severe Osteoarthritis vs. Osteonecrosis

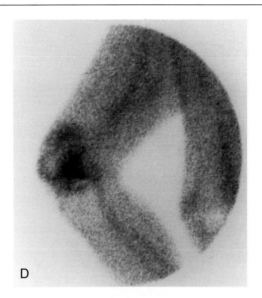

D

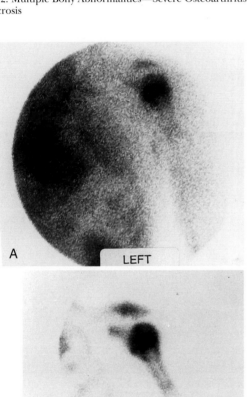

A

LEFT

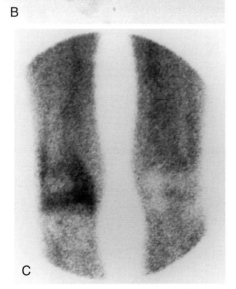

B

C

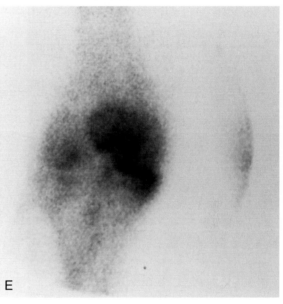

E

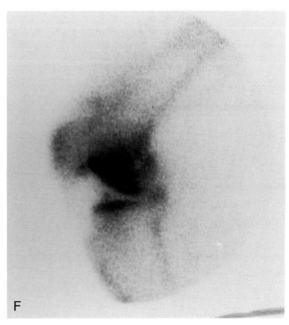

F

TRANSIENT OSTEOPOROSIS

Patient: 38 Year Old Male with 4 Months of Left Hip Pain that Gradually Improved

FIGURE 1–26   A and B.
Anterior and Left Lateral Hip Bone Scans: The superolateral portion of the left femoral head has increased osteogenesis.

FIGURE 1–26   C.
T2 Coronal MRI: There is increased signal in the weight-bearing part of the left femoral head, extending down into the femoral neck. There is no rim of low signal surrounding the "edema," as seen in osteonecrosis.

NOTE 1. Transient osteoporosis or migratory osteoporosis may be indistinguishable from avascular necrosis on radionuclide bone scanning and may be a form of reflex sympathetic dystrophy.

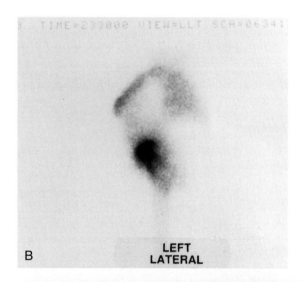

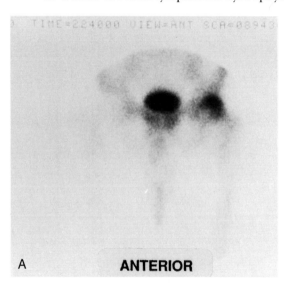

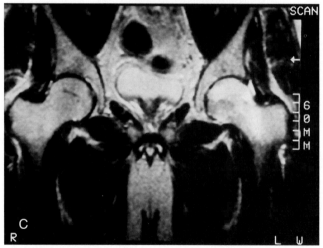

OSTEOID OSTEOMA

Patient 1: 38 Year Old Male

FIGURE 1–27   A and B.
Blood Pool and Delayed Planar Scintigram: There is marked hyperemia and osteogenesis of the ulna.

Patient 2: 42 Year Old Female with Chronic Ankle Pain

FIGURE 1–27   C and D.
Blood Pool and Delayed Lateral Planar Bone Scan of the Left

Foot: There is focal hyperemia and increased osteogenesis in the region of the talocalcaneal joint.

FIGURE 1–27   E and F.
Plain Film X-ray and Tomogram: The tomogram demonstrates the lucent nidus *(arrowhead)* of the osteoma surrounded by sclerotic bone.

Illustration continued on page 32

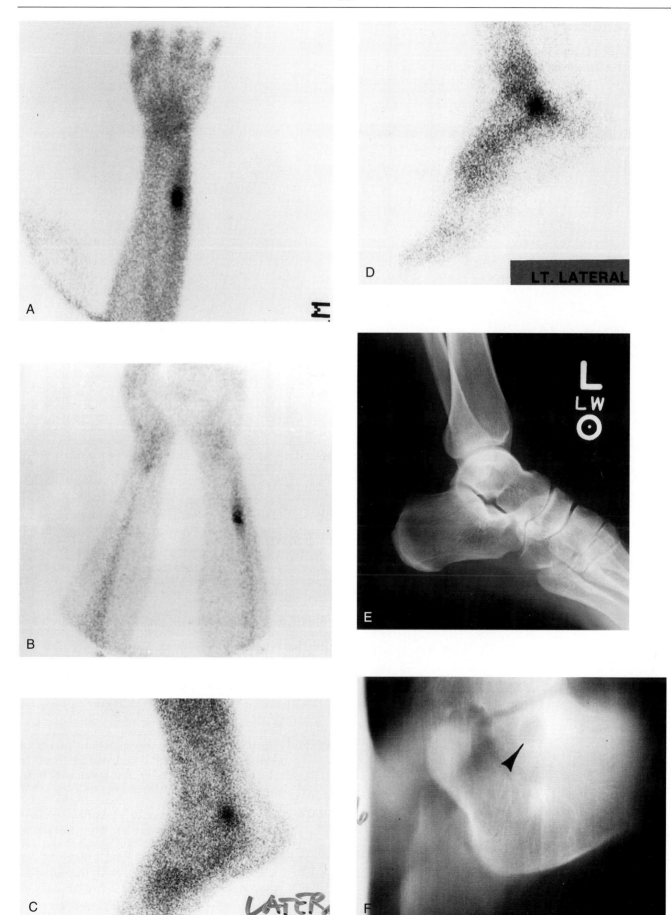

Patient 3: 10 Year Old Female

FIGURE 1–27   G and H.

Blood Pool and Delayed Planar Bone Scan: There is mild hyperemia (*arrow*) and increased activity of the left lesser trochanter and proximal femoral metaphysis.

FIGURE 1–27   I.

Bone SPECT Scan: The apparent greater SPECT scan size of the osteoid osteoma is an artifact of SPECT scanning. (Courtesy of Dr. Michael Kipper, Vista, CA.)

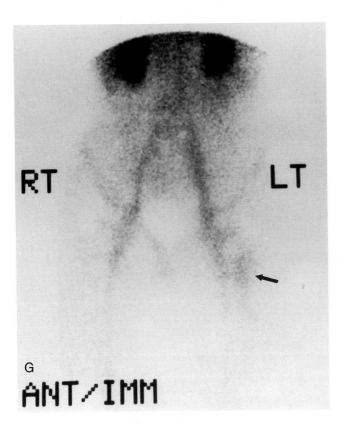

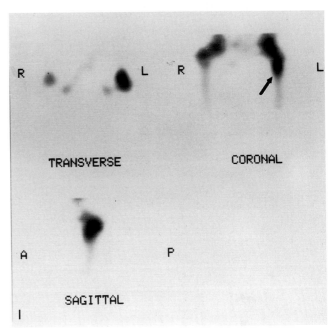

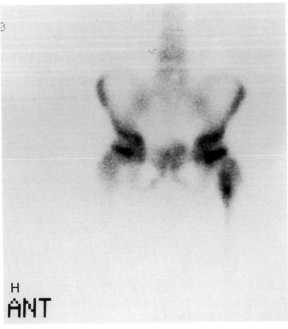

Patient 4

FIGURE 1–27   J.

Pinhole Bone Scan and CT Scan: There is increased osteogenesis of the anterosuperior L2 vertebral body, where dense bone is visualized on CT. The nidus (*arrowhead*) is eccentric. (Courtesy of Dr. Lee Kellerhouse, San Diego, CA.)

NOTE 1. Virtually all osteoid osteomas have increased blood flow, hyperemia, and osteogenesis. In the feet and spine, SPECT scans may best define the location of the lesion.

NOTE 2. The bone scan is particularly helpful in evaluating a sclerotic lesion seen on x-ray. Isointense or minimally increased osteogenesis and the absence of hyperemia suggest a bone island, whereas hyperemia and markedly increased osteogenesis indicate a more active lesion, i.e., osteoid osteoma, blastic metastases, or infection.

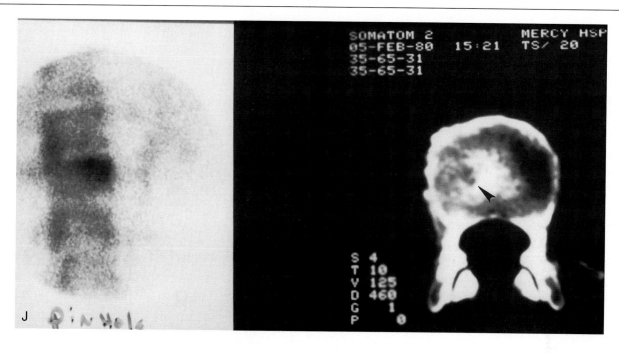

BONE ISLAND

FIGURE 1–28   A.

Plain Film X-ray of Left Ilium: There is a "blastic" lesion just above the left acetabulum.

FIGURE 1–28   B.

Anterior Bone Scan: There is no increased osteogenesis.

NOTE 1. Bone islands are usually inactive on bone scan and do not have increased blood flow or hyperemia.

NOTE 2. Bone islands consist of dense compact bone, have sharp margins, and are usually ovoid or round. Any bone can have bone islands.

NOTE 3. Differential diagnosis of a sclerotic lesion on x-ray includes osteoid osteoma, osteoma, and osteoblastic metastases (prostate and breast mostly), all of which will have hyperemia on blood pool imaging.

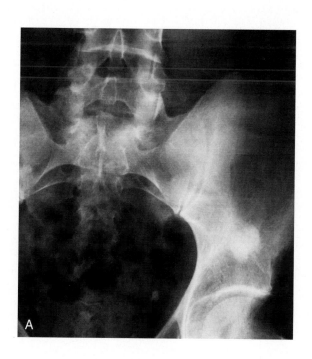

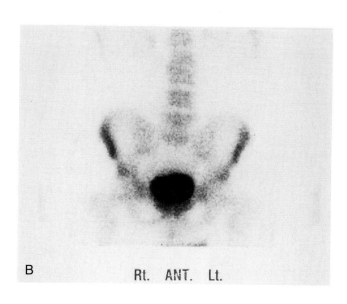

BENIGN FIBROUS CORTICAL DEFECT

Patient 1: 17 Year Old Male with an Active Fibrous Cortical Defect

FIGURE 1–29   A.

Plain Film X-ray: There is a well-circumscribed metaphyseal cortical lesion in the distal femur.

FIGURE 1–29   B.

Delayed Bone Scintigraphy: The increased osteogenesis indicates an active lesion.

Patient 2: 20 Year Old Female with Extensive Abnormality

FIGURE 1–29   C.

Plain Film X-ray: There is an elongated radiolucent lesion, eccentrically involving the cortex of the tibial metaphysis and diaphysis.

FIGURE 1–29   D to F.

Blood Flow, Blood Pool, and Delayed Scans: The increased blood flow, hyperemia, and osteogenesis indicate that this is an active lesion.

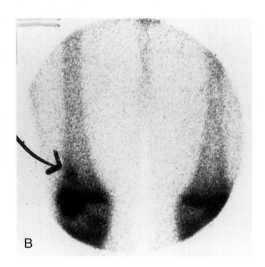

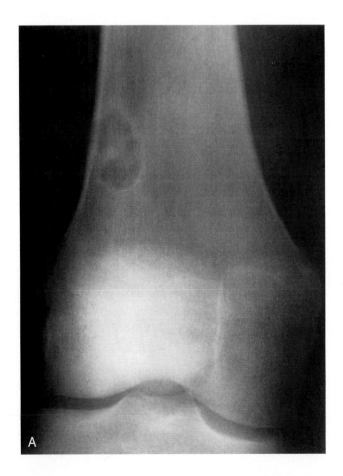

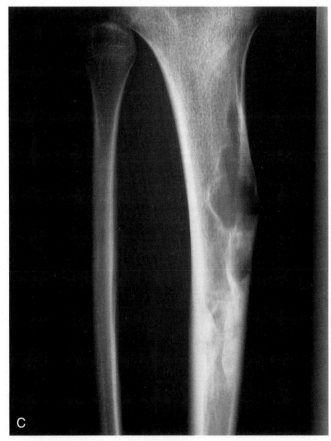

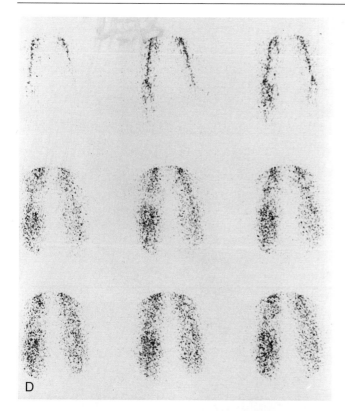

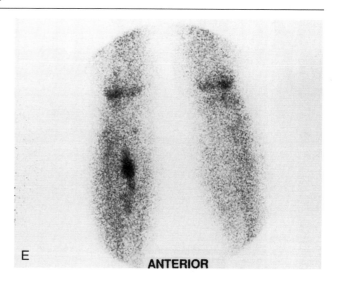

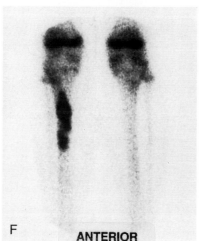

NOTE 2. Nonossifying fibromas are metaphyseal, eccentric, and cortical and have a sclerotic border. They can extend into the diaphysis.

NOTE 3. The hyperemia and increased osteogenesis indicate an active lesion, usually in the "healing" phase. Large lesions can fracture, causing hyperemia and increased osteogenesis.

Illustration continued on following page

Patient 3: 24 Year Old Male with an Almost Healed Fibrous Cortical Defect

FIGURE 1–29   G.

Plain Film X-ray: An ovoid sclerotic rim surrounding a radiolucent center is seen in the metaphysis of the right femur (*white arrow*).

FIGURE 1–29   H and I.

Blood Pool and Delayed Planar Scans: There is no hyperemia and only mildly increased osteogenesis.

NOTE 1. Nonossifying fibromas, or fibrous cortical defects, are usually seen in children and young adults. They "heal" by internal ossification over time.

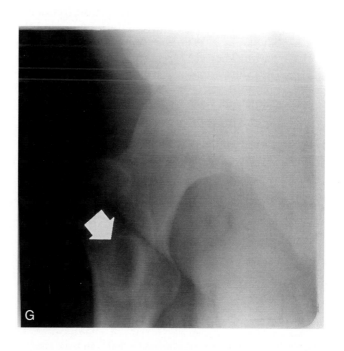

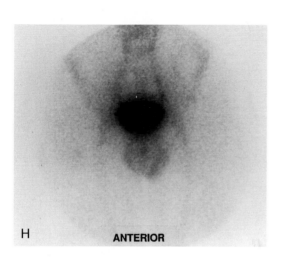

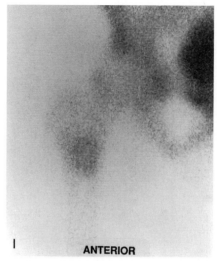

H **ANTERIOR**

I **ANTERIOR**

OSTEOCHONDROMA OF TALUS

FIGURE 1–30   A.

Plain Film X-ray: There is a pedunculated osseous mass extending from the talus *(single arrow)*. The cartilaginous cap cannot be seen. There are also bony spurs of the calcaneus at the Achilles tendon *(black arrow)* and the plantar fascial attachments *(arrowheads)*.

FIGURE 1–30   B.

Planar Bone Scintigram: There is marked increased activity corresponding to the osteochondroma seen on the x-ray. Less intense activity is seen at the calcaneal plantar spur *(arrow)*, the symptomatic site in this patient. The posterior calcaneal spur *(arrowhead)* is even less active.

NOTE 1. Solitary osteochondromas can be "hot" or isointense on bone scan and still be benign. Less than 1 percent degenerate into chondrosarcoma.

NOTE 2. Solitary osteochondromas are most frequently found pointing away from the joint nearest the metaphysis of a long bone, from which they arise. They are rarely symptomatic, except for pressure symptoms. They contain marrow continuous with the marrow of the bone from which they arise.

NOTE 3. Spurs that occur at sites of tendon and ligament attachments, usually secondary to inflammation or trauma, are manifestations of enthesopathies.

NOTE 4. Radiation in childhood can give rise to benign osteochondromas in bones included in the radiation port.

Cross References

Chapter 2: Multiple Bony Abnormalities—Osteochondromas (Exostoses)

Chapter 4: Pelvic Abnormalities—Pelvic Osteochondroma

Chapter 11: Soft Tissue Abnormalities—Tendinitis on Bone Scan

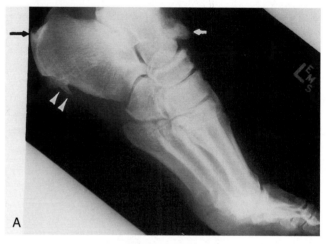

A

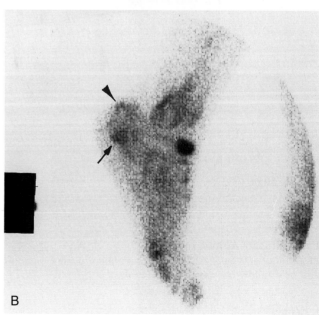

B

BLOOD POOL IMAGING IN BENIGN BONE TUMORS

Patient 1: Osteochondroma of the Ilium

FIGURE 1–31   A.

Plain Film X-ray: There is dense irregular calcification arising in the left SI joint region.

FIGURE 1–31   B.

CT Scan: There is a thin cartilaginous cap *(arrowheads)* over the bony excrescence.

FIGURE 1–31   C and D.

Blood Pool and Delayed Bone Scans: There is no hyperemia and only isointense osteogenesis of the iliac abnormality.

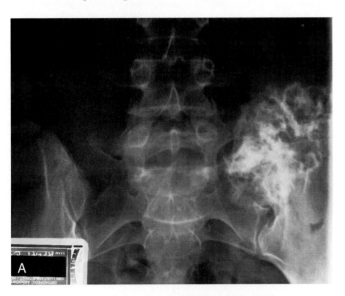

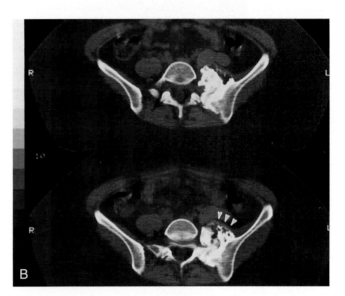

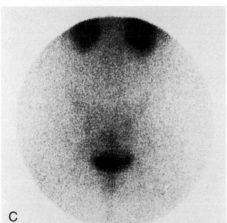

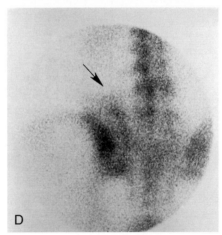

Patient 2: Parosteal Chondroma

FIGURE 1–31   E.

Plain Film X-ray: There is a round mass with a calcified rim arising from the right humeral metaphysis.

FIGURE 1–31   F and G.

Blood Pool and Delayed Planar Scans: There is mild hyperemia and marked osteogenesis of the round mass. The thallium tumor scan was negative.

FIGURE 1–31   H.

Plain Film X-ray 2 Years Later: There are now multiple calcifications in the proximal right upper arm.

FIGURE 1–31   I.

Posterior Internal Rotation Bone Scan: There are multiple masses in the posterior and lateral soft tissues.

NOTE 1. The absence of hyperemia with a bone tumor virtually rules out high-grade primary and secondary malignancies.

NOTE 2. Hyperemia can be seen with either benign or malignant processes.

NOTE 3. Pain, swelling, and tenderness are frequent with parosteal chondromas, despite its benignity. These symptoms are nonspecific but do suggest degeneration of a benign lesion into a more malignant form.

Cross Reference

Chapter 8: Hyperemia—Chondrosarcoma

Illustration continued on following page

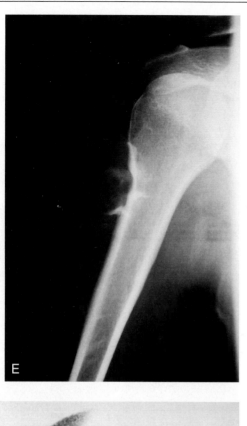

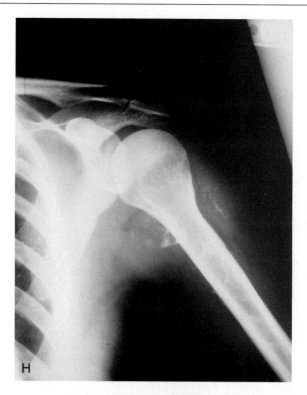

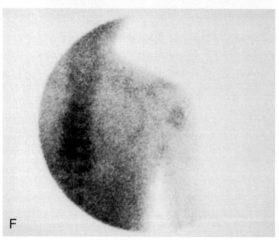

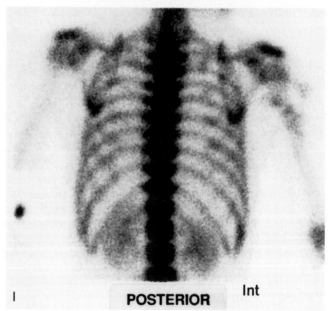

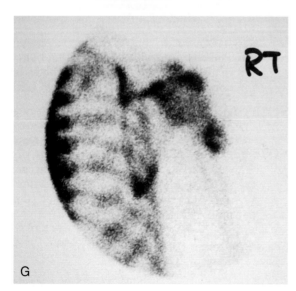

OSTEOSARCOMA

Patient: 17 Year Old Male

FIGURE 1–32   A.
Plain Film X-ray of Left Knee: There is an osteoblastic process in the lateral femoral condyle (p = patella).

FIGURE 1–32   B and C.
Blood Flow and Blood Pool Scintigraphy: There is marked increased blood flow and hyperemia involving the left knee.

FIGURE 1–32   D and E.
Delayed Bone Planar and SPECT Scans: The lateral femoral condyle has increased osteogenesis, with central photopenia.

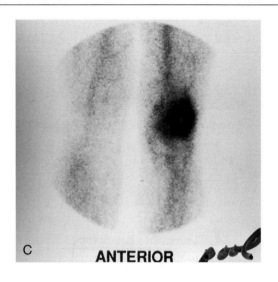

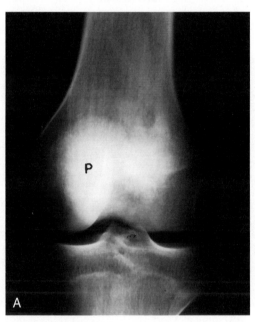

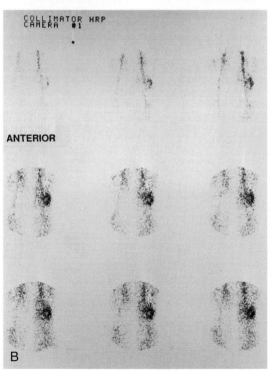

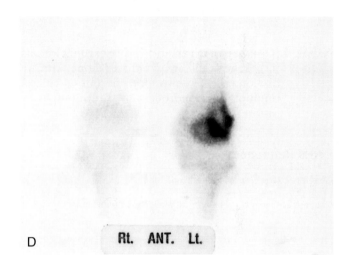

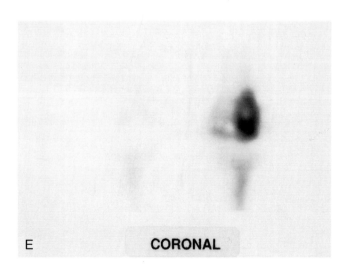

Illustration continued on following page

FIGURE 1–32 F and G.

Thallium Tumor Scan: There is intense thallium accumulation in the anterior lateral femoral condyle, again with a central photopenic zone, suggesting a less active or necrotic portion of tumor.

FIGURE 1–32 H and I.

Axial and Coronal MRI Scans: The destructive mass is well visualized in both its intraosseous and extraosseous components.

NOTE 1. Thallium accumulates intensely in malignant processes, probably based on both growth rate and blood flow.

NOTE 2. Most common sites for osteosarcoma: distal femur, proximal tibia, humerus, and ilium.

NOTE 3. Osteosarcoma arises in teenagers and 20 to 30 year olds.

NOTE 4. Osteosarcoma can arise in pre-existing lesions, i.e., Paget's disease, irradiated bone, chronic osteomyelitis, polyostotic fibrous dysplasia, multiple enchondromatosis, and multiple exostoses.

Cross References

Chapter 8: Hyperemia—Chondrosarcoma

Chapter 72: Tumors—Thallium in Malignant Bone Tumors

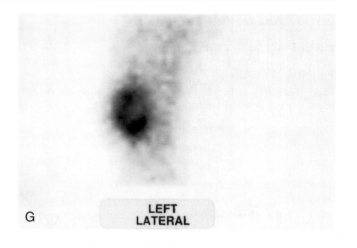

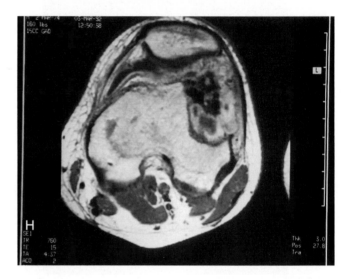

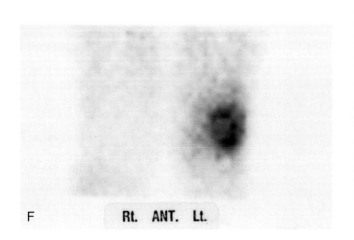

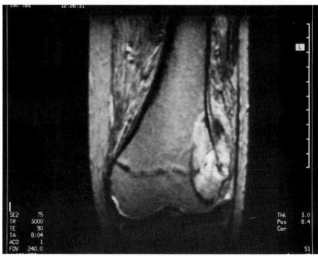

EWING'S SARCOMA

Patient: 17 Year Old Male

FIGURE 1–33.
Anterior and Posterior Scintigrams of the Pelvis: There is a broad vertical area of increased osteogenesis involving the anterior left ilium.

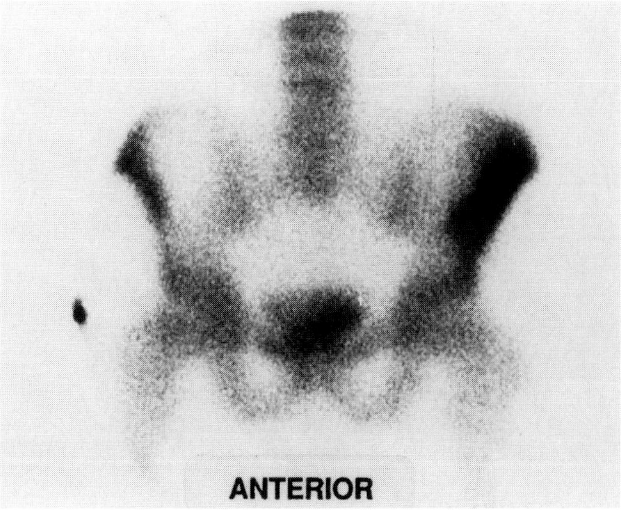

NOTE 1. Ewing's sarcoma is most frequently found in the first and second decades of life. This tumor is most commonly located in the femur, followed by the flat bones (ribs, pelvis, scapula).

Cross Reference

Chapter 72: Tumors—Thallium in Malignant Bone Tumors

ANTERIOR

SOLITARY PLASMACYTOMA

FIGURE 1–34   A.
Plain Film X-ray of Femur: There is a cortical lytic process surrounded by a broad area of sclerosis.

FIGURE 1–34   B.
Blood Pool Scintigram: The "doughnut" hyperemia in the left thigh indicates an active process.

FIGURE 1–34   C.
Delayed Bone Scintigram: There is an ill-defined, elongated region of increased activity with a central area of decreased osteogenesis.

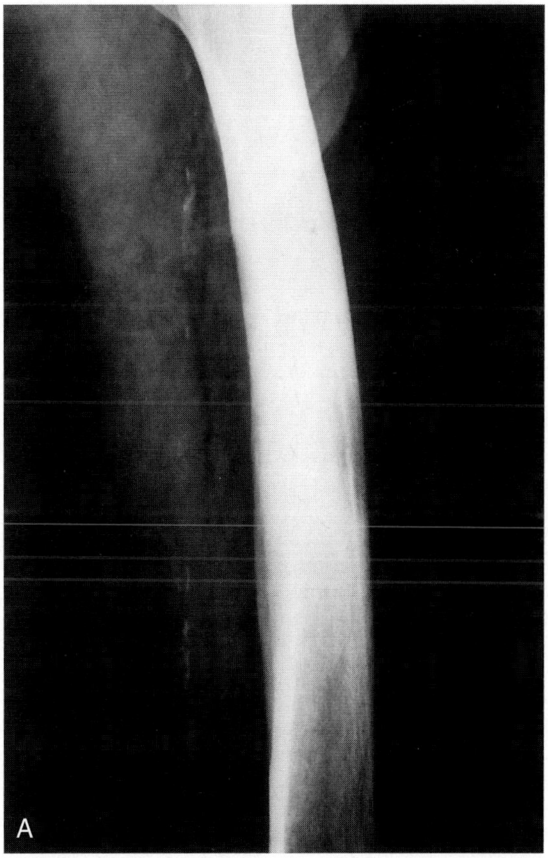

NOTE 1. The hyperemia indicates an active process, versus a static healed lesion with bone sclerosis, i.e., chronic inactive osteomyelitis.

NOTE 2. The "doughnut" sign suggests a central area of necrosis or inactive tumor. Necrosis is probably due to the tumor's outgrowing its blood supply.

NOTE 3. Solitary plasmacytomas can occur in bone, soft tissues (i.e., kidneys), or nasal-paranasal cavities. It can have many radiographic appearances, including osteolysis with or without sclerosis.

Illustration continued on following page

Cross References

Chapter 1: Solitary Bony Abnormalities—Unusual Solitary Metastases

Chapter 72: Tumors—Thallium in Malignant Bone Tumors

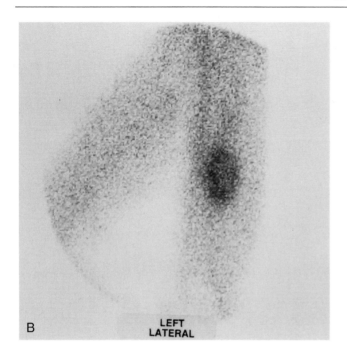

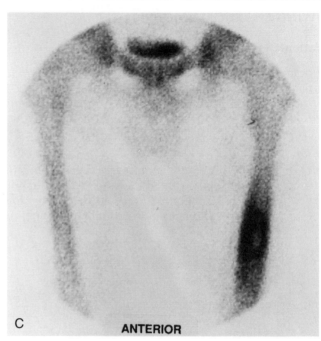

GIANT CELL TUMOR OF THE FEMUR

FIGURE 1–35   A and B.

Anterior and Lateral Plain Film X-rays of the Right Knee: There is an eccentric expansile lytic lesion with areas of broken cortex in the metaphysis and epiphysis.

FIGURE 1–35   C and D.

Blood Flow and Blood Pool Scintigrams: There is marked increased blood flow and hyperemia.

FIGURE 1–35   E and F.

Delayed Bone Scintigrams in Anterior and Lateral Projections: The increased activity involves the metaphysis as well as the medial and lateral femoral condyles down to the joint line.

NOTE 1. The hyperemia does not indicate malignancy. Rapid growth, fracture, or infection can also increase blood flow to a lesion.

NOTE 2. Giant cell tumors occur most frequently in the third and fourth decades, arising in epiphyses, especially in the distal femur. They can degenerate into fibrosarcoma or osteosarcoma.

Cross Reference

Chapter 1: Solitary Bony Abnormalities—Giant Cell Tumor of the Patella

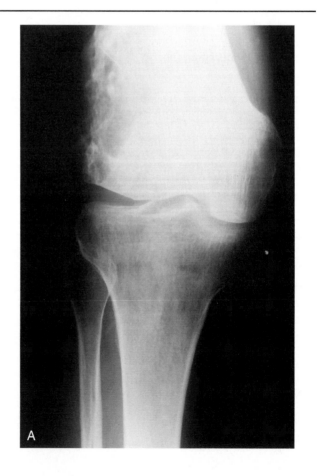

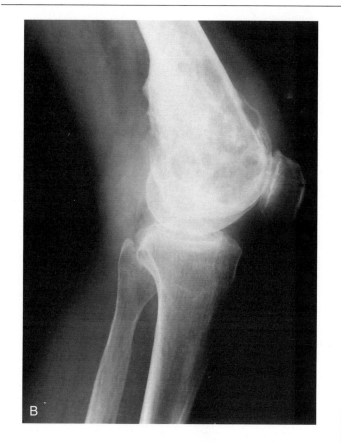

B

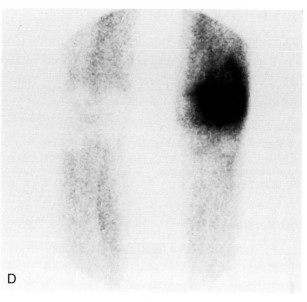

D

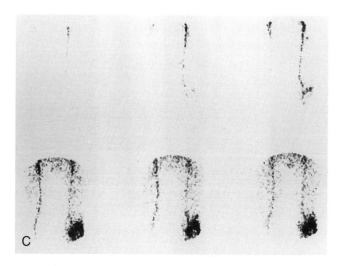

C

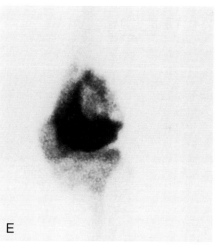

E

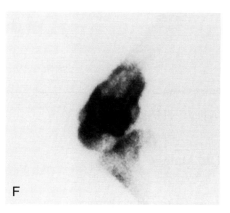

F

LYMPHOMA OF THE THIGH

FIGURE 1–36 A.

Before Radiation Therapy Bone Scan: The soft tissue component of the lymphoma has retained some of the radiopharmaceutical *(arrowheads)*. Note the markedly increased osteogenesis of the femoral cortex adjacent to the tumor.

FIGURE 1–36 B.

After Radiation Therapy Bone Scan: There is no appreciable residual soft tissue activity *(arrow)*, but there is persistent cortical bone or periosteal involvement. A small cortical defect remains along the lateral femur.

Cross References

Chapter 2: Multiple Bony Abnormalities—Hypertrophic Osteoarthropathy

Chapter 9: "Cold" Abnormalities—Primary Lymphoma of Bone

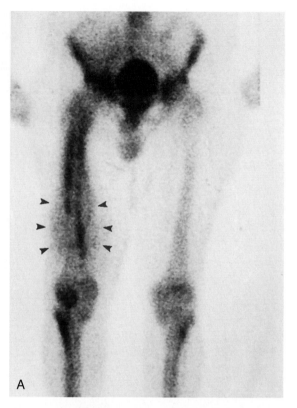

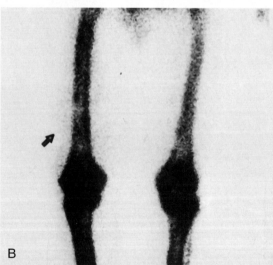

VALUE OF NEGATIVE THALLIUM TUMOR SCAN

Patient: 5 Year Old Male

FIGURE 1–37 A.

Hip X-ray: There is dense periosteal thickening along the proximal left femoral metaphysis.

FIGURE 1–37 B.

CT Scan: The periosteal lamellation suggests Ewing's sarcoma.

FIGURE 1–37 C and D.

Blood Pool and Delayed Bone Scans: There is hyperemia and increased osteogenesis along the left proximal femur.

FIGURE 1–37 E.

Thallium Tumor Scan: There is only minimal increased thallium accumulation, presumably due to the increased blood flow in the region.

NOTE 1. This turned out to be a foreign body reaction, probably due to a DPT vaccination that was placed too deep, beneath the periosteum.

NOTE 2. Negative tumor scanning usually allows for a more conservative approach.

Cross Reference

Chapter 72: Tumors—Thallium in Benign Bone Conditions

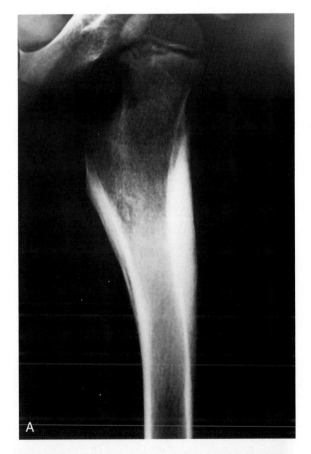

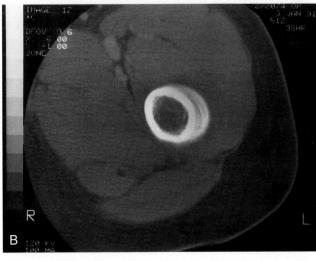

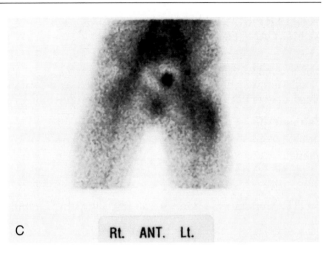

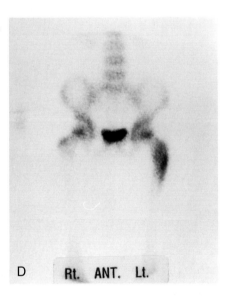

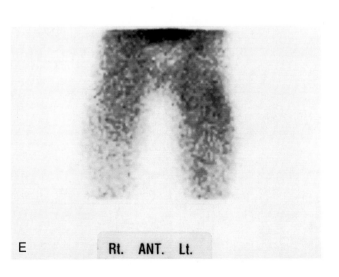

SOLITARY BONE METASTASIS FROM LUNG CANCER

FIGURE 1–38   A and B.

Blood Flow and Blood Pool Scintigrams: There is increased blood flow and hyperemia in the proximal right thigh.

FIGURE 1–38   C.

Delayed Bone Scintigram: There is increased activity in the proximal femoral metaphysis.

NOTE. Metastases to bone are almost always hyperemic.

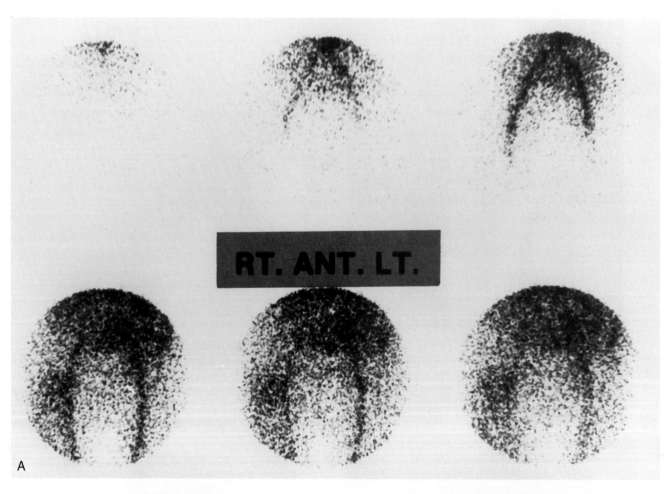

A

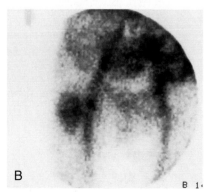

B

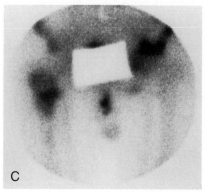

C

CORTICAL METASTASIS FROM LUNG CARCINOMA

FIGURE 1–39   A.
Bone Scintigram: A solitary, elongated lesion involves the left femoral diaphysis.

FIGURE 1–39   B.
Plain X-ray, Coned-Down View: There is a lytic process involving the posterior cortex of the femur.

NOTE 1. Solitary peripheral metastases are unusual.

NOTE 2. By scan appearance, this could be a primary or secondary lesion.

NOTE 3. Direct bone invasion by a soft tissue process can have the same bone scan findings as a primary bone lesion.

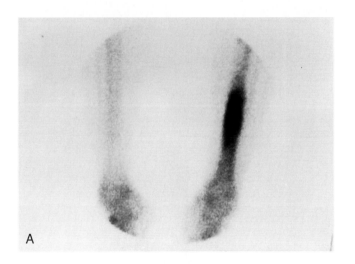

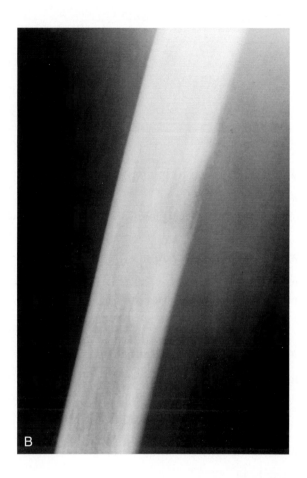

UNUSUAL SOLITARY METASTASES

Patient 1: Lung Carcinoma

FIGURE 1–40   A.
Blood Pool Scintigram: There is marked hyperemia of the ulnar side of the right hand.

FIGURE 1–40   B.
Delayed Planar Scintigram: There is marked increased osteogenesis of the fifth metacarpal, the hamate, and the pisiform bones.

FIGURE 1–40   C.
Plain Film X-ray: The marked destruction of the fifth metacarpal and hamate is evident.

Illustration continued on following page

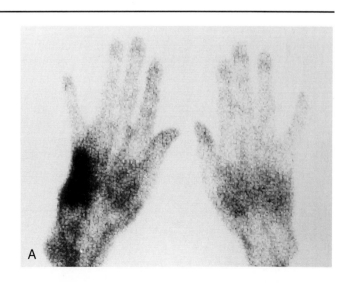

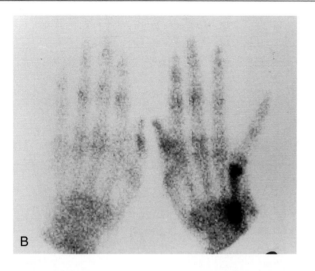

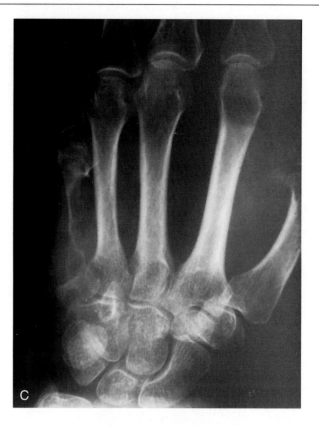

Patient 2: Breast Carcinoma

FIGURE 1–40 D.

Posterior Bone Scan: The right scapula has a focal abnormality.

Patient 3: Breast Carcinoma

FIGURE 1–40 E.

Anterior Bone Scan: The left lesser trochanter has a solitary metastasis.

Patient 4: Prostate Carcinoma

FIGURE 1–40 F.

Anterior Bone Scan: An abnormality can be seen in the right proximal humeral metaphysis.

Patient 5: Renal Cell Carcinoma

FIGURE 1–40 G.

Right Lateral Bone Scan: There is a "cold" lesion surrounded by increased osteogenesis in the right mandible.

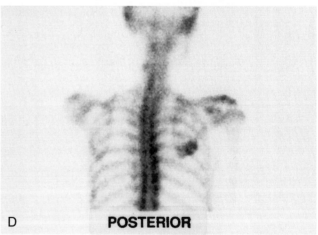

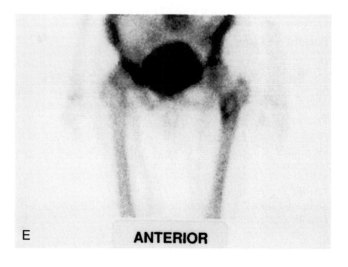

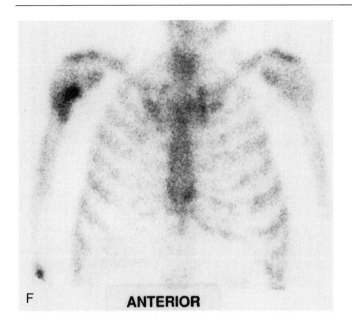

F ANTERIOR

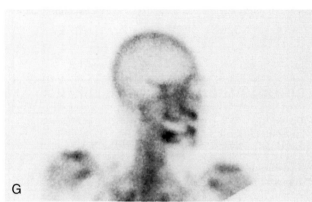

G

GIANT CELL TUMOR OF THE PATELLA

FIGURE 1–41   A.

Blood Flow Scintigraphy: There is marked hyperemia of the left patella.

FIGURE 1–41   B and C.

Delayed Bone Scintigraphy: There is markedly increased osteogenesis of the left patella.

Illustration continued on following page

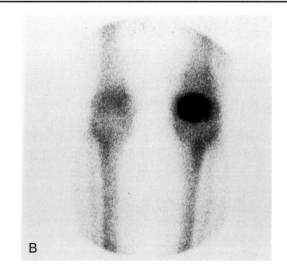

B

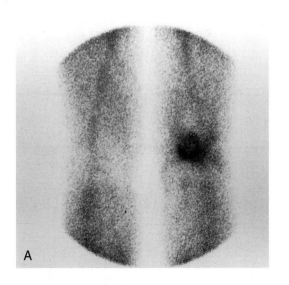

A

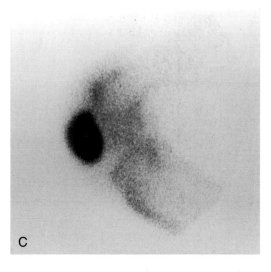

C

FIGURE 1–41 D.
Lateral Plain Film X-ray: The patella is expanded by a septated lytic process.

Cross Reference

Chapter 1: Solitary Bony Abnormalities—Giant Cell Tumor of the Femur

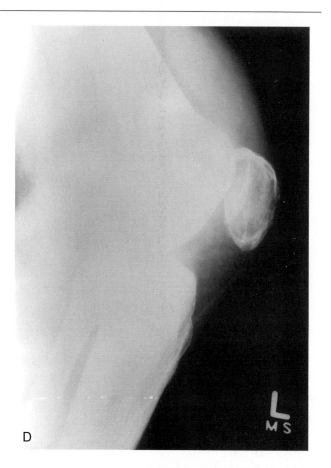

D

DIFFERENTIAL DIAGNOSIS OF "HOT PATELLA"	
Overuse: musculotendinous overload	Patellofemoral arthritis
	Osteomyelitis
Soft tissue or joint hyperemia	Paget's disease
	Hyperparathyroidism
Surgery (should disappear in 18–24 months)	Osteonecrosis
	Neoplasm, primary
Fracture of patella or other knee bone	Neoplasm, secondary
Chondromalacia	"Normal"
Reflex sympathetic dystrophy/regional osteoporosis	Torn knee ligaments

STERNOCLAVICULAR JOINT ARTHRITIS

FIGURE 1–42.
Bone Scan: There is unilateral increased osteogenesis involving both sides of the right sternoclavicular joint.

NOTE. In arthritis the manubrium is affected only at the joint. More diffuse activity suggests metastases or osteomyelitis.

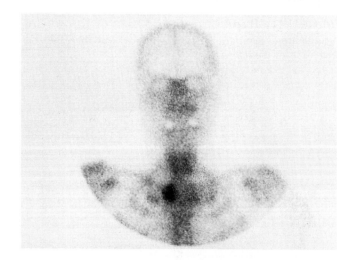

OSTEOMYELITIS OF THE MANUBRIUM AND FIRST RIB

FIGURE 1–43 A.
Bone Scan: There is marked increased osteogenesis of the manubrium extending to involve the right first rib.

FIGURE 1–43 B.
CT Scan: There is destruction of the right first rib–chondromanubrial joint *(arrow)*, with associated soft tissue swelling.

NOTE. Osteomyelitis should be suspected when both sides of a joint are involved and when trauma and arthritis are excluded. Tumor rarely, if ever, involves cartilage, whereas infection readily crosses cartilage.

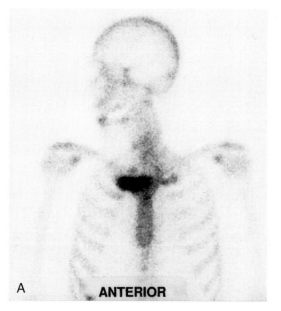

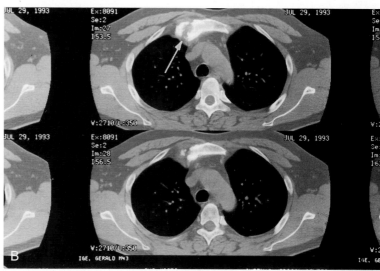

SOLITARY MANUBRIAL METASTASIS FROM BREAST CARCINOMA

FIGURE 1–44   A.

Bone Scintigram: There is focal increased activity in the manubrium and along the superior margin as well as on the manubrial side of the right sternoclavicular joint.

FIGURE 1–44   B.

CT Scan: There is loss of cortex and a lytic process in the right side of the manubrium. A soft tissue mass is associated with the bony abnormality.

NOTE 1. This case demonstrates an asymptomatic metastasis that could be mistaken for sternoclavicular osteoarthritis. However, there is no activity on the clavicular side of the joint, and the manubrial activity extends beyond the right joint margin.

NOTE 2. Solitary metastases in the sternum are often seen with breast carcinoma. Slight oblique views of the sternum may be obtained in otherwise normal bone scans.

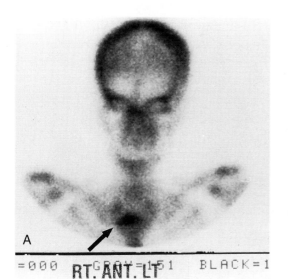

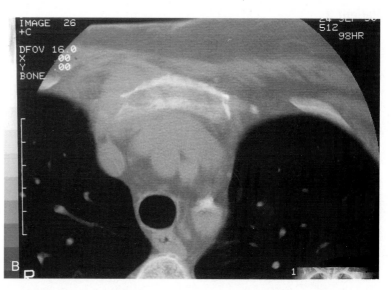

NORMAL STERNOTOMY

FIGURE 1–45   A and B.
Anterior and RAO Bone Scans: The linear, well-defined increased activity in the sternum indicates a normal post-sternotomy.

NOTE. The sternotomy activity may heal to the point where it is barely noticeable.

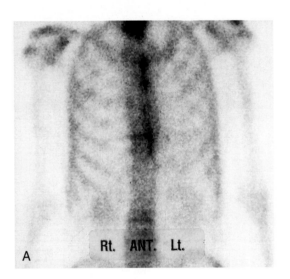

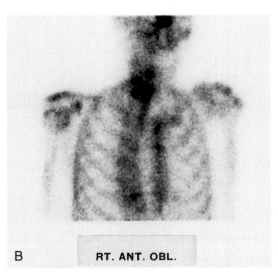

INTRAVENOUS CATHETER ON BONE SCAN

Patient 1

FIGURE 1–46   A and B.
Anterior and RAO Bone Scan: The "hot" spot in the right chest is between the ribs on the oblique view. The vertical extension is the catheter entering the subclavian vein *(arrow).*

Patient 2

FIGURE 1–46   C.
Anterior Chest Bone Scan: There is persistent activity along the entire length of the tubings.

Patient 3

FIGURE 1–46   D.
Anterior Chest Bone Scan: The catheter tip has migrated from the innominate vein up into the jugular vein.

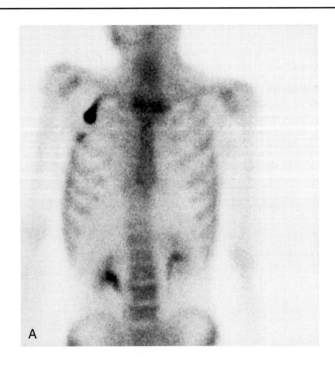

NOTE. Persistent activity in catheters may mean that the tubing was not flushed adequately after injection of the radiopharmaceutical or that there is clot building up along inner walls.

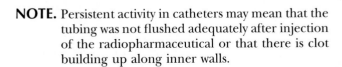

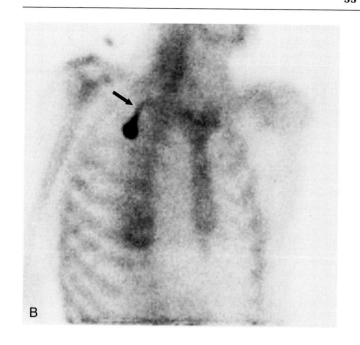

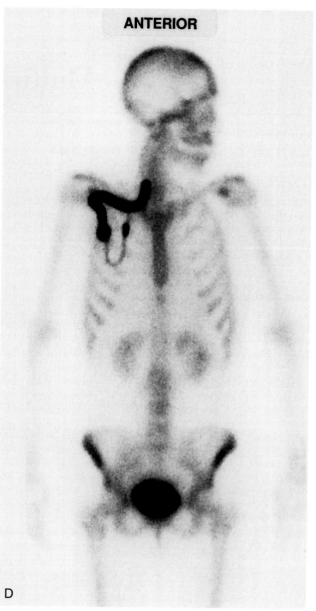

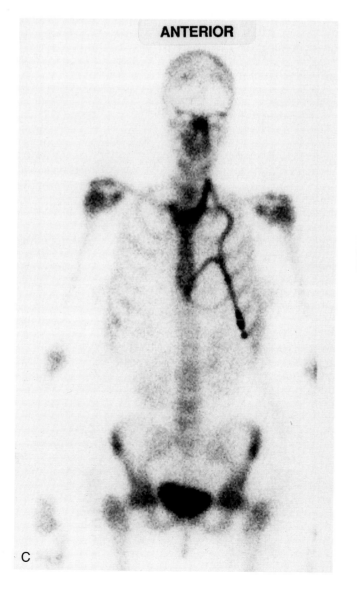

Chapter 2
Multiple Bony Abnormalities

BILATERAL CONGENITAL HIP DYSPLASIA

FIGURE 2–1 A and B.

Anterior and Posterior Pelvic Bone Scan: The right hip is subluxated superiorly, forming a false acetabulum. The left femur has severe coxa vara deformity. The patient also has osteochondral loose bodies about both hips *(arrows)*. The bladder is elevated by a huge prostate gland.

Cross Reference

Chapter 11: Soft Tissue Abnormalities—Impressions on the Bladder; Active Synovial Osteochondromatosis

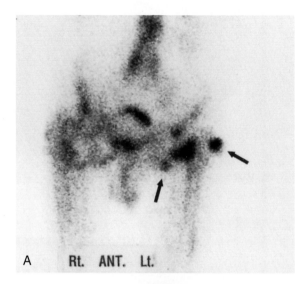

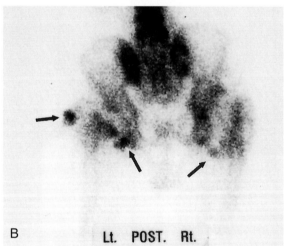

SEVERE OSTEOARTHRITIS
VS. OSTEONECROSIS

Patient 1: 70 Year Old Woman

Figure 2-2 A.

Anterior Bone Scan: There is marked increased activity involving both femoral heads diffusely.

Patient 2: 73 Year Old Woman with Multijoint Complaints

Figure 2-2 B.

Anterior and Posterior Whole Body Bone Scan: There are multiple areas of abnormality in this patient with diffuse osteoarthritis. The shoulders have activity throughout the humeral heads, an appearance similar to that of osteonecrosis.

Figure 2-2 C.

Anterior and Posterior Pelvic Bone Scan: The hip activity is greatest along the joint line, less likely to represent osteonecrosis.

Illustration continued on following page

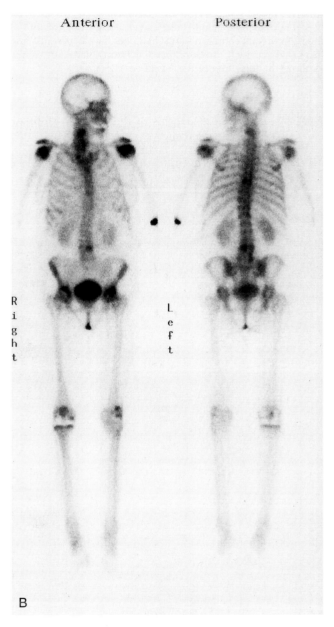

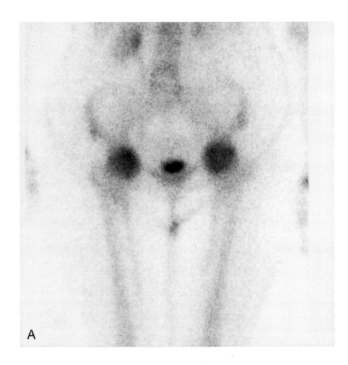

A

B

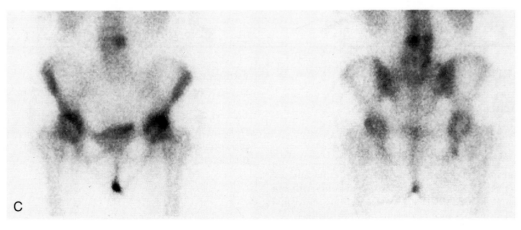

C

Patient 3: 74 Year Old Male with Right Knee Pain, Sent in to Rule Out Osteonecrosis

FIGURE 2–2   D and E.

Anterior Blood Pool and Delayed Bone Scans: There are focal hyperemia and increased osteogenesis along the joint line of the right medial compartment. The knees have hyperemia and increased activity in the suprapatellar bursas bilaterally as well as along the joint line of the left knee.

NOTE 1. Severe osteoarthritis of the hips can simulate avascular necrosis.

NOTE 2. Hyperemia indicates an active process, including degenerative osteoarthritis.

Cross Reference

Chapter 1: Solitary Bony Abnormalities—Late Osteonecrosis; Meniscal Disease and Osseous Changes of the Knee

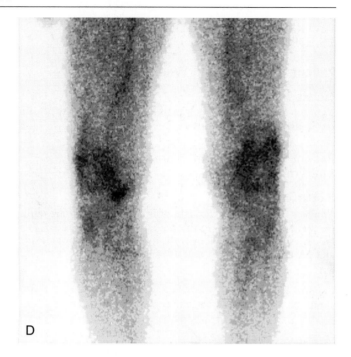

D

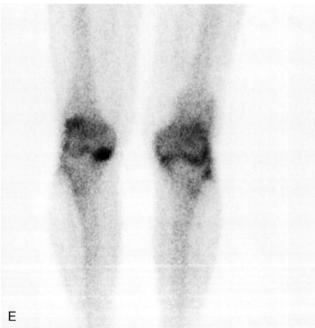

E

RHEUMATOID ARTHRITIS

Various Patients

Hands

FIGURE 2–3   A and B.

Blood Pool and Delayed Bone Scans:The hyperemia and increased osteogenesis involving some of the carpal bones indicate the active rheumatoid joints, whereas other joints are abnormal only on delayed scans because of degenerative arthritis.

FIGURE 2–3   C.

Delayed Bone Scan: The entire carpus is involved.

FIGURE 2–3   D and E.

Delayed Bone Scans: Virtually all the metacarpophalangeal and interphalangeal joints are abnormal, yet the carpal bones are quiescent.

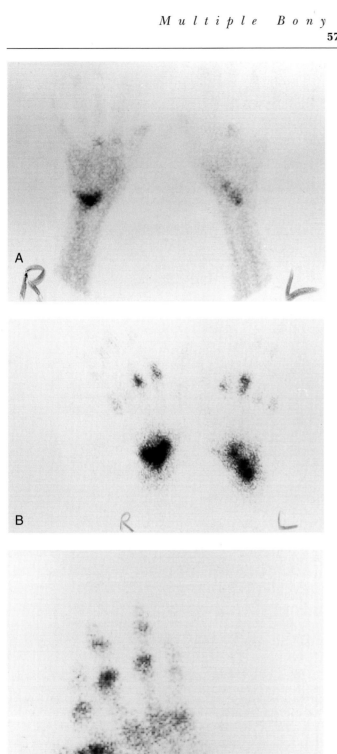

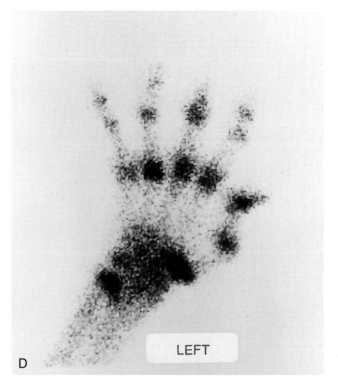

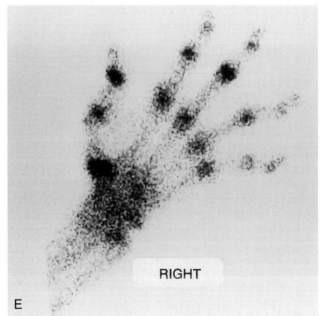

Shoulders

FIGURE 2–3   F.

Delayed Bone Scan: There are fine lines of increased activity in the glenohumeral joints bilaterally as well as symmetric abnormalities of the acromioclavicular joints. The right sternoclavicular joint is abnormal.

FIGURE 2–3   G.

Delayed Bone Scan: Both shoulders have diffuse humeral head activity, reflecting a more advanced and destructive stage of the disease. The symmetric sternoclavicular joint disease suggests rheumatoid arthritis but is nonspecific.

Illustration continued on following page

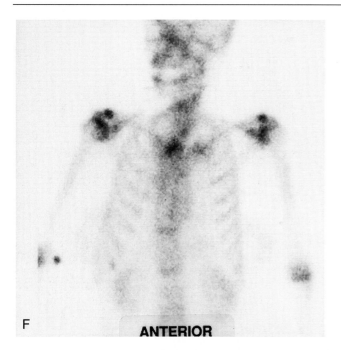

F **ANTERIOR**

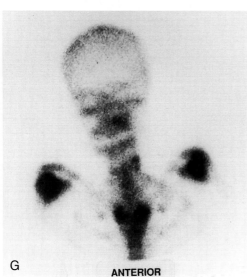

G **ANTERIOR**

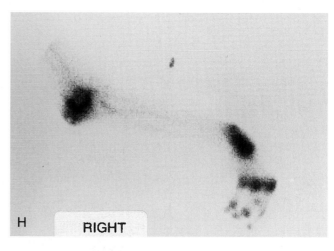

H **RIGHT**

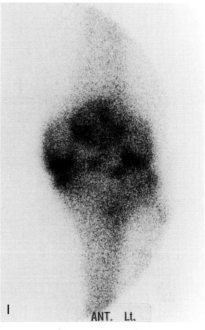

I **ANT. Lt.**

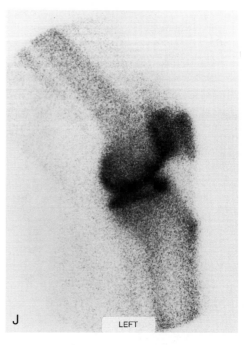

J **LEFT**

Elbow

FIGURE 2–3   H.

Delayed Bone Scan: The elbow is diffusely abnormal.

Knee

FIGURE 2–3   I and J.

Delayed Bone Scan: The medial, lateral, and patellofemoral compartments are involved.

NOTE 1. Rheumatoid arthritis is usually a symmetric arthritis. It involves the joints on both sides, i.e., wrists, fingers, knees, and shoulders, although not all joints are active at the same time.

NOTE 2. Classically, all three compartments of the knee joint are involved in rheumatoid arthritis, as opposed to degenerative arthritis.

ACTIVE RHEUMATOID ARTHRITIS ON WBC SCAN

Patient 1: Urinary Tract Infection

FIGURE 2–4   A and B.

Bone and WBC Scans of Knees: Both the bone radiopharmaceutical and the WBCs concentrate in the right knee.

FIGURE 2–4   C and D.

Bone and WBC Scans of Right Elbow: There is abnormal WBC accumulation in the right elbow and wrist *(arrow)*.

FIGURE 2–4   E and F.

Bone and WBC Scans of the Shoulders: There is no abnormal accumulation of WBCs in the shoulders, indicating no active disease in these joints.

Illustration continued on following page

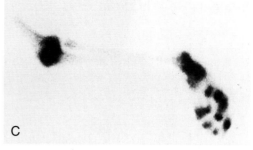

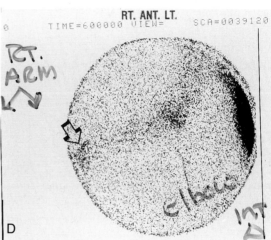

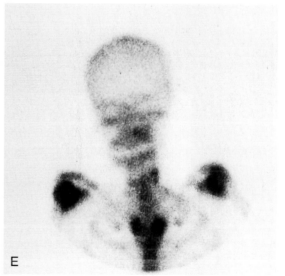

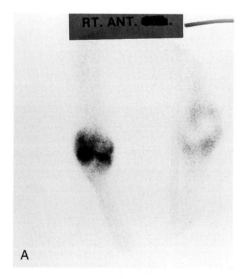

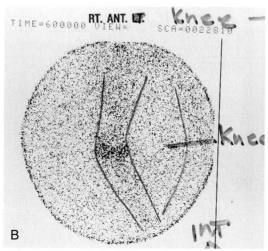

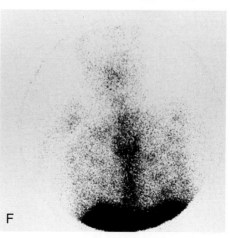

Patient 2: Postoperative WBC Scan

Figure 2–4 G and H.

WBC Scan of the Feet: There are abnormal WBC collections in the subtalar, calcaneocuboid, talonavicular, and possibly tibiotalar joints of the right foot only. The metatarsophalangeal and interphalangeal joints are normal.

Figure 2–4 I and J.

Planar and Lateral Plain X-rays: The fixation wires can be seen in the toes crossing the resected joints. The intertarsal joints are normal at this time.

NOTE. WBCs can accumulate in active rheumatoid joints because of nonspecific inflammation and do not necessarily indicate infection.

Cross References

Chapter 2: Multiple Bony Abnormalities—Multiple Septic Joints

Chapter 7: Hands and Feet—Diabetic Foot: Trauma vs. Infection

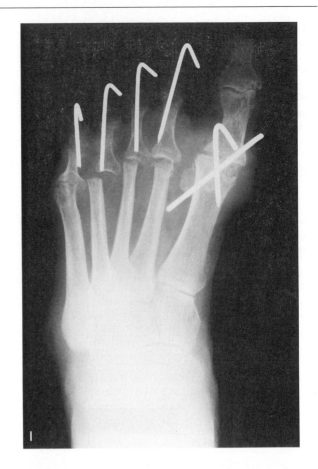

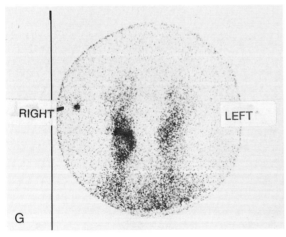

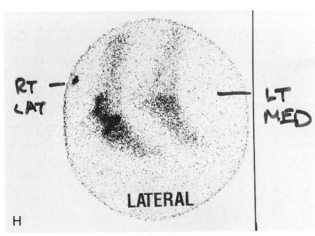

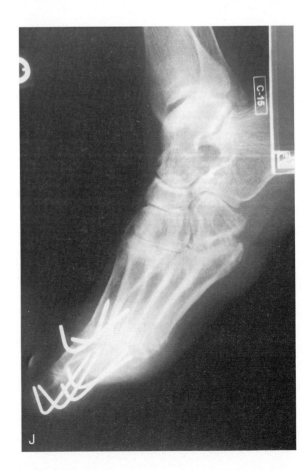

PSORIATIC ARTHRITIS

Patient 1

FIGURE 2–5   A.

Anterior Pelvic Bone Scintigraphy: There is increased activity involving the sacroiliac joints and hips bilaterally.

FIGURE 2–5   B.

RPO Spine Bone Scintigraphy: The apophyseal joints have increased activity at several levels.

Patient 2

FIGURE 2–5   C and D.

Planar Spine Bone Scintigraphy and SPECT Scan: An asymmetric bony outgrowth bridging two vertebrae is present along the right midthoracic vertebral column *(arrow)*. A pedicle, lamina, and spinous process are also abnormal *(arrowhead)* but better defined with SPECT (D).

FIGURE 2–5   E.

Oblique Lumbar Bone Scintigram: The posterior elements have increased activity, including the spinous processes.

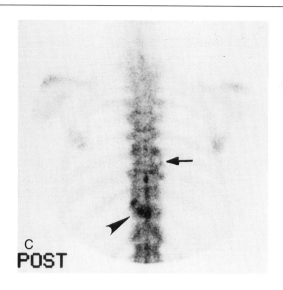

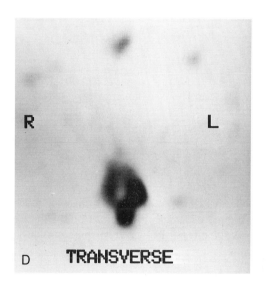

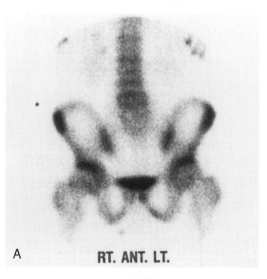

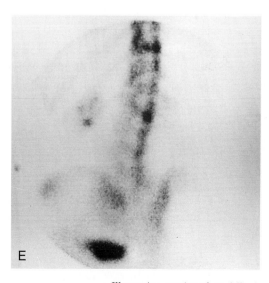

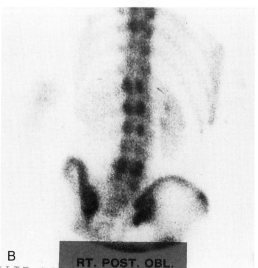

Illustration continued on following page

Figure 2–5 F.

RAO Cervical Spine Bone Scan: There are exuberant osteophytes creating an anterior ankylosis. (Courtesy of Dr. Michael Kipper, Vista, CA.)

NOTE 1. Giant, asymmetric spinal syndesmophytes are common in psoriatic arthritis.

NOTE 2. Spinous process activity may be due to inflammation of the attaching ligaments, muscles, and adjacent bursas. This is seen with rheumatoid arthritis as well.

Cross References

Chapter 3: Spinal Abnormalities—Solitary Osteophyte

Chapter 4: Pelvic Abnormalities—Ankylosing Spondylitis

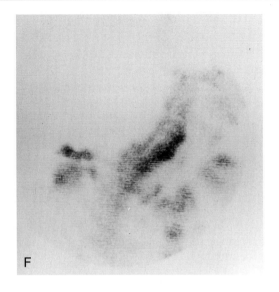

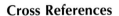

GOUT

Figure 2–6 A.

Bilateral Foot Scan: There is symmetric increased activity involving the great toes and the tarsal bones.

Figure 2–6 B.

Elbow Scan: Gouty tophi can ossify.

NOTE. Gouty changes involve both soft tissues and bones, especially the joints of the feet, hands, wrists, elbows, and, rarely, the spine and hips.

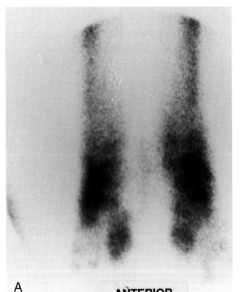

A ANTERIOR

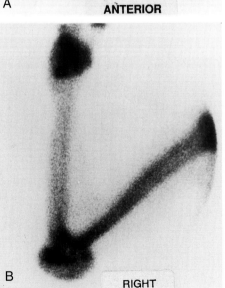

B RIGHT

BROWN TUMORS
IN HYPERPARATHYROIDISM

FIGURE 2–7.

Anterior Delayed Bone Scintigraphy: There are at least four abnormal areas in the distal right humerus as a result of brown tumors from hyperparathyroidism. (Courtesy of Dr. Michael Kipper, Vista, CA.)

NOTE. Brown tumors can be single or multiple, in a single bone or separate bones. They can be eccentric or central.

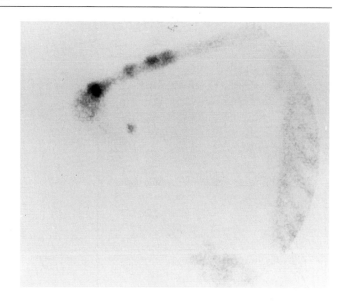

OSTEOMALACIA: PSEUDOFRACTURES IN
VITAMIN D RESISTANT RICKETS

FIGURE 2–8 A.

Anterior Proximal Femur: There are two pseudofractures of the medial left femur.

FIGURE 2–8 B.

Plain Film X-ray: The pseudofractures (Looser's zones) have characteristic findings: perpendicular to the cortex, lucent line bordered by sclerosis, and partial involvement of the shaft.

NOTE. Characteristic sites of involvement include the medial scapula, ribs, medial femur, pubic rami, and posterior proximal ulna.

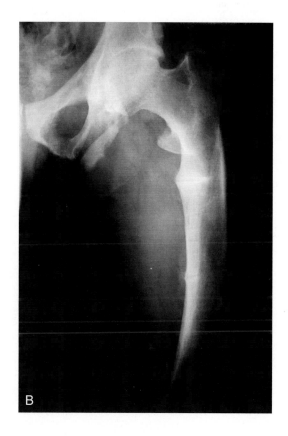

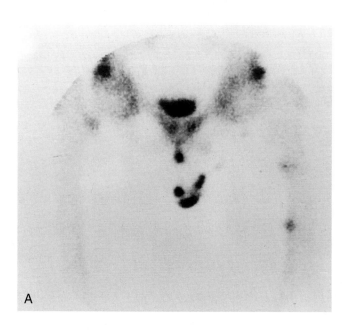

HYPERTROPHIC OSTEOARTHROPATHY

DIFFERENTIAL DIAGNOSIS OF HYPERTROPHIC OSTEOARTHROPATHY
Primary
Pachydermoperiostosis
Secondary
Lung tumors, especially bronchogenic carcinoma and mesothelioma
COPD
Bronchiectasis
Chronic lung infections
Cyanotic heart disease
Inflammatory bowel disease
Abdominal and retroperitoneal neoplasms
Chronic liver disease—cirrhosis, biliary atresia
Thyroid acropachy
Venous stasis
Intrathoracic Hodgkin's disease

Patient 1: Bronchogenic Carcinoma

FIGURE 2–9 A.

Total Body Bone Scan: There are elongated abnormalities along the cortical margins of the lower extremity bones and minimal upper extremity involvement.

Patient 2: Severe Emphysema

FIGURE 2–9 B.

Bone Scan: There is increased cortical activity and irregularity of all the long bones, including the upper extremities.

Cross References

Chapter 1: Solitary Bony Abnormalities—Lymphoma of the Thigh

Chapter 7: Hands and Feet—Osteoarthritis of the Hands

Chapter 8: Hyperemia—Clubbing of the Fingers

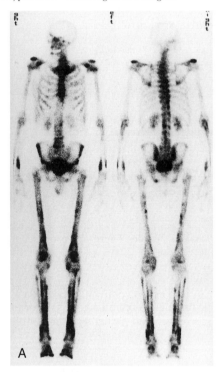

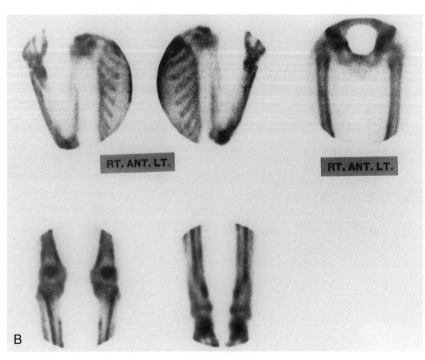

MULTIPLE SEPTIC JOINTS

Patient 1: Sepsis Following Tooth Extraction

FIGURE 2–10   A.
Wrist Bone Scan: All the abnormal joints were infected.

FIGURE 2–10   B.
WBC Scan of the Knees: There is abnormal WBC accumulation in both knee joints, including the suprapatellar bursas.

FIGURE 2–10   C to E.
WBC Scans of the Left Wrist and Elbows: There is abnormal joint, bone, and soft tissue involvement (*arrow,* D). The injection site was in the right antecubital fossa (*arrowhead,* E).

NOTE. Multiple joint infections can be seen in patients with endocarditis, Osler-Weber-Rendu disease, arteriovenous malformations, Lyme disease, mycotic aneurysm, or infected sinus of Valsalva.

Cross References

Chapter 2: Multiple Bony Abnormalities—Active Rheumatoid Arthritis on WBC Scan

Chapter 71: Infectious Diseases—Extremity Soft Tissue Infections

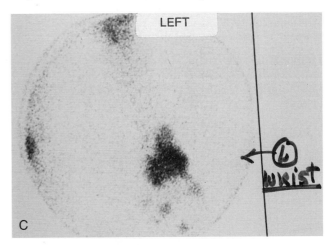

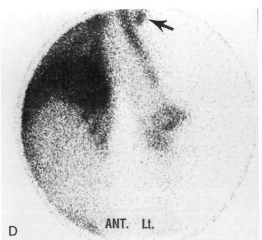

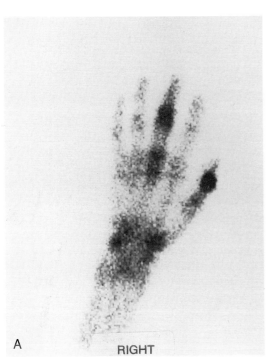

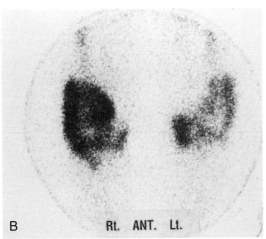

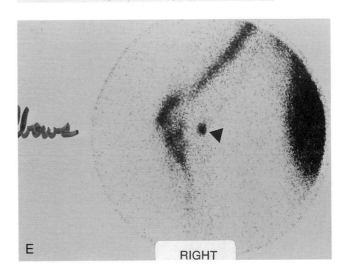

PROGRESSION OF ACUTE OSTEOMYELITIS TO CHRONIC OSTEOMYELITIS

FIGURE 2–11   A.
Lateral Delayed Bone Scan: The initial areas of infection include the fibula and the tibiotalar joint.

FIGURE 2–11   B and C.
Blood Pool and Delayed Bone Scan: One year later there is much more extensive disease.

FIGURE 2–11   D.
WBC Scan: The WBC scan demonstrates infection of the distal tibia, the tibiotalar joint, and the talus.

FIGURE 2–11   E.
WBC Scan: Two years after the initial process, there remains a small focus of infection.

NOTE. There is no clear-cut "best" imaging agent for activity in chronic osteomyelitis. WBC scans may be more accurate than gallium scans because they produce fewer false positive results. MRI is an alternative method of diagnosing reactivation of chronic osteomyelitis.

Cross Reference

Chapter 1: Solitary Bony Abnormalities—Chronic Osteomyelitis

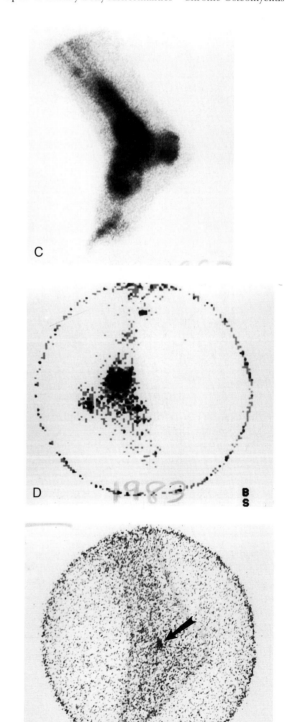

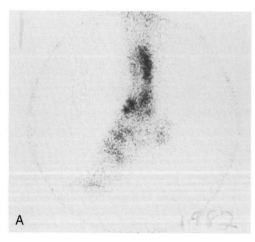

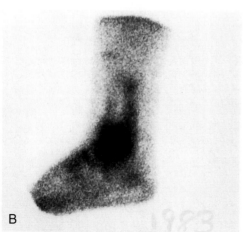

MULTIPLE BENIGN FRACTURES

Patient 1: Automobile Accident

FIGURE 2–12   A to C.

Delayed Bone Scan: There are multiple focal areas of increased osteogenesis whose location and pattern suggest post-traumatic fractures rather than metastatic disease. The spine fracture, called a Chance fracture, is due to the lap seat belt.

Patient 2: Automobile Accident

FIGURE 2–12   D.

Anterior and Posterior Whole Body Bone Scan: There are multiple fractures as well as postoperative changes *(arrowheads)* in this scan done to locate occult fractures. The left femoral fracture is comminuted.

NOTE 1. Rib abnormalities that are focal, rather than elongated and "in line," are more likely to represent benign fractures than metastases. Metastases to the periphery, e.g., tibia, are usually late manifestations.

NOTE 2. Seat belt injuries to the lower thoracic spine are transverse shear injuries.

Cross References

Chapter 1: Solitary Bony Abnormalities—False Negative Bone Scan for Fracture

Chapter 4: Pelvic Abnormalities—Pelvic Fractures

Chapter 6: Rib Abnormalities—Multiple Post-traumatic Rib Fractures

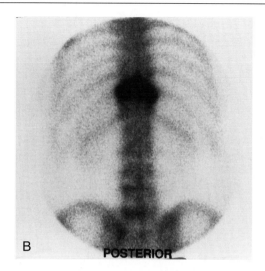

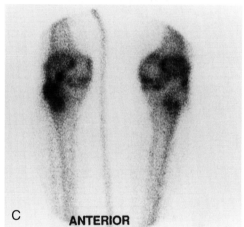

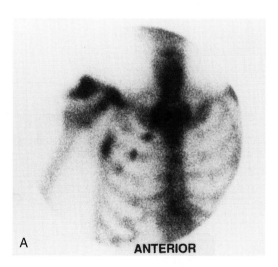

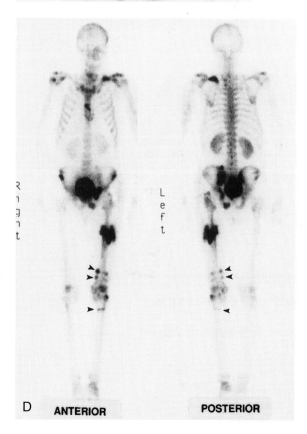

PROGRESSIVE SEVERE OSTEOPOROTIC FRACTURES OVER 2 MONTHS

Figure 2–13   A.
Bone Scan: There are several rib fractures, a thoracic compression fracture, sacral insufficiency fractures, and a lateral tibial plateau fracture.

Figure 2–13   B.
Bone Scan 2 Months Later: There are new right rib fractures, a right lateral tibial plateau fracture, and bilateral talar fractures. The older fractures have shown some healing.

NOTE 1. Osteoporotic fractures can involve any bone but most commonly are recognized in the spine, hip, and wrist.

NOTE 2. Osteoporotic fractures may be relatively asymptomatic or may be confused with avascular necrosis, especially about the knee.

Cross References

Chapter 3: Spinal Abnormalities—Successive Compression Fractures

Chapter 4: Pelvic Abnormalities—Sacral Insufficiency Fractures

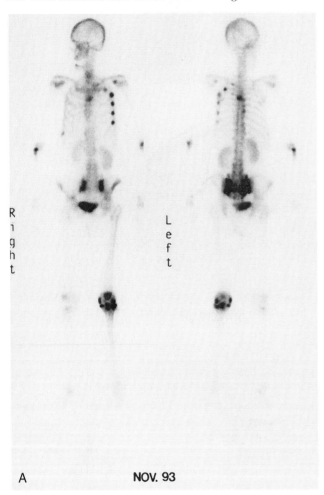

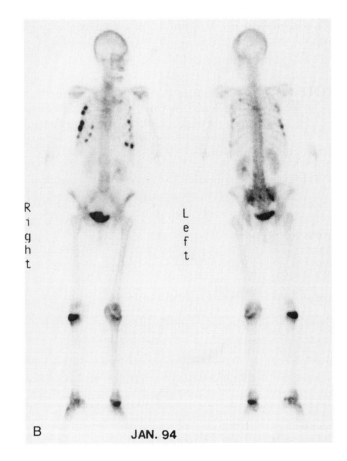

BONY STRESS REACTIONS

Patient 1: Volleyball Player

Figure 2–14   A.
Blood Pool Scan: There are three foci of hyperemia.

Figure 2–14   B to D.
Delayed Bone Scan: There are three slightly elongated foci of increased osteogenesis, two along the posterior right tibia (C) and one along the posterior left tibia (D).

Figure 2–14   E and F.
Left Lateral Plain Film X-rays: Blow-ups of the area involved demonstrate the development of a periosteal reaction over 3 weeks. The right leg had the same course.

Illustration continued on page 70

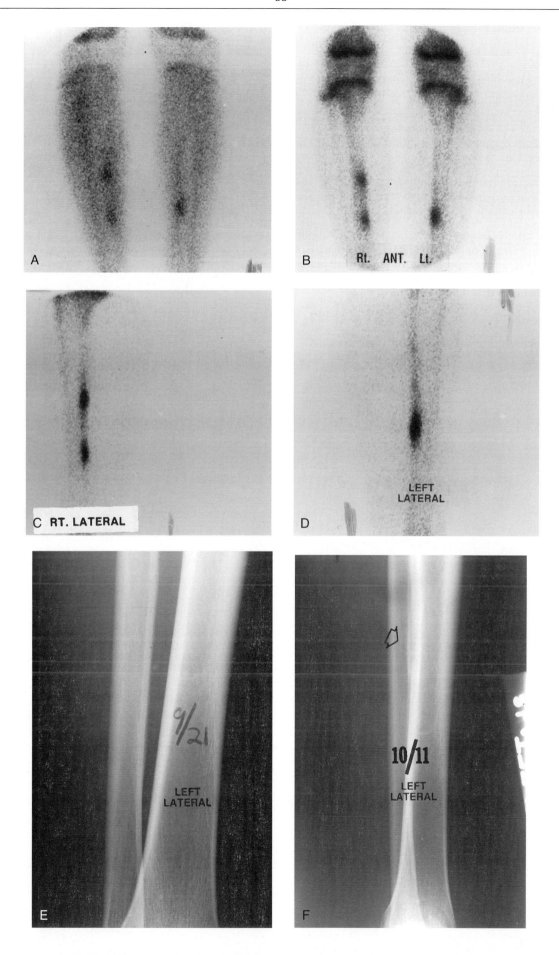

Patient 2: Baseball Player

FIGURE 2–14 G and H.

Anterior and Medial Left Leg Bone Scan: There are three adjacent cortical abnormalities along the proximal left femoral diaphysis. The right femur has a solitary abnormality as well.

NOTE 1. Stress reactions include subperiosteal hemorrhages (''shin splints'') and small cortical fractures (stress fractures).

NOTE 2. It is not always possible to separate subperiosteal hemorrhage from stress fractures, thus the equivocation ''stress reaction.''

NOTE 3. In athletes, scanning of other bones utilized in the sport is helpful to detect other areas of damage. In the lower extremities, the pelvis, femurs, lower legs, ankles, and feet should be checked.

Cross Reference

Chapter 1: Solitary Bony Abnormalities—Solitary Stress Fractures

SHIN SPLINTS

Patient 1: 27 Year Old Runner

FIGURE 2–15 A to C.

Anterior Tibial Bone Scan: There are elongated cortical abnormalities of both tibias. Part of the abnormalities may be chronic, producing cortical thickening.

NOTE. Shin splints occur at muscle insertion sites and are usually elongated abnormalities vs. the more focal stress fractures.

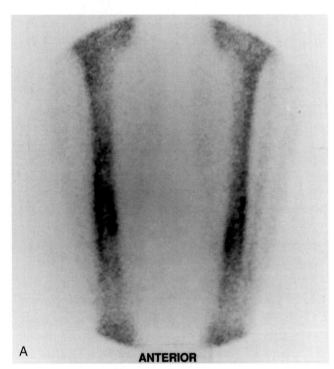

A   **ANTERIOR**

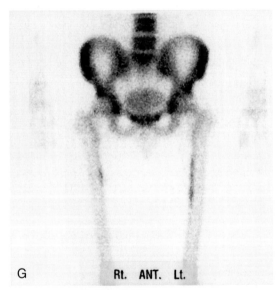

G   **Rt. ANT. Lt.**

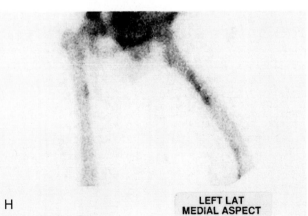

H   **LEFT LAT MEDIAL ASPECT**

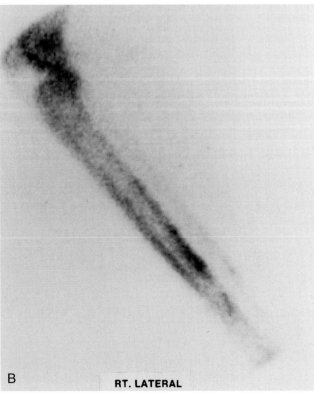

B   **RT. LATERAL**

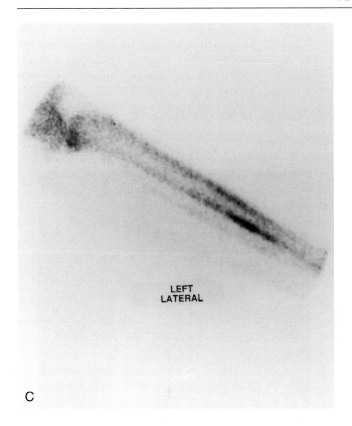

C

LEFT
LATERAL

RECREATIONAL VS. WORK INJURY

Patient: Snowboard and Work Injuries Occurring at Different Times

FIGURE 2–16   A.

Medial Blood Pool Scintigraphy: There is hyperemia involving the left ankle and a mild, very focal abnormality on the right *(arrow)*.

FIGURE 2–16   B.

Medial Delayed Bone Scan: There is intense osteogenesis involving both ankles: the right talus focally and the left more diffusely.

FIGURE 2–16   C.

Anterior Bone Scan: The right talar abnormality is medial, whereas the left is more diffuse.

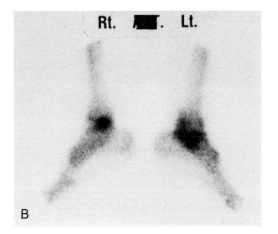

Rt.   Lt.

B

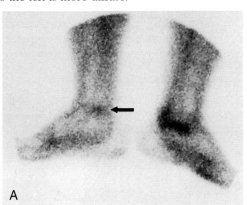

A

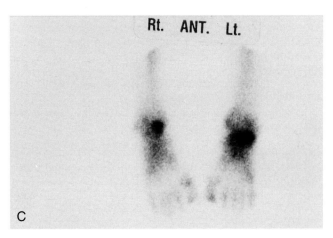

Rt. ANT. Lt.

C

Illustration continued on following page

FIGURE 2–16   D.

Coronal Right Ankle STIR MRI: There is a vertical fracture *(white arrow)* through the talus, with osteochondral injury at the tibiotalar joint.

FIGURE 2–16   E.

Coronal Left Ankle MRI: There is disruption of the tibiotalar joint, with tears of the talofibular ligament.

NOTE 1. The abnormal left talus on bone scan is probably due to the ligamentous avulsion injuries and not fractures. This was a snowboard injury. The right talar fracture occurred at work prior to the snowboard accident.

NOTE 2. Older injuries have little or no hyperemia as compared with acute processes. Dating injuries this way may be important in litigation.

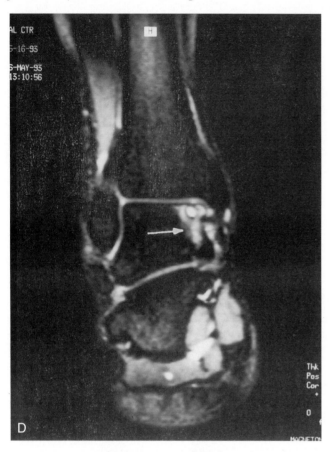

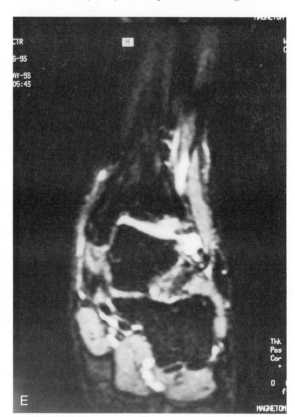

MULTIFOCAL OSTEONECROSIS

Patient 1: Deep Sea Diver

FIGURE 2–17   A.

Blood Pool Scintigraphy: There is decreased blood pool with a surrounding zone of hyperemia in the region of the left hip *(arrow).*

FIGURE 2–17   B.

Delayed Bone Scan: The left femoral head has decreased activity consistent with an early osteonecrosis.

FIGURE 2–17   C.

Delayed Bone Scan: Two months later there is increased activity in the left femoral head and neck, although there is a persistent superior zone with normal activity.

FIGURE 2–17   D.

Right Shoulder Delayed Bone Scan: There is increased activity in the right humeral head, indicating a second site of osteonecrosis.

Patient 2: Renal Transplant

FIGURE 2–17   E and F.

Anterior Blood Pool and Delayed Bone Scan: There is focal hyperemia *(arrowheads)* and increased osteogenesis with superolateral decreased activity in both femoral heads.

NOTE. Patients on steroids or with organ transplants, rheumatoid arthritis, or caisson disease may have more than one bone involved.

Cross Reference

Chapter 1: Solitary Bony Abnormalities—Osteonecrosis

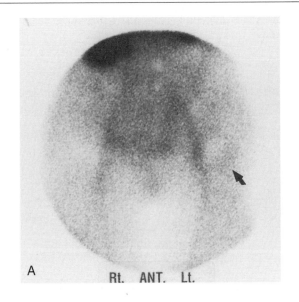

A
Rt. ANT. Lt.

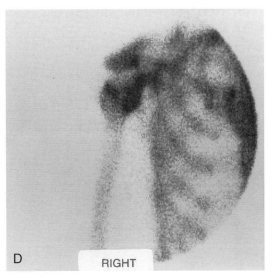

D
RIGHT

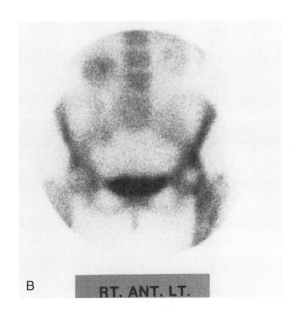

B
RT. ANT. LT.

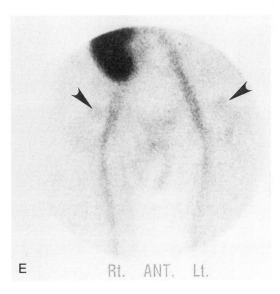

E
Rt. ANT. Lt.

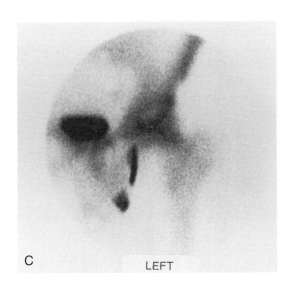

C
LEFT

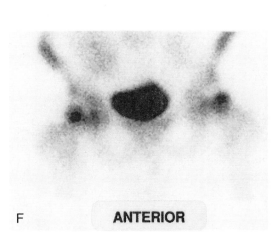

F
ANTERIOR

"COLD" TO "HOT" BONE INFARCTS (SICKLE CELL DISEASE)

FIGURE 2–18   A.

Delayed Bone Scintigraphy: There are several areas of diminished activity involving the femoral metaphyses and diaphyses and the right tibia *(arrows)*.

FIGURE 2–18   B.

Delayed Bone Scintigraphy: One month later there is increased osteogenesis in the regions where there were "cold" abnormalities.

NOTE. Infarcts initially have occluded end-vessels, which either recanalize or are bypassed by ingrowth of new vessels. The dead osteocytes are replaced by osteoclasts and osteoblasts, new bone is formed, and a "hot" spot develops on the bone scan.

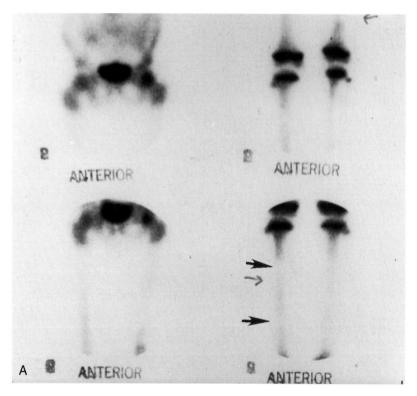

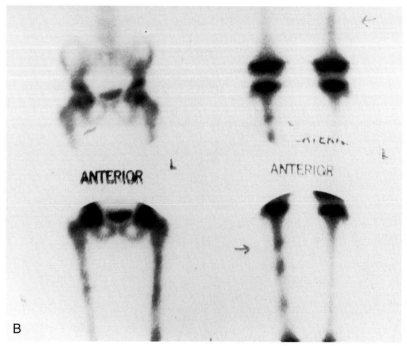

OSTEOCHONDROMAS (EXOSTOSES)

FIGURE 2–19   A.
Plain Film X-ray of Knee: There are bony projections along the medial femoral metaphysis and the proximal tibiofibular joint *(arrowheads)*.

FIGURE 2–19   B.
Blood Pool Scan: There is no hyperemia.

FIGURE 2–19   C.
Delayed Planar Bone Scan: There are very focal areas of mildly increased osteogenesis at each of the sites of exostosis involving both legs.

FIGURE 2–19   D.
Coronal SPECT Scans: The abnormal osteogenesis is more conspicuous on SPECT owing to its inherently increased contrast resolution.

NOTE 1. Osteochondromas can have normal or increased osteogenesis and do not enlarge after closure of the adjacent growth plate.

NOTE 2. Increased activity does not indicate malignant degeneration, although hyperemia should raise some concern, especially in cases of multiple osteochondromatosis.

NOTE 3. There are sporadic as well as hereditary multiple exostoses, an autosomal dominant disease.

Cross References

Chapter 1: Solitary Bony Abnormalities—Osteochondroma of Talus

Chapter 4: Pelvic Abnormalities—Pelvic Osteochondroma

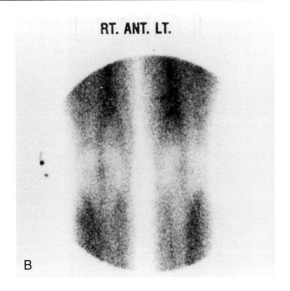

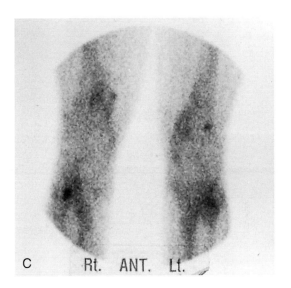

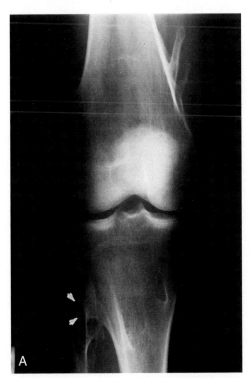

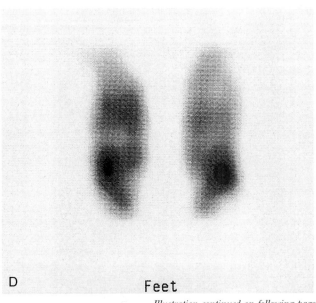

Illustration continued on following page

SUSPECT METASTATIC DISEASE TO BONE

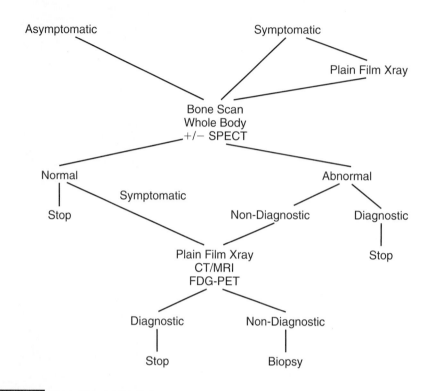

Asymptomatic   Symptomatic

Plain Film Xray

Bone Scan
Whole Body
+/− SPECT

Normal   Abnormal

Symptomatic

Stop   Non-Diagnostic   Diagnostic

Stop

Plain Film Xray
CT/MRI
FDG-PET

Diagnostic   Non-Diagnostic

Stop   Biopsy

X-RAY LYTIC METASTASES ON BONE SCAN

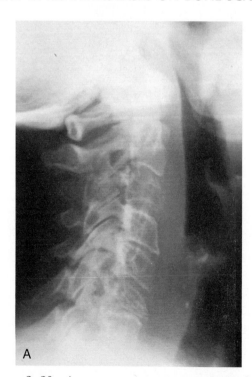

FIGURE 2–20   A.
Plain Film X-ray: The lateral view of the cervical spine demonstrates lytic destruction of C3, C5, and C6.

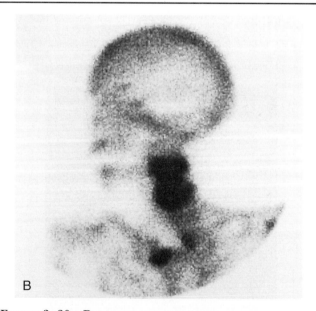

FIGURE 2–20   B.
Delayed Bone Scintigraphy: The cervical spine has several levels of increased activity corresponding to the abnormal levels on x-ray.

NOTE. Bone metastases will have increased osteogenesis whether the x-ray findings are normal or demonstrate lytic or blastic abnormalities.

MULTIPLE MYELOMA

Patient 1

FIGURE 2–21   A.

Bone Scan: There are multiple thoracic and lumbar vertebral abnormalities, especially T6 and L4.

FIGURE 2–21   B.

MRI Scan: Virtually every vertebral body is abnormal.

FIGURE 2–21   C.

CT Scan: There is a lytic metastasis destroying the T6 vertebra.

Illustration continued on following page

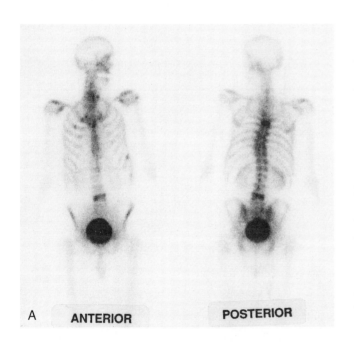

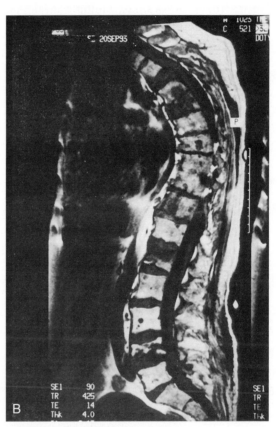

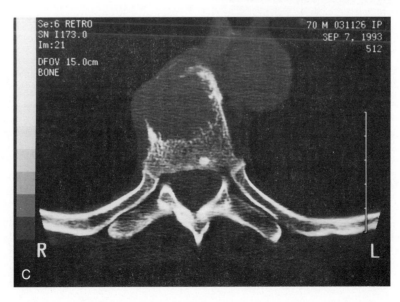

Patient 2

FIGURE 2–21 D.

Anterior Bone Scan: With computer image manipulation, subtle femoral lesions can be detected (*arrow* points to a cold process, *arrowheads* to the cortical/periosteal disease).

NOTE 1. Although multiple myeloma is osteolytic, most bone scans will be abnormal.

NOTE 2. The total body bone scan will be abnormal in marrow processes, i.e., multiple myeloma, leukemias, and intramedullary carcinoma metastases. However, many individual lesions will be missed.

NOTE 3. In metastatic disease, high-count bone scans, magnification, SPECT, and digital image manipulation will help identify more abnormalities than were previously thought to be present.

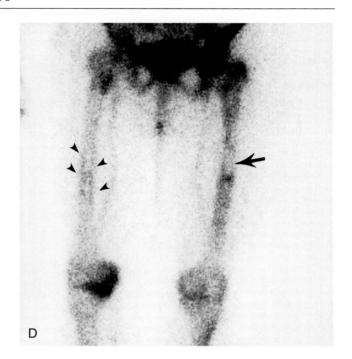

"SUPERSCAN"

DIFFERENTIAL DIAGNOSIS OF A "SUPERSCAN"
Diffuse metastases
Renal osteodystrophy
Osteomalacia
Hypervitaminosis D
Hyperparathyroidism
Paget's disease
Fibrous dysplasia
Chronic familial hyperphosphatemia
Myelofibrosis
Acromegaly
Prostaglandin E-1 therapy
Milk-alkali syndrome

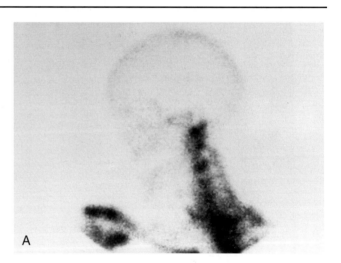

Patient 1: Breast Cancer

FIGURE 2–22 A–D.

Delayed Bone Scintigraphy: There is marked increased osteogenesis involving the axial skeleton, with nonvisualized kidneys, decreased urinary bladder activity, and near nonvisualization of the uninvolved skull.

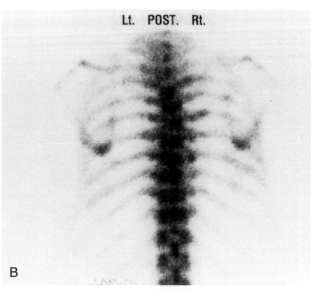

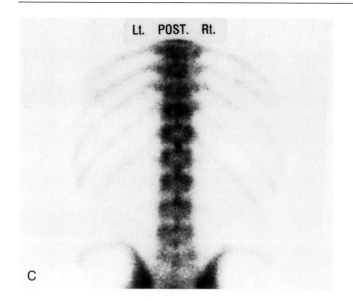

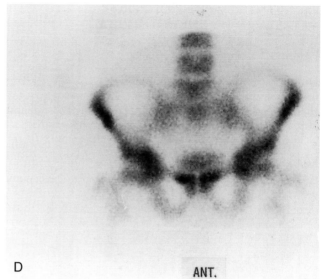

Patient 2: Prostate Cancer

FIGURE 2–22   E.

Total Body Bone Scan: There is nonvisualization of the kidneys as well as poor visualization of uninvolved bone in this patient with multiple bony metastases.

NOTE. The increased osteogenesis due to diffuse metastatic disease can be suspected from the lack of renal visualization (look for kidneys and bladder) and decreased visualization of uninvolved bones.

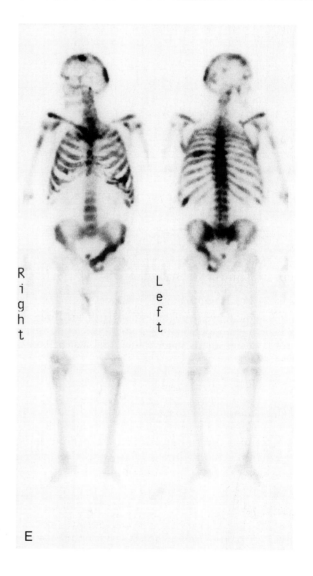

EXCELLENT RESPONSE OF BONE METASTASES TO CHEMOTHERAPY

Patient 1: Breast Carcinoma

FIGURE 2–23 A.

Initial Bone Scan: There are numerous vertebral and pelvic abnormalities indicative of metastases. The marked intensity of the lesions produces a "near-superscan" appearance: no bladder, faint kidney, and faint normal bone activity.

FIGURE 2–23 B.

Bone Scan 6 Months Later: The scan is now normal except for the "hot skull."

NOTE. The "hot skull" does not represent neoplasm and is often seen in breast and lung cancer patients.

Cross Reference

Chapter 5: Skull Abnormalities—Diffusely "Hot" Skull in Breast Carcinoma

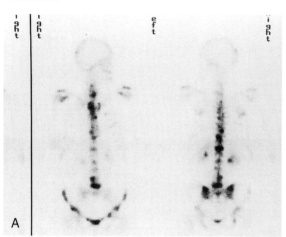

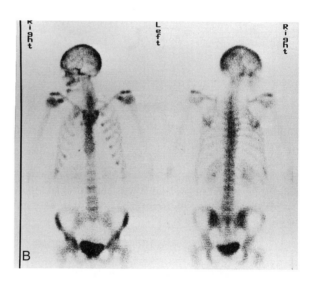

BONE METASTASES DETECTED WITH THALLIUM

FIGURE 2–24 A.

Total Body Bone Scintigraphy: There are multiple bony abnormalities indicative of metastatic disease.

FIGURE 2–24 B and C.

Anterior Pelvic Bone Scintigraphy and Thallium Tumor Scan: The thallium scan was done for a lung mass, but a view over the pelvis demonstrates abnormalities that match those seen on bone scan.

NOTE. Thallium is thought to accumulate, in part, according to both the blood flow and the growth rate of the tumor. Metastases to bone have increased blood flow as demonstrated by the hyperemia seen on blood pool images.

Cross Reference

Chapter 72: Tumors—Thallium in Malignant Bone Tumors

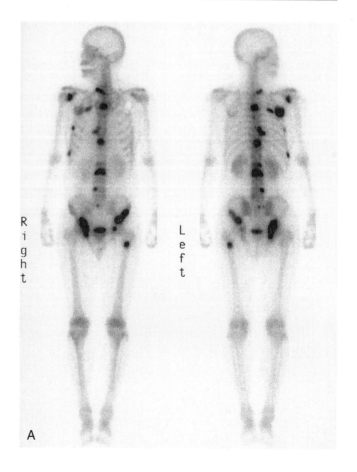

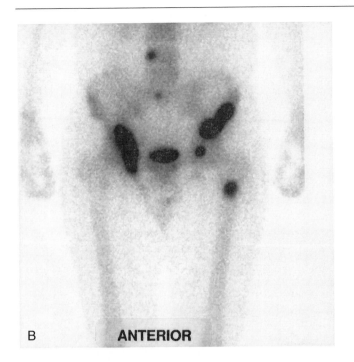

B   **ANTERIOR**

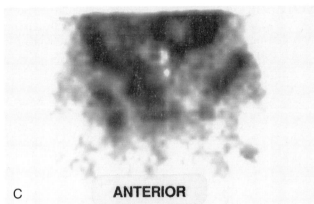

C   **ANTERIOR**

MRI VS. BONE SCAN

FIGURE 2–25 A.

Posterior Bone Scintigraphy: There are several bony abnormalities in this patient with non-Hodgkin's lymphoma, including T6 and T12 "cold" lesions *(arrows)*.

FIGURE 2–25 B.

T1-Weighted MRI of the Thoracic Spine: Virtually every vertebral body has metastatic deposits replacing the normal high signal of the marrow fat.

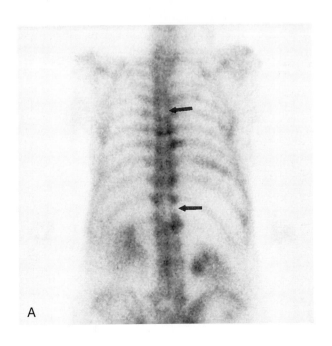

A

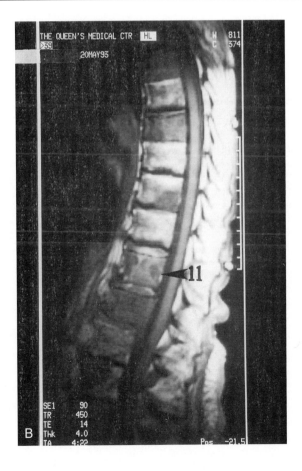

B

Illustration continued on following page

FIGURE 2-25 C.

Cervical Spine Delayed Bone Scintigraphy: C2 is abnormal.

FIGURE 2-25 D.

T2-Weighted MRI of the Cervical Spine: C2 has high signal intensity *(arrow)* indicative of the metastatic involvement.

NOTE. MRI will demonstrate more lesions than will bone scan, especially in vertebrae with small marrow tumors. When the bone scan is abnormal, the MRI will be abnormal.

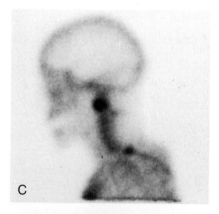

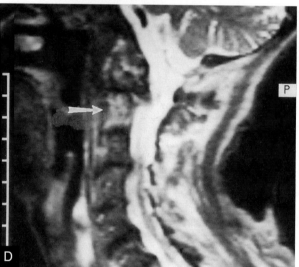

VARYING PATTERNS OF PAGET'S DISEASE

Multiple Patients

FIGURE 2-26 A and B.

Skull Bone Scintigraphy: The thick curvilinear band of increased osteogenesis is asymmetric, being greater posteriorly and on the left side.

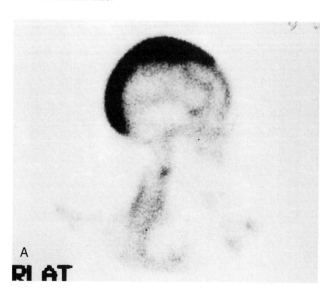

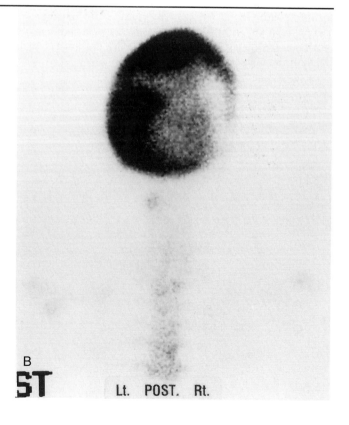

FIGURE 2–26   C and D.
Pelvis Bone Scintigraphy: The anterior (C) scan demonstrates the classic increased osteogenesis involving the iliopubic (iliopectineal) line, whereas the posterior scan (D) demonstrates ilioischial hyperactivity. The sacrum, L4, and L5 are abnormal as well.

FIGURE 2–26   E.
AP Plain X-ray of the Pelvis: The iliopubic line is thickened.

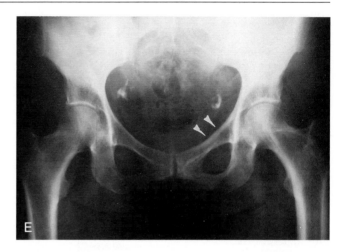

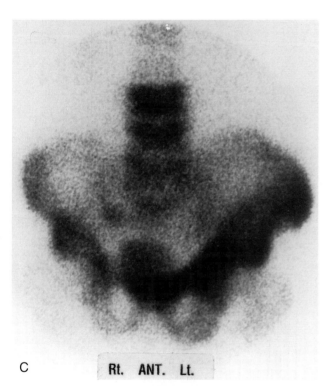

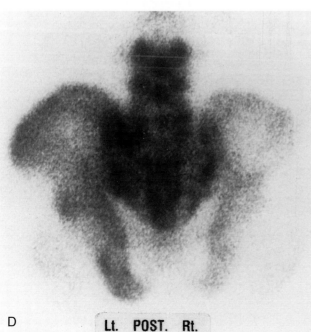

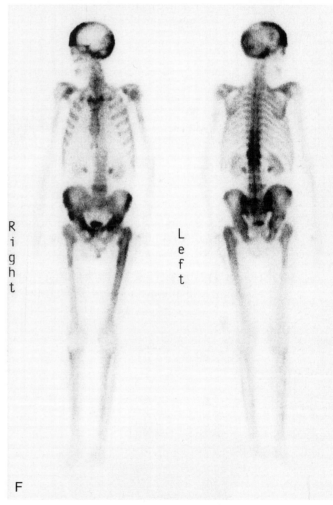

FIGURE 2–26   F.
Whole Body Bone Scan: There are numerous bones with various changes of Paget's disease. The entire pelvis, the left femur, the spine, and the skull have pronounced changes. The proximal left humerus and proximal right femur have more subtle changes.

Illustration continued on following page

FIGURE 2–26   G.

Anterior Spinal and Pelvic Bone Scan: L5 has increased activity along its margins, the so-called picture-frame vertebra *(arrow)*.

FIGURE 2–26   H.

Lateral Plain Film X-ray: L5 has increased density, greatest along its cortical margins.

FIGURE 2–26   I.

Tibia Bone Scintigraphy: The left tibia is expanded and bowed, the latter as the result of bone softening.

FIGURE 2–26   J.

Chest Delayed Bone Scintigraphy: There are abnormalities of a right rib, sternum, and a thoracic vertebra.

FIGURE 2–26   K.

Femur Bone Scintigraphy: There is prominence to the left mid-femoral diaphyseal cortex, the "double-stripe" sign, where the disease is localized.

FIGURE 2–26   L.

Tibia Bone Scan: The increased activity demonstrates a "flame" shape.

FIGURE 2–26   M and N.

Blood Pool and Delayed Planar Image of the Posterior Pelvis Bone Scan: The hyperemia is greater in the right ilium, indicating that this is active Paget's disease, whereas the left ilium, acetabulum, and ischium are more quiescent.

NOTE 1. Increased activity on bone scan can be seen with the radiographic osteolytic phase as well as the blastic phase.

NOTE 2. Hyperemia will be seen with active Paget's disease, but will not be seen in the burnt-out phase.

NOTE 3. Any bone can be involved with Paget's disease, either as a monostotic or as a polyostotic process.

Cross References

Chapter 1: Solitary Bony Abnormalities—Early Paget's Disease of Pelvis

Chapter 4: Pelvic Abnormalities—Pelvic Metastases vs. Paget's Disease

Chapter 5: Skull Abnormalities—Paget's Disease of the Skull

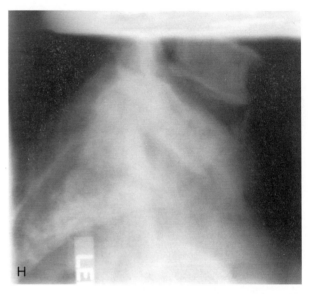

H

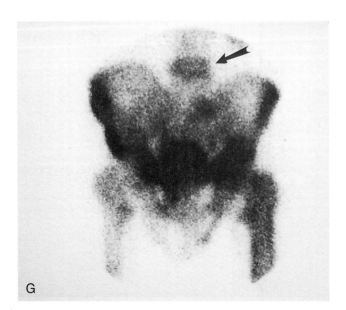

G

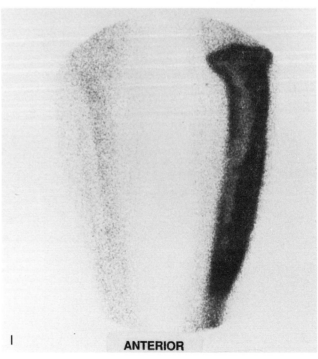

I   **ANTERIOR**

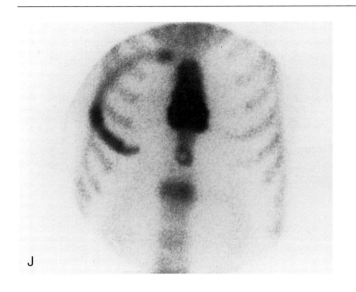

J

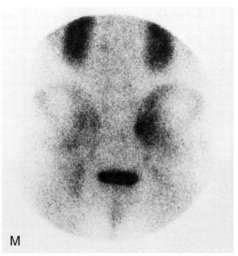

M

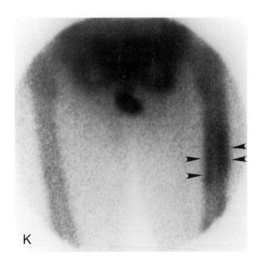

K

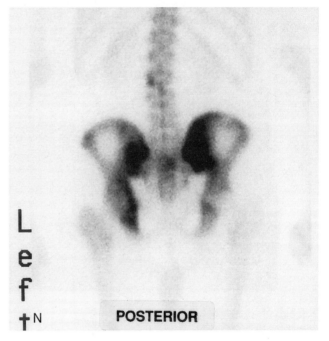

Left

POSTERIOR

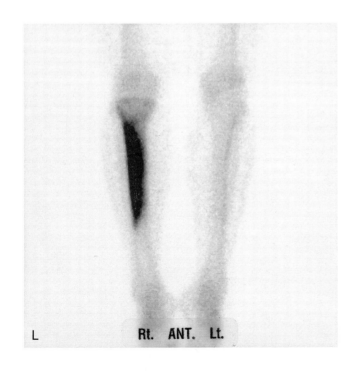

L

Rt. ANT. Lt.

POLYOSTOTIC FIBROUS DYSPLASIA

Patient 1: Limited Disease

FIGURE 2–27   A.

Plain X-ray of the Left Forearm: There is bowing, thickening, and a ground-glass appearance of the radius, sparing the proximal end.

FIGURE 2–27   B.

Bone Scan of the Left Arm: There is increased osteogenesis involving the entire left radius, even the most proximal end.

FIGURE 2–27   C to F.

Blood Flow, Blood Pool, and Delayed Bone Scan of the Left Lower Leg: There is marked hyperemia involving the left tibia and left medial femoral condyle.

FIGURE 2–27   G.

Posterior Pelvic Bone Scan: There is an ischial abnormality *(arrowhead)*.

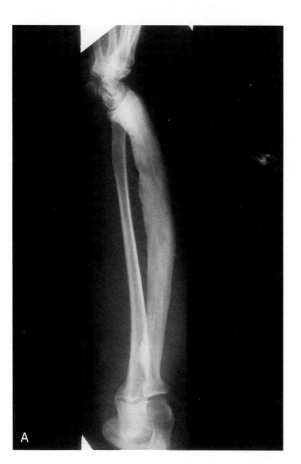

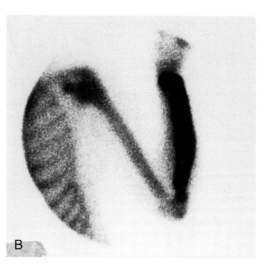

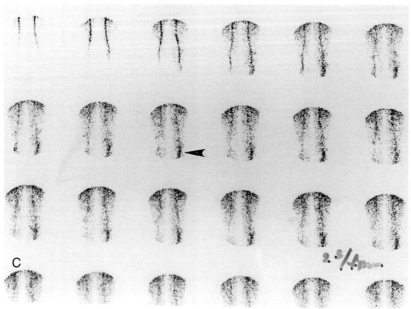

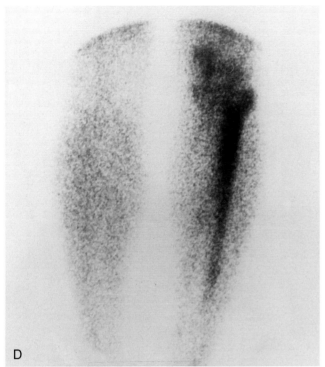

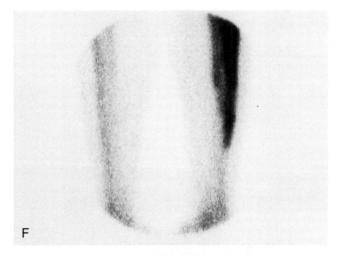

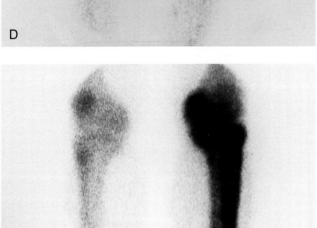

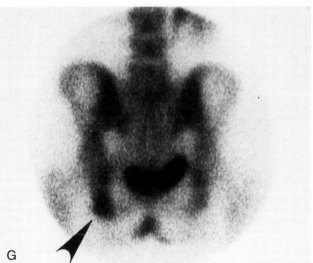

Patient 2: Extensive Disease

FIGURE 2–27 H to J.

Bone Scan: There are multiple bones involved, although the spine is spared.

NOTE 1. The bone scan appearance of fibrous dysplasia is indistinguishable from Paget's disease, with hyperemia, increased osteogenesis, bone expansion, and bowing. Age of onset is usually the distinguishing factor.

NOTE 2. When the cortical activity in the long bones is asymmetric, being longer on one side of the bone than the other (see Fig. 2–27F), one should suspect fibrous dysplasia as opposed to Paget's disease, which is more often symmetric.

NOTE 3. Fibrous dysplasia can be monostotic or polyostotic.

NOTE 4. In fibrous dysplasia the spine is less commonly involved, and the facial bones are involved more often than in Paget's disease.

NOTE 5. Polyostotic fibrous dysplasia may or may not be associated with McCune-Albright syndrome: precocious puberty, cutaneous pigmentation (café-au-lait spots), and polyostotic fibrous dysplasia.

NOTE 6. Malignant degeneration of fibrous dysplasia is rare, constituting less than 1 percent of cases.

Illustration continued on following page

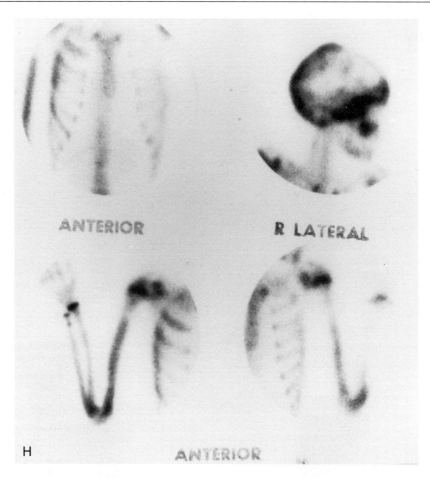

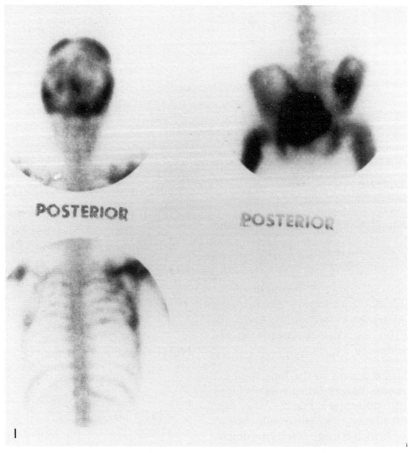

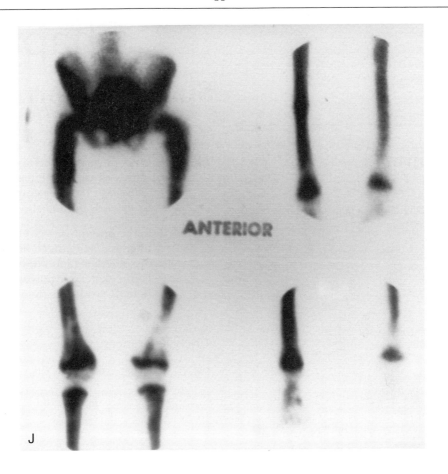

RENAL OSTEODYSTROPHY
FIGURE 2–28.

Anterior and Posterior Whole Body Bone Scan: The kidneys are barely visible, and the bladder has no urine. The "hot" skull can also be seen with renal osteodystrophy.

NOTE. The bone scan can have the appearance of a "superscan," owing to increased bony activity from the secondary hyperparathyroidism or to the renal failure and nonvisualized kidneys and urinary bladder.

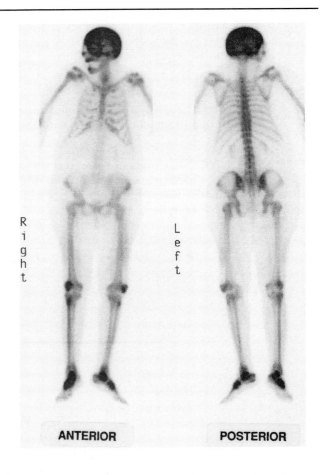

Chapter 3
Spinal Abnormalities

SOLITARY OSTEOPHYTE

FIGURE 3–1.

Posterior Lumbar Spine Scintigram: A large osteophyte bridges L1 and L2 on the right.

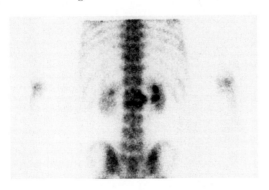

NOTE 1. Osteophytes may be distinguished from metastatic disease by the use of oblique or SPECT scans to find a projection where the abnormality extends beyond the vertebral borders.

NOTE 2. Large osteophytes can be seen after traumatic fractures and infections and in degenerative disk and facet joint disease, disseminated idiopathic skeletal hyperostosis, psoriatic arthritis, Reiter's syndrome, and acromegaly.

Cross References

Chapter 2: Multiple Bone Abnormalities—Psoriatic Arthritis

Chapter 3: Spinal Abnormalities—Spinal Metastasis Simulating Degenerative Disease

ASYMMETRIC THORACIC OSTEOPHYTES

FIGURE 3–2   A and B.

Whole Body and RPO Chest Bone Scintigraphy: There are osteophytes only along the right side of the thoracic spine.

NOTE 1. Left-sided osteophytes are unusual, probably because of the pulsation of the descending thoracic aorta.

NOTE 2. The large osteophytes seen in the thoracic spines of elderly patients are usually due to disseminated idiopathic skeletal hyperostosis (DISH) or Forestier's disease.

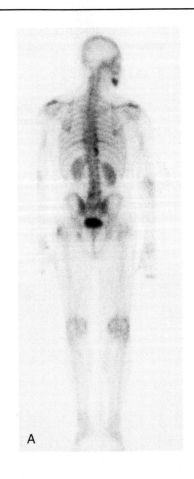

A

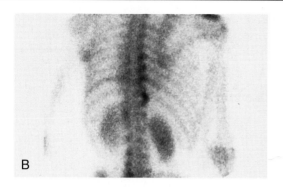

B

DISSEMINATED IDIOPATHIC SKELETAL HYPEROSTOSIS (DISH) OF THE SPINE

Patient: 61 Year Old Male

FIGURE 3–3   A.

Posterior Bone Scan: There are several bony abnormalities projecting off the spine in both the thoracic *(arrows)* and the lumbar regions.

FIGURE 3–3   B.

Lateral Chest X-ray Detail: There is flowing ossification connecting the thoracic vertebrae.

NOTE 1. On the bone scan, DISH can simulate metastatic disease.

NOTE 2. DISH occurs in older patients.

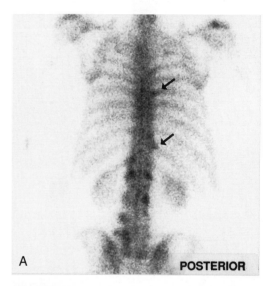

A   **POSTERIOR**

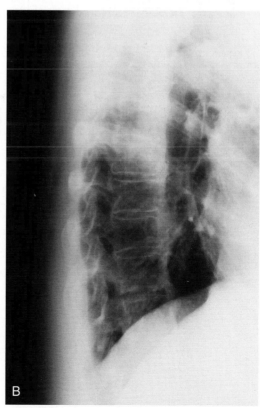

B

LOCALIZED FACET JOINT DISEASE

FIGURE 3–4   A to C.

Delayed Planar Bone Scans: There are focal areas of increased osteogenesis in the region of the L4 facets.

FIGURE 3–4   D.

CT Scan of the Abdomen: A CT scan done for other purposes demonstrates hypertrophy of the facet joints.

NOTE. It can be difficult to distinguish facet (apophyseal) joint disease from pars interarticularis fractures.

Cross Reference

Chapter 3: Spinal Abnormalities—Continued Healing Potential in Pars Interarticularis Fractures

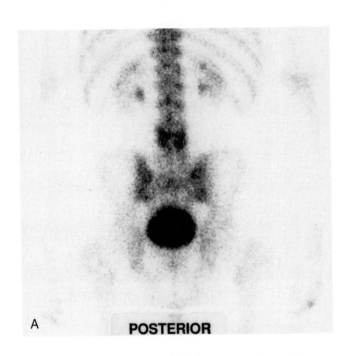

A   **POSTERIOR**

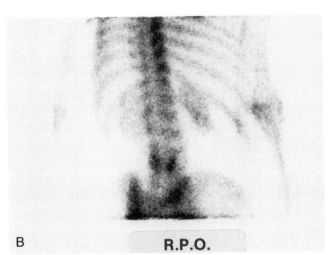

B   R.P.O.

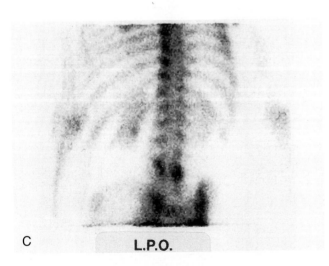

C   L.P.O.

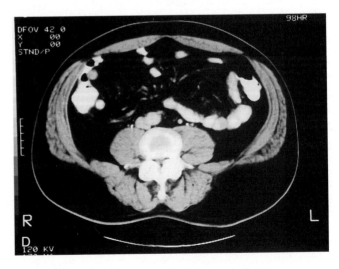

SPINAL METASTASIS SIMULATING DEGENERATIVE DISEASE

Patient 1: Breast Carcinoma

FIGURE 3–5 A and B.
Whole Body Bone Scintigram with Magnification View: There is an eccentric L5 spinal abnormality *(arrow)* suggestive of degenerative change.

FIGURE 3–5 C.
CT of Spine: Biopsy of the destructive lesion of L5 proved it to be a breast metastasis.

FIGURE 3–5 D.
Seven Month Follow-up Bone Scintigram: There are now multiple bony metastases, yet the patient remained asymptomatic.

Illustration continued on following page

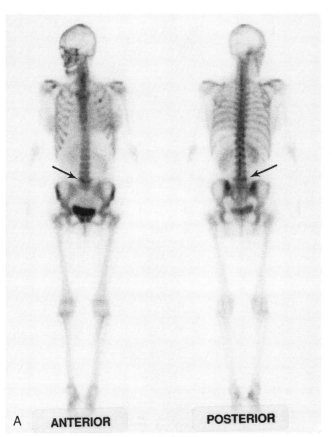

A ANTERIOR   POSTERIOR

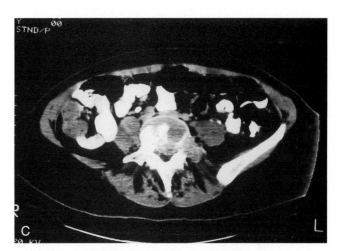

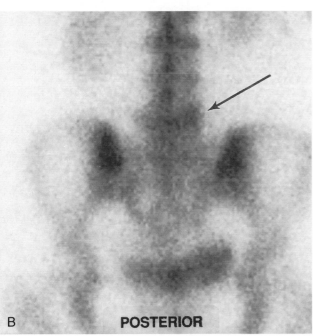

B POSTERIOR

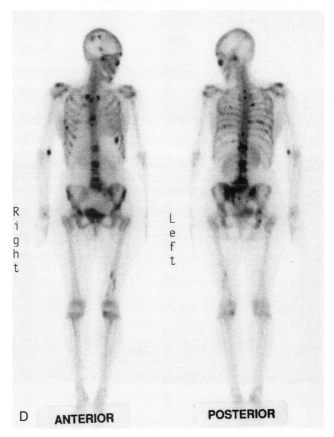

D ANTERIOR   POSTERIOR

Patient 2: Gastric Carcinoma

FIGURE 3–5   E to G.

Posterior, RAO, and LPO Bone Scans: There is a large abnormality simulating an osteophyte involving the right side of L4. The involvement of the posterior elements, as well as the left sacral abnormality, suggests that this may be a metastasis.

FIGURE 3–5   H.

CT Scan of L4: The right pedicle is expanded by a soft tissue mass that invades the vertebral body and transverse process.

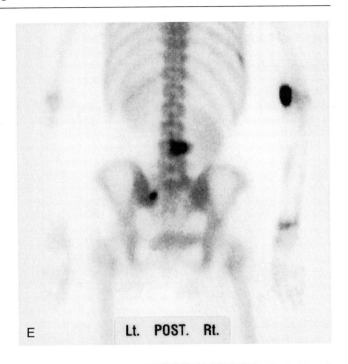

E   **Lt. POST. Rt.**

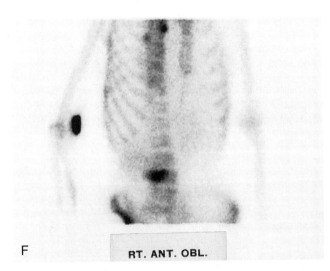

F   **RT. ANT. OBL.**

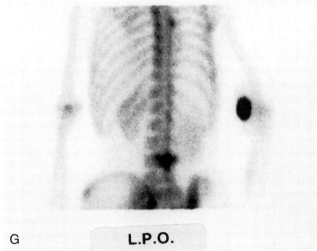

G   **L.P.O.**

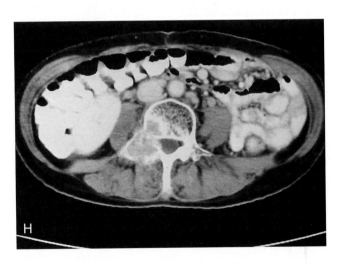

H

NOTE 1. A solitary bony abnormality without degenerative symptoms or history of surgical intervention may require further work-up.

NOTE 2. Osteophytes projecting off the posterior neural arch are rarely seen on bone scan and should raise suspicions of tumor.

NOTE 3. A solitary rib abnormality has only a 10 to 15 percent chance of being a metastasis.

Cross Reference

Chapter 3: Spinal Abnormalities—Benign Compression Fractures vs. Vertebral Metastasis

SUBTLE OSTEOMYELITIS

FIGURE 3–6   A.

Posterior Bone Scan: There is a subtle increase in activity involving L5.

FIGURE 3–6   B.

Magnified Spot Bone Scan: The L5 vertebral body is definitely abnormal.

FIGURE 3–6   C.

Gallium Scan: The vertebral body has intense gallium accumulation.

NOTE. A subtle abnormality can be clarified by magnification, either digitally or with the use of a converging collimator.

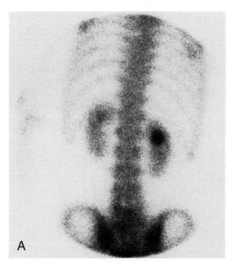

A

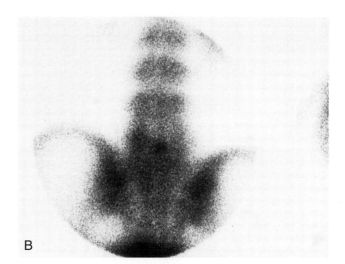

B

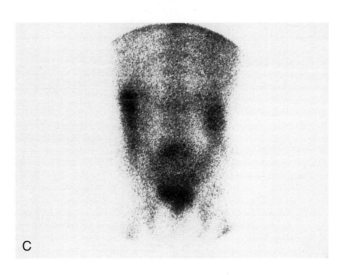

C

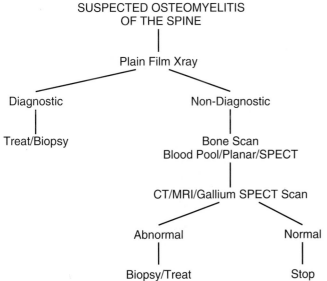

DISKITIS ON BONE SCAN

FIGURE 3–7   A.
October Lumbar Spine Bone Scan: The bone scan is normal.

FIGURE 3–7   B and C.
December Lumbar Spine Blood Pool and Bone Scan: There is hyperemia *(arrow)* and increased activity of L1 and L2.

FIGURE 3–7   D.
May Lumbar Spine Bone Scan: There is persistent increased osteogenesis and loss of the disk interspace. The blood pool scan (not shown) was normal.

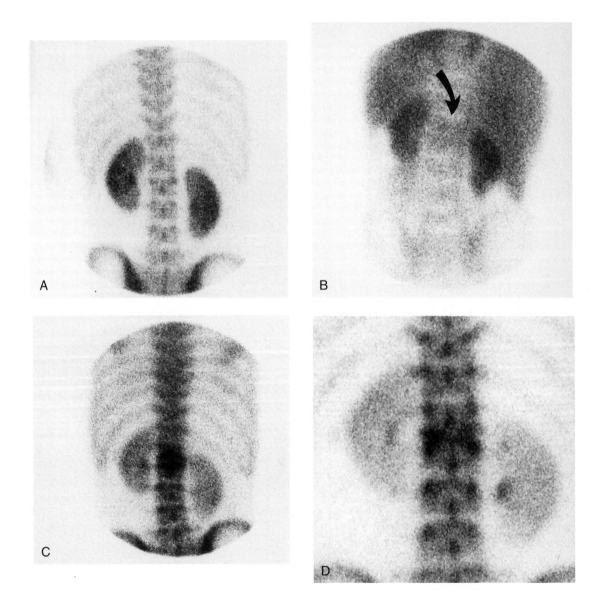

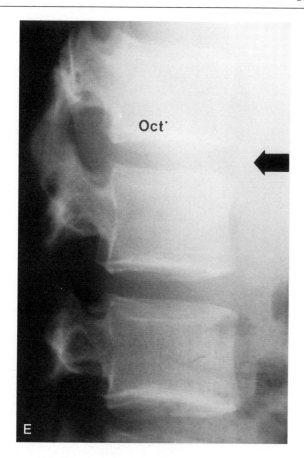

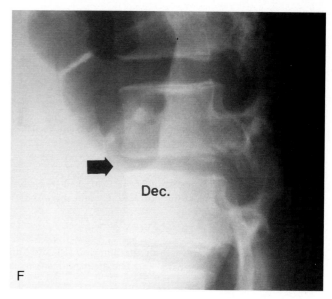

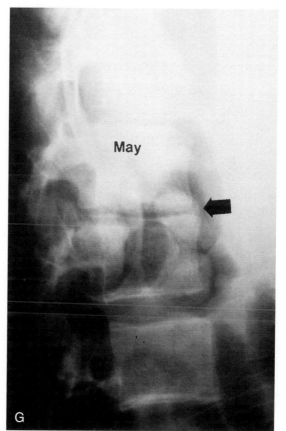

FIGURE 3–7   E to G.
Lateral Plain Film X-rays October, December, and May: There
is progressive loss of the L1–L2 disk interspace *(arrow)* due to
the diskitis, which was treated medically.

NOTE. Tumor rarely, if ever, crosses or destroys disk
material or cartilage, whereas infections do so
more readily.

VALUE OF SPECT IN GALLIUM SCANNING FOR SPINAL OSTEOMYELITIS AND DISKITIS

Patient 1

FIGURE 3–8   A and B.

Planar Lumbar Spine Bone Scan: There is increased osteogenesis of L5 vertebral body, best seen on the right lateral view *(arrow)*. The patient had had a laminectomy 3 years earlier, accounting for the apparent "cold" spot at L4.

FIGURE 3–8   C and D.

Lumbar Spine SPECT Bone Scan: There is marked increased osteogenesis of L5 seen in the coronal (C) and sagittal (D) planes.

FIGURE 3–8   E and F.

Planar Gallium Scintigraphy: Both the anterior (E) and the posterior (F) views are normal at L5. The decreased activity is due to the laminectomy.

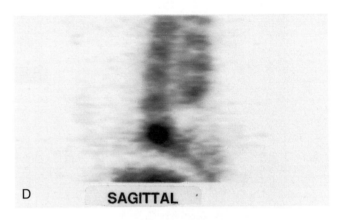

D   SAGITTAL

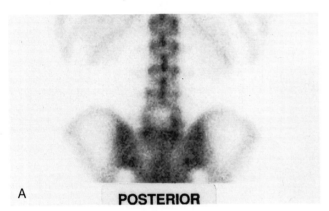

A   POSTERIOR

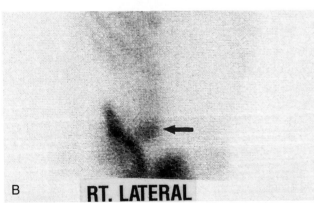

B   RT. LATERAL

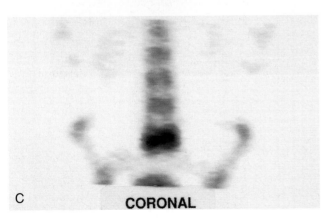

C   CORONAL

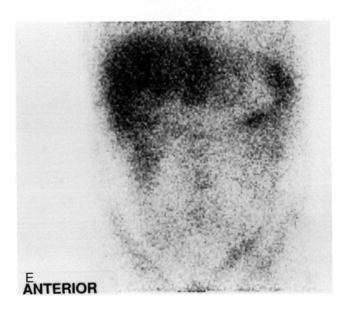

E ANTERIOR

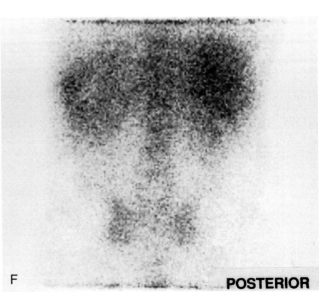

F   POSTERIOR

FIGURE 3–8   G and H.

SPECT Gallium Scan: The coronal (G) and sagittal (H) tomograms demonstrate increased gallium *(arrow)* in L5, indicative of osteomyelitis (surgically proven).

FIGURE 3–8   I.

Lateral Plain Film X-ray: There is narrowing of the L5–S1 disk interspace with sclerosis of L5.

FIGURE 3–8   J.

CT Scan: Gas is seen in the disk and L5 vertebral body.

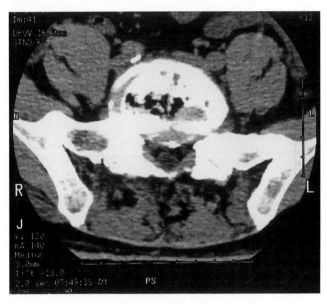

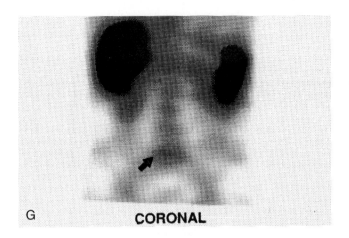

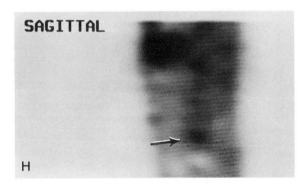

Patient 2: Fever and Low Back Pain 2 Days Following Facet Steroid Injection

FIGURE 3–8   K.

Sagittal T2 MRI Scan: The scan was indeterminate for recurrent extruded disk material vs. an epidural abscess *(arrow)*. There is high signal intensity of the remaining disk material.

FIGURE 3–8   L.

18 Hour Posterior Planar Gallium Scan: There is abnormal gallium accumulating at the level of L5, but whether it represents an epidural abscess or an osteomyelitis and diskitis cannot be determined.

FIGURE 3–8   M to O.

SPECT Scans of the Lumbosacral Spine: The L5 vertebral body has marked gallium accumulation, indicating an osteomyelitis as well as the probable epidural abscess.

NOTE. An early gallium scan, as early as 3 hours post injection, can be attempted. If positive, later scans are unnecessary, and considerable time can be saved in initiating therapy.

Cross Reference

Chapter 71: Infectious Diseases—Paraspinal Abscess

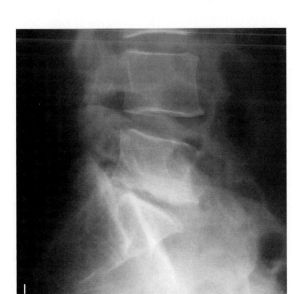

Illustration continued on following page

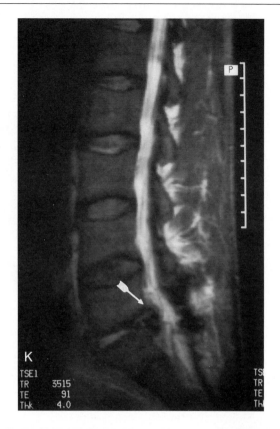

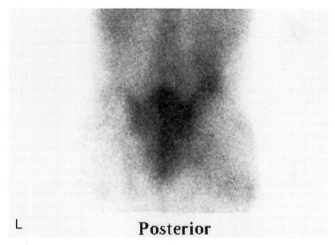

L   **Posterior**

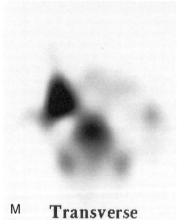

M   **Transverse**

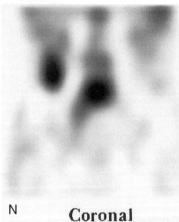

N   **Coronal**

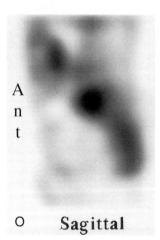

O   **Sagittal**

DECREASED WBC, INCREASED GALLIUM IN SPINAL OSTEOMYELITIS

Patient 1

FIGURE 3–9 A.

Delayed Bone Scan: There is increased activity involving L5 and S1.

FIGURE 3–9 B.

WBC Scan: There is decreased WBC accumulation at L5 and S1.

FIGURE 3–9 C.

Gallium Scan: There is an intense focus of gallium accumulation at L5–S1.

FIGURE 3–9 D.

CT Scan: There is a destructive process involving S1, with holes and sclerosis of the anterior vertebral body.

Patient 2

FIGURE 3–9 E.

WBC Scan: There is a subtle decrease in the WBC accumulation in the lower cervical spine *(arrowhead)*.

FIGURE 3–9 F.

Gallium Scan: There is increased gallium accumulation at C6 and C7 five days after the WBC scan.

Illustration continued on page 102

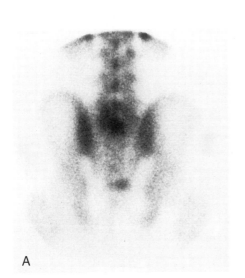

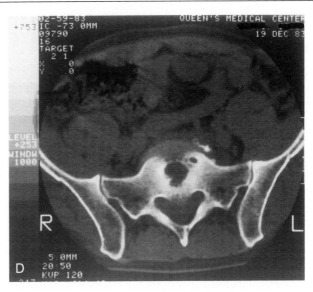

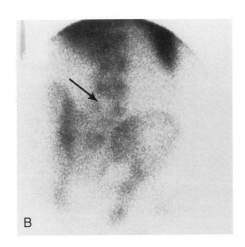

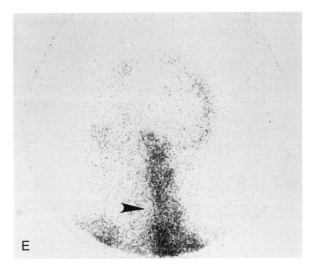

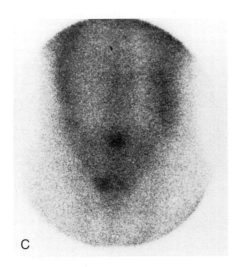

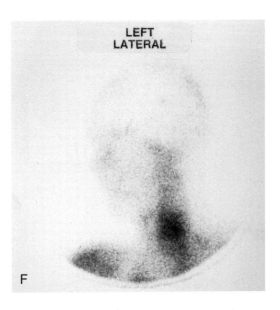

Patient 3: 67 Year Old Female with Back Pain and 102°F Fever, with Degenerative Changes on CT Scan

FIGURE 3-9 G.

Bone Scan: There are several abnormalities, including T11–T12, the right side of L3, and the left side of L4 and L5.

FIGURE 3-9 H.

WBC Scan: T11–T12 have mildly increased WBC accumulation. The lumbar vertebrae have areas of decreased activity as well as normal activity.

FIGURE 3-9 I.

Posterior Planar Gallium Scan: All the abnormalities on the bone scan have corresponding areas of increased gallium accumulation.

FIGURE 3-9 J and K.

Coronal and Sagittal Gallium Scans: The abnormalities are more clearly identified, especially the extension into the posterolateral soft tissues.

NOTE 1. In spinal osteomyelitis there can be an increase or a decrease in the white cell accumulation. Gallium SPECT scans may be easier to interpret.

NOTE 2. "Cold" defects with WBC scans include vertebral osteomyelitis, sites of marrow replacement, surgical bone defect, radiation therapy, metastases, lymphoma, metal artifacts, metallic fixation devices (e.g., Harrington rods), and joint prostheses.

NOTE 3. Decreased accumulation of white cells in spinal infections may be due to vascular congestion and stasis.

Cross Reference

Chapter 71: Infectious Diseases—Psoas Abscess; Decreased WBCs with Osteomyelitis

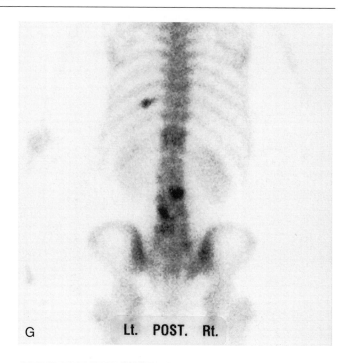

G   **Lt. POST. Rt.**

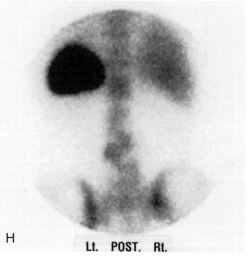

H   **Lt. POST. Rt.**

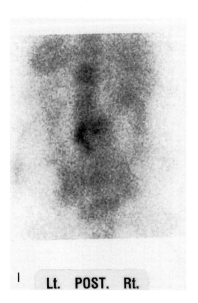

I   **Lt. POST. Rt.**

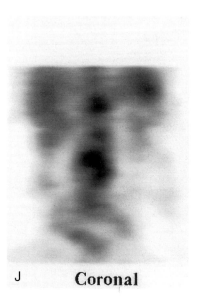

J   **Coronal**

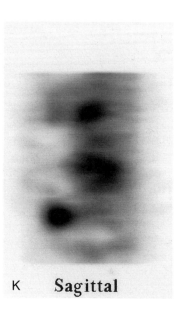

K   **Sagittal**

INCREASED WBCs IN SPINAL OSTEOMYELITIS

FIGURE 3–10   A and B.

Anterior and Posterior WBC Scans: There is increased WBC accumulation in L4.

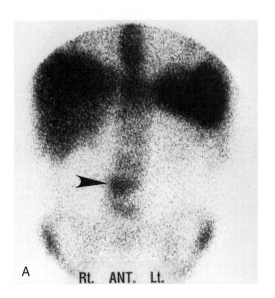
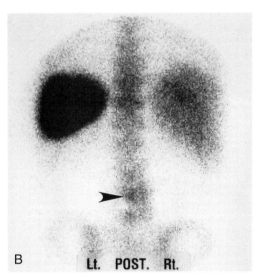

SPINAL OSTEOMYELITIS ASSOCIATED WITH HYDRONEPHROSIS

FIGURE 3–11.

Delayed Bone Scan: There is increased osteogenesis of L2 *(arrow)* and hydronephrosis of the left kidney.

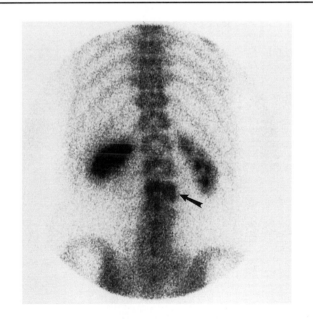

NOTE 1. An infected hydronephrotic kidney can be associated with spinal osteomyelitis, probably because of lymphatic drainage.

NOTE 2. *Mycobacterium tuberculosis*, which can cause renal obstruction, and *Escherichia coli*, which can infect an already obstructed kidney, are the two most common organisms in spinal osteomyelitis associated with hydronephrosis.

Cross References

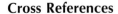

Chapter 36: Unilateral Abnormalities—Urinary Obstruction with "Flip-Flop" Function

Chapter 59: Venous Thrombosis—WBCs in Deep Venous Thrombosis

Chapter 71: Infectious Diseases—Psoas Abscess

CONTINUED HEALING POTENTIAL IN PARS INTERARTICULARIS FRACTURES

Patient 1: 16 Year Old Male with Acute Pain Playing Soccer

FIGURE 3–12   A to C.

Planar Delayed Bone Scintigraphy: There are bilateral focal L5–S1 pars interarticularis abnormalities.

FIGURE 3–12   D and E.

Planar Delayed Bone Scan: Eight months later there is still significant pars interarticularis activity on the left, indicating nonunion. The right side has healed.

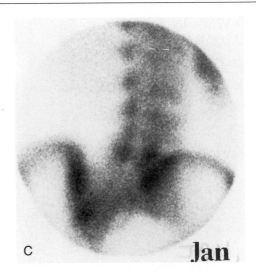

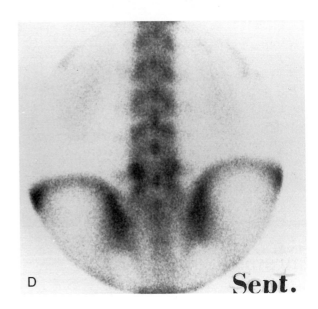

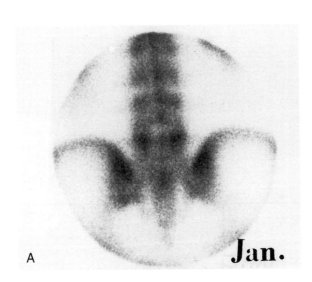

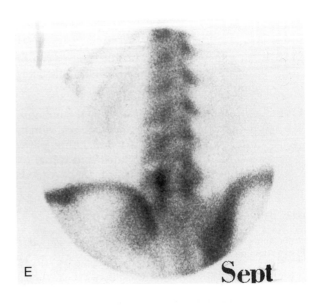

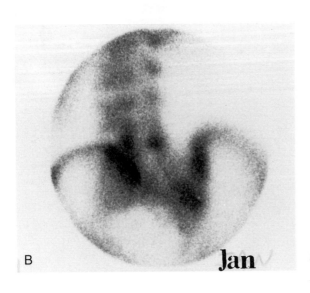

Patient 2

FIGURE 3–12 F to H.

SPECT Bone Scan: There is marked uptake of both pars interarticularis regions with persistent post-traumatic back pain. Coronal (F), sagittal (G), transverse (H).

NOTE 1. Increased activity, especially hyperemia, indicates continued potential for healing. Absence of increased osteogenesis indicates that spontaneous healing is unlikely.

NOTE 2. It may be difficult to distinguish between facet disease and pars interarticularis fractures on the bone scan alone. History and x-ray correlation must be made.

NOTE 3. Pars interarticularis fractures should be suspected with spondylolisthesis, especially in young males. In older patients, facet joint degenerative disease, with ligamentous laxity, can cause spondylolisthesis.

NOTE 4. Pars defects are probably not congenital fibrous nonfusions but are due to acute or repeated trauma and should be considered fractures.

Cross Reference

Chapter 3: Spinal Abnormalities—Localized Facet Joint Disease

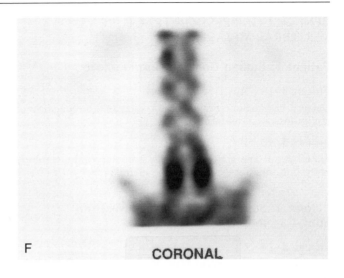

F   **CORONAL**

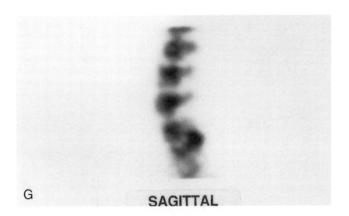

G   **SAGITTAL**

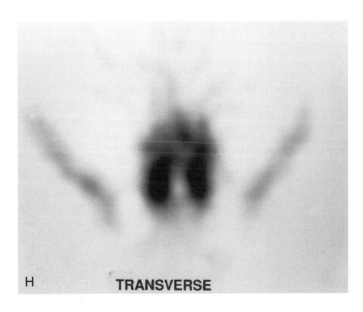

H   **TRANSVERSE**

BENIGN COMPRESSION FRACTURE VS. VERTEBRAL METASTASIS

Patient 1: Benign Compression Fracture

FIGURE 3–13   A.

Delayed Planar Bone Scan: There is increased osteogenesis of a midthoracic vertebral body.

FIGURE 3–13   B.

SPECT Scan: The abnormal activity is limited to the vertebral body and does not extend into the neural arch.

Patient 2: Solitary Spinal Metastasis from Lung Carcinoma

FIGURE 3–13   C.

Delayed Planar Bone Scan: There is increased activity in a midthoracic vertebra.

FIGURE 3–13   D.

SPECT Scan: The abnormal activity extends into the left pedicle *(arrow)*.

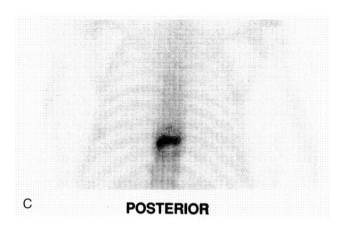

C   **POSTERIOR**

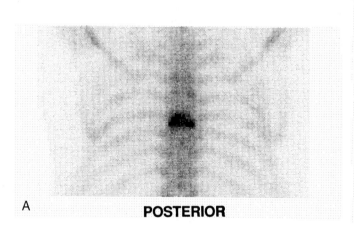

A   **POSTERIOR**

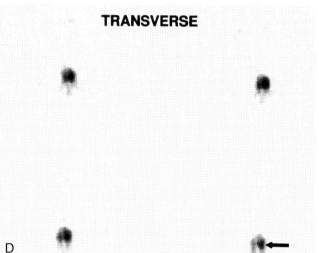

TRANSVERSE

D

TRANSVERSE

B

Patient 3: Post-traumatic Benign Compression Fracture Extending into the Pedicles

FIGURE 3–13   E and F.

Anterior and Posterior Planar Bone Scans: The superior endplate of L3 has increased activity.

FIGURE 3–13   G.

Transverse SPECT Scan: Both pedicles and the right transverse process are involved in the fracture.

Patient 4: Entire Vertebral Body Involved with a Compression Fracture

FIGURE 3–13   H.

Posterior Planar Bone Scan: L4 *(arrow)* is diffusely abnormal, while L1 and L2 *(arrowheads)* have inferior end-plate fractures.

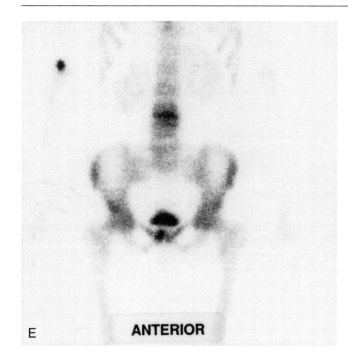

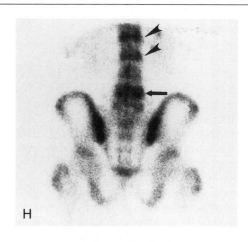

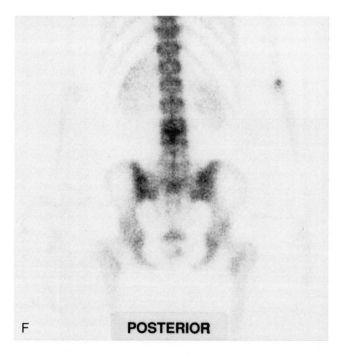

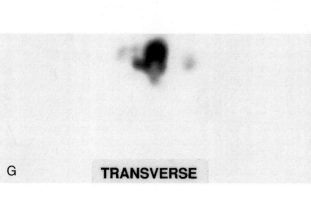

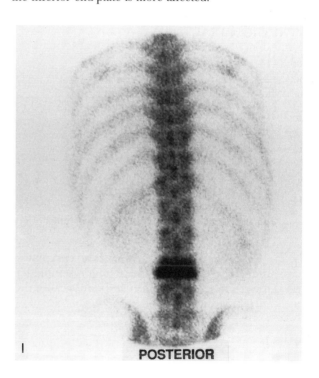

Patient 5: Solitary Spinal Metastasis

FIGURE 3–13 I.
Posterior Planar Bone Scan: L3 is diffusely abnormal, although the inferior end-plate is more affected.

NOTE 1. Benign compression fractures can be seen as end-plate or entire vertebral body abnormalities. The fractures may extend into the neural arch.

NOTE 2. In cases in which there is difficulty distinguishing between benign and malignant spinal abnormalities, CT or MRI may be helpful. When these are equivocal, biopsy or a repeat bone scan in 2 to 3 months can be helpful.

Cross Reference

Chapter 3: Spinal Abnormalities—Solitary Spinal Metastasis Simulating Degenerative Disease

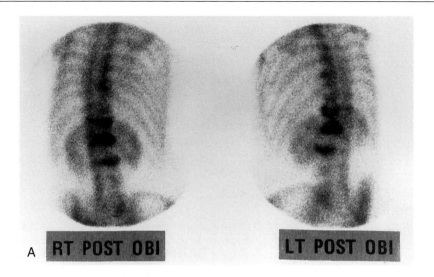

"FISH VERTEBRAE" AS COMPRESSION FRACTURES

FIGURE 3–14 A.
Oblique Spine Bone Scintigraphy: There are several concave vertebral abnormalities.

FIGURE 3–14 B.
X-ray: There are multiple depressed vertebral end-plates and an L1 compression fracture.

NOTE 1. Osteoporotic and weakened vertebral bodies will allow the nucleus pulposus to expand, depressing the vertebral end-plates.

NOTE 2. "Fish vertebrae" have biconcave end-plates; they are so called because of their resemblance to vertebrae found in fish and not because the vertebrae look like fish.

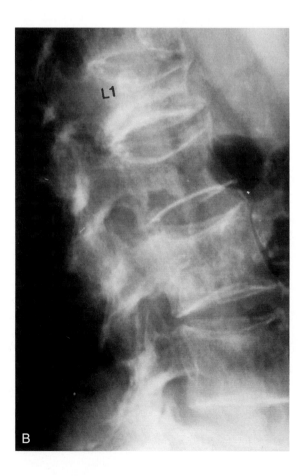

SUCCESSIVE COMPRESSION FRACTURES

FIGURE 3–15   A.

Delayed Bone Scintigraphy: There is a solitary T11 abnormality *(open arrow)*.

FIGURE 3–15   B and C.

Delayed Bone Scintigraphy: Three months later there is a second abnormality at the L3 superior end-plate *(solid arrow)*.

FIGURE 3–15   D and E.

Delayed Bone Scintigraphy: After an additional year there are more fractures: T7, T8, and L2. There is healing of the previous fractures.

NOTE. It may take up to 1 year for a compression fracture to collapse and become evident on plain film x-ray, although it will be abnormal on bone scan within 72 hours.

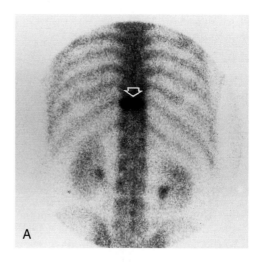

A

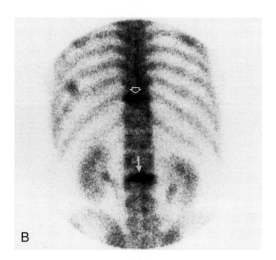

B

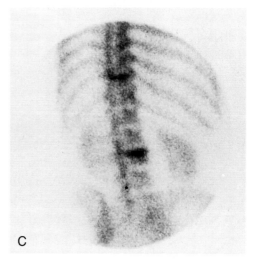

C

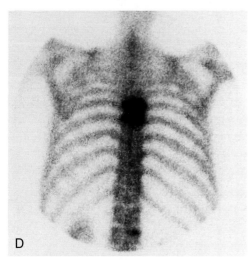

D

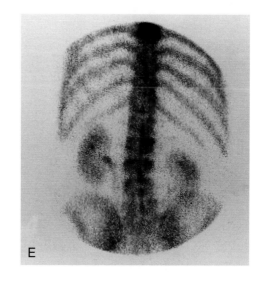

E

Cross Reference

Chapter 2: Multiple Bony Abnormalities—Progressive Severe Osteoporotic Fractures over 2 Months

FRACTURE OF SPINOUS PROCESS

FIGURE 3–16   A.
Delayed Planar Bone Scan: There is increased activity involving the T6 spinous process.

FIGURE 3–16   B.
SPECT Bone Scan: The posterior activity is well defined in the sagittal plane. (Courtesy of Dr. Michael Kipper, Vista, CA.)

NOTE 1. Spinous process fractures can occur from direct blows or hyperextension ("kissing fractures"), where two spinous processes bang against one another.

NOTE 2. Musculotendinous trauma (enthesopathy) to the rotator muscles of the spine, which attach to the laminae and the spinous processes, can cause bone scan changes.

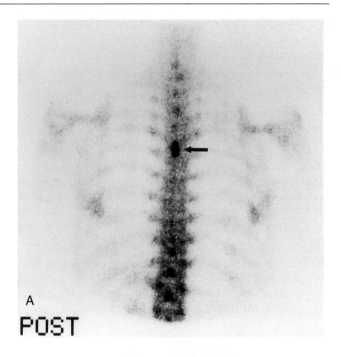

A
POST

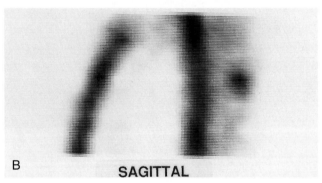

B   SAGITTAL

NORMAL SPINAL FUSION

Patient: Low Back Pain 5 Years After Spinal Fusion

FIGURE 3–17   A and B.

Planar Posterior and Coronal SPECT Lumbosacral Bone Scans: There is homogeneous activity involving the bridging fusion from L4 to S1.

NOTE. The increased activity in the left sacroiliac joint may be symptomatic, probably representing abnormal motion and stress due to the fusion.

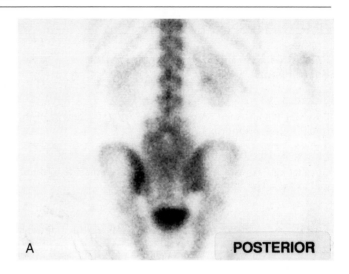

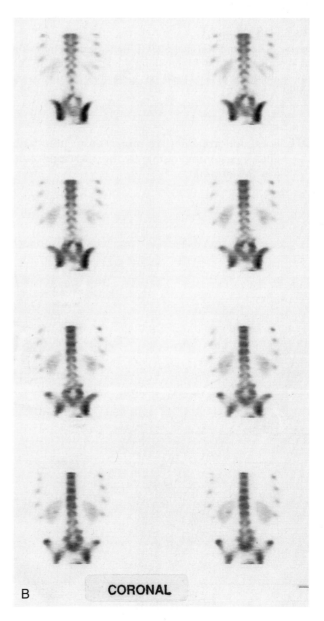

FRACTURED SPINAL FUSION

Patient 1: Low Back Pain 2 Years After Back Fusion

FIGURE 3–18   A.

Posterior Planar Bone Scan: The left sacral attachment of the spinal fusion is abnormal *(arrow)*.

FIGURE 3–18   B and C.

Coronal and Transverse SPECT Scans: The right side is abnormal as well. The SI joints are normal.

Patient 2

FIGURE 3–18   D.

Posterior Blood Pool Scan: There is focal hyperemia adjacent to the left side of L4 *(arrow)*.

FIGURE 3–18   E and F.

Posterior Planar and Coronal SPECT Bone Scans: There is a focal abnormality in the fusion along the left side of L4. The fusion is also loose at the L5–S1 level bilaterally, best seen on the SPECT scan.

NOTE. Focal abnormalities are more conspicuous with SPECT scanning owing to the increased contrast resolution.

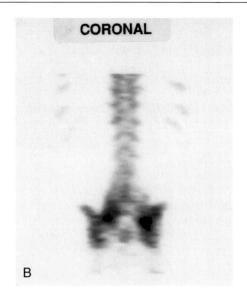

B

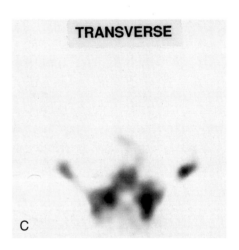

C

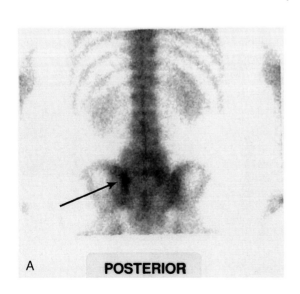

A

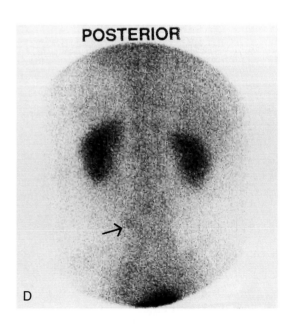

D

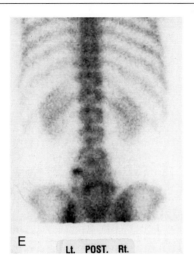

E   Lt. POST. Rt.

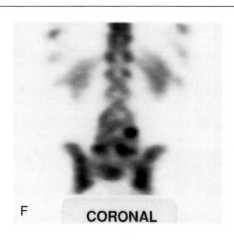

F   CORONAL

Chapter 4

Pelvic Abnormalities

NORMAL PELVIS/SACRUM

Patient 1: 8 Year Old Male

FIGURE 4–1   A and B.
Anterior and Posterior Bone Scans: The femoral growth plates are quite prominent.

Patient 2: Adult Male

FIGURE 4–1   C and D.
Anterior and Posterior Bone Scans: Subcapital activity of a mild degree is usually seen from young adulthood through middle age.

NOTE 1. Activity should be symmetric for the sacroiliac (SI) joints, the iliac spines, the symphysis pubis, and the acetabula.

NOTE 2. The sacral neural foramina should be well seen.

NOTE 3. Planar images should be obtained immediately after voiding. SPECT scans of the pelvis should be done with a bladder catheter in place.

Illustration continued on following page

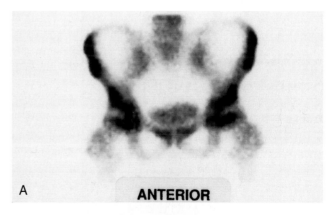

A   ANTERIOR

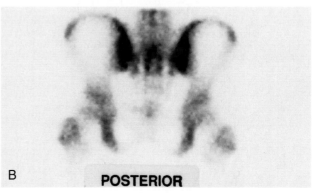

B   POSTERIOR

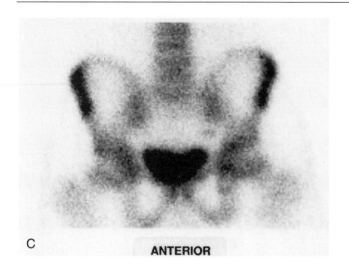

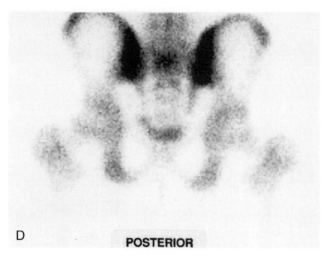

SEPTIC SYMPHYSIS PUBIS

FIGURE 4–2.

Bone Scan: The pubic symphysis has increased osteogenesis extending vertically, with irregular cortical margins medially.

NOTE. True osteitis pubis is most often seen after pelvic surgery and is believed to be inflammatory. Sclerosis of the pubic bones is frequent after childbirth but does not have the joint space narrowing seen with osteitis pubis.

Cross Reference

Chapter 4: Pelvic Abnormalities—Stress Fracture of Symphysis Pubis

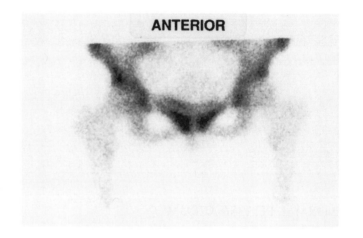

OSTEITIS CONDENSANS ILII

FIGURE 4–3 A.

Delayed Bone Scintigraphy: There is bilateral increased activity in the inferior aspect of both ilii in a triangular configuration.

FIGURE 4–3 B.

Plain Film X-ray: demonstrates sclerotic bone in the inferior ilii adjacent to the SI joints.

NOTE. Osteitis condensans ilii is seen in multiparous women. It is bilateral but may have asymmetric activity on bone scan despite symmetric appearances on x-ray.

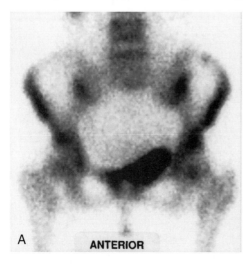

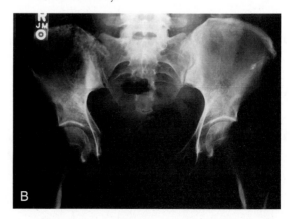

SACROILIAC JOINT OSTEOARTHRITIS

FIGURE 4–4.
Delayed Bone Scan: There is increased activity at the lower edges of the SI joints.

NOTE 1. The increased activity is in the same area as the small spurs commonly seen on x-rays.

NOTE 2. Any activity above this level indicates other disease processes: other arthritides (Reiter's, psoriatic, ankylosing spondylitis), trauma, infection, neoplasm, inflammatory bowel disease.

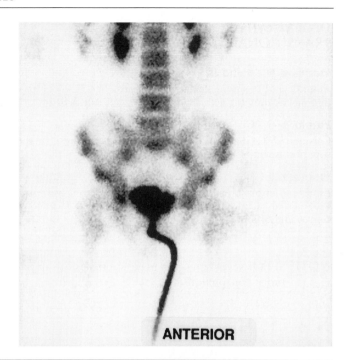

ANTERIOR

ANKYLOSING SPONDYLITIS

FIGURE 4–5   A to C.
Posterior Blood Pool and Delayed Anterior and Posterior Pelvic Scans: The right SI joint is hyperemic and has increased osteogenesis, as does the lower lumbar spine.

NOTE. Ankylosing spondylitis starts in the SI joints and is classically symmetric but can initially be asymmetric on bone scan.

Cross Reference

Chapter 2: Multiple Bony Abnormalities—Psoriatic Arthritis

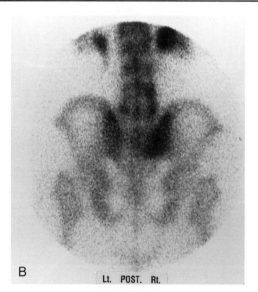

B   Lt. POST. Rt.

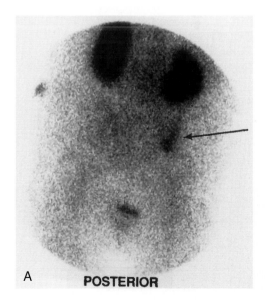

A   POSTERIOR

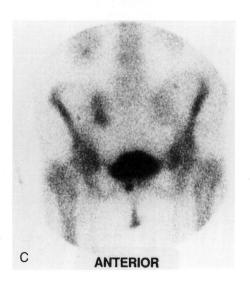

C   ANTERIOR

DEGENERATIVE CHANGES OF THE TRANSITIONAL VERTEBRA

FIGURE 4–6   A and B.

Anterior and Posterior Planar Bone Scans: The SI joints have minimal asymmetry, with slightly greater left side activity.

FIGURE 4–6   C.

Coronal SPECT Scan: There is abnormal osteogenesis at the superior aspect of the left SI joint *(arrow)*.

FIGURE 4–6   D.

Anteroposterior Pelvis X-ray Detail: L5 is a transitional vertebra, with partial sacralization and sclerosis of the left facet joint *(arrow)* and SI joint.

NOTE. SPECT scans can often make subtle lesions much more conspicuous.

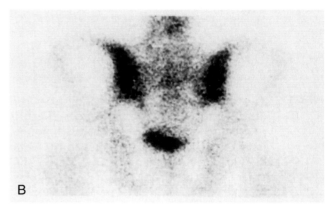

B

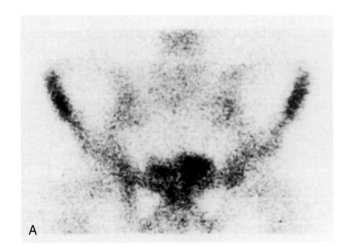

A

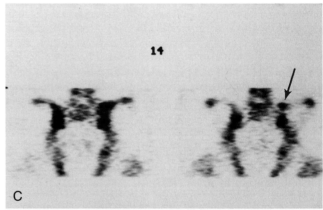

C

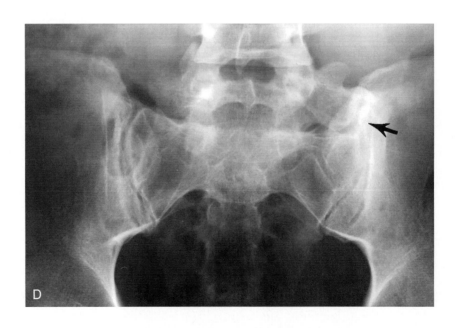

D

SACROILIAC JOINT INFECTION

FIGURE 4–7 A and B.

Posterior Blood Pool and Delayed Posterior Pelvis Scans: The left SI joint is hyperemic and has increased osteogenesis, extending into S1 and S2.

FIGURE 4–7 C.

Posterior 24 Degree Gallium Scan: There is increased gallium overlying the left SI joint, sacrum, and soft tissues.

NOTE 1. Sacral infections can be seen in IV drug users and patients with decubitus ulcers, psoas abscess extension, or any hematogenous infection.

NOTE 2. SI joint diseases on bone scan cannot be distinguished from post-traumatic fractures, insufficiency fractures, and septic or inflammatory arthritis, e.g., ankylosing spondylitis, Reiter's disease.

NOTE 3. A gallium scan may be positive as early as 3 hours but may require 24 to 48 hours to be diagnostic.

Cross Reference

Chapter 1: Solitary Bony Abnormalities—Brodie's Abscess of Ilium

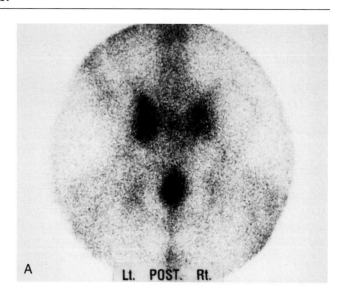

A   Lt. POST. Rt.

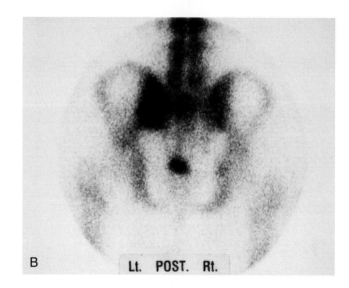

B   Lt. POST. Rt.

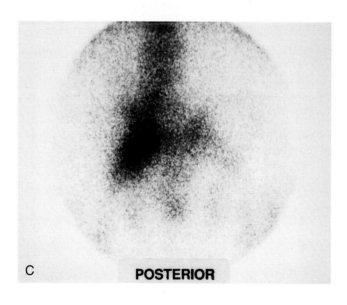

C   POSTERIOR

SACRAL INSUFFICIENCY FRACTURES

Patient 1

FIGURE 4–8   A and B.

Anterior and Posterior Pelvis Delayed Bone Scan: There is increased osteogenesis involving both SI joints and seen across the midsacral body ("Honda sign").

Patient 2

FIGURE 4–8   C to E.

Blood Pool, Posterior Pelvic and T.O.D. Scans: There is hyperemia and increased activity of both SI joints without a sacral body fracture. (T.O.D. = "tush-on-detector" or seated view.)

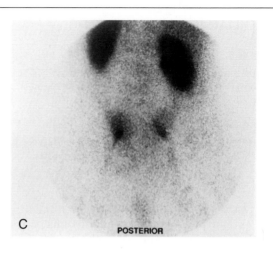

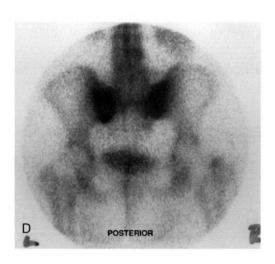

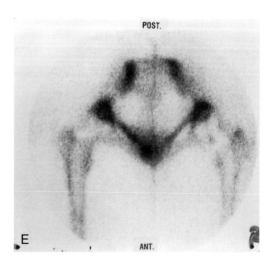

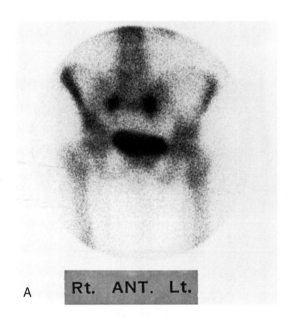

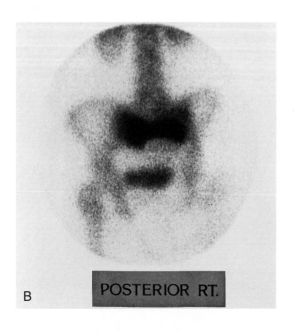

Patient 3

FIGURE 4–8   F.
Posterior Sacral Bone Scan: There is vertical increased activity involving S1 through S4 vertebral bodies, along with the sacral alae.

NOTE 1. Hyperemia indicates an acute injury.

NOTE 2. T.O.D. views are especially valuable when the bladder cannot be adequately emptied.

NOTE 3. Insufficiency fractures can occur with osteoporosis, any osteopenic state, chemotherapy, and immobilization.

Cross Reference

Chapter 2: Multiple Bony Abnormalities—Progressive Osteoporotic Fractures over 2 Months

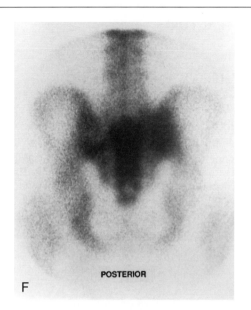

POST-TRAUMATIC SACRAL FRACTURE

FIGURE 4–9   A and B.
Posterior and Left Lateral Bone Scan: There is a horizontal fracture of the midsacrum due to a fall from a horse.

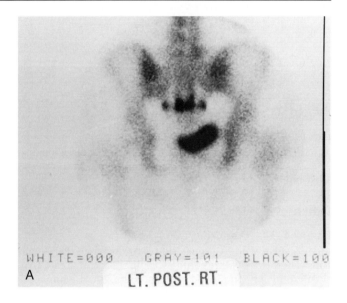

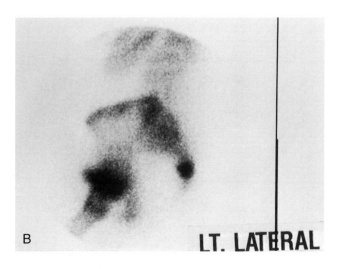

PELVIC FRACTURES

Patient 1

FIGURE 4–10 A.

Blood Pool Scintigraphy: There are several areas of hyperemia including both ischii *(arrows)*, the left symphysis pubis *(arrowhead)*, and the right lateral superior pubic ramus *(arrowhead)*.

FIGURE 4–10 B.

Delayed Bone Scan: There are multiple bony abnormalities consistent with fractures, including the left SI joint. The bladder is displaced to the right by an intrapelvic hematoma.

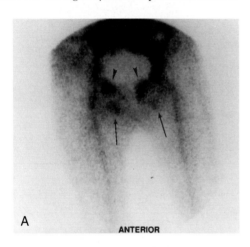

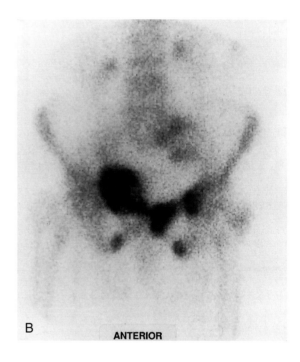

Patient 2

FIGURE 4–10 C.

Anterior Pelvic Bone Scan: There is a vertical iliac wing fracture *(arrowheads)* as well as acetabular and pubic bone fractures and a left hip fracture.

Patient 3

FIGURE 4–10 D and E.

Anterior Planar and Coronal SPECT Scans of the Pelvis and Hips: There are fractures of the left hip, the right greater trochanter, the left symphysis pubis, and the right SI joint.

NOTE. Pelvic fractures usually number two or more because of the rigid pelvic ring structure. SI joints or symphysis pubis separation may be part of the ring breaks.

Cross Reference

Chapter 1: Solitary Bony Abnormalities—False Negative Bone Scan for Fracture

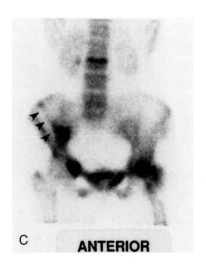

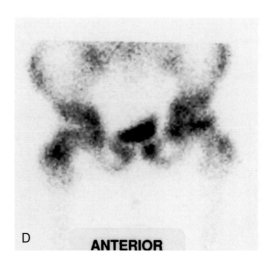

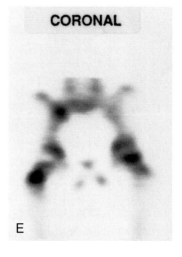

STRESS FRACTURE OF SYMPHYSIS PUBIS

Patient: Football Player

FIGURE 4–11.

Anterior Pelvic Bone Scan: There is asymmetric increased activity involving the right symphysis pubis and right superior pubic ramus.

NOTE. The symphysis pubis should have symmetric activity.

Cross Reference

Chapter 4: Pelvic Abnormalities—Septic Symphysis Pubis

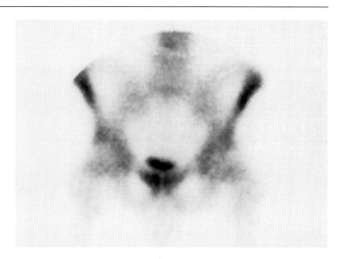

ABNORMALITIES HIDDEN BY FULL BLADDER

Patient 1: Elderly Patient Who Fell

FIGURE 4–12   A.

Delayed Bone Scintigraphy: The prevoid film does not adequately evaluate the hips because of scatter from the bladder, despite the bladder shield.

FIGURE 4–12   B.

Delayed Bone Scintigraphy After Voiding: The hip fracture *(arrow)* can now be seen.

Illustration continued on following page

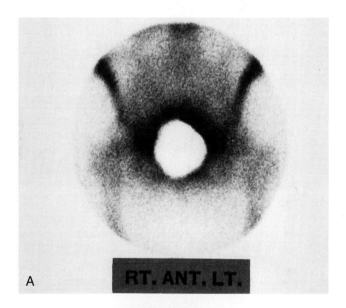

A · RT. ANT. LT.

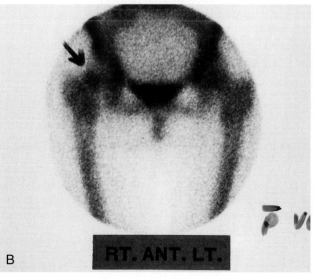

B · RT. ANT. LT.

Patient 2: Lung Cancer Metastases

FIGURE 4–12   C and D.
Bone Scan: There is a large urinary bladder in a patient with metastatic lung carcinoma.

FIGURE 4–12   E and F.
Pelvic Bone Scan After Bladder Catheterization: There are sacral metastases at S1–S2 and S5.

NOTE 1. Bladder emptying is essential in the evaluation of the hips, with catheterization especially necessary for SPECT. The bladder may need to be flushed even after catheterization.

NOTE 2. T.O.D. views can be helpful for sacral and pelvic abnormalities.

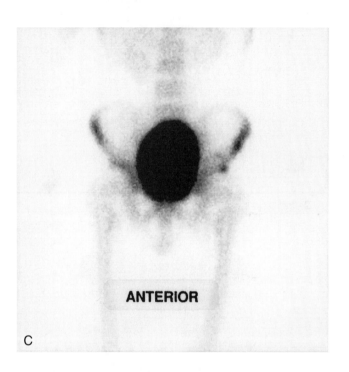

C   ANTERIOR

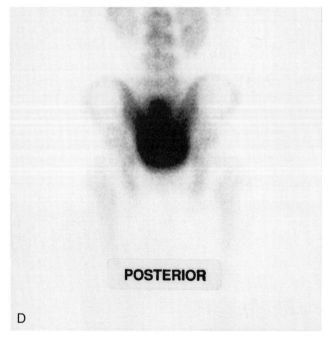

D   POSTERIOR

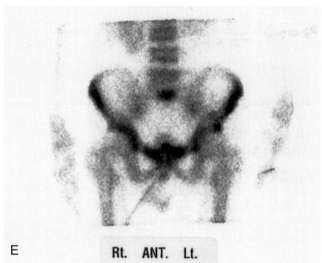

E   Rt.   ANT.   Lt.

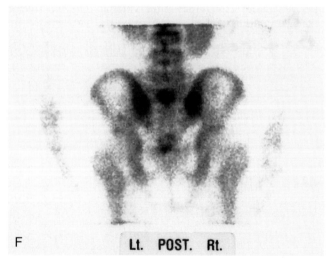

F   Lt.   POST.   Rt.

PELVIC OSTEOCHONDROMA

FIGURE 4–13.

Anterior Pelvic Bone Scan: There is a large protruding bony excrescence arising from the left ilium.

NOTE. The most common benign tumor of the ilium is the osteochondroma.

Cross References

Chapter 1: Solitary Bony Abnormalities—Osteochondroma of Talus

Chapter 2: Multiple Bony Abnormalities—Osteochondromas (Exostoses)

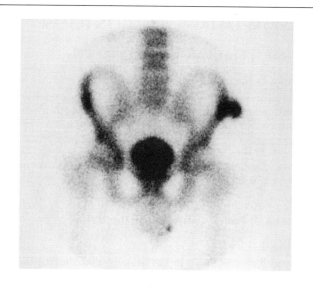

PELVIC CHONDROSARCOMA AND ABNORMAL WEIGHT BEARING

FIGURE 4–14   A.

Posterior Planar Bone Scan: There is an irregular zone of increased osteogenesis within the right iliac wing.

FIGURE 4–14   B.

Anteroposterior Pelvis X-ray: There are irregular areas of increased density involving the right ilium *(arrowhead)*.

FIGURE 4–14   C.

Delayed Bone Scan: The right leg has less activity than the left.

NOTE 1. Diffusely decreased activity on bone scan can be seen with immobilized bone or reduced blood flow. Increased activity results from increased weight bearing or usage or from increased blood flow.

NOTE 2. The most common primary malignancies of the ilium (innominate bone) are osteosarcomas and chondrosarcomas.

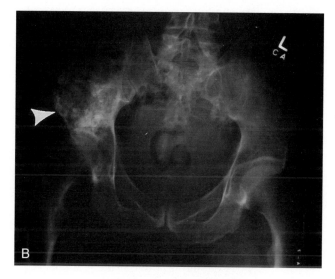

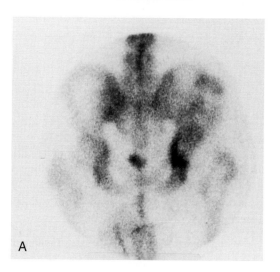

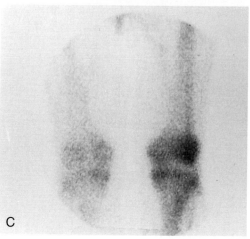

PELVIC METASTASES VS. PAGET'S DISEASE

Patient 1: Breast Metastases to the Pelvis

FIGURE 4–15   A and B.

Anterior and Posterior Pelvic Bone Scans: The increased activity extends along the iliopectineal line. The abnormality was new in this patient, who was being followed for breast cancer.

FIGURE 4–15   C.

X-ray of the Right Pelvis: There are numerous blastic metastases, best seen in the ischium.

Patient 2: Paget's Disease of the Pelvis

FIGURE 4–15   D.

Anterior Pelvic Bone Scan: The intensity of the osteogenesis is so great that the normal bones of the pelvis are virtually absent.

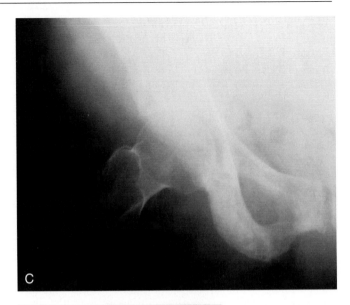

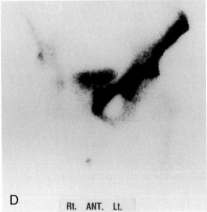

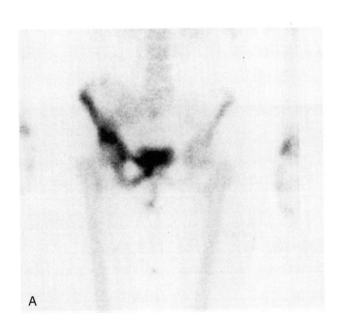

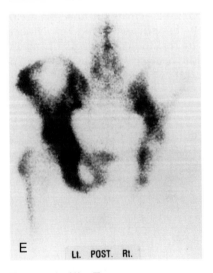

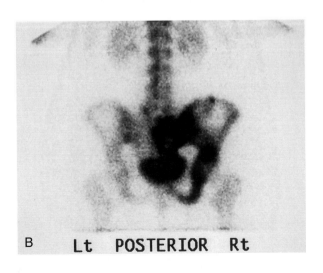

FIGURE 4–15   E.

Posterior Pelvic Bone Scan: There are multiple abnormalities that have been stable over years in this patient without cancer. (Courtesy of Dr. Michael Kipper, Vista, CA.)

Cross Reference

Chapter 2: Multiple Bony Abnormalities—Varying Patterns of Paget's Disease

Skull Abnormalities

BENIGN FOCAL ABNORMALITIES OF THE SKULL

Patient 1

FIGURE 5–1 A.
Bone Scan: The focal abnormality in the region of the frontal suture was stable for 4 years.

Patient 2: Paget's Disease

FIGURE 5–1 B and C.
Vertex and Lateral Skull Bone Scans: There is a focal, solitary skull abnormality, surgically proven to be Paget's disease *(arrow)*. (Courtesy of Dr. Arnold Jacobson, Seattle, WA.)

NOTE 1. Benign focal abnormalities of the skull have increased osteogenesis but remain unchanged over time. They are common in the frontal and lambdoidal sutures and may include hemangiomas or histiocytosis X or unknown entities.

NOTE 2. Solitary metastases are unusual. A biopsy, a CT scan, or a follow-up bone scan in 4 months may help.

Cross Reference

Chapter 5: Skull Abnormalities—Paget's Disease of the Skull

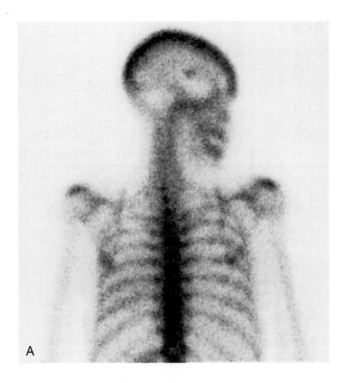

A

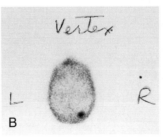

B

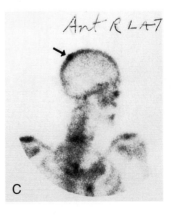

C

HYPEROSTOSIS FRONTALIS INTERNA

Patient 1

FIGURE 5-2   A.

Anterior Bone Scan: The increased osteogenesis of each frontal bone is separated by normal activity.

FIGURE 5-2   B.

Lateral Skull Bone Scan: As part of a total body bone scan, the frontal bone activity could resemble a malignant abnormality.

Patient 2

FIGURE 5-2   C and D.

Anterior and Left Lateral Skull WBC Scans: The WBC activity in the areas of hyperostosis indicates that bone marrow is present.

NOTE. A continuous abnormality crossing the midline suggests a meningioma or a metastatic deposit. Hyperostosis frontalis interna never crosses the midline.

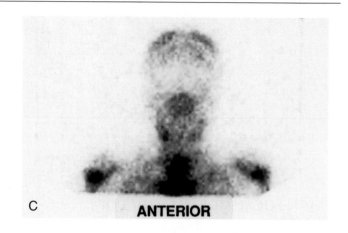

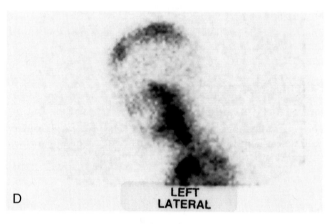

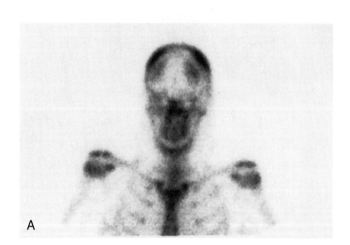

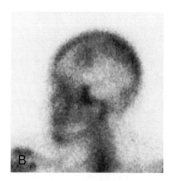

BIPARIETAL THINNING ON BONE SCAN

FIGURE 5–3.
Anterior Skull Bone Scan: There is symmetric thinning of the parietal bones *(arrowheads)*.

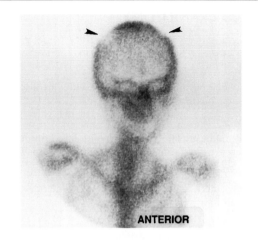

NOTE 1. In the elderly there may be thinning of the outer table of the cranium, apparent only in the parietal bones.

NOTE 2. Persistent parietal foramina, congenital defects in the skull, may not fuse and will appear as either unilateral or bilateral "cold" skull defects.

TEMPOROMANDIBULAR JOINT SYNDROME

FIGURE 5–4   A and B.
Bone Scan: There is increased activity involving the right temporomandibular joint (TMJ).

FIGURE 5–4   C and D.
Bone Scan 1 Year Later: After splinting was applied, the right TMJ returned to normal.

NOTE. Rest will often reduce abnormal bony reaction.

Cross Reference

Chapter 10: Prostheses—Reduced Loosening of Hip Prosthesis

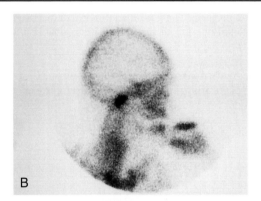

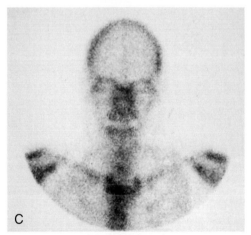

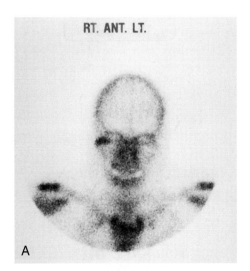

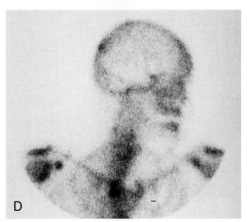

INFECTED CRANIOTOMY

Patient 1

FIGURE 5–5 A.
Blood Pool Scintigraphy: There is hyperemia involving the left parietal bone (arrow = marker).

FIGURE 5–5 B.
Delayed Bone Scan: The craniotomy site has a photon deficit. There is an area anterior to it that has increased activity.

FIGURE 5–5 C.
WBC Scan: There is abnormal WBC accumulation in the infected craniotomy.

Patient 2: Normal Craniotomy

FIGURE 5–5 D.
Delayed Bone Scan: There is only a thin rim of increased activity in the frontal bone in this patient, 1 week after craniotomy.

NOTE. A normal recent craniotomy should have a discrete margin of increased osteogenesis.

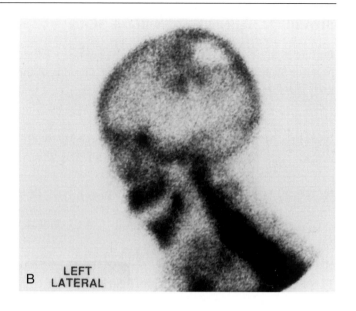

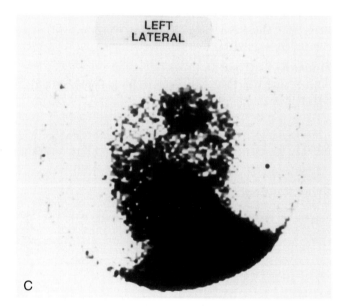

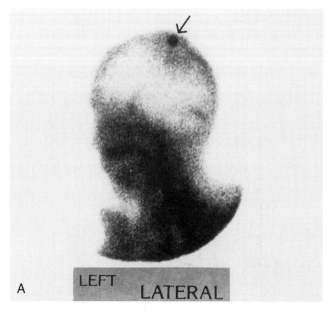

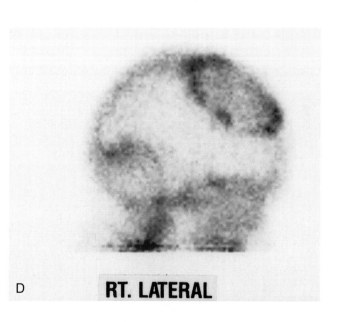

MALIGNANT OTITIS EXTERNA

Patient 1

FIGURE 5–6   A and B.
Left Lateral and Posterior Bone Scans: There is increased osteogenesis involving the left temporal bone.

Patient 2

FIGURE 5–6   C and D.
Bone Scan: There is extensive involvement from the external auditory canal anteriorly to involve the temporal squamosa, posteriorly to the occipital bone, and medially to cross over to the right side.

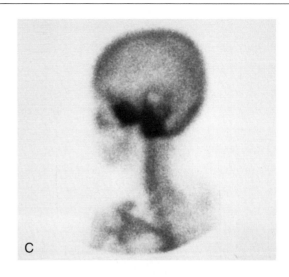

C

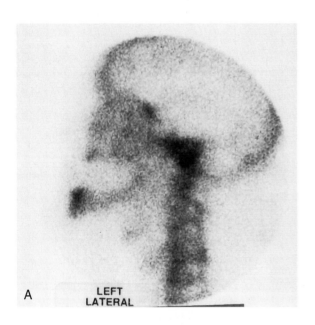

A   LEFT LATERAL

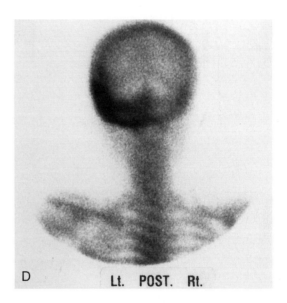

D   Lt. POST. Rt.

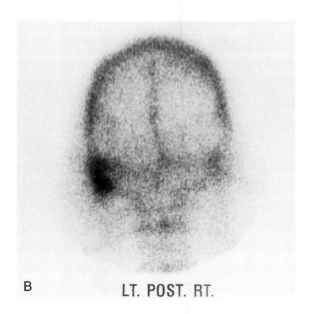

B   LT. POST. RT.

FIGURE 5–6   E and F.
Gallium Scan: The soft tissue and bone involvement with infection is extensive.

Patient 3

FIGURE 5–6   G and H.
Transverse Bone and Gallium SPECT Scans: The infection has extended along the entire length of the left petrous ridge.

NOTE. SPECT scans are also valuable in malignant otitis media to determine the depth of involvement.

Illustration continued on following page

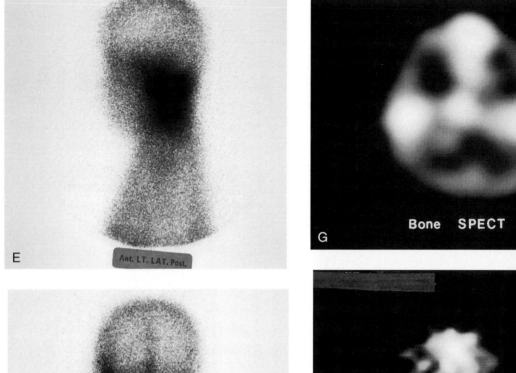

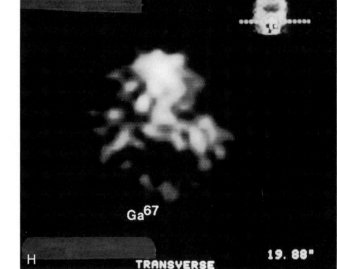

SICKLE CELL SKULL

FIGURE 5–7   A and B.

Bone Scan: The skull is diffusely "hot" owing to the extramedullary hematopoiesis.

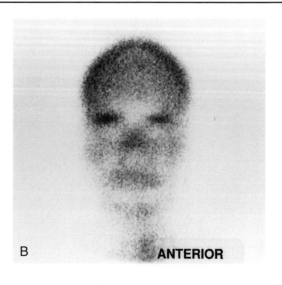

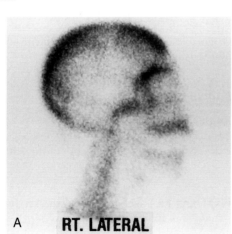

ETHMOID-FRONTAL OSTEOMA

FIGURE 5–8.

Multiple Views of Bone Scan: There is intense osteogenesis in the ethmoid sinuses extending into the frontal bone.

NOTE. Osteomas of the paranasal sinuses, most frequently seen in the frontal sinus, are usually asymptomatic.

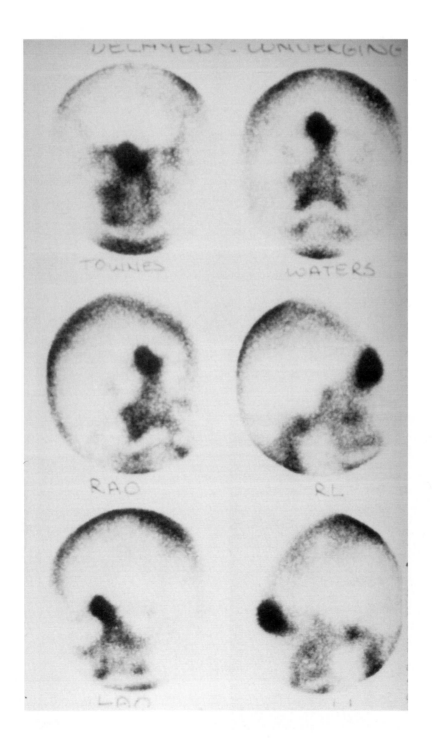

HISTIOCYTOSIS X

Patient 1

FIGURE 5–9   A.
Plain Film of Skull: The multicentric lytic lesions in the skull are characteristic of histiocytosis X.

FIGURE 5–9   B.
Bone Scintigram: There is increased activity *(arrowheads)* indicating the active parts of the lesion.

Patient 2

FIGURE 5–9   C.
Bone Scintigram: There is increased osteogenesis in the mandible and the maxilla before treatment.

FIGURE 5–9   D.
Post-therapy Bone Scintigram: The mandible and maxilla are now normal.

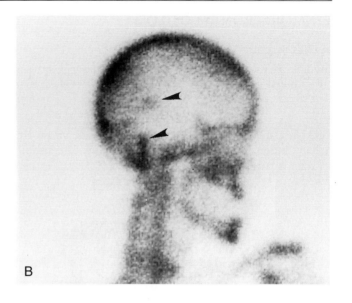

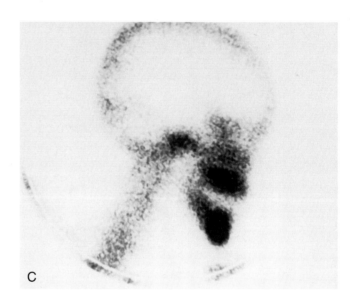

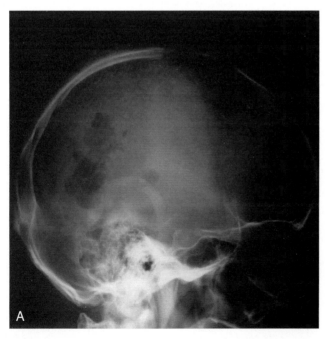

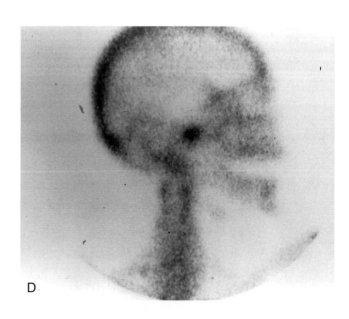

Patient 3

FIGURE 5–9 E.
Lateral Skull Scintigram: The mandible and petrous bones are involved.

NOTE 1. The skull, especially the posterior aspect, and the mandible, spine, pelvis, and femurs are most commonly involved.

NOTE 2. There are three histiocytosis X syndromes: eosinophilic granuloma, Hand-Schüller-Christian disease, and Letterer-Siwe disease. The more bones involved, the worse the prognosis.

Cross Reference

Chapter 9: "Cold" Abnormalities—Histiocytosis X on Bone Scan

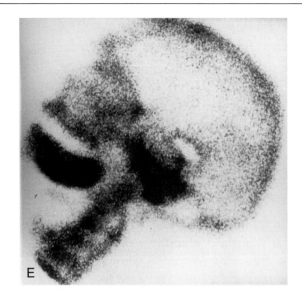

SKULL METASTASES

Patient 1: Breast Carcinoma

FIGURE 5–10 A.
Right Lateral Skull Bone Scan: There is a solitary abnormality involving the occipitomastoid region.

FIGURE 5–10 B.
Lateral Plain Film X-ray: There is a lytic lesion in the occipitomastoid skull *(arrow)*.

Illustration continued on following page

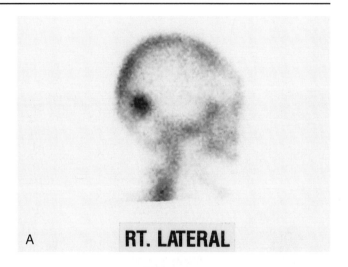

A **RT. LATERAL**

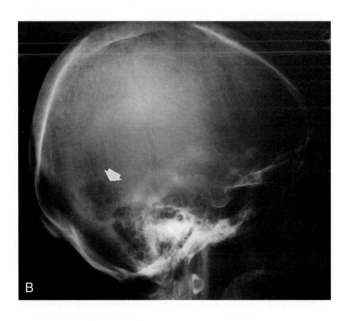

B

Patient 2: Prostate Carcinoma

FIGURE 5–10   C and D.

Bone Scan: There are several "hot" spots in the skull, including doughnut lesions.

Patient 3: Breast Carcinoma

FIGURE 5–10   E.

Bone Scan: The skull metastases are more "solid." The skull base is also involved.

NOTE. Skull base involvement should be noted, since cranial nerve involvement may occur.

Cross Reference

Chapter 9: "Cold" Abnormalities—"Doughnut" Lesions of the Bone

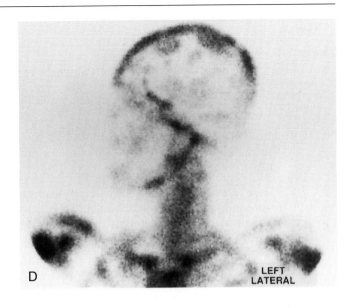

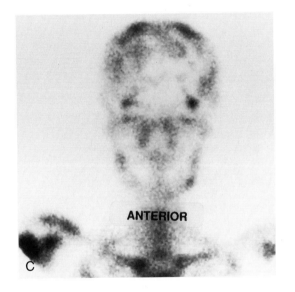

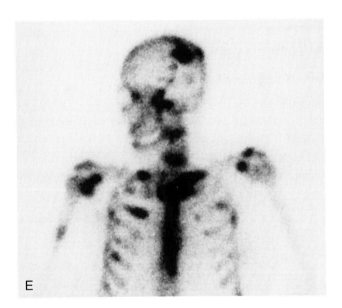

DIFFUSELY "HOT" SKULL IN BREAST CARCINOMA

FIGURE 5–11.

Bone Scan: The skull has diffuse increased osteogenesis.

NOTE. In breast and sometimes other malignant neoplasms, e.g., lung cancer, the skull has diffuse increased osteogenesis. The cause and significance are still uncertain, but it does not indicate metastases.

Cross Reference

Chapter 2: Multiple Bony Abnormalities—Renal Osteodystrophy

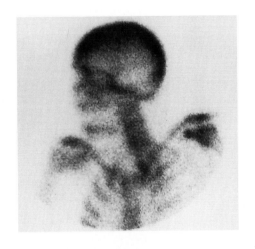

PAGET'S DISEASE OF THE SKULL

Patient 1: Blastic Phase

FIGURE 5–12   A and B.

Anterior and Right Lateral Skull Bone Scans: The intense activity and diffuse pattern, as well as the skull enlargement, are characteristic of Paget's disease.

Patient 2: Osteolytic Phase (Osteoporosis Circumscripta)

FIGURE 5–12   C and D.

Anterior and Left Lateral Bone Scan: There is asymmetric involvement of the skull. The left side has increased activity diffusely.

FIGURE 5–12   E.

Plain Film Skull X-ray: There is increased lucency of the right frontal, parietal, and temporal bones, where Paget's disease is in its osteolytic phase.

Illustration continued on following page

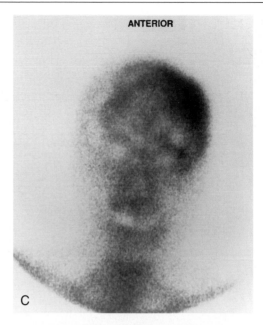

C

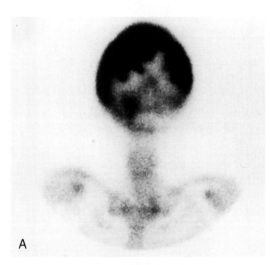

A

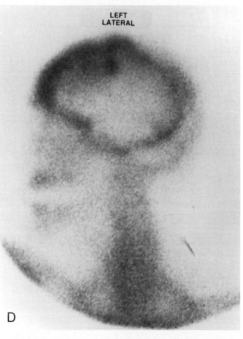

D

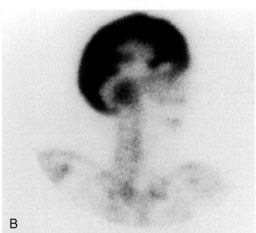

B

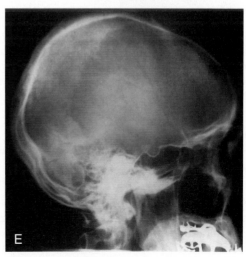

E

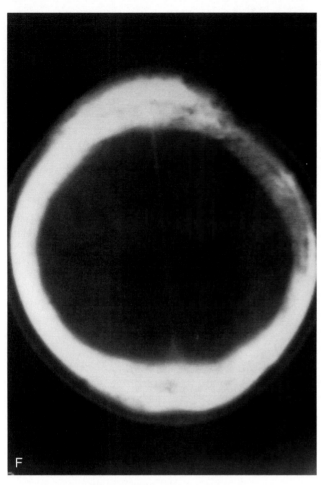

FIGURE 5–12 F.

CT of Paget's Skull: There is decreased density and thinning of the pagetoid bone.

Patient 3

FIGURE 5–12 G.

Anterior Bone Scan: The bilateral involvement here is across the base of the skull.

NOTE 1. Paget's disease begins with an osteoporotic phase followed by a blastic stage. The abnormally thickened pagetoid bone has less calcified osteoid per cm^3 than normal bone. It is also highly vascular.

NOTE 2. Paget's disease of the skull starts at one end or side and may progress to the opposite side.

NOTE 3. Pagetoid bone is softer than normal, resulting in settling of the skull and basilar invagination. The flattened, elongated shape of the skull has been described as resembling the Scottish hat tam-o'-shanter.

Cross References

Chapter 2: Multiple Bony Abnormalities—Varying Patterns of Paget's Disease

Chapter 5: Skull Abnormalities—Benign Focal Abnormalities of the Skull

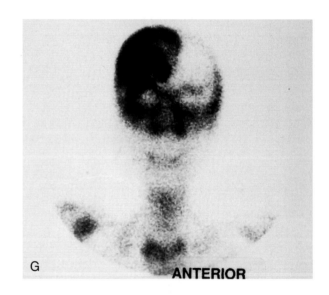

VIABLE EYE PROSTHESIS

FIGURE 5–13 A to C.

Anterior and Both Lateral Skull Scans: The hydroxyapatite prothesis *(arrow)* has MDP activity, indicating that it has an intact vasculature.

FIGURE 5–13 D.

Coronal SPECT Scan: The right eye prosthesis has homogeneous activity.

NOTE. A normal viable prosthesis has diffuse ingrowth of blood vessels and should have homogeneous accumulation of the bone scanning agent.

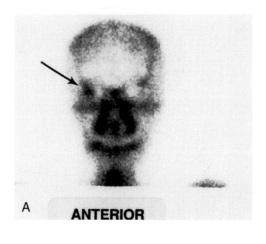

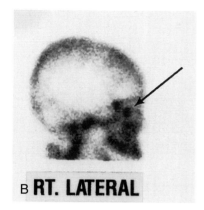

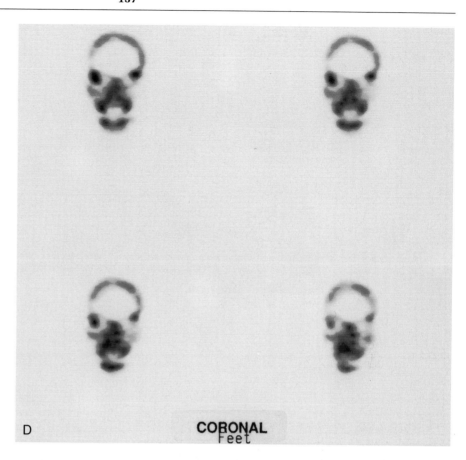

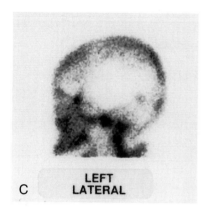

PARANASAL SINUSITIS

Patient 1

FIGURE 5–14   A.

Plain Film X-ray: There is opacification of the right maxillary sinus antrum.

FIGURE 5–14   B and C.

Anterior and Right Lateral Delayed Bone Scans: There is bony involvement of the right antrum.

FIGURE 5–14   D.

Gallium Scan: There is intense right maxillary sinus activity as well as inflammatory cervical lymph nodes.

Illustration continued on following page

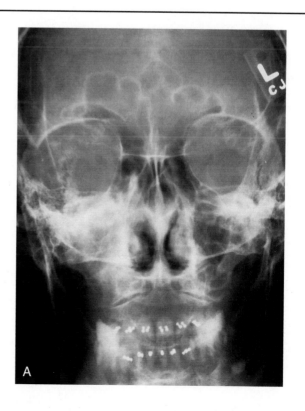

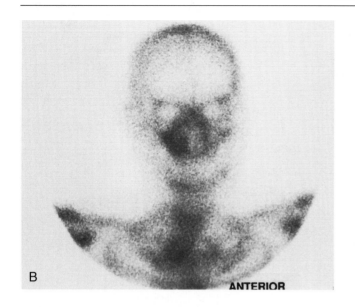

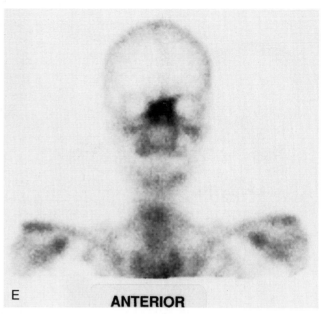

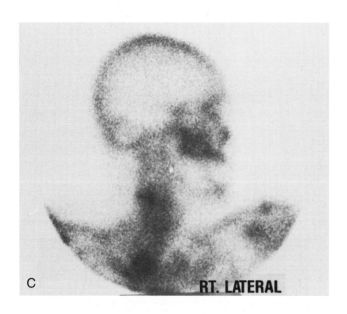

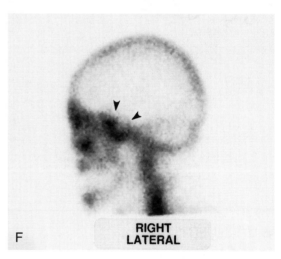

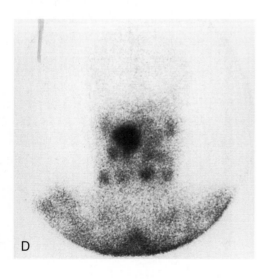

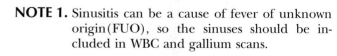

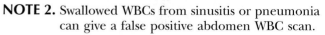

Patient 2

FIGURE 5–14   E and F.
Anterior and Right Lateral Delayed Bone Scans: There is a bony abnormality at the base of the skull, outlining the sphenoid sinus *(arrowheads)*.

Patient 3

FIGURE 5–14   G and H.
Anterior and Left Lateral WBC Scans: There is active bilateral maxillary, right ethmoid, and right frontal sinusitis.

NOTE 1. Sinusitis can be a cause of fever of unknown origin (FUO), so the sinuses should be included in WBC and gallium scans.

NOTE 2. Swallowed WBCs from sinusitis or pneumonia can give a false positive abdomen WBC scan.

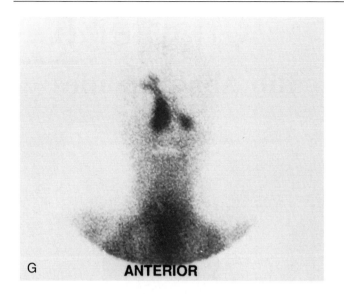

G   **ANTERIOR**

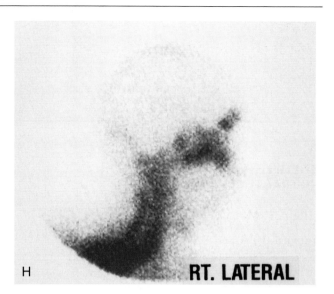

H   **RT. LATERAL**

NOTE 3. Frontal sinusitis is still a high-risk disease for meningitis and brain abscess, because the infection can break through the thin inner table of the skull.

NOTE 4. Increased activity of a sinus on bone scan indicates mucoperiosteal infection. The patient should be treated with a more intensive course of antibiotics.

NOTE 5. Sinusitis cannot be distinguished from tumor with bone scans, gallium scans, or WBC scans. These are usually abnormal owing to the presence of infection in most sinus tumors.

Cross Reference

Chapter 33: Gastrointestinal and Abdominal Infections—Swallowed WBCs

MAXILLARY CARCINOMA

FIGURE 5–15   A and B.

Anterior and Lateral Planar Bone Scans: The right maxillary antrum, the nasal cavity, and the superior left antrum are markedly abnormal.

NOTE. Tumors of the sinuses, both benign and malignant, often present after bony involvement.

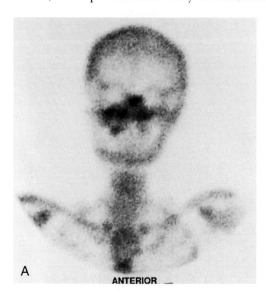

A   **ANTERIOR**

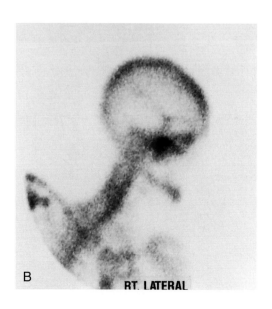

B   **RT. LATERAL**

Chapter **6**
Rib Abnormalities

MULTIPLE POST-TRAUMATIC RIB FRACTURES

Patient 1: Motor Vehicle Accident

FIGURE 6–1   **A and B.**
Anterior and RAO Bone Scans: Multiple focal rib abnormalities are present.

Patient 2: Flail Chest

FIGURE 6–1   **C and D.**
Right Lateral and RPO Bone Scans: There are post-traumatic fractures of ribs, two on each rib, creating a flail chest.

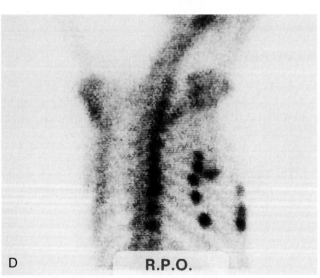

C   **RT. LATERAL**

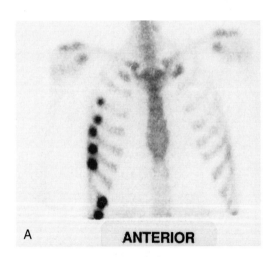

A   **ANTERIOR**

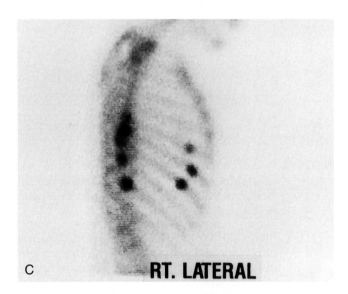

D   **R.P.O.**

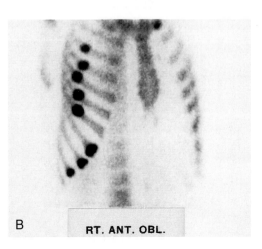

B   **RT. ANT. OBL.**

NOTE. Post-traumatic rib fractures are usually in a line and focal. Metastases are random and most often elongated.

COSTOVERTEBRAL FRACTURES

FIGURE 6–2   A.

Posterior Thoracic Bone Scan: There are four focal abnormalities along the lower right margin of the thoracic spine.

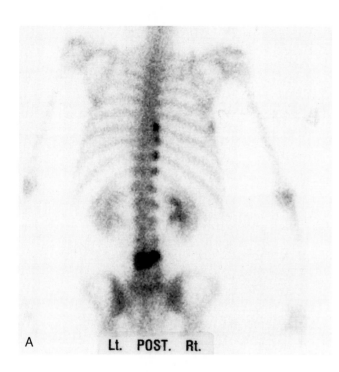

FIGURE 6–2   B.

Left Posterior Oblique Thoracic Bone Scan: The abnormalities are slightly separated from the vertebrae and remain posterior on this obliquity, whereas hypertrophic spurs would have rotated anteriorly and overlapped the vertebral bodies.

NOTE. These fractures are most commonly seen after thoracotomies but also may result from blunt chest trauma.

Cross Reference

Chapter 3: Spinal Abnormalities—Asymmetric Thoracic Osteophytes

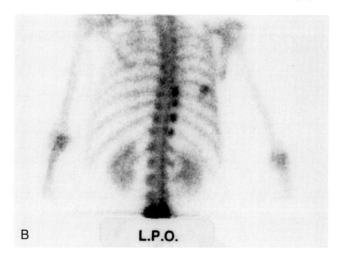

POST-TRAUMATIC CARTILAGE OSSIFICATION

FIGURE 6–3   A and B.

Left Anterior Oblique Bone Scans: A solitary ossification is presumed to be an old fracture of a costal cartilage.

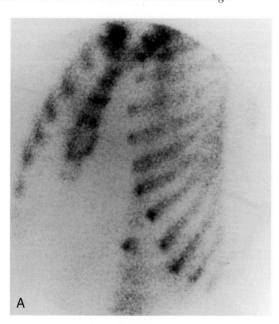

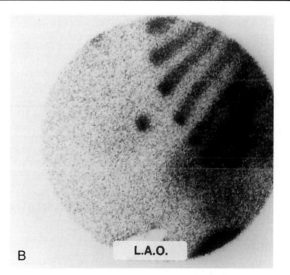

RIB RESECTIONS

Patient 1

FIGURE 6–4 A.

Posterior Bone Scan: The right eleventh and twelfth ribs have been removed in their entirety.

Patient 2

FIGURE 6–4 B.

Anterior Bone Scan: A short segment of rib has been removed.

Cross Reference

Chapter 9: "Cold" Abnormalities—"Cold" Bone Lesion due to Direct Invasion by Tumor

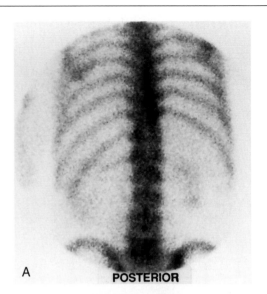

A **POSTERIOR**

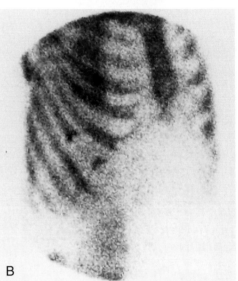

B

RIB METASTASES

Patient 1: Breast Carcinoma

FIGURE 6–5 A.

Posterior Chest Bone Scan: There are multiple abnormalities, including elongated lesions of the ribs.

FIGURE 6–5 B.

Coned-down View from Lateral Chest X-ray: Blastic metastases may be subtle, with increased density of a rib seen on end *(arrow)*.

Patient 2: Prostate Carcinoma

FIGURE 6–5 C.

Posterior Chest Bone Scan: The rib metastases are more focal than elongated but are random rather than in line.

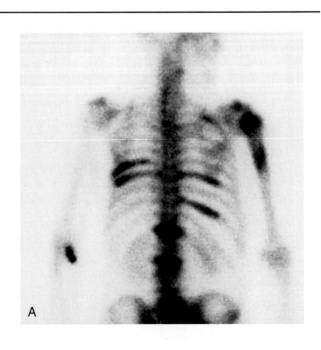

A

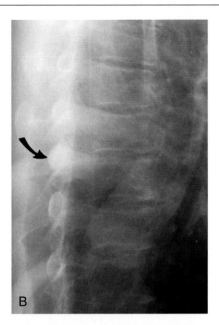

B

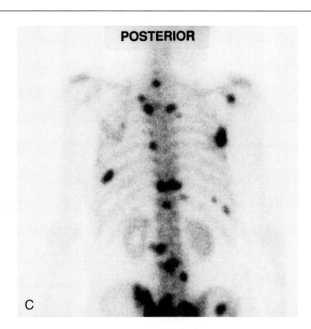

POSTERIOR

C

DIRECT INVASION OF RIB BY TUMOR

Patient 1

FIGURE 6–6   A.
Posterior Bone Scan: There is a large photon-deficient area of bone destruction involving T2 and T3 vertebrae and the left second and third ribs.

Patient 2

FIGURE 6–6   B.
Anterior Bone Scan: The right first rib has subtle increased activity *(arrow)* from a Pancoast tumor.

Illustration continued on following page

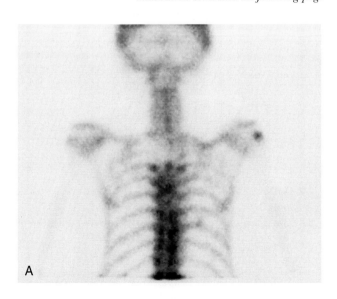

A

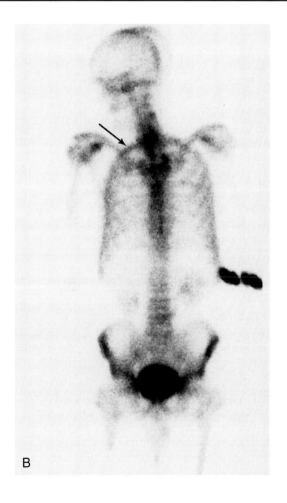

B

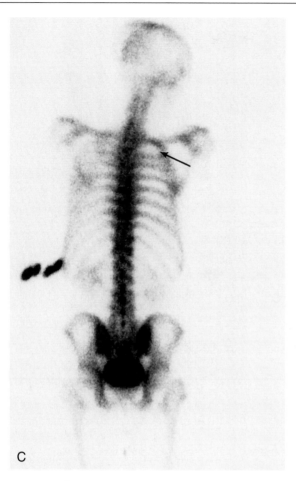

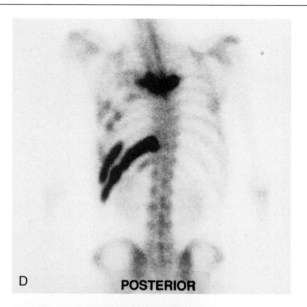

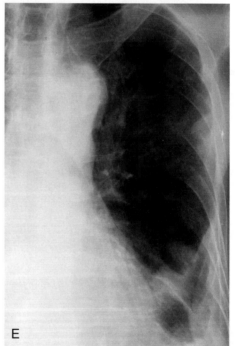

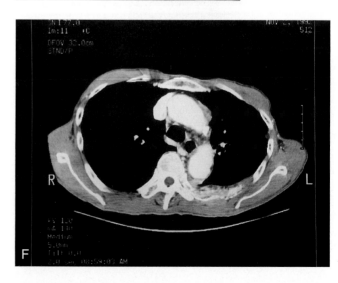

FIGURE 6–6   C.

Posterior Bone Scan: The right second rib is missing *(arrow)* as a result of direct invasion by tumor.

Patient 3

FIGURE 6–6   D.

Posterior Bone Scan: There are multiple rib abnormalities, some due to direct invasion by pleural tumors on the left side.

FIGURE 6–6   E.

PA Chest X-ray: There are multiple pleural masses on the left side.

FIGURE 6–6   F.

CT Scan: The pleura is thickened, and there is rib destruction posteriorly.

NOTE 1. Direct invasion, like metastases, can produce increased or decreased activity on bone scan.

NOTE 2. Direct invasion of ribs occurs in approximately 10 percent of peripheral lung tumors.

Cross Reference

Chapter 9: ''Cold'' Abnormalities—''Cold'' Bone Lesion Due to Direct Invasion by Tumor

ELONGATED RIB ABNORMALITIES

Patient 1

FIGURE 6–7   A.
Posterior Bone Scan: fibrous dysplasia.

Patient 2

FIGURE 6–7   B.
Right Posterior Oblique Bone Scan: Paget's disease of rib.

Patient 3

FIGURE 6–7   C.
Right Posterior Oblique Bone Scan: metastatic breast cancer to the rib as well as spine.

NOTE. Elongated rib abnormalities may be caused by metastatic disease, trauma, Paget's disease, fibrous dysplasia, infection, surgery, and primary rib tumor.

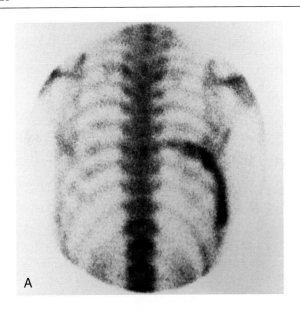

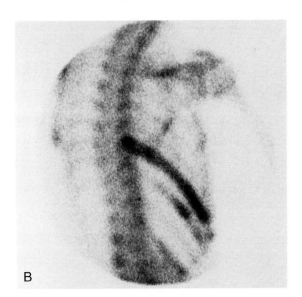

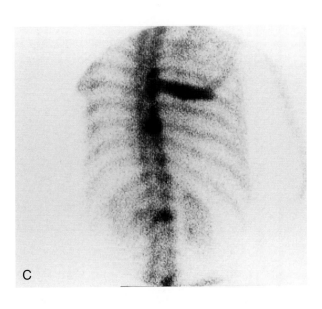

Chapter 7
Hands and Feet

NORMAL HANDS AND FEET

FIGURE 7–1 A and B.
Palmar and Dorsal Hand Bone Scan: The dorsal scan allows
for better carpal bone and radiocarpal differentiation.

FIGURE 7–1 C to E.
Blood Pool and Delayed Foot Bone Scans: normal plantar and
right lateral views.

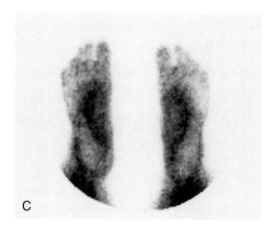
C

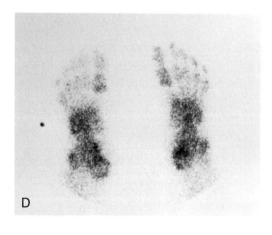
D

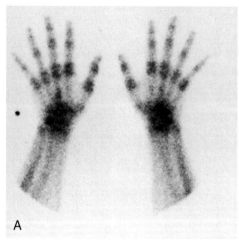
A

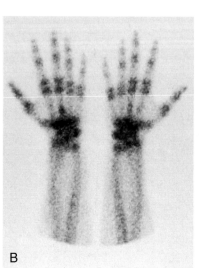
B

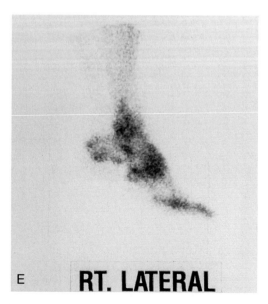
E RT. LATERAL

OSTEOARTHRITIS OF THE HANDS

Patient 1: Early Osteoarthritis

FIGURE 7–2   A and B.

Blood Pool and Delayed Bone Scans: The first interphalangeal (IP) joint and the third proximal IP joint are hyperemic and demonstrate increased activity. The first and second metacarpophalangeal (MCP) and second proximal IP joints are less active, having normal blood pools but abnormal osteogenesis.

Patient 2

FIGURE 7–2   C.

Bone Scan: Symmetric Heberden's nodes are present in this patient with hypertrophic osteoarthropathy.

Patient 3

FIGURE 7–2   D.

Bone Scan: The IP joints and the first carpometacarpal (CMC) joints are common sites of osteoarthritis.

NOTE 1. The distal interphalangeal (DIP) joints can have an aggressive form of osteoarthritis known as erosive osteoarthritis.

NOTE 2. As with most bone diseases, osteoarthritic changes appear earlier on bone scans than on x-rays.

NOTE 3. The active sites of osteoarthritis will be hyperemic.

Cross Reference

Chapter 8: Hyperemia—Active Rheumatoid Arthritis

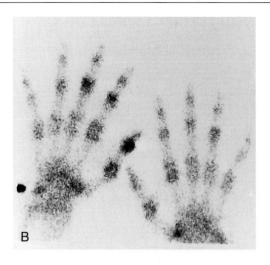

B

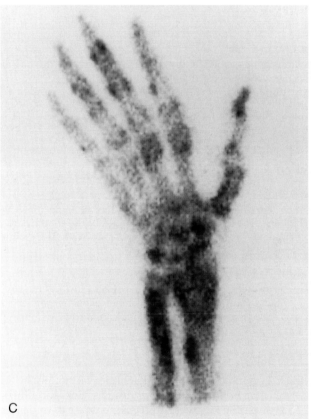

C

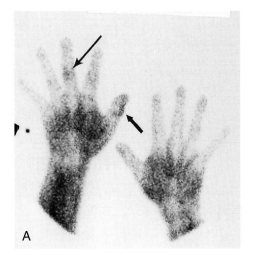

A

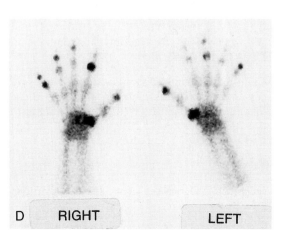

D   RIGHT   LEFT

DIABETIC FOOT: TRAUMA VS. INFECTION

Patient 1: Osteomyelitis of Multiple Bones

FIGURE 7–3   A.
Blood Pool Scan: There is hyperemia involving the tarsal bones and the second and third metatarsophalangeal (MTP) joints.

FIGURE 7–3   B.
Delayed Bone Scan: The areas of hyperemia have increased osteogenesis.

FIGURE 7–3   C.
Gallium Scan: The bony abnormalities have increased gallium accumulation. (Courtesy of Dr. Michael Kipper, Vista, CA.)

Patient 2: Neuropathic Fractures

FIGURE 7–3   D.
Blood Pool Scan: There is hyperemia of the distal first toe.

FIGURE 7–3   E.
Delayed Bone Scan: The distal tuft of the first toe, the tarsus, and the calcaneus are all abnormal.

FIGURE 7–3   F.
Gallium Scan: The fractured toe and other bones of the foot do not accumulate gallium.

Patient 3: Osteomyelitis

FIGURE 7–3   G.
Plantar Bone Scan: There is a focal abnormality at the fifth MTP joint. The less intense abnormalities of the foot are due to hyperemia from cellulitis. The first and fourth MTP joints are abnormal.

FIGURE 7–3   H.
Plantar ^{111}In-WBC Scan: The only abnormality involves the fifth MTP joint. Biopsy revealed an osteomyelitis *(Staphylococcus aureus)*. The first and fourth MTP joints are normal. (Courtesy of Dr. Arnold Jacobson, Seattle, WA.)

NOTE 1. Bone and joint abnormalities on bone scan in diabetic patients are usually due to neuropathic changes. A positive WBC scan indicates an active infection.

NOTE 2. If the bone scan/WBC scan is equivocal, and clinical suspicion for osteomyelitis remains, an MRI can be performed.

NOTE 3. Gallium can accumulate in post-traumatic processes such as acute fractures, including those of neuropathic joints. WBCs are less likely to do so.

Cross References

Chapter 2: Multiple Bony Abnormalities—Active Rheumatoid Arthritis on WBC Scan

Chapter 71: Infectious Diseases—Gallium Uptake in Benign Fractures

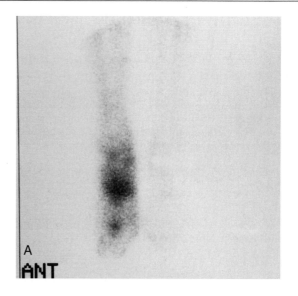

A
ANT

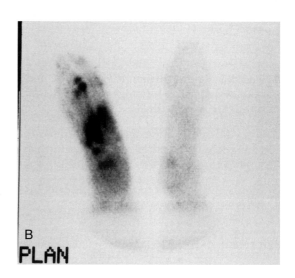

B
PLAN

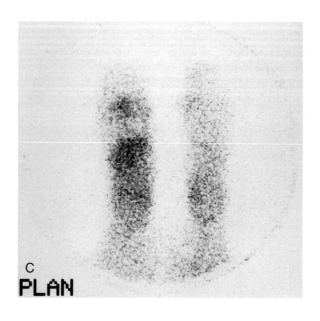

C
PLAN

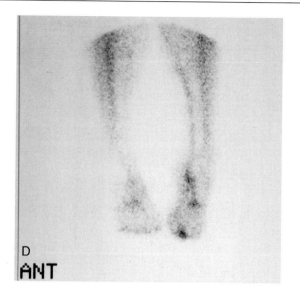

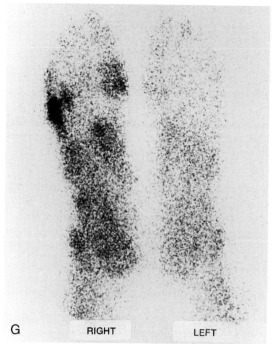

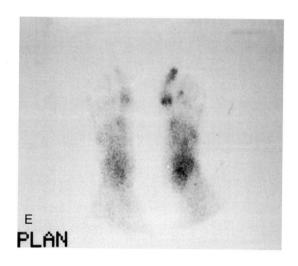

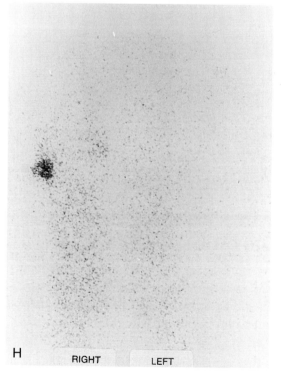

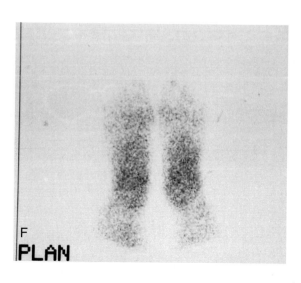

PERIOSTITIS

FIGURE 7–4   A.

Blood Pool Scintigraphy: The bones of the right foot are hyperemic. The overlying soft tissues are normal.

FIGURE 7–4   B and C.

Delayed Scintigraphy: The plantar (B) and lateral (C) projections demonstrate marked increased osteogenesis of the distal tibia, the talus, calcaneus and tarsal bones. At surgery this proved to be a periostitis rather than osteomyelitis.

NOTE. A large number of contiguous bones involved in an initial infection is more suggestive of cellulitis with periostitis, rather than osteomyelitis from a hematogenous origin.

Cross Reference

Chapter 7: Hands and Feet—Reflex Sympathetic Dystrophy Syndrome

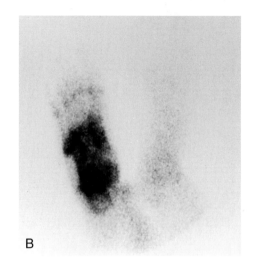

B

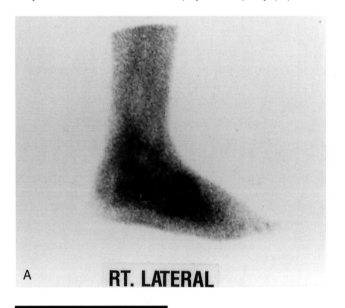

A   RT. LATERAL

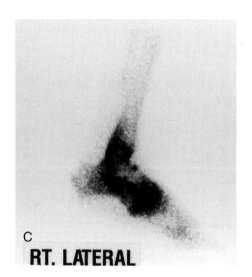

C   RT. LATERAL

INCREASED OSTEOGENESIS DUE TO SOFT TISSUE ABSCESS

FIGURE 7–5   A to C.

Blood Flow and Blood Pool Scans: There is increased blood flow and hyperemia of the right foot.

FIGURE 7–5   D and E.

Delayed Bone Scan: There is increased osteogenesis of the entire right foot, without an intense focal abnormality.

FIGURE 7–5   F and G.

Gallium Scan: Although it would appear that there is increased gallium in the first metatarsal (MT) bone on the plantar view (F), the medial view clearly shows that the abnormal collection is in the soft tissues.

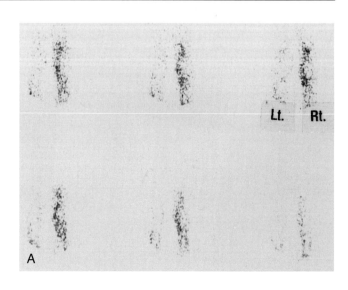

Lt.   Rt.

A

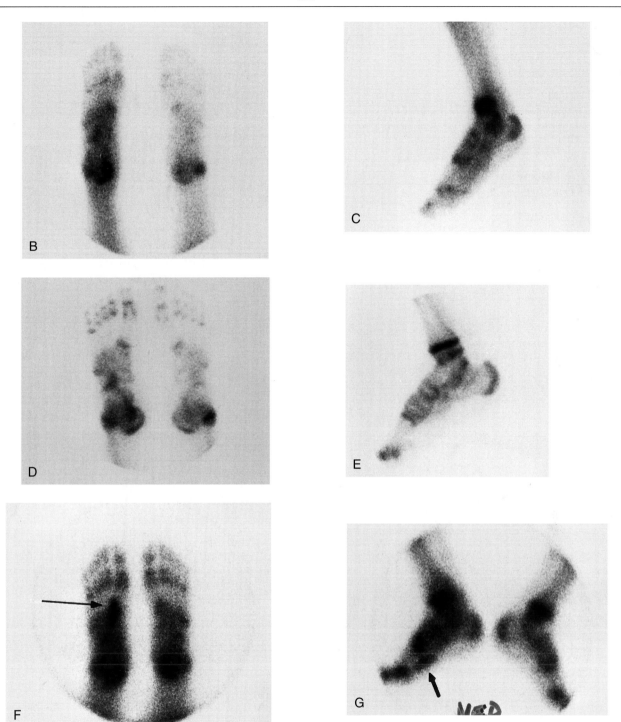

NOTE 1. Increased blood flow and hyperemia of soft tissues will produce a mild to moderate increase in the osteogenesis of all adjacent bones.

NOTE 2. Marked osteogenesis of several bones suggests a periostitis or osteomyelitis.

Cross Reference

Chapter 8: Hyperemia—Cellulitis Without Osteomyelitis; Thigh Abscess on Bone Scan

HAND AND FOOT FRACTURES

Patient 1: Ballet Dancer; Talar Fracture Simulating an Os Trigonum

FIGURE 7–6   A.

Medial Foot Bone Scan: The increased activity at the posterior talus *(arrow)* represents a talar fracture rather than a normal os trigonum. There is also a navicular fracture.

Patient 2: Jackhammer Operator; Scaphoid Fracture

FIGURE 7–6   B and C.

Blood Flow and Blood Pool Scans: There is focal increased blood flow and hyperemia in the radial aspect of the left wrist.

FIGURE 7–6   D.

Delayed Bone Scan: The scaphoid has marked increased activity.

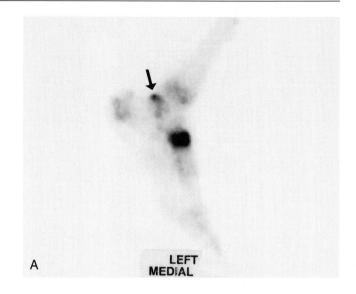

A   LEFT MEDIAL

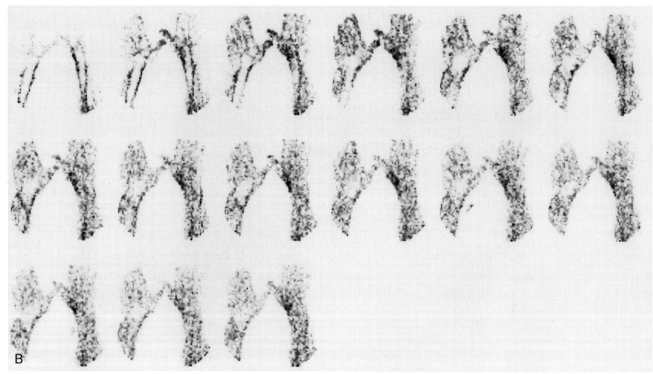

B

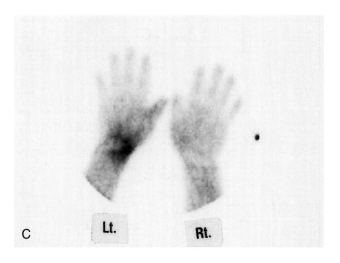

C   Lt.   Rt.

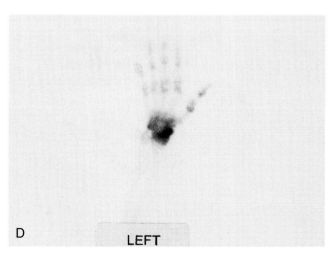

D   LEFT

Patient 3: 63 Year Old Male with Wrist Pain After Fall on Outstretched Hand

FIGURE 7–6   E and F.

Blood Pool and Delayed Bone Scans: There is hyperemia *(arrow)* and increased osteogenesis involving the right lunate bone.

NOTE 1. An os trigonum is an unfused secondary ossification center for the talus.

NOTE 2. Fractures of the posterior talus may be seen more often in ballet dancers, from standing en pointe.

NOTE 3. Hyperemia indicates an acute process.

Cross Reference

Chapter 1: Solitary Bony Abnormalities—Solitary Stress Fractures

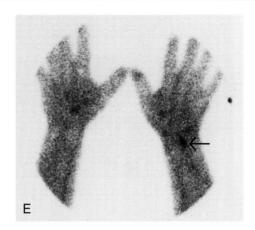

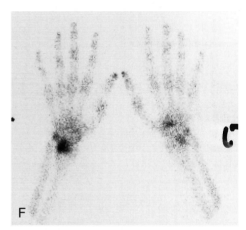

CHARCOT JOINTS (NEUROPATHIC JOINTS)

Patient 1

FIGURE 7–7   A.

Plantar Foot Bone Scans: There are bilateral tarsal bone abnormalities.

Patient 2

FIGURE 7–7   B and C.

Plantar and Medial Bone Scans: The right foot has tarsal and distal joint abnormalities.

NOTE 1. Diabetic neuropathy involves tarsal and carpal bones. Syringomyelia patients have upper extremity joint involvement. Syphilis involves spine, hips, and knees. Leprosy has small joint involvement. Alcoholic neuropathy involves distal joints, especially the feet. Congenital indifference to pain involves ankle and tarsal bones. Amyloid involves large joints, e.g., knee and ankle.

NOTE 2. The scan appearance of neuropathic joints can be worse on one side than the other, because of either asymmetric trauma or infections.

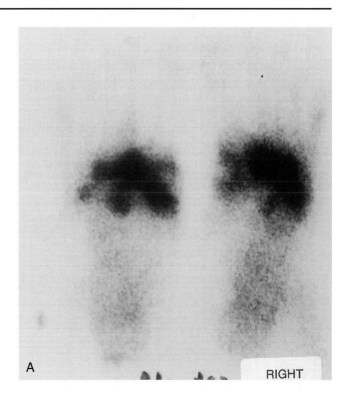

Illustration continued on following page

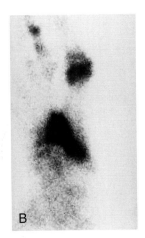
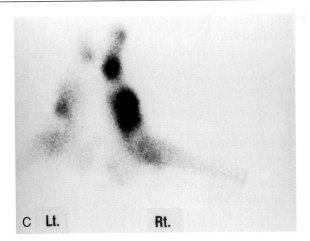

REFLEX SYMPATHETIC DYSTROPHY SYNDROME

FIGURE 7–8   A and B.
Blood Flow and Blood Pool Scintigraphy: There is increased blood flow and hyperemia involving the right foot.

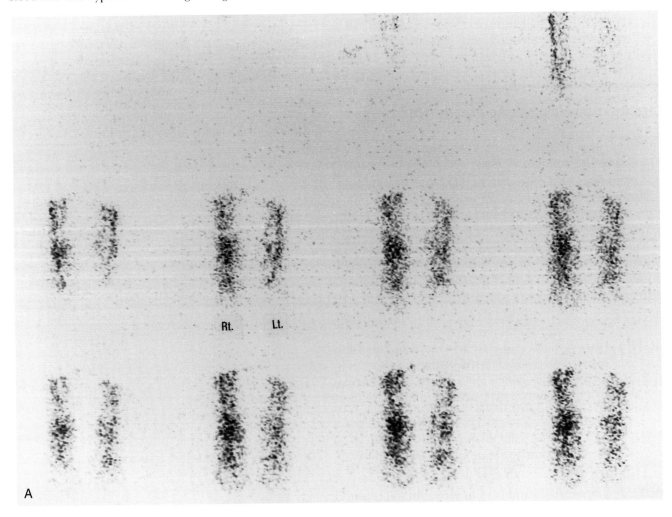

FIGURE 7–8   **C and D.**

Delayed Bone Scintigraphy: There are multiple bones of the right foot with increased osteogenesis. (Courtesy of Dr. Michael Kipper, Vista, CA.)

Cross Reference

Chapter 8: Hyperemia—Reflex Sympathetic Dystrophy Syndrome

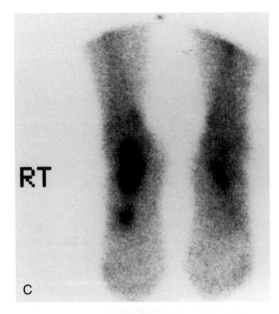

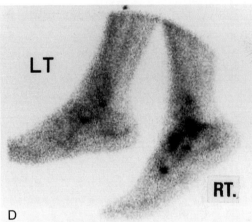

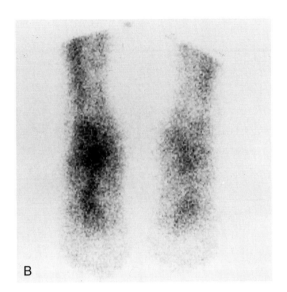

BONE AND SOFT TISSUE HEMANGIOMA OF THE FOOT

FIGURE 7–9   **A and B.**

Bone Scan: There is diffuse increased activity of the left bony tarsus.

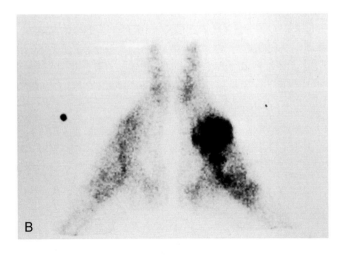

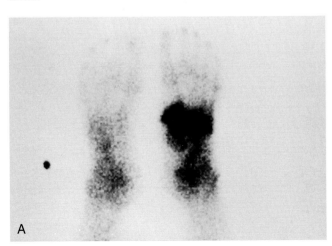

Illustration continued on following page

FIGURE 7–9   C.

Plain Film X-ray: There are soft tissue calcifications and phlebo-liths characteristic of a hemangioma *(arrows).*

Cross References

Chapter 1: Solitary Bony Abnormalities—Unusual Solitary Metastases

Chapter 11: Soft Tissue Abnormalities—Hemangioma

Chapter 15: Solitary Liver Defects—Hemangioma

Chapter 17: Multiple Liver Defects—Multiple Hepatic Hemangiomas

Chapter 59: Venous Thrombosis—Leg Hemangioma on Tagged RBC Scan

Chapter 72: Tumors—Giant Hemangioma (Kasabach-Merritt Syndrome)

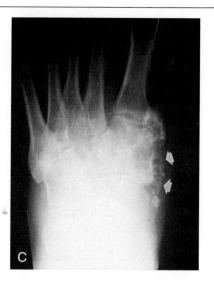

Chapter **8**

Hyperemia

OSTEOMYELITIS

FIGURE 8–1   A and B.

Blood Flow and Blood Pool Scintigraphy: There is increased blood flow to the right hand, especially the distal thumb.

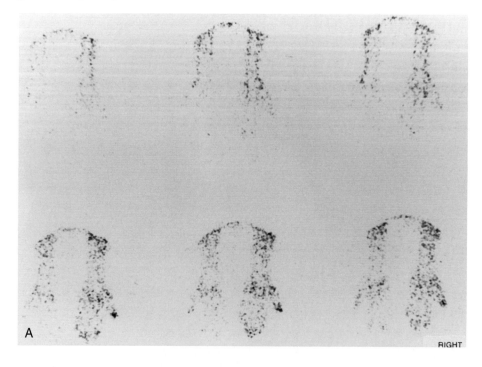

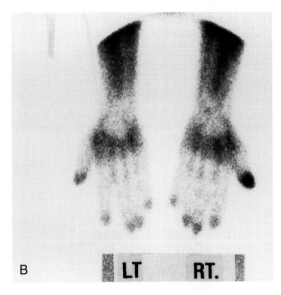

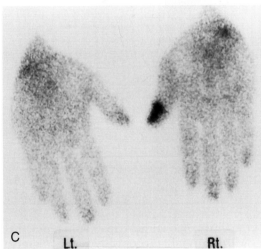

DIFFERENTIAL DIAGNOSIS OF HYPEREMIA ON BONE SCAN

1. Recent post-traumatic injury (0–8 weeks or ongoing "repair")

    A. Subperiosteal hemorrhage or reaction, enthesopathy

    B. Stress fracture

    C. Fracture

    D. Osteochondral injuries (osteochondritis dissecans)

2. Neoplasm

    A. Metastases

    B. Primary bone tumors

        a. Benign, e.g., osteoid osteoma

        b. Malignant, e.g., osteosarcoma, chondrosarcoma

    C. Soft tissue neoplasms and vascular malformations

    D. Active heterotopic bone

3. Infection

    A. Acute osteomyelitis and active chronic osteomyelitis

    B. Cellulitis

    C. Septic arthritis

    D. Synovitis—may also be "cold"

4. Osteonecrosis

    A. Avascular necrosis—late stage

    B. Legg-Perthes disease—late stage

    C. Bone infarcts—during early repair

    D. Reflex sympathetic dystrophy—late stage

5. Postoperative reparative process

6. Synovial osteochondroma

7. Paget's disease—active phases

8. Active arthritides, growing osteophytes

9. Growing or maturing fibrous cortical defect

10. Normal growth plates

FIGURE 8–1   C.
Delayed Bone Scan: The distal phalanx of the right thumb is markedly abnormal.

NOTE 1. Acute osteomyelitis is always hyperemic.

NOTE 2. This patient also has hyperemia with minimally increased osteogenesis of the tips of all fingers due to clubbing from chronic bronchitis.

Cross Reference

Chapter 8: Hyperemia—Clubbing of the Fingers

HYPEREMIA VS. EXTENT OF BONE ACTIVITY IN OSTEOMYELITIS

FIGURE 8–2   A and B.
Blood Pool and Delayed Bone Scintigraphy: The hyperemia in the bone is less extensive than the increased osteogenesis.

NOTE 1. The extent of hyperemia is often less than the bony reaction, probably reflecting the active portions of the lesions.

NOTE 2. The soft tissue extent of the hyperemia is due to the associated cellulitis seen in almost all cases of osteomyelitis.

Cross Reference

Chapter 1: Solitary Bony Abnormalities—Metaphyseal Hyperemia and Osteomyelitis; Osteomyelitis and Cellulitis

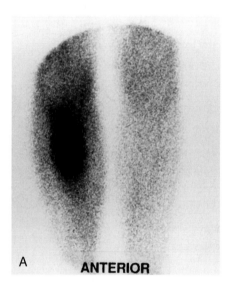

A **ANTERIOR**

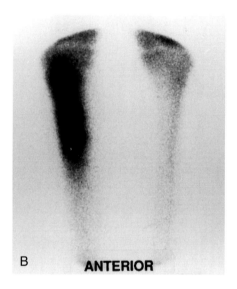

B **ANTERIOR**

OSTEOCHONDRITIS DISSECANS

FIGURE 8–3   A.
Blood Pool Scintigraphy: There is localized hyperemia along the articular surface of the left medial femoral condyle *(arrow).*

FIGURE 8–3   B.
Delayed Bone Scan: There is increased activity of the subchondral bone of the left medial femoral condyle.

NOTE. Arthroscopic surgery may either pin the loose cartilage and bone or remove the fragment. MRI scanning is valuable to define the integrity of the cartilage.

Cross Reference

Chapter 1: Solitary Bony Abnormalities—Osteochondritis Dissecans

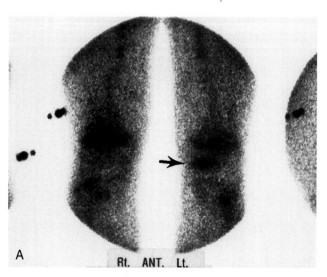

A **Rt. ANT. Lt.**

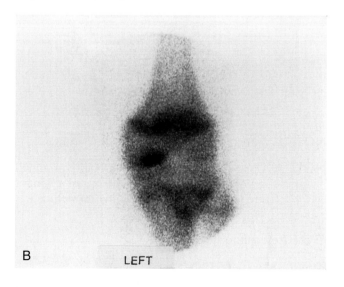

B **LEFT**

CHONDROSARCOMA

FIGURE 8–4   A.

Plain Film X-ray: There is smooth cortical thickening along the medial distal diaphysis and metaphysis of the left femur.

FIGURE 8–4   B.

Medial Knee Blood Pool Scintigram: There is marked hyperemia of the abnormality, indicating an active process.

FIGURE 8–4   C and D.

Anterior and Medial Scintigrams: There is increased osteogenesis corresponding to the distribution of the bony density on x-ray.

NOTE. The presence of hyperemia in an abnormality that appears indolent on x-ray should be suspect for a more active process, e.g., benign or malignant neoplasm, infection, or trauma.

Cross Reference

Chapter 1: Solitary Bony Abnormalities—Blood Pool Imaging in Benign Bone Tumors; Osteosarcoma

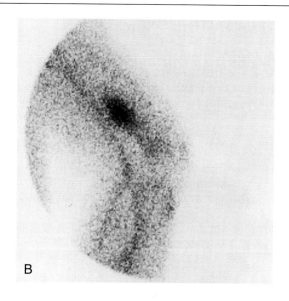

B

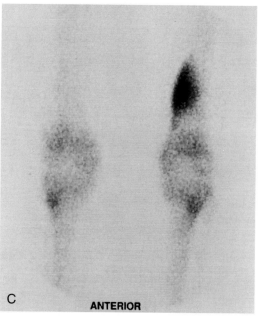

C   **ANTERIOR**

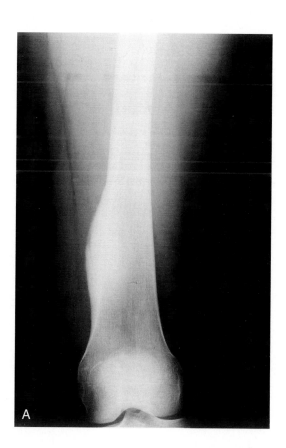

A

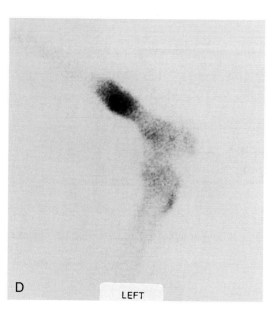

D   LEFT

HYPEREMIA WITH BONE METASTASES

FIGURE 8–5   A and B.
Blood Pool and Delayed Bone Scintigraphy: There are areas of hyperemia that match the bony abnormalities seen on the delayed scan. Other areas of hyperemia matched the lower pelvic lesions on bone scan.

NOTE. Bone metastases from virtually all tumors appear to be hyperemic on the blood pool image, whether they are lytic or blastic on x-ray.

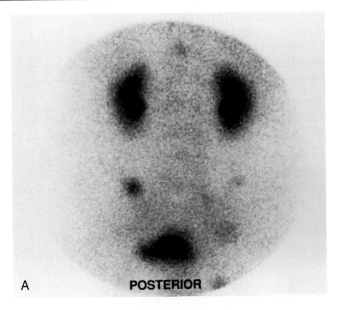

A   POSTERIOR

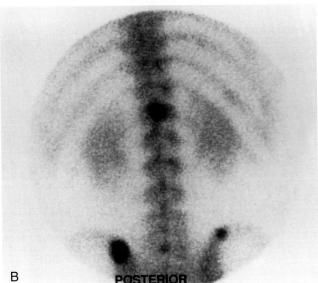

B   POSTERIOR

DIFFUSE SKELETAL "HYPEREMIA" VS. DIFFUSE METASTASES

Patient: Cholangiocarcinoma

FIGURE 8–6   A and B.
Two- to Five-Minute Blood Pool Scan: These scans were obtained immediately after injection because of back pain. The appearance could be confused with a delayed bone scan.

FIGURE 8–6   C.
Two-Hour Whole Body Scan: There are multiple metastatic foci, yet with the intense bladder activity, this scan would not be called a "superscan."

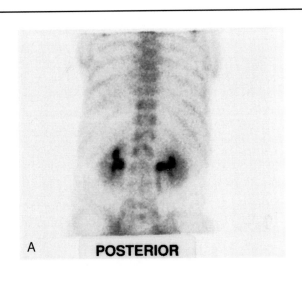

A   POSTERIOR

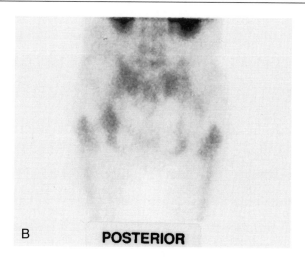

B POSTERIOR

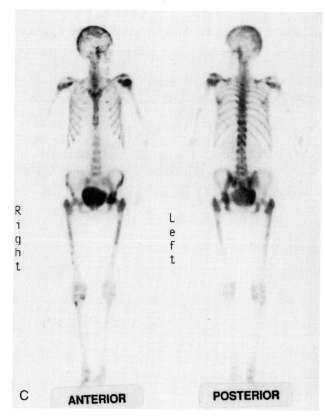

C   ANTERIOR   POSTERIOR

Right   Left

STAGE 1 REFLEX SYMPATHETIC DYSTROPHY SYNDROME (RSDS)

FIGURE 8–7   A.

Blood Flow Scan: There is decreased blood flow to the symptomatic right wrist and hand.

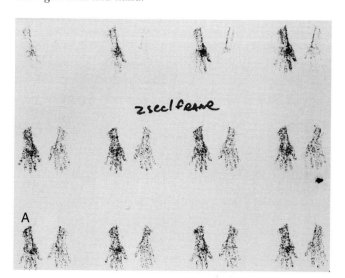

A

STAGES OF REFLEX SYMPATHETIC DYSTROPHY	
Blood Flow	**Delayed Scan**
Scan	
Stage 1: ↓	nl or ↓
Stage 2: ↑ ↑	↑ ↑ ↑
Stage 3: nl	↑
Clinical	
Stage 1: Pain, stiffness, tenderness, swelling, and weakness (probably due to sympathetic stimulation)	
Stage 2: Resolution of swelling, skin atrophy, pigmentation changes (resolution of sympathetic stimulation but vasomotor instability)	
Stage 3: Further skin atrophy	

Illustration continued on following page

FIGURE 8–7   B and C.
Blood Pool and Delayed Bone Scan: There is no significant
difference between the two extremities.

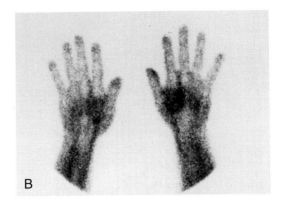

NOTE 1. After trauma, the vasoconstriction from increased sympathetic tone is thought to cause
hypoxic bone damage (stage 1).

NOTE 2. In RSDS, hyperemia and increased osteogenesis will be seen prior to any changes
on plain film.

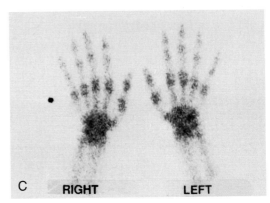

STAGE 2 REFLEX SYMPATHETIC DYSTROPHY SYNDROME (RSDS)

Patient 1

FIGURE 8–8   A and B.
Blood Flow and Blood Pool Scans: There is hyperemia involving
the left wrist.

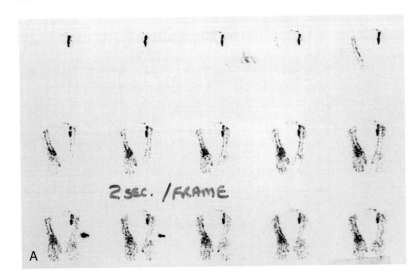

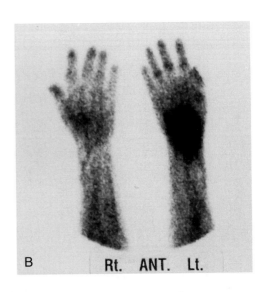

FIGURE 8–8 C.

Delayed Bone Scan: The increased osteogenesis involves all the bones of the left wrist and hand.

Patient 2

FIGURE 8–8 D.

Blood Pool: There is hyperemia of the left wrist.

FIGURE 8–8 E.

Delayed Bone Scan: The left wrist demonstrates changes of RSDS, the right has degenerative changes to the first metacarpophalangeal (MCP) joint.

NOTE 1. After the vasoconstriction is relieved, bony repair begins and induces hyperemia and increased osteogenesis.

NOTE 2. RSDS is associated with trauma, but not all trauma produces an RSDS.

NOTE 3. The distal radius and ulna are involved with all wrist RSDS.

Cross Reference

Chapter 7: Hands and Feet—Reflex Sympathetic Dystrophy Syndrome

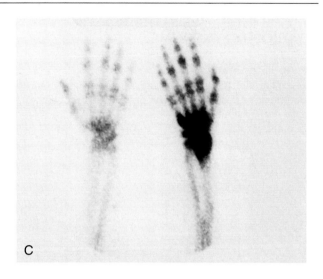

C

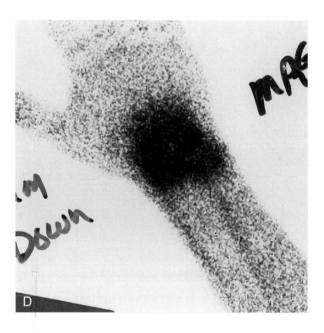

D

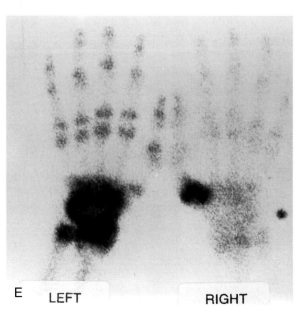

E   LEFT   RIGHT

STAGE 3 REFLEX SYMPATHETIC DYSTROPHY SYNDROME

FIGURE 8–9 A and B.
Blood Flow and Blood Pool Scans: There is slightly increased blood flow and blood pool of the right hand, but these are still within normal limits.

FIGURE 8–9 C.
Delayed Bone Scan: There is diffuse, increased osteogenesis of the right wrist finger joints. (Courtesy of Dr. Michael Kipper, Vista, CA.)

NOTE. At this stage, the blood flow has returned to normal but the bone repair is still ongoing.

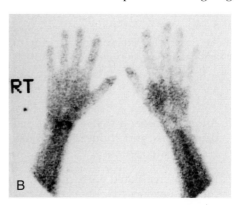

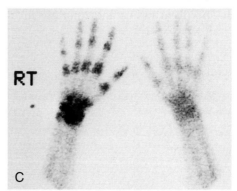

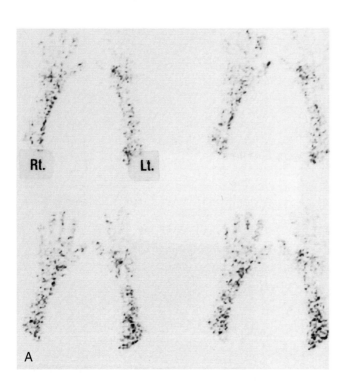

RSDS: SHOULDER-HAND SYNDROME

Patient: 40 Year Old Female Crane Operator with No Injury

FIGURE 8–10 A and B.
Blood Pool Scans: The left shoulder and wrist are hyperemic.

FIGURE 8–10 C to E.
Delayed Bone Scan: The left humeral head, the scapula, and the entire wrist and hand have increased osteogenesis. The right side is normal.

NOTE. Reflex sympathetic dystrophy can occur in many bones, usually in the distal extremities, but the combination of the shoulder and hand (wrist) is not uncommon.

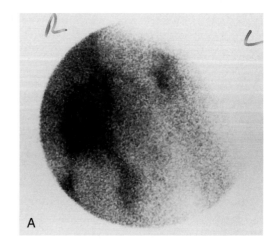

Cross Reference

Chapter 11: Soft Tissue Abnormalities—Differential Diagnosis of Muscle Uptake on Bone Scan

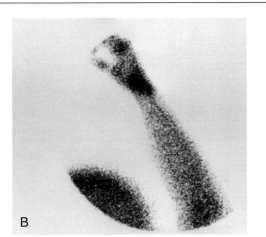

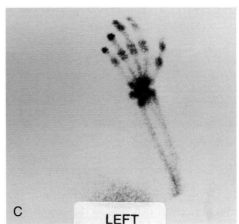

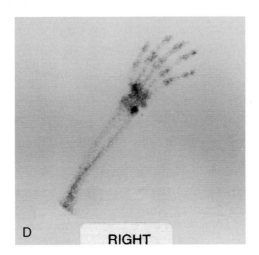

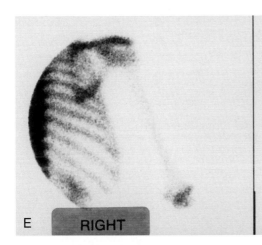

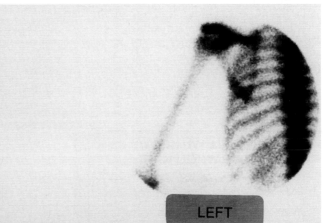

ACTIVE RHEUMATOID ARTHRITIS

FIGURE 8–11   A.
Blood Pool Scan of the Hands: There is hyperemia involving the carpal bones diffusely in the left wrist, whereas the right wrist has radiocarpal joint and ulnar styloid activity. The small bone joints are asymmetrically involved.

FIGURE 8–11   B.
Blood Pool Scan of the Feet: The involvement is more symmetric except for the solitary tarsometatarsal disease on the right.

FIGURE 8–11   C.
Delayed Bone Scan of the Hand: The asymmetric pattern persists. There are no abnormalities now present that did not have hyperemia. Note that the ulnar styloid activity is distinct from the radiocarpal and radioulnar activity.

FIGURE 8–11   D.
Delayed Bone Scan of the Foot: The same lesions seen on the blood pool scan are evident.

NOTE 1. Hyperemia indicates an active process.

NOTE 2. Bony activity may be due to the hyperemia of the hypertrophic synovium rather than to frank bone erosion.

NOTE 3. Rheumatoid arthritis is radiographically symmetric in most cases, whereas the bone scan demonstrates which joints and bones are active at the moment.

NOTE 4. Radiocarpal joint and ulnar styloid activity may be seen early, before the rest of the carpal compartments become involved.

Cross Reference

Chapter 7 Hands and Feet—Osteoarthritis of the Hands

HYPEREMIA WITHOUT BONY PATHOLOGY
1. Cellulitis
2. Septic arthritis—low grade
3. Clubbing secondary to COPD
4. Capsulitis
5. Soft tissue tumor, vascular malformation
6. Soft tissue trauma, muscle necrosis
7. Heterotopic bone, myositis ossificans
8. Dermatomyositis, polymyositis
9. Active muscular dystrophy
10. Gravid or menstruating uterus

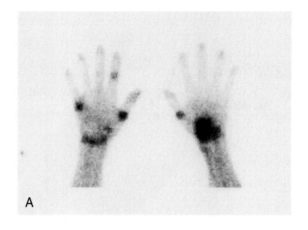

A

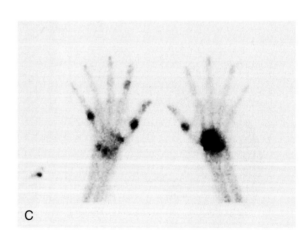

B

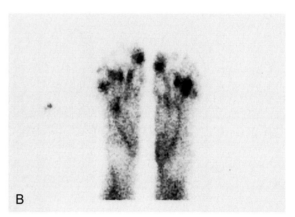

C

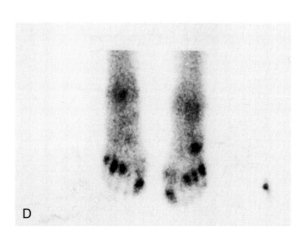

D

HYPEREMIA IN SEPTIC ARTHRITIS

FIGURE 8–12 A.
Blood Pool Scan of the Knees: There is bilateral marked hyperemia.

FIGURE 8–12 B.
Delayed Bone Scan: The increased osteogenesis is diffuse and involves all intracapsular bone.

NOTE. Increased blood flow will increase delivery of the scanning agent and cause a diffusely "hot" bone(s).

Cross Reference

Chapter 1: Solitary Bony Abnormalities—Septic Arthritis

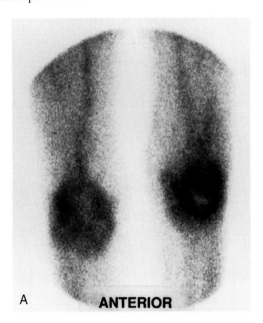

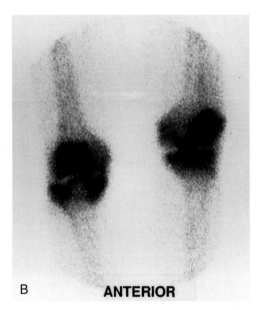

CELLULITIS WITHOUT OSTEOMYELITIS

FIGURE 8–13 A and B.
Blood Flow and Blood Pool Scintigraphy: There is marked increased flow to the right foot with hyperemia.

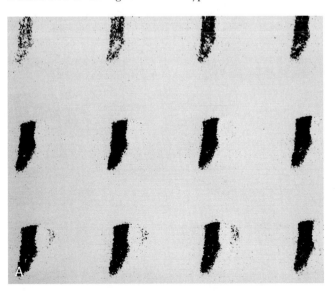

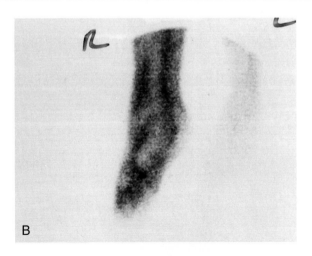

Illustration continued on following page

FIGURE 8–13   C and D.

Delayed Bone Scintigraphy: There is diffuse increased activity in the lateral soft tissues *(arrowheads)*.

FIGURE 8–13   E and F.

Gallium Scintigraphy: The accumulation of the gallium is in the soft tissues overlying the bones. The tibia and fibula were not infected.

NOTE. Hyperemia in soft tissues will increase osteogenesis.

Cross References

Chapter 1: Solitary Bony Abnormalities—Osteomyelitis and Cellulitis

Chapter 7: Hands and Feet—Increased Osteogenesis due to Soft Tissue Abscess

Chapter 11: Soft Tissue Abnormalities—Cellulitis on Bone Scan

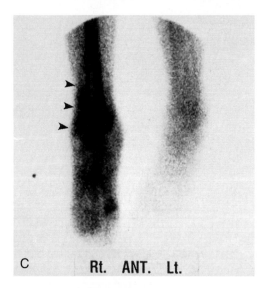

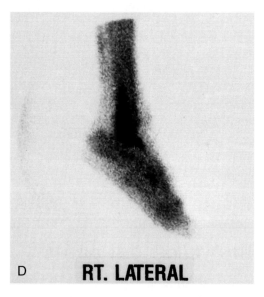

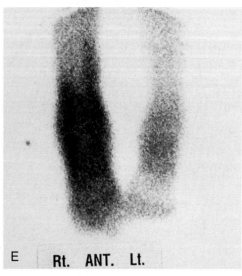

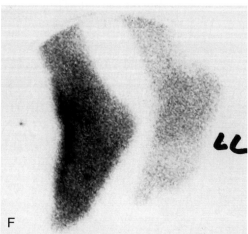

THIGH ABSCESS ON BONE SCAN

FIGURE 8–14   A and B.

Blood Flow and Blood Pool Scintigraphy: There is marked increased blood flow in the right upper thigh.

FIGURE 8–14   C.

Delayed Bone Scintigraphy: There is diffuse uptake in the soft tissues of the right thigh but only mildly increased osteogenesis of the proximal right femur.

FIGURE 8–14   D.

Gallium Scan: The thigh abscess has intense gallium accumulation, with surrounding cellulitis.

Cross Reference

Chapter 7: Hands and Feet—Increased Osteogenesis due to Soft Tissue Abscess

Chapter 11: Soft Tissue Abnormalities—Muscle Necrosis on Bone Scan

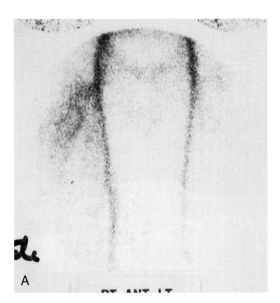

A

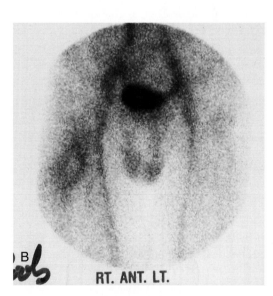

B   RT. ANT. LT.

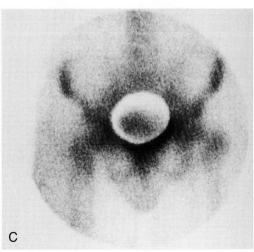

C

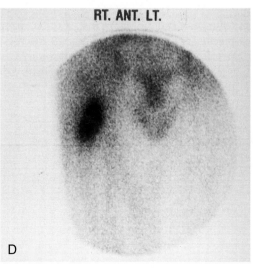

RT. ANT. LT.

D

SHOULDER CAPSULITIS

Patient: Adhesive Capsulitis

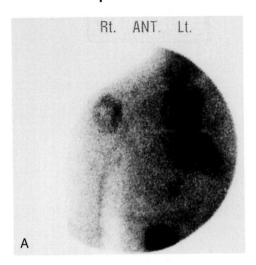

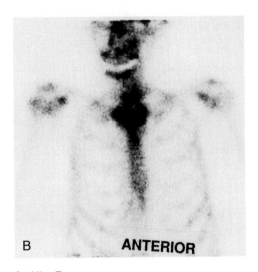

FIGURE 8–15 A.

Blood Pool Scintigraphy: There is a halo of hyperemia involving the right shoulder.

FIGURE 8–15 B.

Anterior Planar Bone Scan: There is minimal increased osteogenesis involving the right humeral head.

CLUBBING OF THE FINGERS

FIGURE 8–16 A.

Blood Pool Scan: There is marked hyperemia of the finger tufts.

FIGURE 8–16 B.

Delayed Bone Scan: There are minimal distal phalangeal changes due to hyperemia.

NOTE. Clubbing can be seen with COPD, lung neoplasms, congenital cyanotic heart disease (right-to-left shunt), A-V fistulas, sarcoidosis, cirrhosis, inflammatory bowel disease (Crohn's disease, ulcerative colitis), endocarditis, aortitis, and esophageal and colon carcinoma.

Cross Reference

Chapter 8: Hyperemia—Osteomyelitis

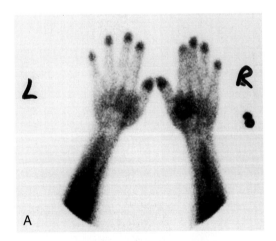

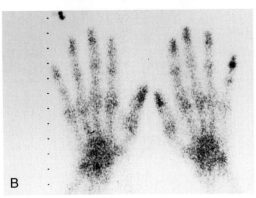

SKIN FOLDS SIMULATING LYMPH NODES

FIGURE 8–17.

Anterior Blood Pools: The top images have focal areas of hyperemia in both axillae. These disappear when the arms are raised, eliminating the skin folds.

NOTE. Whenever axillary lymph nodes are seen with gallium or WBC, the arms must be abducted to avoid falsely identifying skin folds as inflammatory or neoplastic lymph nodes.

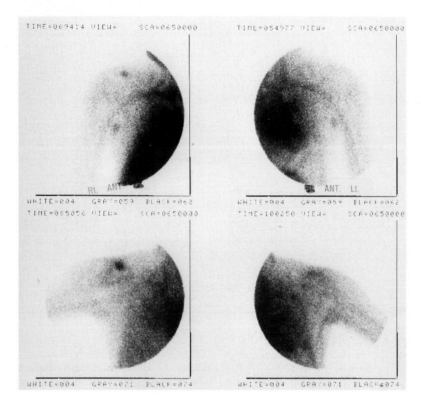

UTERINE HYPEREMIA

Patient: 26 Year Old with Same Day Onset of Menses

FIGURE 8–18 A.

Blood Flow Scan: There is markedly increased blood flow within the pelvis.

Illustration continued on following page

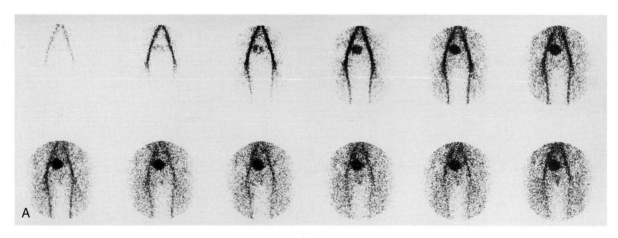

A

FIGURE 8–18   B.
Blood Pool Scan: The hyperemic uterus indents the dome of the bladder.

NOTE. The markedly increased blood flow is usually seen only during menses or pregnancy or with vascular tumors.

Cross Reference

Chapter 11: Soft Tissue Abnormalities—Impressions on the Bladder

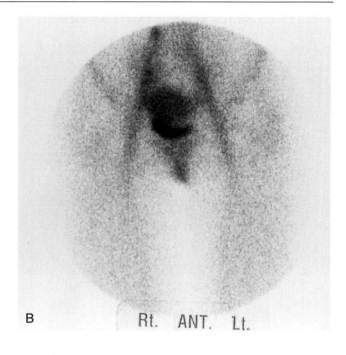

CLAUDICATION SIMULATING HYPEREMIA IN THE OPPOSITE LEG

Patient: 74 Year Old Female with Left Leg Pain

FIGURE 8–19   A.
Blood Flow Bone Scan: The blood flow down the right leg is far faster than that of the left.

FIGURE 8–19   B and C.
Plantar and Anterior Blood Pool Scans: The right ankle and lower leg have greater activity than the left.

FIGURE 8–19   D and E.
Delayed Plantar and Anterior Bone Scans: The osteogenesis of the two feet and lower legs are markedly dissimilar. There is no pathologic process evident in either lower extremity.

NOTE. Osteogenesis is directly proportional to blood flow. A decrease in the blood flow in one leg can make the normal side appear hyperemic.

Cross Reference

Chapter 60: Arterial Disease—Thallium Perfusion Scanning in Claudication

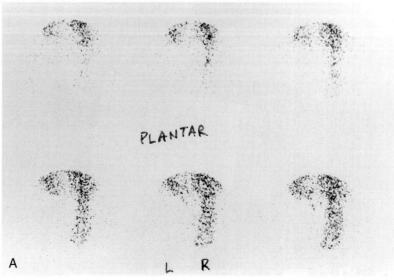

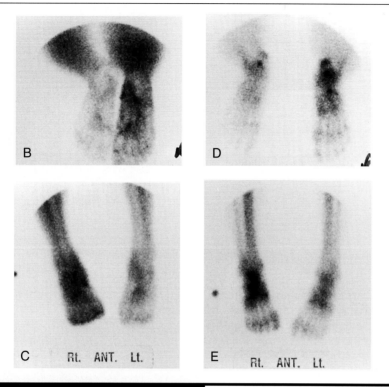

Chapter 9

"Cold" Abnormalities

<table>
<tr><td>

DIFFERENTIAL DIAGNOSIS OF DECREASED ACTIVITY ON BONE SCAN BLOOD POOL

1. Vascular insufficiency

    A. Early avascular necrosis

    B. Early infarct

    C. Early Legg-Perthes disease

    D. Early reflex sympathetic dystrophy

    E. Slipped capital femoral epiphysis

    F. Arterial compromise (e.g., atherosclerosis, vasculitis, post-traumatic occlusion)

2. Infection—synovitis with tense joint capsule secondary to fluid

3. Prostheses

4. Metal artifacts

5. Ice treatment to extremity

6. Stomach filled with gas or food

7. Methylmethacrylate spacers

</td></tr>
</table>

METAL ARTIFACT ON BONE SCAN

Patient 1: Pacemaker

FIGURE 9–1 A.

Anterior Thoracic Bone Scan: The pacemaker creates a photon-deficient artifact in the left chest *(arrow)*.

Illustration continued on following page

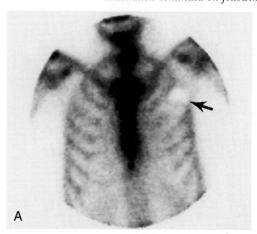

Patient 2: Belt Buckle

FIGURE 9–1 B.

Anterior Bone Scan: The belt buckle defect can be seen over the right sacroiliac (SI) joint.

Patient 3: Necklace

FIGURE 9–1 C.

Thoracic Spine Bone Scan: The patient's metal medallion was tossed behind him, causing the "cold" defect of T3.

Patient 4: Keys

FIGURE 9–1 D.

Anterior Pelvic Bone Scan: The key artifact partially obscures the right hip stress fracture.

NOTE. Common "cold" artifacts include necklaces, pacemakers, buckles, zippers, metal buttons, coins or keys in pockets, and barium from gastrointestinal studies.

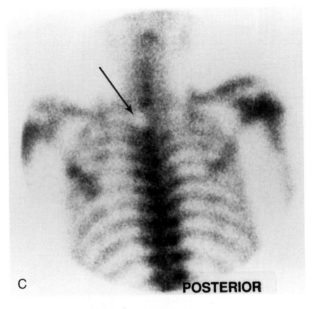

C   POSTERIOR

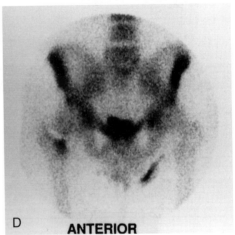

D   ANTERIOR

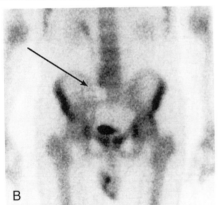

B

"COLD" LESION IN SPINE DUE TO METHYLMETHACRYLATE

FIGURE 9–2 A and B.

Anterior and Posterior Lumbar Spine Bone Scans: There is a "cold" defect involving L2 and L3.

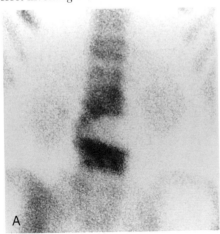

A

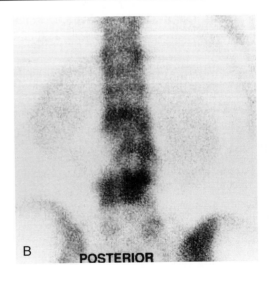

B   POSTERIOR

Figure 9–2 C.

Plain X-ray of Spine: There is a radiopaque spacer in the lumbar spine used because of the destruction from thyroid carcinoma.

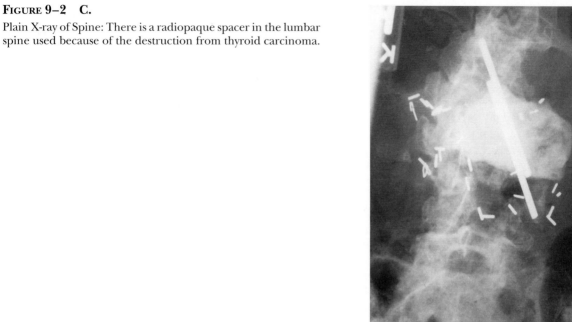

"COLD" OSTEOMYELITIS OF THE SPINE

Figure 9–3 A.

Lumbar Spine Bone Scan: There is decreased activity *(arrowheads)* involving the left side of L2, L3, and L4.

Figure 9–3 B.

CT of Spine: There is a destructive process involving the vertebral body, associated with a prevertebral soft tissue mass.

NOTE. Infections can cross cartilage and disks, affecting contiguous bones.

Cross Reference

Chapter 71: Infectious Diseases—Psoas Abscess

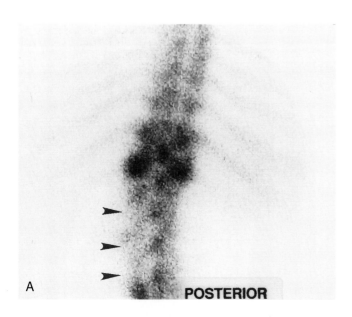

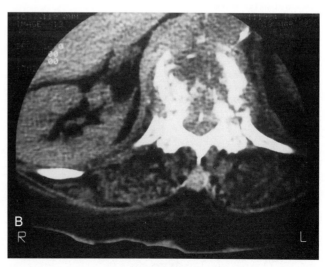

"COLD" TO "HOT" OSTEOMYELITIS ON BONE SCAN

Patient 1

FIGURE 9–4 A.

Arm Bone Scan: The right humeral diaphysis is not seen at all, and the humeral head has decreased osteogenesis.

FIGURE 9–4 B.

Arm Bone Scan: Two and one-half weeks later there is extensive increased activity involving the entire right humerus with the exception of the proximal metaphysis, where a bone abscess was found.

NOTE 1. Most missed osteomyelitis cases are in newborns and young children, but subtle findings, including hyperemia on blood pool images, decreased activity of a bone, and asymmetry of the growth plates and epiphyses, can help reduce false negative results.

NOTE 2. Repeat bone scans at 24 hours or delaying the first scan for 24 hours may be necessary to rule out osteomyelitis in young children.

Cross References

Chapter 1: Solitary Bony Abnormalities—Metaphyseal Hyperemia and Osteomyelitis

Chapter 2: Multiple Bony Abnormalities—"Cold" to "Hot" Bone Infarcts (Sickle Cell Disease)

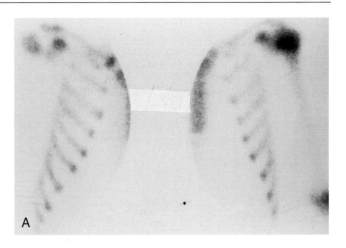

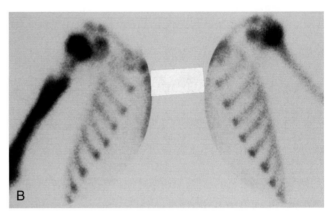

"COLD" ABNORMALITY IN EARLY OSTEONECROSIS OF THE HIP

Patient 1

FIGURE 9–5 A and B.

Blood Pool and Delayed Bone Scans: On the delayed scan there is decreased activity in the left femoral head, although there is some activity on the blood pool image *(curved arrows)*. The left femoral fracture of 24 hours has increased activity on blood pool and delayed scan.

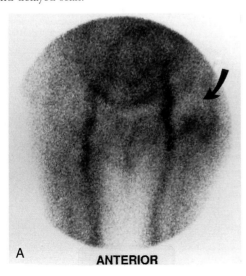

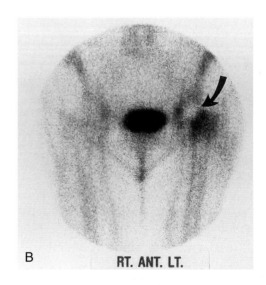

RT. ANT. LT.

ANTERIOR

Patient 2

FIGURE 9–5   C and D.

Blood Pool and SPECT Scans: There is normal blood supply but decreased osteogenesis *(arrow)* in the right femoral head. The left hip is normal, with mild but definite activity.

FIGURE 9–5   E.

Repeat Planar Bone Scan After 6 Weeks: There is markedly increased activity in the right superolateral femoral head and more mildly increased osteogenesis throughout the femoral head.

NOTE 1. Scintigraphic stages of osteonecrosis (also known as aseptic necrosis and avascular necrosis) are shown in the table.

NOTE 2. A "cold" femoral head on early scanning of femoral fractures can be due to early osteonecrosis or joint fluid (blood).

NOTE 3. MRI scanning and bone scintigraphy are about equal in sensitivity (80 percent) for osteonecrosis.

Cross Reference

Chapter 1: Solitary Bony Abnormalities—Early Osteonecrosis

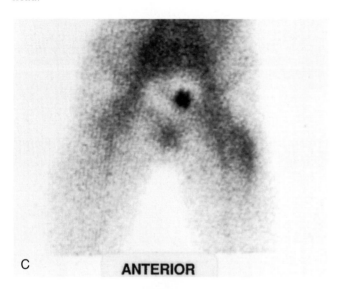

C   **ANTERIOR**

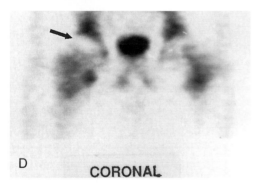

D   **CORONAL**

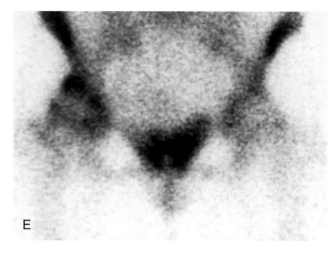

E

SCINTIGRAPHIC STAGES OF OSTEONECROSIS
1. Early (0–2 weeks): normal or decreased blood flow/ blood pool, "cold" on delayed scan. Normal x-ray.
2. Intermediate: normal or increased blood flow with normal delayed scan. Crescent sign or normal x-ray.
3. Late (6–8 weeks): increased blood flow and marked increased osteogenesis. Crescent sign or increased density/fragmentation on x-ray.

HISTIOCYTOSIS X ON BONE SCAN

FIGURE 9–6   A.

Anterior Pelvic Bone Scan: There is irregular decreased osteogenesis of the right pubic bone *(arrow)*.

Illustration continued on following page

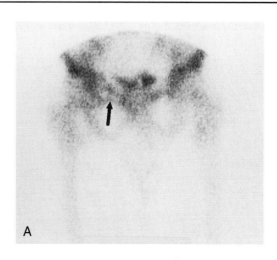

A

FIGURE 9–6   B.

Plain Film X-ray: The right pubic bone is replaced by a lytic process that has a benign appearance (sclerotic margins).

FIGURE 9–6   C.

Anterior Skull Bone Scan: An additional lesion in this patient was found in the left mandible *(arrow)*.

NOTE. Histiocytosis X can be either "hot" or "cold" on bone scan.

Cross Reference

Chapter 5: Skull Abnormalities—Histiocytosis X

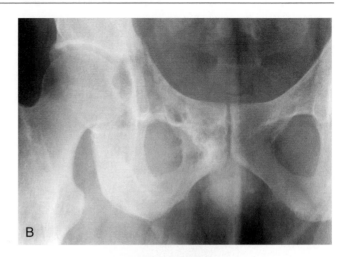

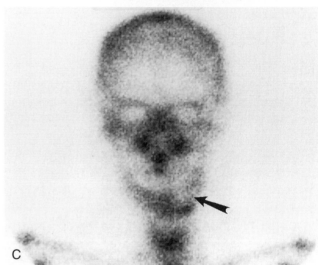

PRIMARY LYMPHOMA OF BONE

FIGURE 9–7.

Bone Scan: There are bilateral femoral and tibial areas of increased osteogenesis surrounding foci of normal activity and "cold" lesions *(arrowheads)*.

NOTE. Lymphoma has a tendency to present with elongated abnormalities, in both homogeneous and heterogeneous patterns.

Cross Reference

Chapter 1: Solitary Bony Abnormalities—Lymphoma of the Thigh

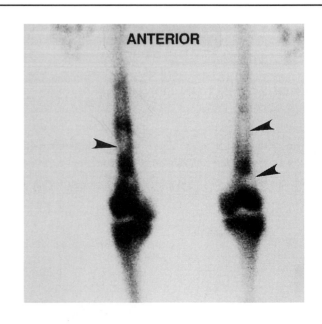

RADIATION THERAPY OF LYMPHOMA OF THE BONE

Patient 1

FIGURE 9–8   A.

Anterior Hip Bone Scan: The right femoral head and neck have increased activity.

FIGURE 9–8   B.

Plain Film X-ray: The right hip is moth-eaten, a pattern highly suspect for malignant disease.

FIGURE 9–8   C.

CT Scan: There is a destructive lesion arising within the right femur.

FIGURE 9–8   D.

Coronal T1 MRI Scan: The marrow of the right femur *(asterisk)* has abnormally low signal intensity extending down to the proximal femoral diaphysis.

FIGURE 9–8   E.

Five Months Post Radiation Therapy Pelvic Bone Scan: The right femoral head and neck are "cold," and the femoral head has collapsed. The surgical specimen was free of tumor.

Illustration continued on following page

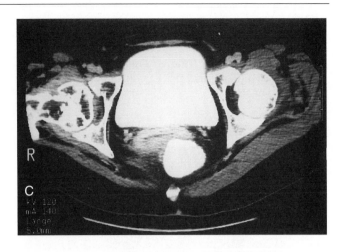

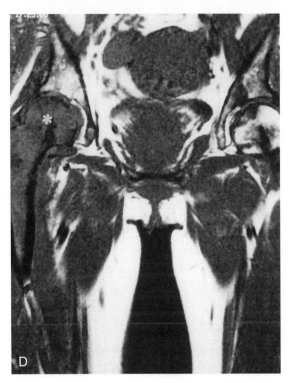

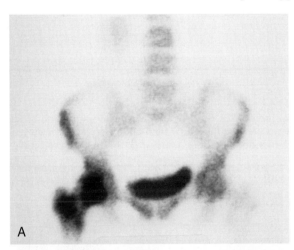

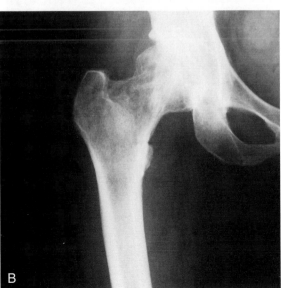

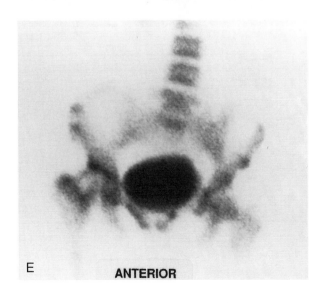

Patient 2

FIGURE 9–8   F.

PostRadiation Bone Scan: There is a photon-deficient mass replacing the right humerus following radiation therapy for solitary lymphoma in bone.

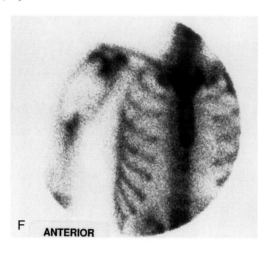

FIGURE 9–8   G.

PostRadiation Gallium Scan: The gallium accumulated only in the periphery of the mass. Several biopsies have remained negative for recurrence.

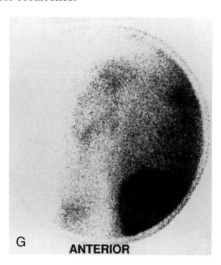

RADIATION CHANGE ON BONE SCAN

Patient 1: Lung Cancer

FIGURE 9–9   A.

Thoracic Spine Bone Scan: There is a broad sharply demarcated area of decreased osteogenesis in the upper thorax, both spine and ribs, delineating the radiation therapy field.

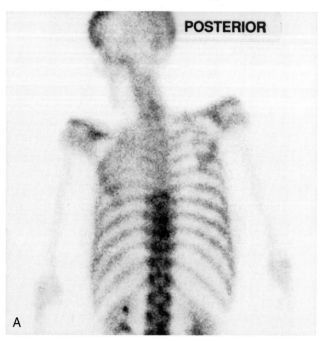

FIGURE 9–9   B.

T1-Weighted MR Scan of the Thoracic Spine: The radiation changes are manifested by increased high signal fat replacing the hematopoietic bone marrow of the upper vertebrae.

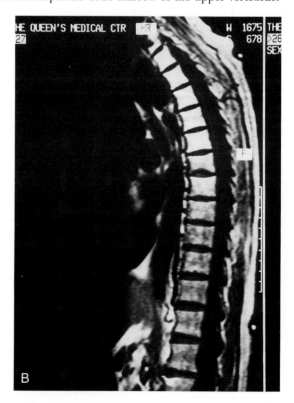

Patient 2: Prostate Cancer

FIGURE 9–9   C.

WBC Scan of the Lumbar Spine and Pelvis: There is markedly decreased uptake of ^{111}In-labeled WBCs by the marrow in the area of the radiation port. The nonirradiated lumbar spine accumulates white cells in the marrow.

NOTE. A colloid marrow scan would also demonstrate decreased activity in the radiation port.

Cross Reference

Chapter 33: Gastrointestinal and Abdominal Infections—Abdominal Abscess in Immunosuppression and After Radiation Therapy

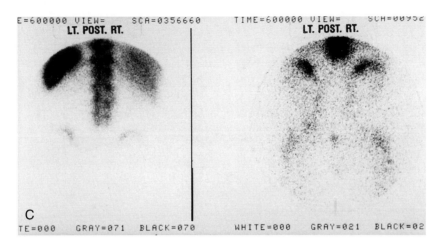

C

"COLD" METASTASES ON BONE SCAN

Patient 1: Nasopharyngeal Carcinoma

FIGURE 9–10   A.

Posterior Chest Bone Scan: There are multiple "cold" or photon-deficient abnormalities of the spine and ribs.

Patient 2: Renal Cell Carcinoma

FIGURE 9–10   B.

Posterior Lumbar Spine Bone Scan: T11, L4, and S1 vertebrae *(arrow)* have decreased activity.

NOTE. "Cold" metastases can be seen with any metastatic process, although most commonly with lung, breast, prostate, and renal carcinomas.

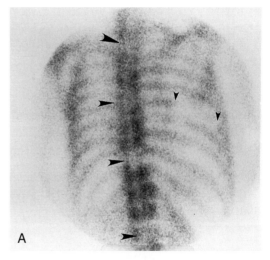

A

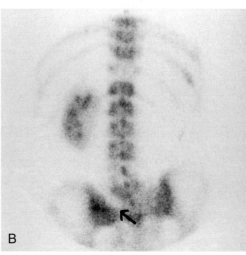

B

"COLD" BONE LESION DUE TO DIRECT INVASION BY TUMOR

Patient 1: Lung Carcinoma

FIGURE 9-11   A.

Posterior Thorax Bone Scan: There is no bony activity involving the posterior right upper ribs and T5 vertebra *(arrowheads)*.

FIGURE 9-11   B.

Chest X-ray: There is a huge mass in the right upper lobe of the lung. It is difficult to evaluate the ribs fully. An "overpenetrated" film is necessary.

FIGURE 9-11   C.

CT of Chest: The large mass has grown into the chest wall, with destruction of ribs and erosion of the lateral vertebral body.

Patient 2: Bronchogenic Carcinoma

FIGURE 9-11   D.

Posterior Thoracic Spine Bone Scan: There is increased osteogenesis along the right side of T3 and T4 vertebrae. The left side has a subtle decrease in activity.

FIGURE 9-11   E.

Sagittal Bone SPECT Scan: The left sides of the T3 and T4 vertebrae have decreased activity.

FIGURE 9-11   F.

CT Scan with Parasagittal Reconstruction: There is destruction of vertebral bone by a soft tissue mass.

NOTE 1. Chest wall invasion occurs in approxiately 10 percent of peripheral lung tumors.

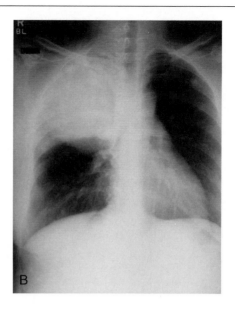

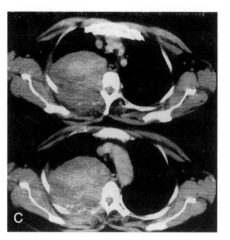

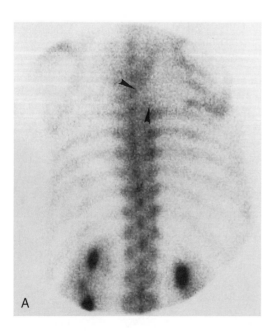

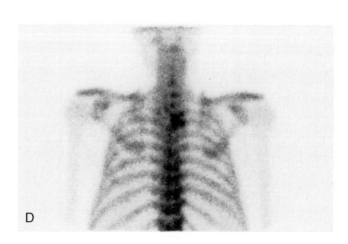

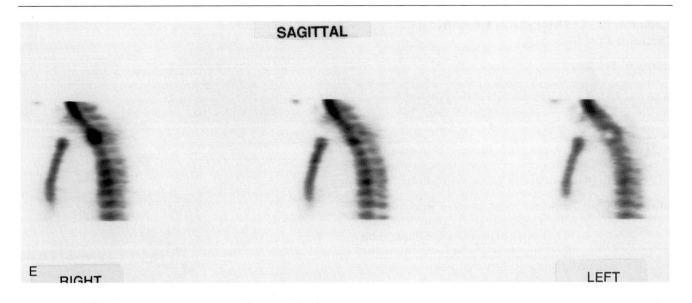

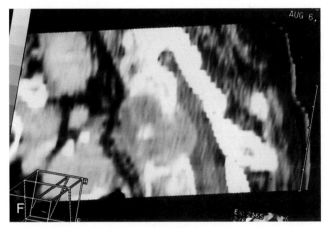

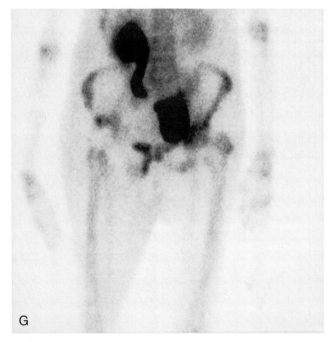

Patient 3: Non-Hodgkin's Lymphoma

FIGURE 9–11   G.

Bone Scan: The right ischium and pubic bones are not visualized. The ischium is displaced inferiorly. There is a right hip prosthesis.

FIGURE 9–11   H.

Scout Film from CT: The bone destruction is evident.

Illustration continued on following page

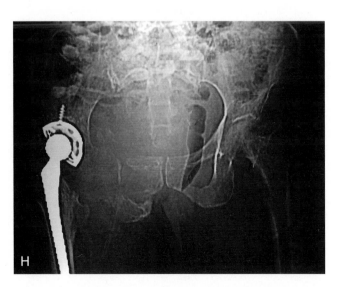

Patient 4: "Cold" Metastases from Breast Carcinoma on Bone Scan

FIGURE 9–11 I to L.

Lumbar Spine Bone Scan: There are photon-deficient lesions of L3 and L4 along the anterior side of the vertebral bodies.

NOTE 1. Tumor involving two adjacent vertebrae does so by growing around rather than through the disk. Only infection can cross cartilage.

NOTE 2. "Cold" abnormalities can occur from any rapidly growing neoplasm. The photon deficiency is thought to be due to invasion or compression of the blood supply to the bone, and/or the lack of a stimulatory factor to incite osteoblasts.

Cross Reference

Chapter 6: Rib Abnormalities—Rib Resections; Direct Invasion of Rib by Tumor

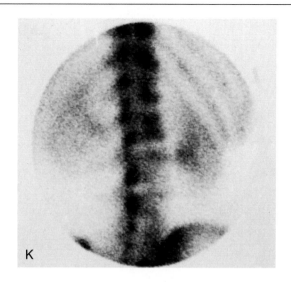

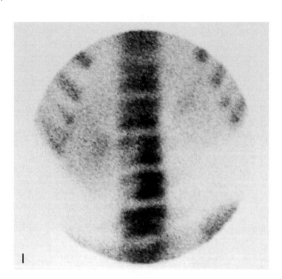

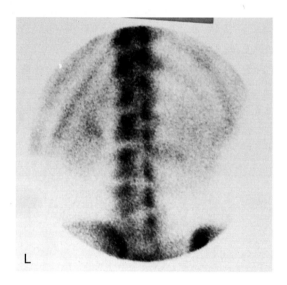

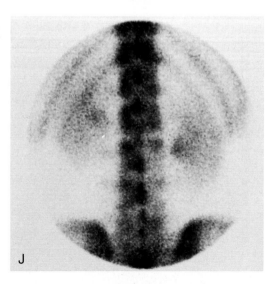

"COLD" TO "HOT" BONE LESIONS FROM LUNG CARCINOMA

FIGURE 9–12 A.

Thoracic Spine Bone Scan: The T8 vertebra has decreased osteogenesis.

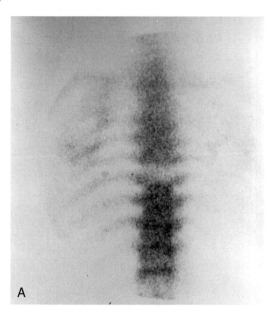

FIGURE 9–12 B.

Thoracic Spine Bone Scan: One month later the lesion has increased osteogenesis.

NOTE. "Cold" metastases develop into the more usual "hot" abnormality after 2 to 4 weeks.

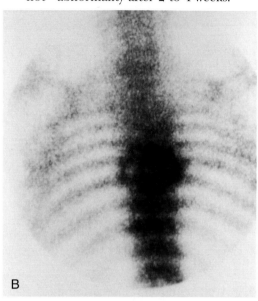

"DOUGHNUT" LESIONS OF THE BONE

Patient 1: Lung Carcinoma

FIGURE 9–13 A.

Bone Scan: The large lytic metastasis in the skull has two rims of increased osteogenesis. This may be due to differential invasion of the inner and outer tables.

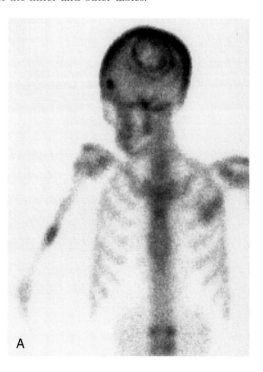

Patient 2: Prostate Carcinoma

FIGURE 9–13 B.

Posterior Bone Scan: The left femur, the right ischium, and the sacrum have "doughnut" metastases.

NOTE 1. Any aggressive tumor can have central areas of diminished activity surrounded by increased osteogenesis.

NOTE 2. Some infections may also present with a "doughnut" appearance.

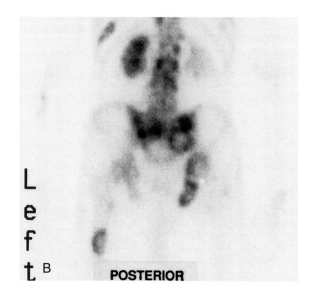

Chapter 10
Prostheses

NORMAL HIP PROSTHESIS

FIGURE 10–1.

Planar Bone Scan: There is no increased activity along the edges of the femoral component. The increased activity along the margins of the acetabular component is due to degenerative or reactive changes, not loosening. (The patient has insufficiency fractures of the left symphysis and sacroiliac (SI) joints.)

NOTE 1. Cementless prostheses may have mild increased activity postoperatively for a prolonged period compared with prostheses using cement.

NOTE 2. When studying hip prostheses, the entire length of the femoral component, which is variable, must be scanned.

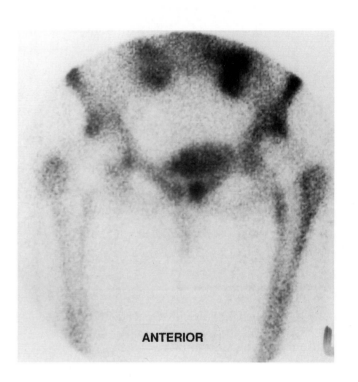

ANTERIOR

NORMAL KNEE PROSTHESES

FIGURE 10–2 A to D.

Four Views of the Knees: There is only a fine line of increased activity along the right tibial plateau. The left knee demonstrates diffuse increased activity due to severe osteoarthritis.

FIGURE 10–2 E.

Plain Film X-ray in Different Patient: There is no stem to this prosthesis, and the tibial component is radiolucent.

FIGURE 10–2 F.

Anterior Planar Knee Bone Scan: The tibial components have intramedullary stems of different lengths.

FIGURE 10–2 G.

Lateral Plain Film X-ray: Note that the tibial prosthetic stem is radiopaque.

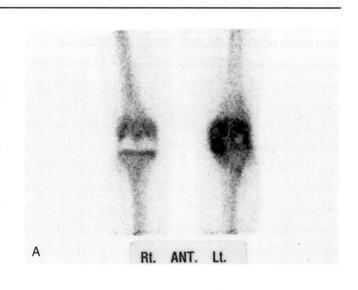

A

Rt. ANT. Lt.

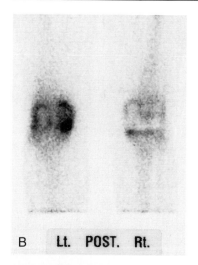

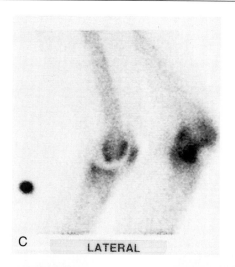

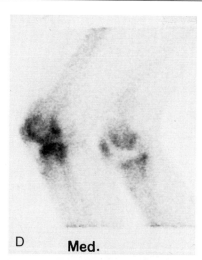

B   **Lt. POST. Rt.**

C   LATERAL

D   **Med.**

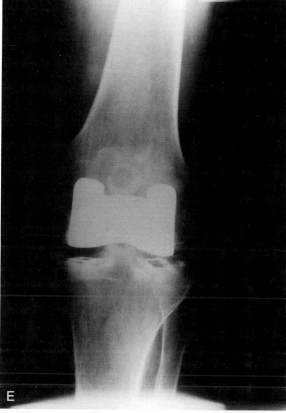

E

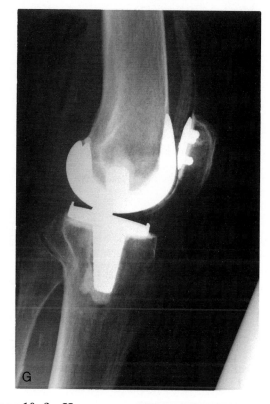

G

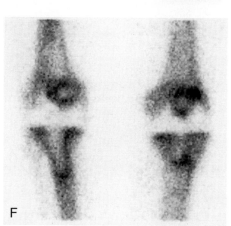

F

FIGURE 10–2   H.

Anterior ^{99m}Tc-colloid and ^{111}In-WBC Scans: The white blood cells and colloid accumulate equally in the bone marrow.

Illustration continued on following page

NOTE 1. There are numerous variations in knee prostheses, so review of the x-rays is important in interpreting the scans.

NOTE 2. Radiocolloid in the marrow precludes an active infection. It is often necessary to do a dual-isotope scan, with visual and computer subtraction, to determine whether the white cell accumulation is in normal marrow or represents infection.

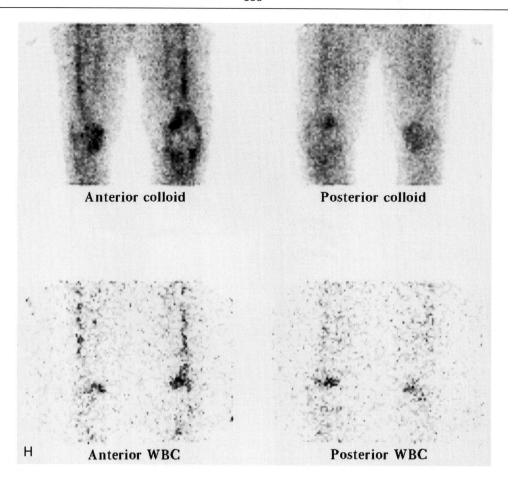

Anterior colloid   Posterior colloid

H   Anterior WBC   Posterior WBC

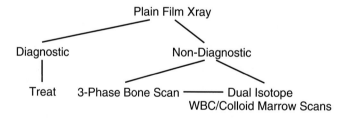

SUSPECTED INFECTION OF
METALLIC PROSTHESIS
OR FIXATION DEVICE

Plain Film Xray

Diagnostic   Non-Diagnostic

Treat   3-Phase Bone Scan ——— Dual Isotope
                                    WBC/Colloid Marrow Scans

INFECTED PROSTHETIC HIP

Patient 1

FIGURE 10–3 A and B.

Anterior Bone Scan: There is diffuse increased activity of the proximal right prosthesis and the distal tip. The left hip prosthesis is a good normal control.

FIGURE 10–3 C and D.

Anterior Gallium Scan: There is abnormal gallium accumulation along the right femoral stem and about the femoral neck.

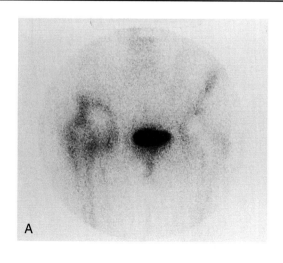

A

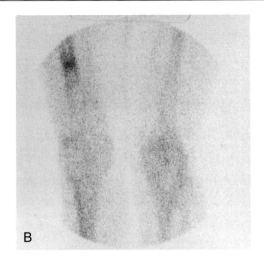

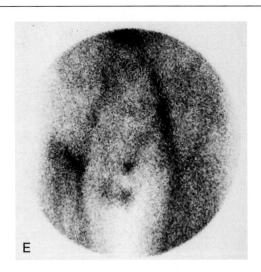

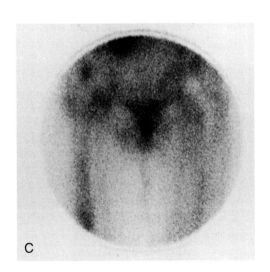

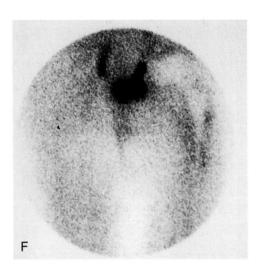

Illustration continued on following page

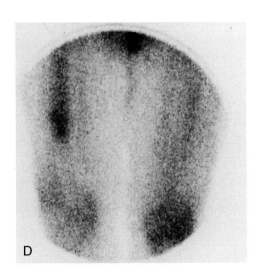

Patient 2

FIGURE 10–3 E to H.
Blood Pool and Delayed Bone Scans: There is hyperemia and increased activity involving the prosthetic stem.

NOTE 1. Diffuse increased activity surrounding a prosthesis should raise concern for infection. Hyperemia occurs more often with infection than with loosening but may not be seen with either.

NOTE 2. Either WBC/colloid marrow scan or gallium scan can be used to identify infected prostheses. However, fractures and granulation tissue may cause false positive gallium scans.

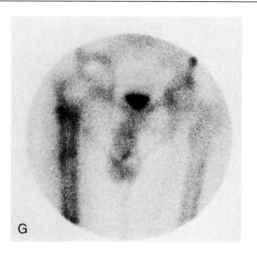

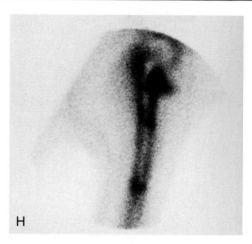

G

H

INFECTED KNEE PROSTHESIS

Patient 1

FIGURE 10–4   A.

Anterior Bone Scan: There is a large area of left tibial activity at the distal end of a long tibial component stem. The right prosthesis is normal. This configuration could represent a fracture or infection.

FIGURE 10–4   B.

Anterior Gallium Scan: The intense gallium accumulation indicates an active infection (biopsy proven).

Patient 2

FIGURE 10–4   C and D.

Anterior and Lateral WBC Scan: There is intense WBC accumulation in the proximal tibia, where the intramedullary stem of the prosthesis is located.

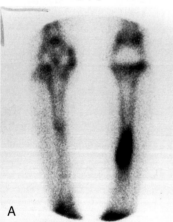

A

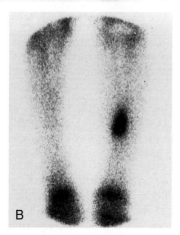

B

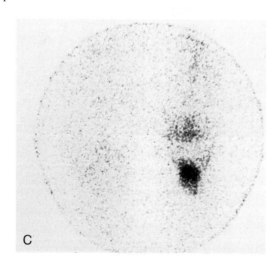

C

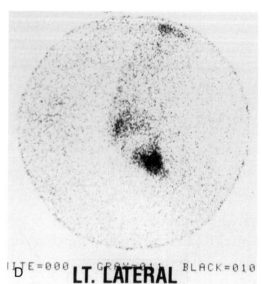

D   LT. LATERAL

SPECT OF INFECTED KNEE PROSTHESIS

FIGURE 10–5   A.
Planar Anterior Knee Bone Scan: There is diffuse increased activity about the knee prosthesis but no definite activity around the intramedullary components.

FIGURE 10–5   B.
Planar Gallium Scan: It is difficult to determine if the gallium is within the joint or around the prosthesis.

FIGURE 10–5   C and D.
Bone SPECT Scan of the Knees: There is increased activity surrounding the right tibial prosthesis.

FIGURE 10–5   E and F.
Gallium SPECT Scan of the Knees: The area of increased gallium activity is under the prosthesis along the tibial plateaus and prosthetic stem.

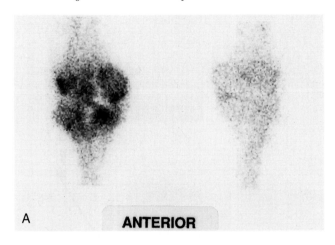

A **ANTERIOR**

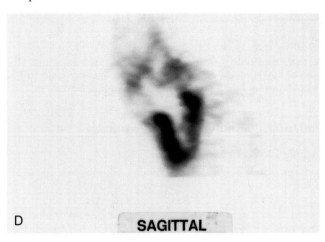

D **SAGITTAL**

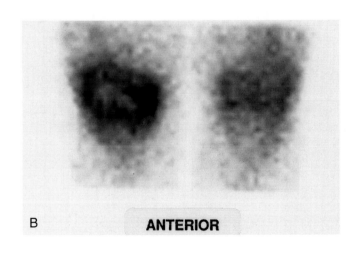

B **ANTERIOR**

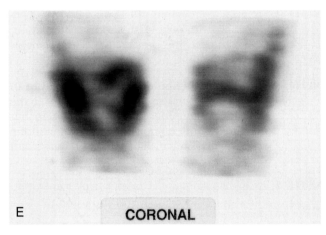

E **CORONAL**

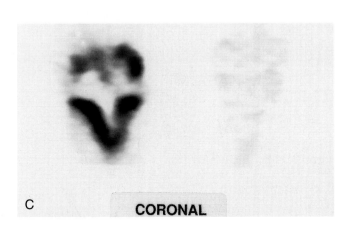

C **CORONAL**

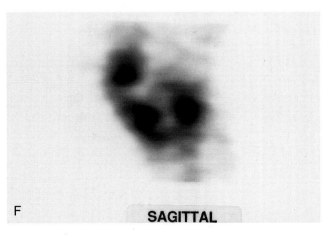

F **SAGITTAL**

MARROW COMPRESSION WITH NORMAL HIP PROSTHESIS

Patient: Bilateral Hip Prostheses with Pain on the Right

FIGURE 10–6   A to C.
Anterior and Both Lateral Femoral WBC Scans: The midfemoral diaphyses have increased WBC accumulations.

FIGURE 10–6   D to F.
Anterior and Both Lateral Femoral Colloid Marrow Scans: The marrow in the midfemoral diaphyses also has increased radiocolloid accumulation in the same distribution.

Patient 2. Painful Right Hip Prosthesis

FIGURE 10–6   G and H.
Anterior ^{111}In-WBC and ^{99m}Tc-Albumin Colloid Scans: The small isolated focus of WBCs has marrow present.

NOTE 1. As the prosthesis is pushed into the bone, it compresses the normal marrow ahead of it. Normal bone marrow will accumulate both radiolabeled WBCs and colloid.

NOTE 2. In areas of infection, there will be WBC accumulation without radiocolloid accumulation. This is due to the destruction of the marrow by the infection.

NOTE 3. A marrow scan should be done if the WBC scan demonstrates increased activity adjacent to the prosthesis. Computer subtraction will help, but the patient must not move if the scans are done sequentially rather than simultaneously with dual-energy windows.

NOTE 4. Using dual-energy windows, the acquisition allows for exact comparison and computer subtraction.

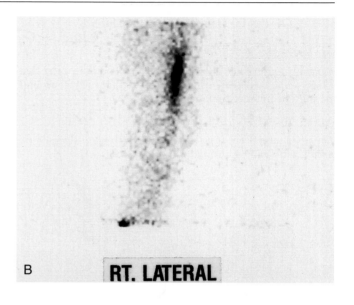

B **RT. LATERAL**

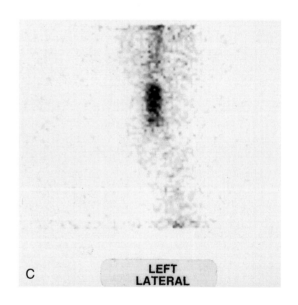

C **LEFT LATERAL**

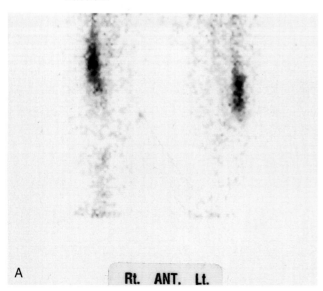

A **Rt. ANT. Lt.**

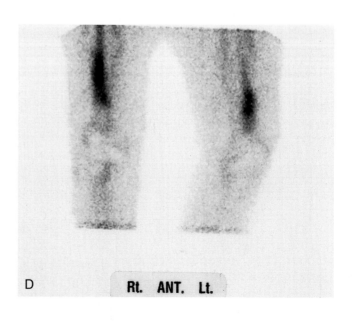

D **Rt. ANT. Lt.**

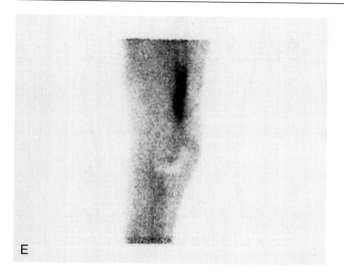

E

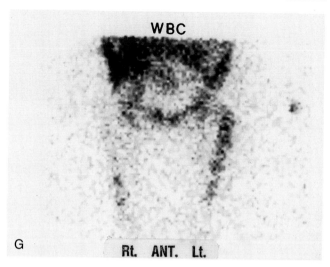

WBC

G

Rt. ANT. Lt.

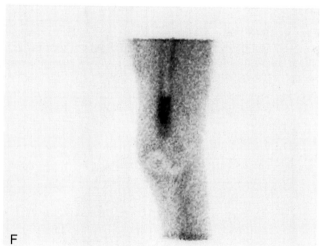

F

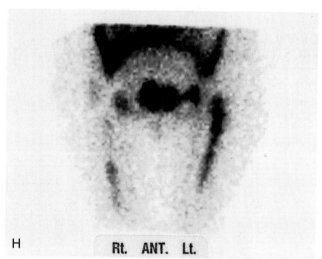

H

Rt. ANT. Lt.

WBC/COLLOID SUBTRACTION IN PROSTHETIC INFECTION

FIGURE 10–7 A.

Anterior Knee WBC Scan: There is a focal WBC accumulation in the proximal left tibial metaphysis and more diffuse activity in the joint space.

FIGURE 10–7 B.

Anterior Knee Albumin Colloid Scan: The radiocolloid in the inflamed joint covers the entire knee.

FIGURE 10–7 C.

Computer Subtraction of WBC/Colloid Scans: There are WBCs in the tibia, indicating prosthetic infection.

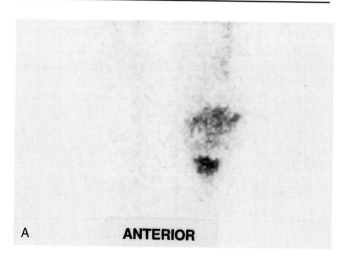

A

ANTERIOR

Illustration continued on following page

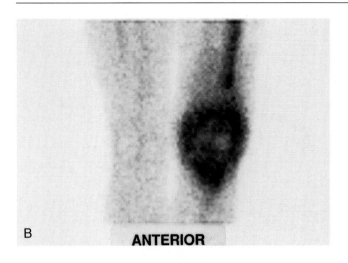

B   **ANTERIOR**

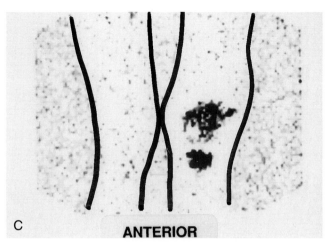

C   **ANTERIOR**

GRANULATION TISSUE WITH PROSTHETIC HIP

FIGURE 10–8   A.

Anterior Bone Scan: There is diffuse increased activity along the right femoral prosthesis.

FIGURE 10–8   B.

Anterior Gallium Scan: There is only mild gallium accumulation along the right femoral prosthesis.

NOTE. Sterile granulation tissue can create a diffuse, mildly abnormal gallium scan.

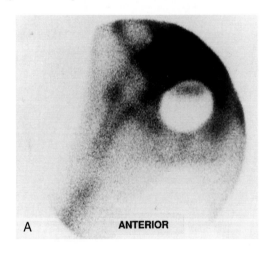

A   **ANTERIOR**

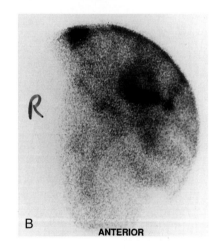

B   **ANTERIOR**

LOOSE HIP PROSTHESIS

FIGURE 10–9.

Anterior Bone Scan: There is increased activity at the tip of the left hip prosthesis.

NOTE 1. The most reliable bone scan sign of loosening in a cemented femoral component is increased activity at the distal tip.

NOTE 2. With cementless hips, increased activity at the medial aspect of the distal tip of the prosthesis is most diagnostic of loosening.

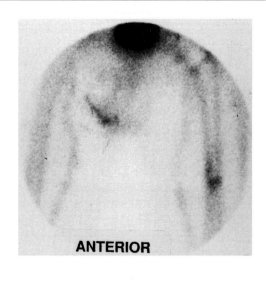

ANTERIOR

PROGRESSIVE LOOSENING OF HIP PROSTHESIS

FIGURE 10–10   A and B.

Blood Pool Scintigraphy: There is no hyperemia involving the right hip prosthesis.

FIGURE 10–10   C and D.

Anterior Delayed Bone Scan: There are focal areas of increased activity at the greater and lesser trochanters, lateral midshaft, and distal tip. The acetabular component is normal.

FIGURE 10–10   E to G.

Two Years Later, Anterior and Right Lateral Bone Scan: The entire intramedullary portion of the femoral prosthesis is surrounded by increased osteogenesis, as is the acetabular component. Heterotopic bone is present as well.

NOTE. Increased lesser trochanteric activity may persist for 1 to 2 years, especially with a calcar graft.

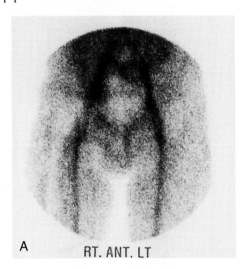

A   RT. ANT. LT

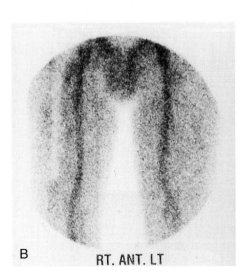

B   RT. ANT. LT

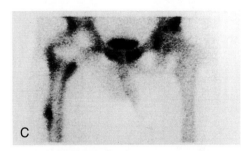

C

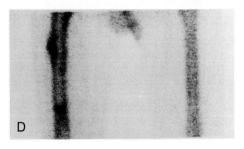

D

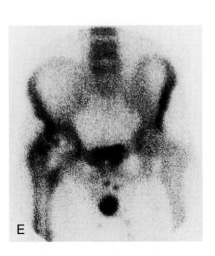

E

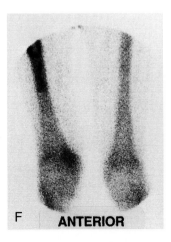

F   ANTERIOR

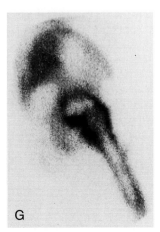

G

REDUCED LOOSENING OF HIP PROSTHESIS

FIGURE 10–11 A.

Anterior Delayed Bone Scan: The increased activity at the distal tip of the left hip prosthesis indicates loosening.

FIGURE 10–11 B.

Anterior Delayed Bone Scan 1 Year Later: The activity is unchanged.

FIGURE 10–11 C.

Anterior Delayed Bone Scan 2 Years Later: The loosening has diminished with use of a wheelchair by the patient.

NOTE. Decreased physical activity may allow stabilization of a loose prosthesis.

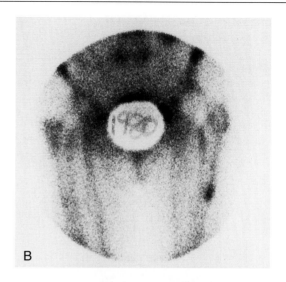

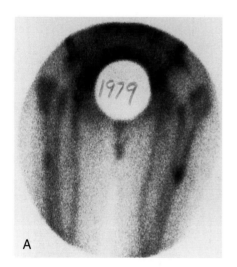

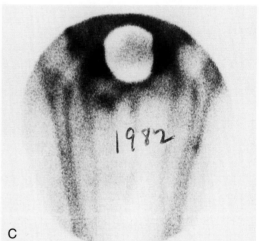

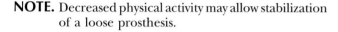

LOOSE FEMORAL PROSTHESIS WITH NUCLEAR ARTHROGRAM

FIGURE 10–12 A.

Planar Delayed Bone Scan: There is increased activity along the entire margin of the right femoral prosthesis. The left prosthesis is normal. Both hip acetabular components are abnormal, suggesting loosening.

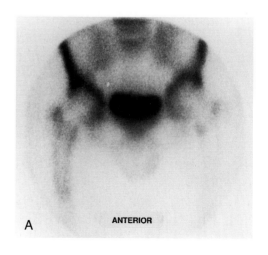

FIGURE 10–12   B.

Hip Arthrogram: After an intra-articular injection of 100 μCi ^{99m}Tc-albumin colloid, there is migration of the radiopharmaceutical between the prosthesis and the femoral cortex, indicative of loosening. Despite the bone scan abnormality, the acetabular component does not appear to be loose.

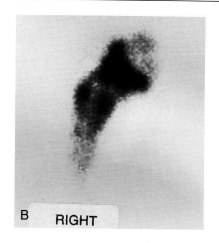

NOTE 1. Activity along the entire intramedullary component may be seen with either loosening or infection.

NOTE 2. At the time of contrast arthrography, it is easy to inject ^{99m}Tc-macroaggregated albumin or a ^{99m}Tc-colloid. The patient should walk or exercise before scanning is done. Any dissection alongside the intramedullary component indicates loosening.

LOOSE ACETABULAR PROSTHESES

FIGURE 10–13.

Bone Scan: The increased activity of the acetabular component on the right corresponded to the patient's symptoms and to the contrast arthrogram. The left acetabular component was loose as well, but asymptomatic.

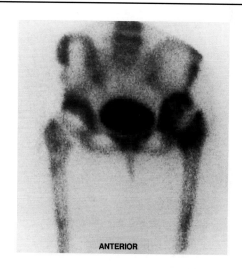

NOTE. The bone scan is less accurate with acetabular component loosening than with femoral component loosening.

LOOSE KNEE PROSTHESIS

FIGURE 10–14.

Anterior Bone Scan: The right proximal tibia has diffuse increased activity along the prosthetic stem. The left knee prosthesis is normal.

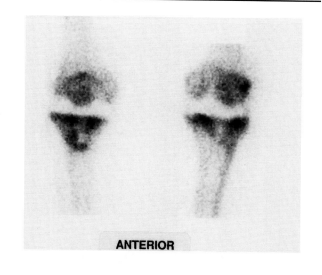

NOTE 1. It may be difficult to diagnose knee prosthetic loosening because of the residual increased activity beneath the tibial plateaus and sometimes along the stem. A knee arthrogram would then be helpful.

NOTE 2. The presence of broad areas of activity extending out from the prosthesis is definitely abnormal.

STRESS FRACTURE WITH PROSTHESIS

Patient 1: Three Years After Hip Prosthesis Revision

FIGURE 10–15   A.

Blood Pool Scintigraphy: There is focal hyperemia in the distal femoral diaphysis.

FIGURE 10–15   B.

Delayed Bone Scan: The focal increased osteogenesis at the distal tip of the prosthesis extends to the lateral femoral cortex.

Patient 2: Two Years After Knee Prosthesis

FIGURE 10–15   C.

Blood Pool Scintigraphy: There is linear hyperemia across the proximal right tibia.

FIGURE 10–15   D and E.

Anterior and Lateral Bone Scans: There is linear increased activity across the proximal right tibia.

NOTE. The hyperemia indicates that the fractures are relatively acute.

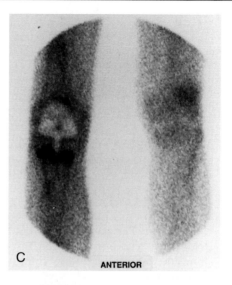

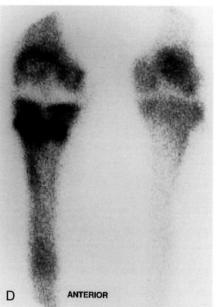

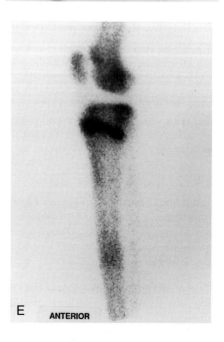

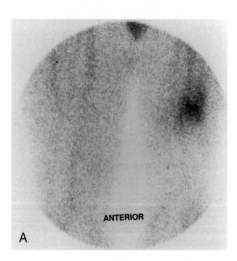

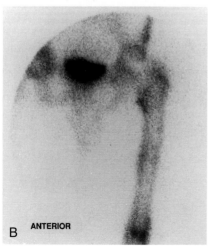

PROSTHETIC HIP DISLOCATION

Patient: 28 Year Old Male with Long-standing Juvenile Rheumatoid Arthritis and Secondary Dwarfism

FIGURE 10–16   A and B.

Anterior and Posterior Pelvic Bone Scans: The left hip prosthesis has dislocated posteriorly and has rotated laterally. The right prosthesis is in a higher position than normal due to a surgically constructed acetabulum.

FIGURE 10–16   C.

Anteroposterior Pelvis X-ray: The location of the prostheses is exactly like that seen on the bone scan.

FIGURE 10–16   D.

Whole Body Bone Scan: The short stature and multiple prostheses are evident.

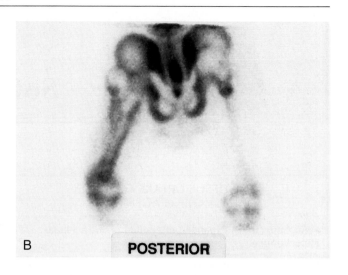

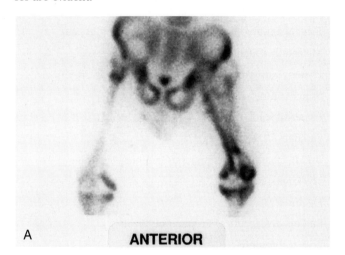

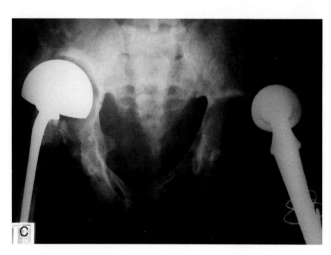

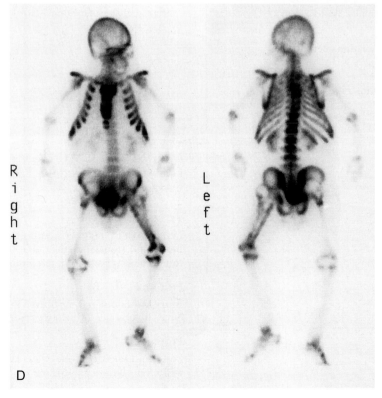

Chapter 11
Soft Tissue Abnormalities

See also Chapter 64: Normal Thyroid/Normal Variants—Free Technetium Distribution.

SOFT TISSUE UPTAKE OF BONE SCANNING AGENTS

Fluid Collections, Expanded Interstitial or Intracellular Fluid Volume

Pleural effusions, especially malignant

Pericardial effusions, especially malignant

Ascites

Infection, inflammation, neoplasms, especially mucin-secreting adenocarcinomas

Lymphedema, anasarca

Renal failure

Rhabdomyolysis, delayed-onset muscle strain, trauma

Thyroid, Graves' disease, or "hot" nodule

Ossification and Dystrophic Calcification

Muscle necrosis or severe ischemia, including myocardial infarction

Myositis ossificans (heterotopic bone formation)

Muscular dystrophy

Vascular calcification (especially Mönckeberg's), hemangiomas

Post chemotherapy, post radiation therapy

Surgical scars

Brain, splenic, other organ infarcts

Scleroderma, dermatomyositis

Trauma

Calcific tendinitis

Gouty tophi

Hematomas

Falx cerebri

Cartilage

Amyloidosis

SOFT TISSUE UPTAKE OF BONE SCANNING AGENTS *Continued*

Malignant New Bone Formation

Osteosarcoma

Chondrosarcoma

Fetal or embryonic tissue, teratomas, dermoid cysts

Metastatic Calcification

Hyperparathyroidism

Renal failure

Hypercalcemia

Sarcoid

Breast, small cell or squamous cell lung carcinoma

Myeloma

Oxalosis

Radiopharmaceutical Preparation Error

Free technetium

See also Chapter 64: Normal Thyroid/Normal Variants—Free Technetium Distribution.

Adapted from Worsley DF, Lentle B: J Nucl Med 34:1614, 1993.

METASTATIC CALCIFICATION FROM FUNCTIONING PARATHYROID CARCINOMA

FIGURE 11–1 A.

Left Anterior Oblique Chest Bone Scan: There is marked lung, heart, and stomach activity due to calcium deposition by the functioning parathyroid carcinoma *(arrow)*.

FIGURE 11–1 B.

Anterior Abdomen Bone Scan: The stomach has intense activity. Note the absence of urinary bladder activity.

FIGURE 11–1 C.

Posterior Low Back Bone Scan: The cortices of the kidneys are well seen, without calyceal or renal pelvic activity.

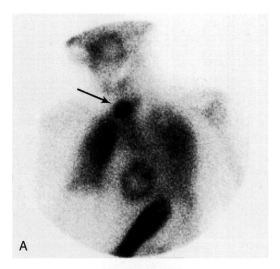

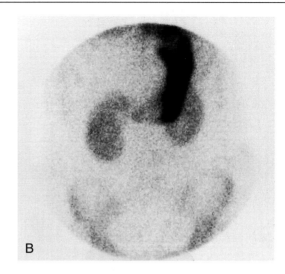

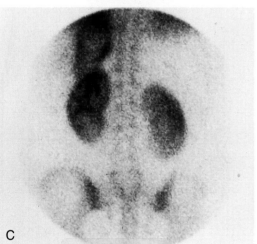

NOTE. Any process that causes marked osteogenesis or calcium deposition far beyond normal may "use up" all the available bone scanning agent so that there is none left for urinary excretion. Examples include diffuse metastatic disease, Paget's disease, fibrous dysplasia, and severe hyperparathyroidism.

Cross References

Chapter 2: Multiple Bony Abnormalities—Superscan

Chapter 69: Parathyroid Diseases—Functioning Parathyroid Carcinoma

SOFT TISSUE CALCIFICATION DUE TO ELEVATED PARATHORMONE FROM SQUAMOUS CELL CARCINOMA

FIGURE 11–2   A.

Anterior Chest Bone Scan: There is diffuse lung uptake of the bone scanning agent due to microcalcification. The stomach can also be seen *(arrow)*.

Illustration continued on following page

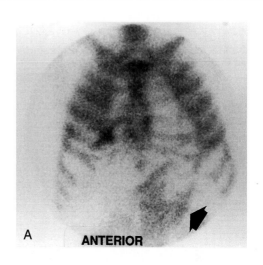

FIGURE 11–2 B.

Right Lower Leg Bone Scan: There is a metastatic mass expanding the midtibia with a central photon-deficient necrotic area surrounded by increased osteogenesis in the margins.

FIGURE 11–2 C.

Right Shoulder Bone Scan: The deltoid muscle *(arrow)* has abnormal accumulation of the bone scanning agent.

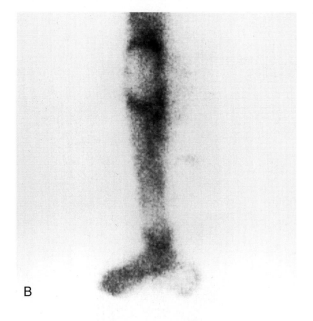

B

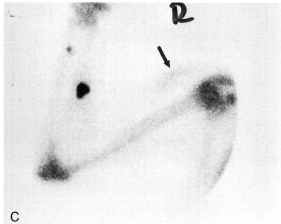

C

MULTIPLE SOFT TISSUE METASTASES WITH MUCIN-SECRETING COLON CARCINOMA ON BONE SCAN

FIGURE 11–3.

Posterior Bone Scan: There is bilateral upper lobe and/or pleural accumulation of the bone scanning agent. The liver and left adrenal *(arrow)* also take up the methylene diphosphonate (MDP) owing to metastatic involvement. The liver activity is homogeneous and is separated from the abdominal wall *(arrowheads)* by ascites.

NOTE. It is of interest to note that mucin-secreting tumor metastases may have abnormal uptake on bone scanning, probably owing to their calcium-binding capacity.

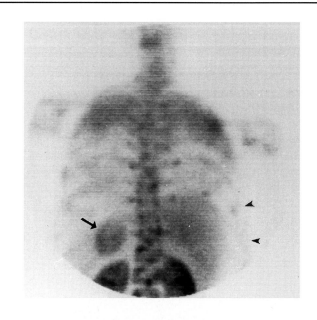

FALX CEREBRI OSSIFICATION

FIGURE 11–4 A.

Bone Scan: There is bony activity in the midline of the skull.

FIGURE 11–4 B.

Plain Film X-ray: The falx is seen in the midline as a thick area of calcium.

FIGURE 11–4 C.

CT Scan: The CT was done for metastatic thyroid papillary carcinoma seen as destructive lesions in the skull. The falx ossification can be seen anteriorly.

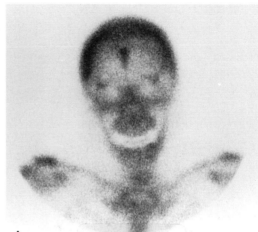

A **ANTERIOR**

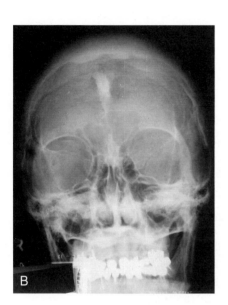

B

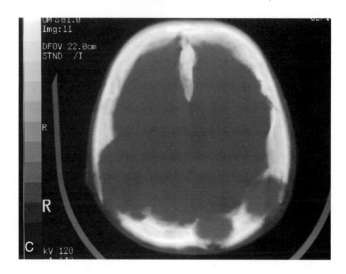

C

CALCIFIED CHRONIC SUBDURAL HYGROMA ON BONE SCAN

FIGURE 11–5 A.

Lateral Skull Delayed Bone Scan: There is a "doughnut" lesion in the posterior head.

FIGURE 11–5 B.

Posterior Skull Delayed Bone Scan: The subdural hematoma has calcified (or ossified) and now is biconvex, its classified appearance.

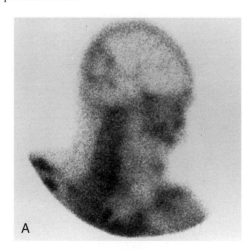

A

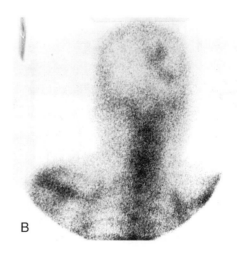

B

CEREBRAL INFARCT ON BONE SCAN

FIGURE 11–6   A.
Lateral Skull Delayed Bone Scan: There is irregular activity over the posterior temporoparietal region of the brain or skull.

FIGURE 11–6   B.
Anterior Skull Delayed Bone Scan: The fan-shaped, or wedge-like, abnormality is seen to be within the brain.

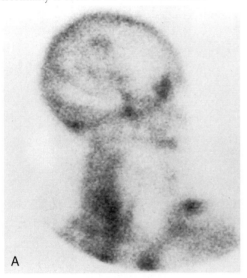

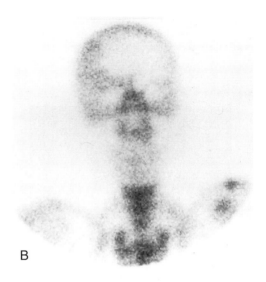

THYROID CARTILAGE OSSIFICATION

Patient 1

FIGURE 11–7   A to C.
Anterior and Oblique Bone Scans: The focal increased activity in the thyroid cartilage is a normal finding in virtually all scans.

Patient 2

FIGURE 11–7   D and E.
Lateral Bone Scans: The calcified thyroid cartilage is clearly anterior to the cervical spine.

Patient 3

FIGURE 11–7   F.
Oblique Bone Scan: There is hyoid bone ossification and minimal thyroid cartilage ossification.

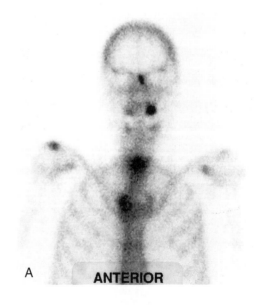

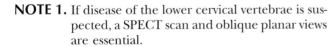

NOTE 1. If disease of the lower cervical vertebrae is suspected, a SPECT scan and oblique planar views are essential.

NOTE 2. Bone scanning agents can accumulate in diffuse toxic goiters.

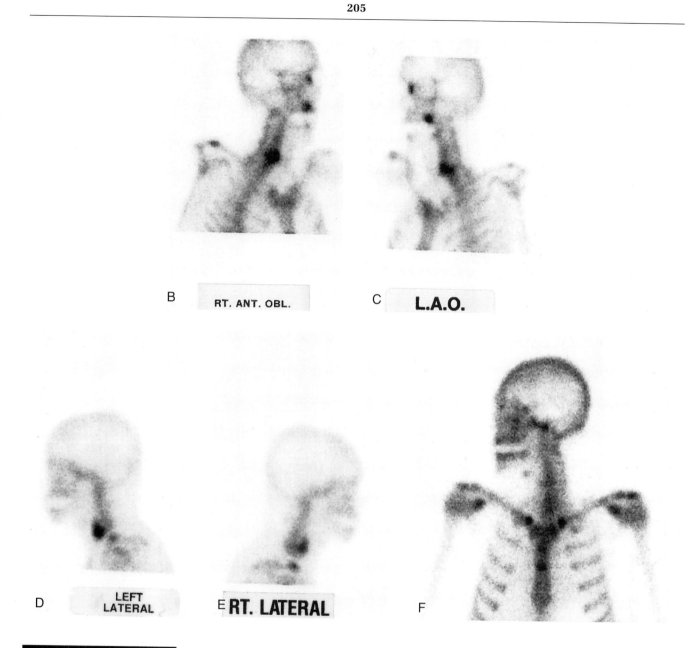

B   RT. ANT. OBL.   C   L.A.O.

D   LEFT LATERAL   E   RT. LATERAL   F

SUPRACLAVICULAR NODES ON BONE SCAN

Patient 1: Hodgkin's Disease

FIGURE 11–8 A.

Anterior Bone Scan: A left upper lobe pulmonary mass and supraclavicular lymph nodes *(arrowhead)* take up the bone scanning agent. (Courtesy of Dr. Michael Kipper, Vista, CA.)

Illustration continued on following page

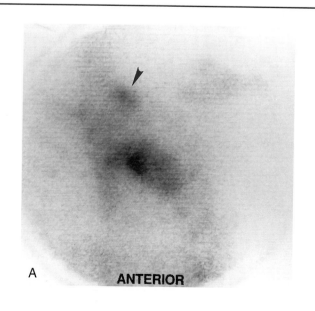

A   ANTERIOR

Patient 2: Colon Carcinoma

FIGURE 11–8 B.

Anterior Bone Scan: The supraclavicular lymph nodes are well seen, along with the left lobe of the liver metastasis *(arrow)*.

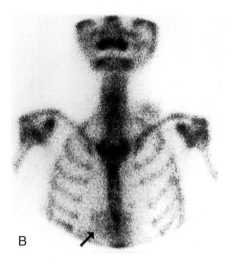

COSTOCHONDRAL OSSIFICATION

FIGURE 11–9 A.

Delayed Bone Scan: The female costocartilage ossifies with a single central line of bone, a "male" configuration.

FIGURE 11–9 B.

Delayed Bone Scan: The costocartilage in the male has a "female" configuration. It has two lines of ossification.

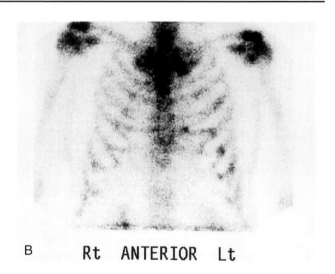

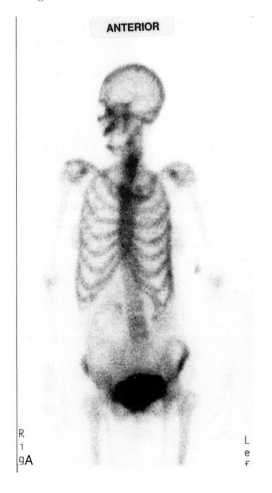

CHRONIC OBSTRUCTIVE LUNG DISEASE ON BONE SCAN

FIGURE 11–10 A.
Posterior Chest Blood Pool Scan: The pulmonary arteries are prominent, and the diaphragms are flattened.

FIGURE 11–10 B.
Anterior Chest Bone Scan: The thorax is barrel-shaped.

FIGURE 11–10 C.
Chest X-ray: There is hyperinflation of the lungs, or barrel chest, and flattened diaphragms.

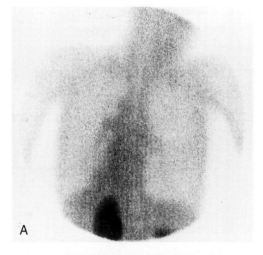

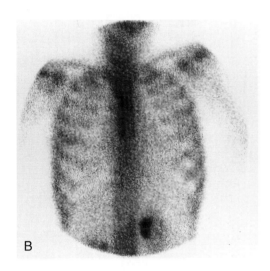

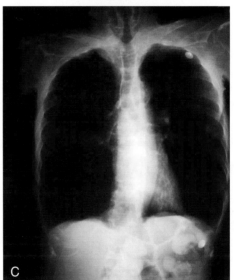

PULMONARY MICROLITHIASIS ON BONE SCAN

FIGURE 11–11 A.
Anterior Chest Bone Scan: There is intense accumulation of the bone radiopharmaceutical in the lungs. There is attenuation at the bases due to fluid from congestive heart failure.

FIGURE 11–11 B and C.
Chest X-ray with Magnified View of the RUL: There are multiple fine nodules in the lungs.

Illustration continued on following page

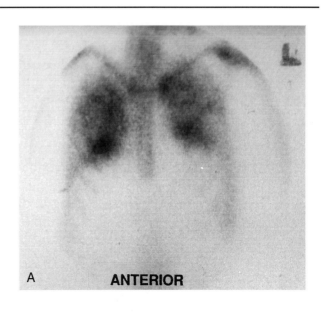

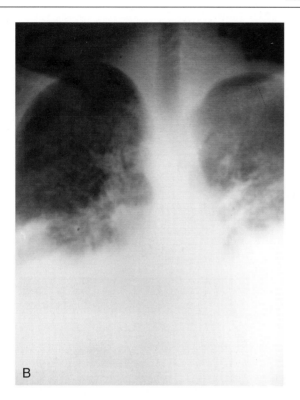

B

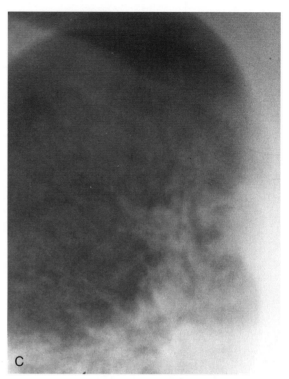

C

METASTATIC OSTEOSARCOMA

Patient 1: 21 Year Old Male

FIGURE 11–12   A.
Delayed Bone Scan: There are several pulmonary metastases accumulating the bone scanning agent.

Patient 2: 17 Year Old Male

FIGURE 11–12   B.
Delayed Bone Scan: There are right chest wall and pulmonary metastases.

NOTE. Metastatic osteosarcoma frequently has active osteogenesis and will take up the bone scanning radiopharmaceutical.

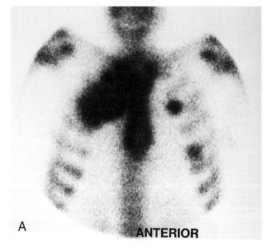

A

ANTERIOR

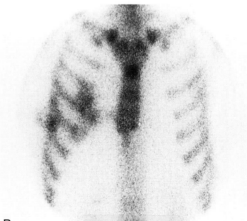

B

ANTERIOR

LUNG TUMOR ON BONE SCAN

Patient 1: Bronchogenic Carcinoma

FIGURE 11–13   A.

Posterior Chest Bone Scan: The primary bronchogenic carcinoma of the lung takes up the bone scanning agent *(arrow)*. A renal infarct is also seen *(arrowhead)*.

FIGURE 11–13   B.

CT of Chest: The lung carcinoma is seen in the posterior right lung against pleura.

Patient 2: Multifocal Bronchogenic Carcinoma

FIGURE 11–13   C and D.

Anterior and Posterior Bone Scans: There is a subtle abnormality *(arrows)* between the ribs on the right.

FIGURE 11–13   E and F.

SPECT Scan of Thorax with ^{99m}Tc-MDP: There are several areas of uptake that proved to be multiple tumors.

Illustration continued on following page

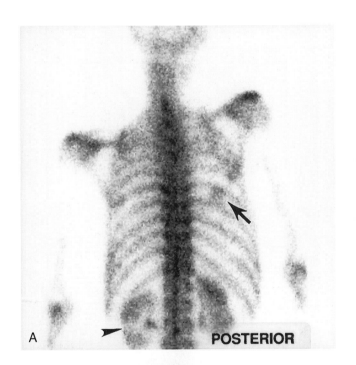

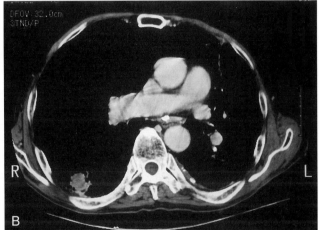

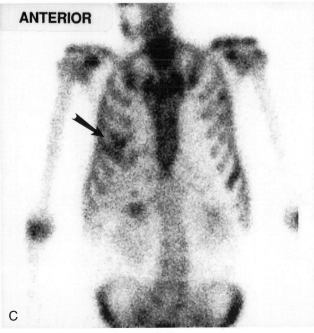

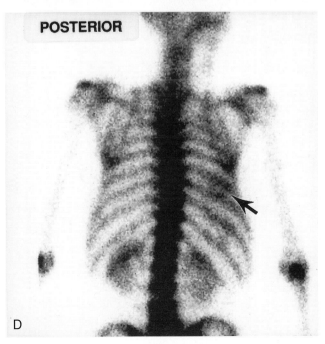

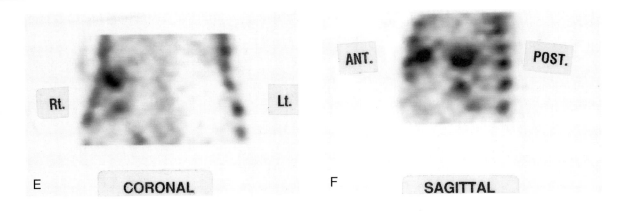

E   **CORONAL**   F   **SAGITTAL**

MEDIASTINAL NODAL UPTAKE ON BONE SCAN

Patient: Metastatic Seminoma

FIGURE 11–14.

Computer-Enhanced Delayed Bone Scan: There is mild diffuse activity in the mediastinum thought to be in metastatic lymph nodes. The scan was done 4 hours after injection, so this should not represent blood pool. Enlarged retroperitoneal lymph nodes are partially obstructing the ureters.

NOTE. Seminomas have a predilection for anterior mediastinal as well as retroperitoneal lymph node spread.

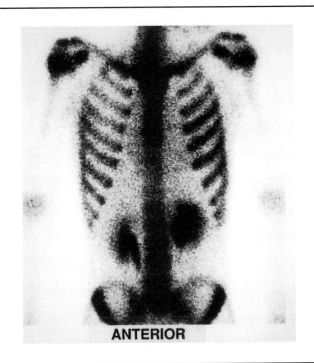

ANTERIOR

PLEURAL METASTASES

Patient 1

FIGURE 11–15 A.

Posterior Bone Scan: There is diffuse increased activity over the left hemithorax.

Patient 2

FIGURE 11–15 B.

Posterior Bone Scan: There is a left lower thoracic accumulation of the tracer in a loculated pleural effusion.

Patient 3

FIGURE 11–15 C.

Posterior Bone Scan: There is diffuse right upper pleural disease, with direct invasion of the spine *(arrow)* and several ribs by tumor.

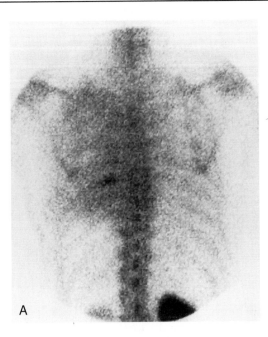

A

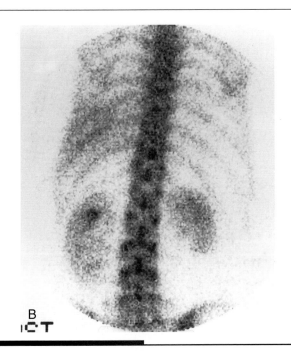

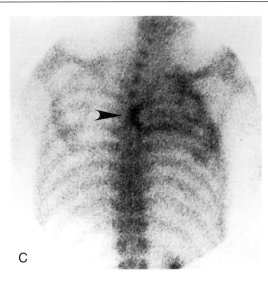

NOTE. If there is accumulation of the bone scanning agent in a pleural effusion, it is almost always malignant.

MALIGNANT PERICARDIAL EFFUSION

Patient 1

FIGURE 11–16 A.

Delayed Bone Scintigraphy: There is accumulation of the bone scanning radiopharmaceutical in the region of the heart *(arrowheads)*, in the known malignant pericardial effusion.

Patient 2

FIGURE 11–16 B.

Delayed Bone Scan: There is a broad linear-appearing soft tissue accumulation of the bone scanning agent across the bottom of the heart.

FIGURE 11–16 C.

SPECT Scan: The activity outlines the heart, suggesting pericardial disease.

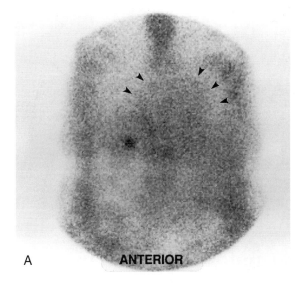

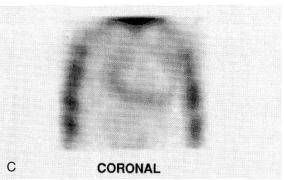

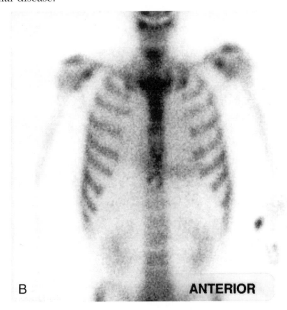

Illustration continued on following page

FIGURE 11–16   D.

Contrast-Enhanced CT Scan: There is a thick soft tissue density rim around the contrast-enhanced heart blood pool indicative of a dense pericardial effusion. Bilateral pleural effusions are also present.

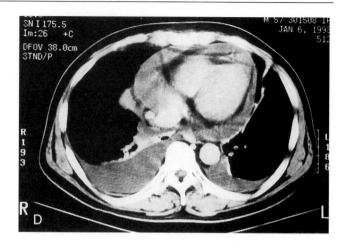

UPTAKE OF BONE SCANNING AGENTS IN THE HEART
1. Myocardial infarction
2. Hypercalcemia, including hyperparathyroidism
3. Amyloidosis
4. Myocarditis
5. Pericardial effusions, especially malignant
6. Myocardial contusion

MYOCARDIAL INFARCT WITH MDP

FIGURE 11–17.

Delayed Bone Scan: There is a curvilinear accumulation of the MDP in a 10 day old myocardial infarct.

NOTE. MDP is not as infarct avid as pyrophosphate and should not be used for myocardial infarct scanning.

Cross Reference

Chapter 53: Myocardial Infarction—Acute Myocardial Infarct on ^{99m}Tc-Pyrophosphate Scans

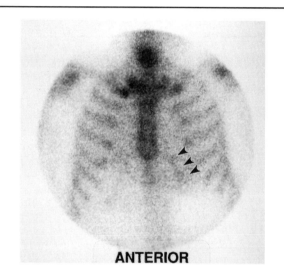

ANTERIOR

SENILE AMYLOID OF THE HEART ON BONE SCAN

FIGURE 11–18   A and B.

Anterior and LAO Chest Bone Scan: The entire heart accumulates the bone scan agent (^{99m}Tc-MDP).

NOTE. Senile amyloidosis is most often asymptomatic and has no clinical signs or ECG abnormalities.

Cross Reference

Chapter 54: ^{99M}Tc-Pyrophosphate Scanning—Cardiac Amyloidosis

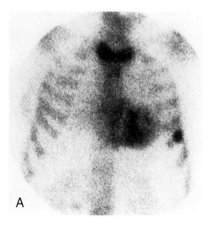

A

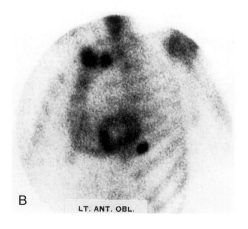

B   LT. ANT. OBL.

MALIGNANT ASCITES

Patient 1

FIGURE 11–19 A.

Supine Delayed Bone Scan: There is accumulation of the bone scan radiopharmaceutical at the periphery of the peritoneum (including the paracolic gutter) with bowel floating centrally.

Patient 2

FIGURE 11–19 B.

Total Body Bone Scan: The ascites can be seen within the abdomen as a round halo.

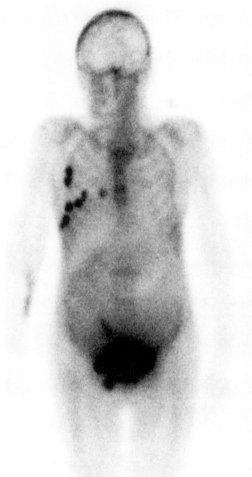

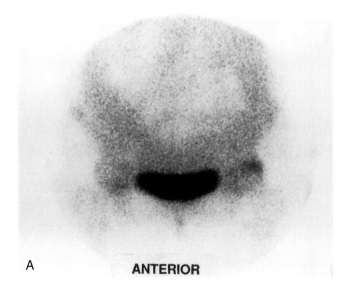

ADENOCARCINOMA METASTASES TO LIVER

Patient 1: Lung Carcinoma

FIGURE 11–20 A.

Anterior Chest and Abdomen Bone Scan: A metastasis to the liver retains the bone scan agent.

Patient 2: Colon Carcinoma

FIGURE 11–20 B.

Posterior Bone Scan: The ^{99m}Tc-MDP accumulates in the right lobe of the liver *(arrow)*.

FIGURE 11–20 C.

Posterior Liver Colloid Scan: There is a focal defect in the same area *(arrow)*.

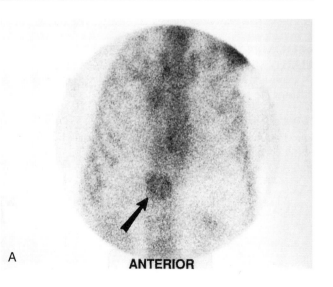

Illustration continued on following page

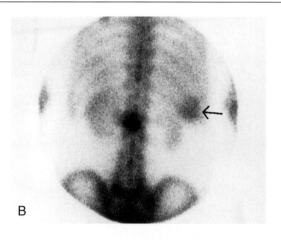

B

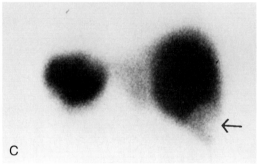

C

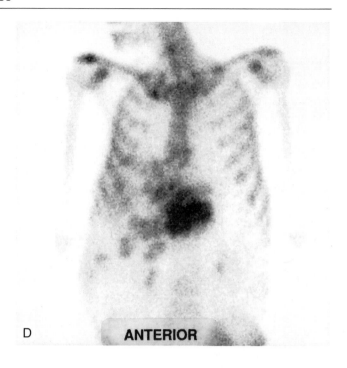

D

ANTERIOR

Patient 3: Colorectal Carcinoma

FIGURE 11–20   D.

Anterior Bone Scan: There are numerous metastases to the liver.

FIGURE 11–20   E.

CT Scan Without Contrast: There are multiple calcified metastases in both lobes of the liver.

NOTE. Liver metastases from mucin-secreting carcinomas (e.g., adenocarcinoma of the colon) are the most likely to take up the bone scanning agent.

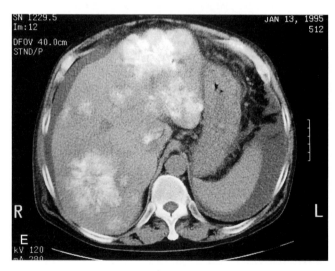

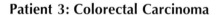

ABDOMINAL LYMPH NODES AND ADRENAL METASTASES ON BONE SCAN

Patient 1: Hodgkin's Disease

FIGURE 11–21   A.

Anterior Bone Scan: Areas of decreased activity are present within the abdomen.

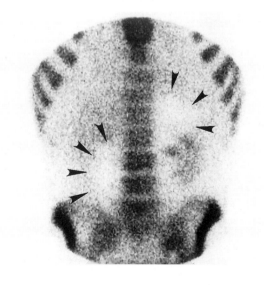

A

FIGURE 11–21   B.

CT Scan: There are bilateral enlarged para-aortic lymph nodes.

Patient 2: Lung Carcinoma

FIGURE 11–21   C.

Posterior Bone Scan: The "cold" adrenal metastases *(arrowheads)* distort and displace the kidneys.

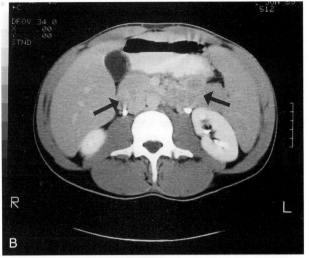

DIFFUSE LIVER ACTIVITY ON BONE SCAN
1. Artifact from very recent liver scan
2. Ischemia, anoxic damage
3. Amyloidosis
4. Iron overload, IV iron therapy
5. Chemotherapy
6. Elevated serum aluminum
7. Faulty radiopharmaceutical preparation (colloid formation)
8. Contrast media: sodium diatrizoate, iohexol
9. Liver necrosis

From Poulton TB, Rauchenstein JN, Murphy WD: Clin Nucl Med 11:864, 1992.

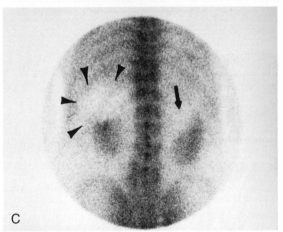

DIFFUSE LIVER ACTIVITY ON BONE SCAN

Patient 1: Ischemic Liver Necrosis

FIGURE 11–22   A.

Anterior Bone Scan: There is mild diffuse liver activity.

Patient 2: Chemotherapy Damage to Liver

FIGURE 11–22   B.

Anterior Bone Scan: The liver necrosis from chemotherapy is thought to have caused the uptake of the bone scanning agent.

Illustration continued on following page

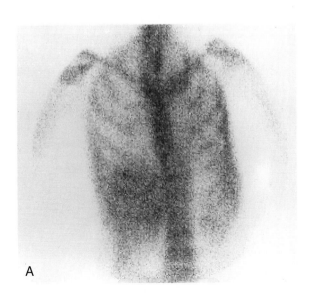

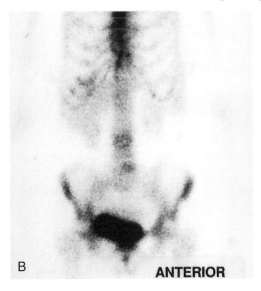

Patient 3: Amyloidosis

FIGURE 11–22   C.
SPECT ^{99m}Tc-Pyrophosphate Scan: There is diffuse liver activity in this patient examined for myocardial infarction.

NOTE. Liver necrosis can be seen with bone marrow transplantation, presumably the result of veno-occlusive disease.

Cross References

Chapter 14: Liver Dysfunction—Amyloid Liver Disease

Chapter 54: ^{99M}Tc-Pyrophosphate Scanning—Cardiac Amyloidosis

C   **CORONAL**

PTOTIC KIDNEY ON BONE SCAN

FIGURE 11–23   A.
Blood Pool Scan: In the left decubitus position, the right kidney overlies the lower spine, simulating a hyperemic abnormality.

FIGURE 11–23   B.
Bone Scan: In the supine position, the right kidney is higher and more lateral.

NOTE 1. From supine to upright, a ptotic kidney will move inferiorly.

NOTE 2. A ptotic kidney is almost always on the right side.

Cross Reference

Chapter 35: Normal/Normal Variants—Ptotic Kidney

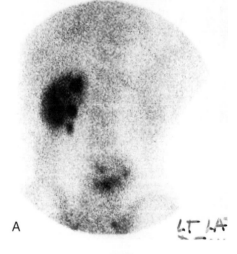

A

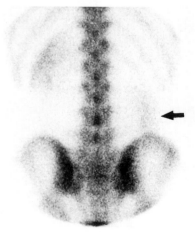

B

PELVIC KIDNEY

FIGURE 11–24   A.

Whole Body Bone Scan: There is increased activity over the lower lumbar spine on the anterior view.

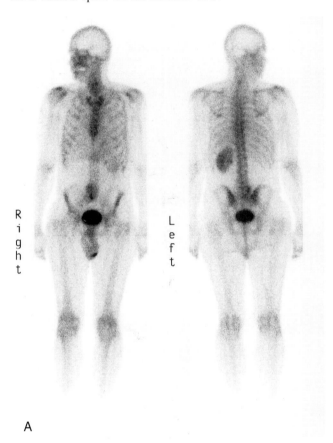

A

FIGURE 11–24   B and C.

Sagittal and Transverse SPECT Bone Scans: The increased activity represents the right kidney with its pelvis anterior.

Cross Reference

Chapter 35: Normal/Normal Variants—Pelvic Kidneys

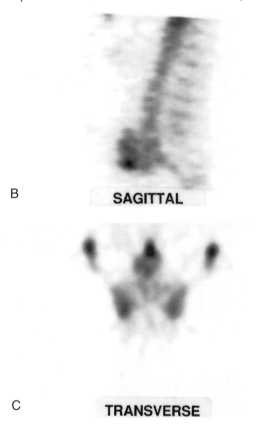

B   **SAGITTAL**

C   **TRANSVERSE**

TRANSPLANTED KIDNEY ON BONE SCAN

FIGURE 11–25.

Anterior Delayed Bone Scan: The transplanted kidney, with normal-appearing calyces, is seen in the right pelvis.

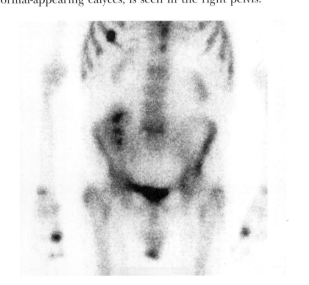

DIFFERENTIAL DIAGNOSIS OF "HOT" KIDNEYS ON BONE SCAN
1. Urinary obstruction
2. Chemotherapeutic, radiation, and antibiotic therapies
3. Acute renal failure (acute tubular necrosis)
4. Hypercalcemia (metastatic calcification)
5. Multiple myeloma
6. Leukemia
7. Lymphoma
8. Sickle cell anemia
9. Amyloidosis
10. Renal artery stenosis
11. Renal vein thrombosis
12. Lupus nephritis
13. Myoglobinuria, rhabdomyolysis
14. Idiopathic

"HOT" KIDNEYS ON BONE SCAN

Patient 1: Sickle Cell Anemia

FIGURE 11–26   A.

Bone Scan: There is intense renal activity in this patient during sickle cell crisis. The kidneys appear enlarged.

Patient 2: Breast Carcinoma Treated with Doxorubicin

FIGURE 11–26   B.

Initial Scan: The kidneys had excreted virtually all the ^{99m}Tc-MDP by the time the scan was obtained.

FIGURE 11–26   C and D.

Bone Scan 2 Months Later: There is intense activity within both kidneys, which appear enlarged.

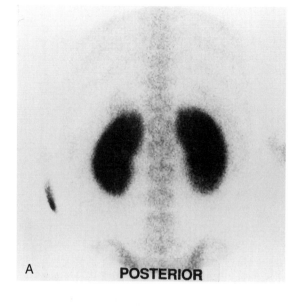

A   **POSTERIOR**

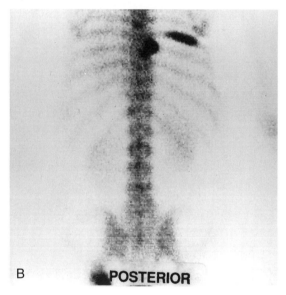

B   **POSTERIOR**

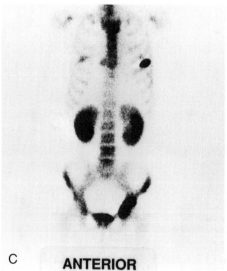

C   **ANTERIOR**

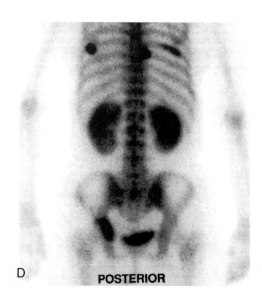

D   **POSTERIOR**

URINARY OBSTRUCTION ON BONE SCAN

Patient 1

FIGURE 11–27   A.

Posterior Pelvis Bone Scan: The right kidney has intense activity in the massively dilated renal collecting system.

Patient 2

FIGURE 11–27   B.

Posterior Lumbar Spine Bone Scan: The right kidney is hydronephrotic. In this case, a rim of functioning cortex can be seen surrounding the dilated collecting system.

Cross Reference

Chapter 36: Unilateral Abnormalities—Urinary Obstruction due to Retroperitoneal Tumor

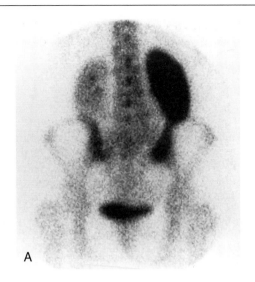

A

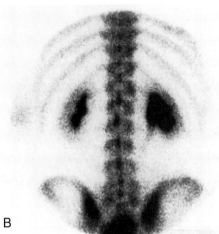

B

OBSTRUCTED LOWER POLE CALYX

FIGURE 11–28   A to C.

Anterior, Posterior, and Oblique Bone Scan: The left lower pole calyx is abnormally dilated.

Illustration continued on following page

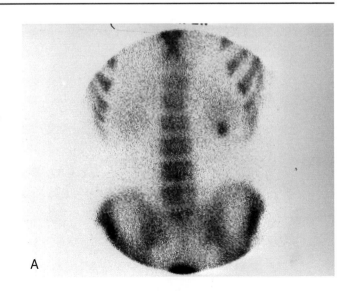

A

FIGURE 11–28 D.

AP Plain Film X-ray: A calcification is seen in the lower pole of the left kidney, which subsequently proved to be a stone obstructing the calyx.

NOTE. The lower pole of each kidney is more anterior than the upper pole. It should not be distended in the supine position. Distention of the upper pole calyx is normal when studies are done supine. The opposite is true for upright scans.

Cross Reference

Chapter 36: Unilateral Abnormalities—Lower Pole Calyceal Obstruction

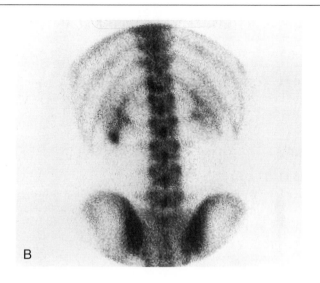

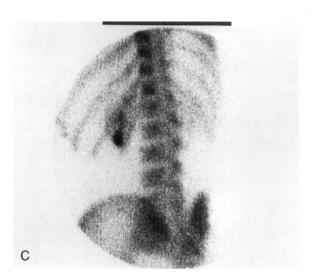

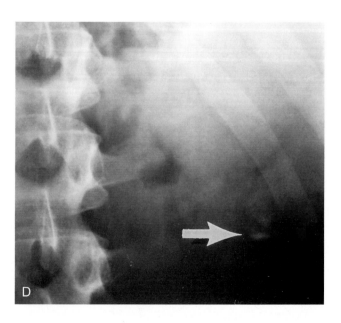

URINOMA ON BONE SCAN

FIGURE 11–29   A and B.

Whole Body Bone Scan Detail: There is a dense urine collection behind the left kidney, with extravasated urine dissecting down the left paracolic gutter.

Cross Reference

Chapter 36: Unilateral Abnormalities—Urinoma

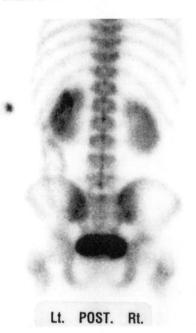

A   **Lt. POST. Rt.**

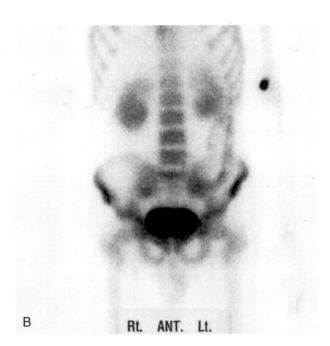

B   **Rt. ANT. Lt.**

RENAL CYST ON BONE SCAN

Patient 1: Giant Renal Cyst

FIGURE 11–30   A.

Blood Pool Scintigraphy: The left kidney *(arrow)* is displaced and compressed medially toward the spine. There is a large photon-deficient area *(arrowheads)* where the normal kidney should reside.

Illustration continued on following page

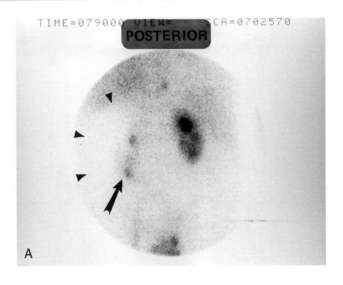

A

FIGURE 11–30   B.

Delayed Bone Scan: The left kidney is not seen.

FIGURE 11–30   C.

CT Scan: There is a huge simple cyst displacing the left kidney anteromedially.

Patient 2: Solitary Renal Cyst

FIGURE 11–30   D.

Delayed Bone Scintigraphy in the Right Posterior Oblique: A round defect in the midpole of the right kidney represents the mass effect of a large renal cyst.

Patient 3: Multiple Renal Cysts

FIGURE 11–30   E.

LPO Enhanced Bone Scan: There are at least three cysts in the left kidney and two in the right.

Cross Reference

Chapter 39: Renal Defects—Unilateral Simple Cysts

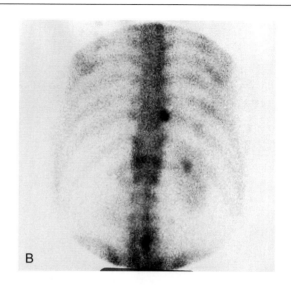

B

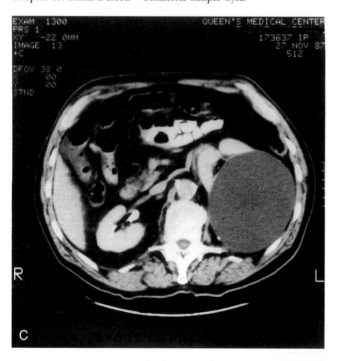

C

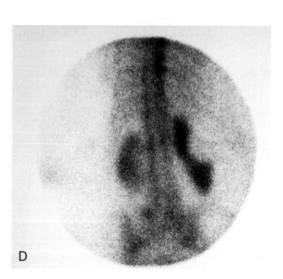

D

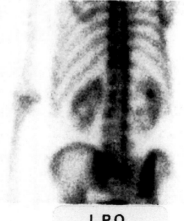

E   L.P.O.

LYMPHOMA IN BONE AND KIDNEY

FIGURE 11–31   A.

Posterior Enhanced Lumbar Bone Scan: The left kidney is large and retains the radiopharmaceutical. There is a "cold" abnormality involving the L2 vertebra *(arrow)*.

FIGURE 11–31   B.

Anterior Lumbar Bone Scan: The "cold" abnormality is better seen *(arrow)*.

NOTE 1. Lymphoma in the kidney may present as a general enlargement of the kidney rather than discrete mass lesions, probably owing to diffuse infiltration.

NOTE 2. Lymphoma of the kidneys is most often secondary and bilateral.

NOTE 3. Enlarged retroperitoneal lymph nodes may obstruct the ureters.

Cross References

Chapter 11: Soft Tissue Abnormalities—Mediastinal Nodal Uptake on Bone Scan

Chapter 72: Tumors—Gallium-Avid Lymphomas

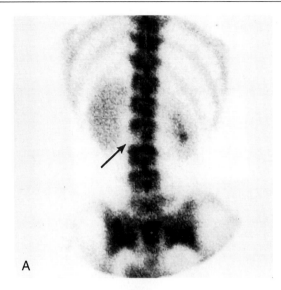

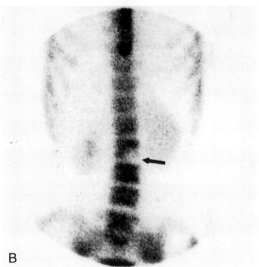

RENAL CELL CARCINOMA ON BONE SCAN

Patient 1

FIGURE 11–32   A.

Posterior Bone Scan: The primary tumor has no appreciable accumulation of the bone agent *(arrowheads)* and appears as a defect in the kidneys. There are pleural metastases that do take up the radiopharmaceutical *(arrows)*.

Illustration continued on following page

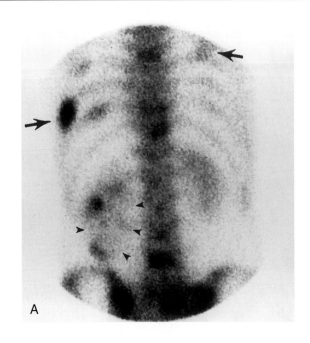

Patient 2

FIGURE 11–32 B.

Delayed Bone Scan: The right kidney *(arrow)* is displaced and tipped inferiorly by an upper pole mass. This is not a ptotic kidney.

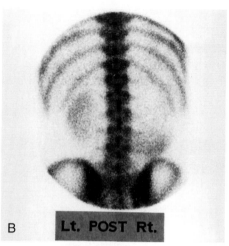

B Lt. POST Rt.

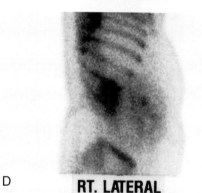

D RT. LATERAL

Patient 3

FIGURE 11–32 C and D.

Anterior and Lateral Bone Scan: The large abdominal mass retains the bone scanning agent.

FIGURE 11–32 E.

CT Scan: The mass arises from the right kidney.

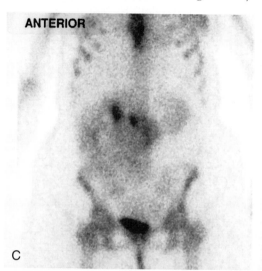

ANTERIOR

C

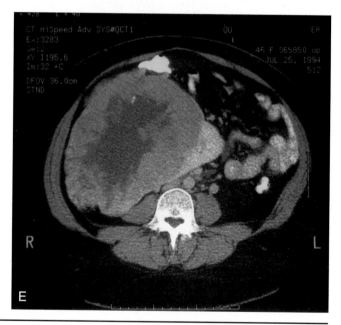

E

TERATOMA ON BONE SCAN

FIGURE 11–33.

Anterior Bone Scan: There is a bilobed mass taking up the bone scanning agent overlying the sacrum and the right sacroiliac (SI) joint region. The tiny foci of greater activity are presumed to be in teeth and bone. Another nodule is seen just inferior to the mass on the right.

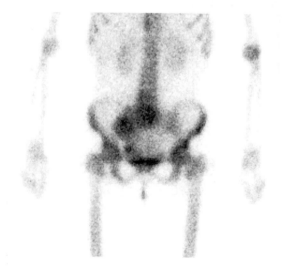

ILEAL LOOP ON BONE SCAN

FIGURE 11–34.

Anterior Pelvic Bone Scan: There is no normal urinary bladder. The collection of radioactive urine in the right pelvis represents an ileal loop. The stoma *(arrow)* is on the left.

Cross Reference

Chapter 37: Bilateral Abnormalities—Ileal Loop

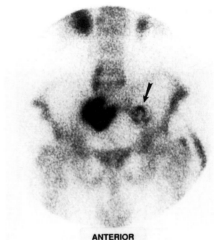

ANTERIOR

ENTEROVESICAL FISTULA ON BONE SCAN

Patient: Crohn's Disease

FIGURE 11–35.

Anterior Pelvic Bone Scan: The small bowel *(arrowhead)* connects to the bladder through a wide fistula *(arrow)*.

NOTE. Causes of enterovesical fistulas include Crohn's disease, diverticulitis, radiation therapy, and carcinomatous fistulas.

Cross Reference

Chapter 33: Gastrointestinal and Abdominal Infections—Inflammatory Bowel Disease

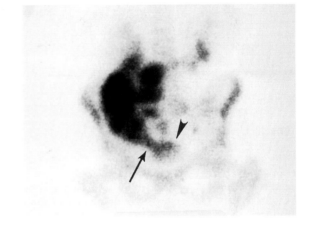

NEUROGENIC BLADDER

FIGURE 11–36 A.

Posterior Bone Scan: The urinary bladder is markedly distended.

Illustration continued on following page

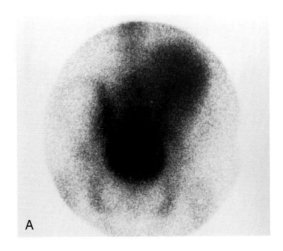

A

FIGURE 11–36   B.

Intravenous Urogram: Massive distention of the neurogenic bladder can be seen.

Cross Reference

Chapter 40: Bladder Abnormalities—Neurogenic Bladder with Secondary Hydronephrosis

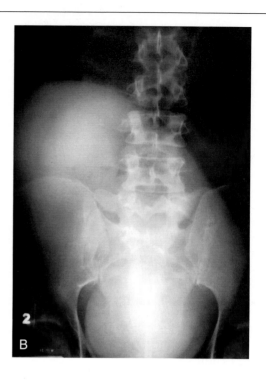

BLADDER DIVERTICULUM ON BONE SCAN

Patient 1: Urinary Tract Infection

FIGURE 11–37   A and B.

Anterior and Posterior Pelvic Bone Scans: The increased intensity of the radiopharmaceutical within the bladder is due to summation of urine radioactivity in both the diverticulum and the bladder.

FIGURE 11–37   C.

Posterior WBC Scan: There are WBCs in the region of the bladder diverticulum *(arrow)*, indicating the presence of an inflammatory process. The left SI joint is also abnormal.

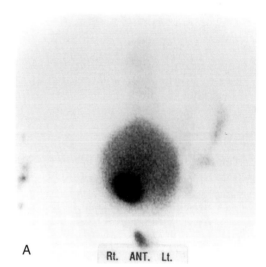

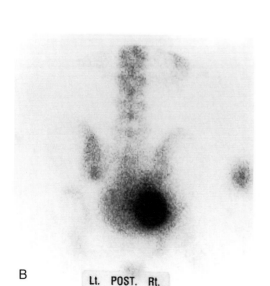

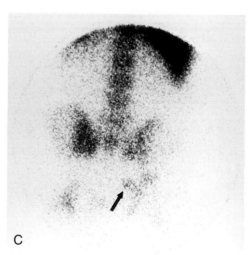

Patient 2: Hutch Diverticulum and Metastatic Lung Cancer

FIGURE 11–37 D.

Posterior Bone Scan: There is a small bladder diverticulum in the region of the left trigone without ureteral obstruction.

NOTE 1. Bladder diverticula can develop stones and infections, presumably owing to stasis of urine.

NOTE 2. Hutch diverticula are seen in the region of the trigone, most often in paraplegics, and can be a cause of ureteral stasis.

Cross Reference

Chapter 40: Bladder Abnormalities—Bladder Diverticulum

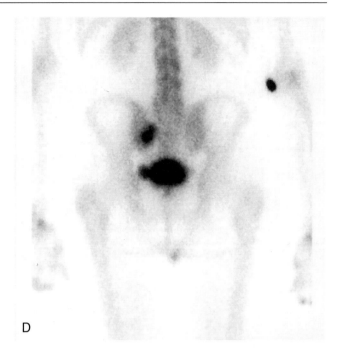

D

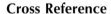

IMPRESSIONS ON THE BLADDER

Patient 1: Enlarged Prostate

FIGURE 11–38 A.

Posterior Pelvic Bone Scans: There is an extrinsic impression on the inferior bladder wall.

Illustration continued on following page

EXTRINISTIC PRESSURE DEFORMITY ON THE BLADDER
1. Prostate enlargement
2. Uterine enlargement (pregnancy, tumors)
3. Colonic distention, small bowel distention
4. Pelvic abscess
5. Hematoma
6. Lymphadenopathy
7. Pelvic fibrolipomatosis
8. Retroperitoneal tumor
9. Venous collaterals
10. Ovarian tumor or cyst
11. Other neoplasms

A   **POSTERIOR**

See also Chapter 40: Bladder Abnormalities—Bladder Hematoma.

Patient 2: Prostate Carcinoma Invading the Pelvis

FIGURE 11–38   B and C.
Anterior and Posterior Pelvic Bone Scans: There is an impression upon the bladder from the left side.

FIGURE 11–38   D and E.
Anterior and Posterior Pelvic Bone Scan 1 Year Later: The bladder now has a small capacity, and the left ureter is obstructed in the pelvis.

Patient 3: Prostate Cancer Invading the Pelvic Floor

FIGURE 11–38   F.
Anterior Bone Scan: The bladder is elevated out of the pelvic floor by tumor. A Foley catheter is in place.

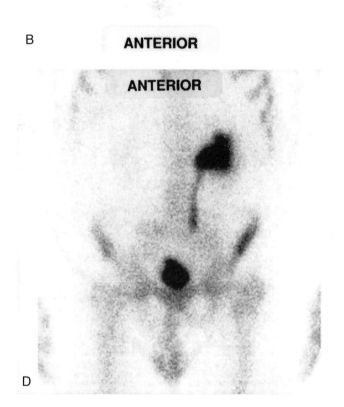

B   **ANTERIOR**

ANTERIOR

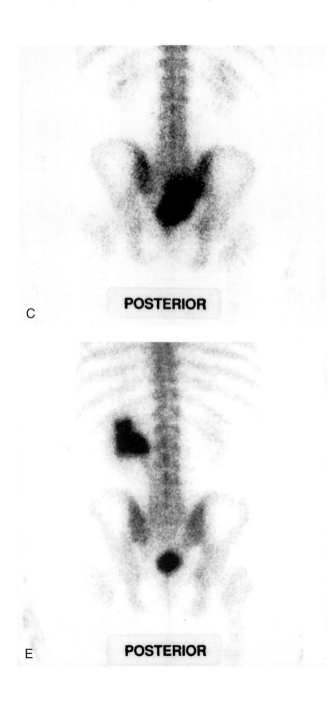

C   **POSTERIOR**

D

E   **POSTERIOR**

Patient 4: Uterine Blush

FIGURE 11–38   G.
Blood Pool Scintigraphy: There is a round vascular blush above and to the left of the urinary bladder.

FIGURE 11–38   H.
Delayed Bone Scintigraphy: The impression upon the bladder dome from the uterus can be seen as decreased activity, since the vascular phase has cleared.

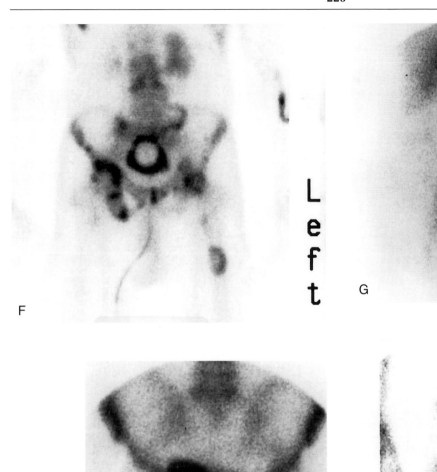

F

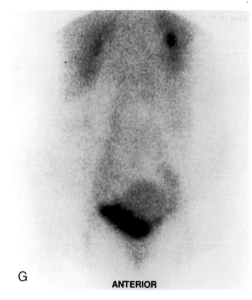

L e f t

G

ANTERIOR

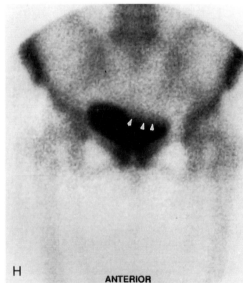

H   **ANTERIOR**

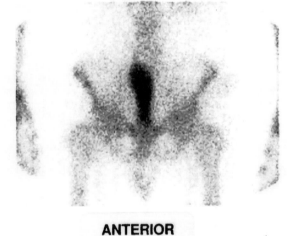

I   **ANTERIOR**

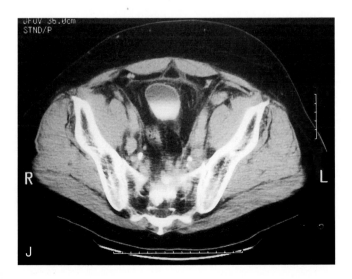

J

Patient 5: Pelvic Fibrolipomatosis

FIGURE 11–38   I.
Anterior Bone Scan: The bladder is constricted from both sides.

FIGURE 11–38   J.
Pelvic CT: The bladder is surrounded by an abnormal amount of fat.

NOTE 1. Impressions on the bladder can also be from the colon, usually the cecum, and small bowel.

NOTE 2. The prostatic impression is best seen on the posterior view when scanning the supine patient.

Cross References

Chapter 2: Multiple Bony Abnormalities—Congenital Hip Dysplasia

Chapter 4: Pelvic Abnormalities—Pelvic Fractures

Chapter 8: Hyperemia—Uterine Hyperemia

HYDROCOELE ON BONE SCAN

FIGURE 11–39.

Anterior Pelvic Bone Scan: There is a photon-deficient area in the right scrotum that represents a hydrocoele *(arrowhead).* (Courtesy of Dr. Michael Kipper, Vista, CA.)

NOTE. Any mass can present as a "cold" area on bone scan if it is avascular or hypovascular.

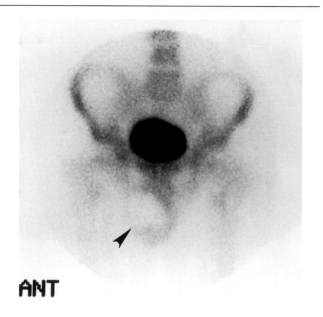

ANT

CELLULITIS ON BONE SCAN

FIGURE 11–40.

Delayed Bone Scan: The inflamed soft tissues of the left calf accumulate the bone scanning agent. Biopsy of the tibia was negative for infection.

NOTE 1. Cellulitis causes diffuse, mildly increased osteogenesis, whereas osteomyelitis usually has localized, intense osteogenesis.

NOTE 2. Cellulitis will accompany osteomyelitis.

Cross References

Chapter 1: Solitary Bony Abnormalities—Stump Infection

Chapter 8: Hyperemia—Cellulitis without Osteomyelitis

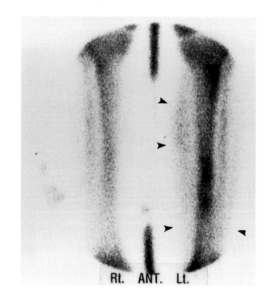

Rt. ANT. Lt.

TENDINITIS ON BONE SCAN

Patient 1

FIGURE 11–41 A.

Blood Pool Scintigraphy: There is localized hyperemia involving the distal Achilles tendon.

FIGURE 11–41 B.

Delayed Bone Scan: The distal Achilles tendon has intense activity.

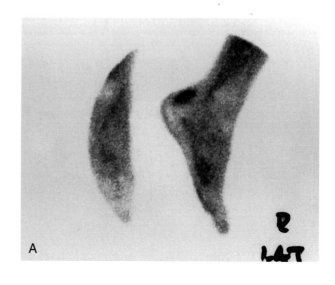

A

LAT

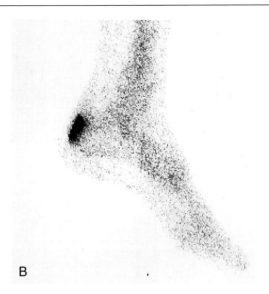

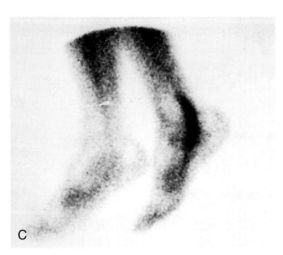

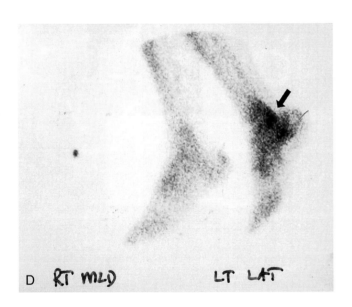

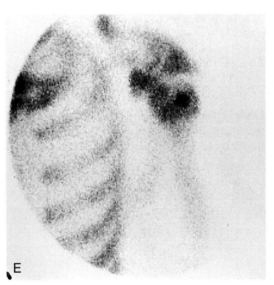

Patient 2

FIGURE 11–41   C.

Blood Pool Scintigraphy: There is marked hyperemia along the peroneal tendons.

FIGURE 11–41   D.

Delayed Bone Scan: There is a small focus of increased osteogenesis that may present a calcific deposit within the peroneal tendons or reactive bone changes from the hyperemia.

Patient 3

FIGURE 11–41   E and F.

Delayed Shoulder Bone Scan in External Rotation (E) and Internal Rotation (F): There is increased activity in the left subscapularis tendon in calcific tendinitis *(arrowhead)*. The area of increased activity moves medially with internal rotation, demonstrating the anterior location of the subscapularis tendon. If it moved laterally it would be the supraspinatus tendon.

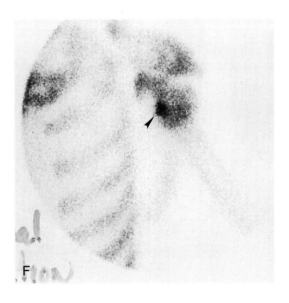

NOTE. In tendinitis, the bone scanning agent accumulates in the tendon, whereas in an enthesopathy, the abnormality is along the surface of the bone where the tendon or ligament attaches.

Cross Reference

Chapter 1: Solitary Bony Abnormalities—Osteochondroma of Talus; Ischial Enthesopathy

DELAYED ONSET MUSCLE STRAIN (DOMS)

Patient 1: Beginner Surfer

FIGURE 11–42   A and B.

Anterior and Posterior Bone Scan: The deltoid muscles have ^{99m}Tc-MDP accumulation.

Patient 2: Weightlifter

FIGURE 11–42   C and D.

Anterior and RPO Lower Leg Bone Scan: The gastrocnemius muscle is abnormal owing to overuse.

NOTE. DOMS is due to overuse of unconditioned muscles, which hurt for several days after exercise. The scan can remain positive after the relief of pain.

DIFFERENTIAL DIAGNOSIS OF MUSCLE UPTAKE ON BONE SCAN
1. Direct trauma causing acute or delayed necrosis
2. Overuse (DOMS)
3. Electrical injury
4. Infection
5. Frostbite
6. Polymyositis, dermatomyositis
7. Active muscular dystrophy
8. Injections
9. Hyperparathyroidism/hypercalcemia

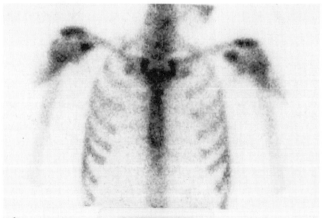

A   **ANTERIOR**

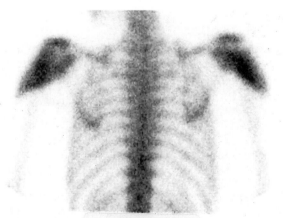

B   **POSTERIOR**

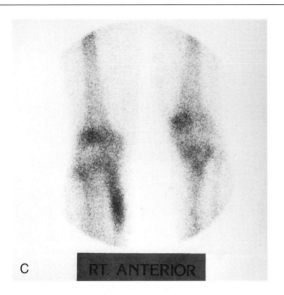

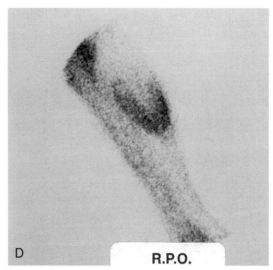

MUSCLE NECROSIS ON BONE SCAN

FIGURE 11–43   A to C.

Blood Flow and Blood Pool Scintigraphy: There is marked increased blood flow and hyperemia involving the anterolateral right thigh.

FIGURE 11–43   D.

Delayed Bone Scan: The soft tissue of the right thigh retains some of the bone scanning agent. The increased activity of the femur was due to a femoral fracture 5 years earlier, along with a response of the bone to the soft tissue hyperemia.

FIGURE 11–43   E.

T1 with Gadolinium Axial MR Scan of the Thigh: There is marked contrast enhancement of the vastus lateralis with central low signal, which was due to necrotic tissue.

NOTE. Muscle necrosis can develop immediately after an acute insult, or after several years.

Illustration continued on following page

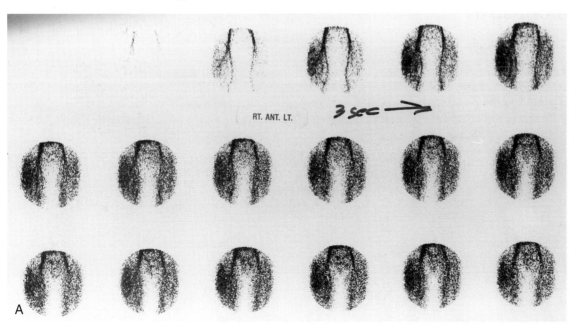

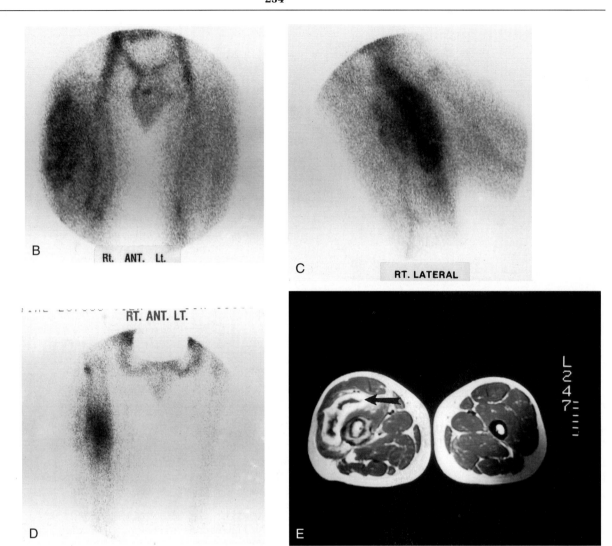

MYOSITIS OSSIFICANS (HETEROTOPIC BONE)

Patient 1: C7 Paraplegic

FIGURE 11–44   A.

Blood Pool Scintigraphy: There is hyperemia involving soft tissue areas. The left femoral metaphysis has increased blood pool from a recent fracture *(arrowhead)*.

FIGURE 11–44   B.

Delayed Bone Scan: The intense soft tissue activity in this patient proved to be myositis ossificans. The fracture *(arrowhead)* is partially covered by the myositis.

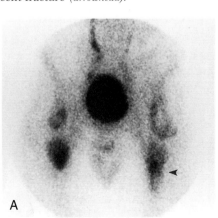

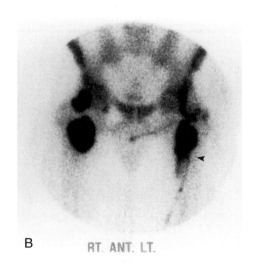

Patient 2: Post-traumatic

FIGURE 11–44   C.

Delayed Bone Scan: The right hip is obscured by the massive heterotopic bone.

FIGURE 11–44   D.

Delayed Bone Scan 8 Months Later: The myositis ossificans is no longer as evident, since it is not as active.

Patient 3: 11 Year Old Girl

FIGURE 11–44   E.

Delayed Bone Scan: There is a round extraosseous focus of increased osteogenesis adjacent to the right proximal humeral diaphysis. This was surgically removed and proved to be myositis ossificans.

NOTE. Hyperemia indicates that the myositis is active.

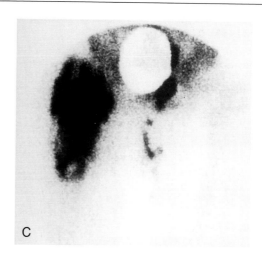

C

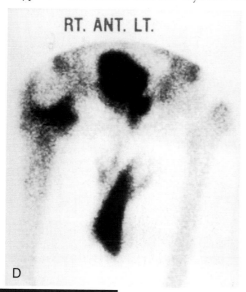

D

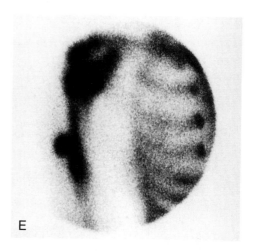

E

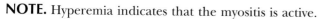

ACTIVE SYNOVIAL OSTEOCHONDROMATOSIS

FIGURE 11–45   A and B.

Anterior and Posterior Blood Pool Scans: There is mild hyperemia surrounding the left hip extending beyond the joint capsule.

Illustration continued on following page

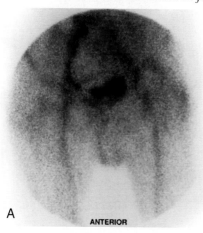

A

ANTERIOR

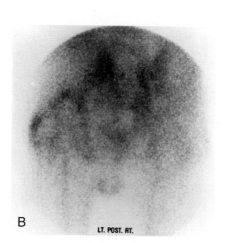

B

LT. POST. RT.

FIGURE 11–45   C and D.

Anterior and Posterior Pelvic Delayed Bone Scan: There is intense activity over the left hip superiorly and posteriorly.

FIGURE 11–45   E.

Plain Film X-ray: An osteochondral loose body *(arrow)* is seen in the same location as the scan abnormality.

NOTE. The extensive hyperemia is probably due to a synovitis or capsulitis.

Cross Reference

Chapter 2: Multiple Bony Abnormalities—Bilateral Congenital Hip Dysplasia

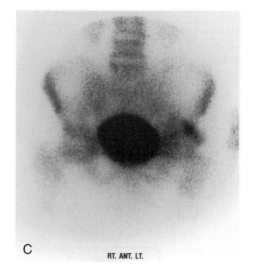

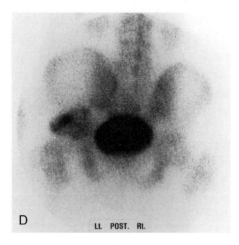

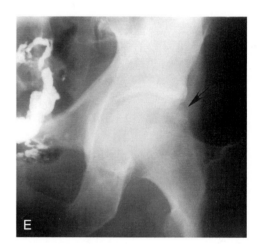

POLYMYOSITIS ON BONE SCAN

FIGURE 11–46   A and B.

Delayed Bone Scans: There is fairly symmetric uptake in the deltoid and triceps muscles as well as the adductor muscles of the thighs.

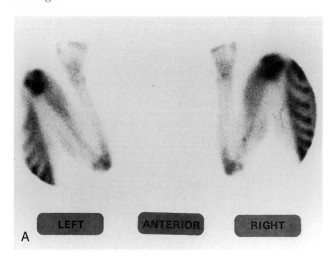

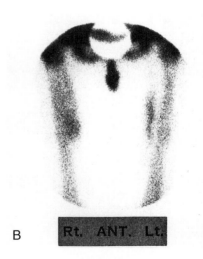

PORPHYRIA CUTANEA TARDA

FIGURE 11–47   A and B.

Anterior Hip Bone Scans: There is linear soft tissue activity in the fascia lata.

FIGURE 11–47   C.

Anterior Thigh Bone Scan: The skin activity is abnormal.

NOTE. The bone scanning agent may accumulate in the cutaneous scars that form in porphyria.

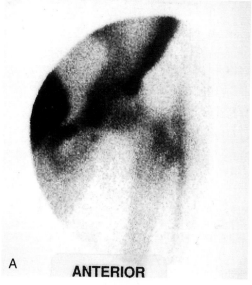

A   **ANTERIOR**

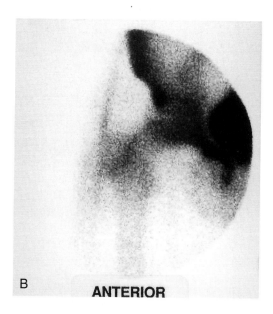

B   **ANTERIOR**

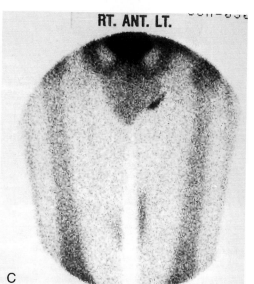

RT. ANT. LT.

C

INJECTION "EXTRAVASATION" SEEN ON BONE SCAN

FIGURE 11–48.

Posterior Bone Scintigraphy: There is a broad collection of the bone scanning agent in the left buttock owing to dispersion of an intramuscular injection of dextran several weeks earlier. The injected material spread out beyond the confines of the muscle into the subcutaneous tissue *(arrow)*.

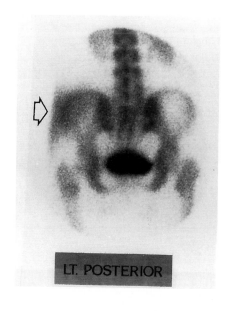

LT. POSTERIOR

HEMATOMA ON BONE SCAN

FIGURE 11–49   A.

Planar Bone Scan: There are at least two intense collections of the bone scanning agent overlying L4 and L5.

FIGURE 11–49   B and C.

Transverse and Sagittal SPECT Scan: The abnormal collections are posterior *(arrow)* in post-traumatic hematomas.(Courtesy of Dr. Michael Kipper, Vista, CA.)

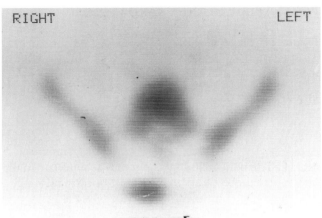

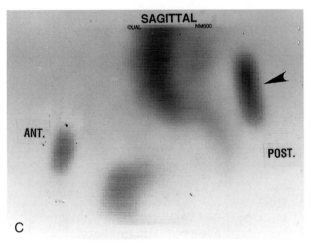

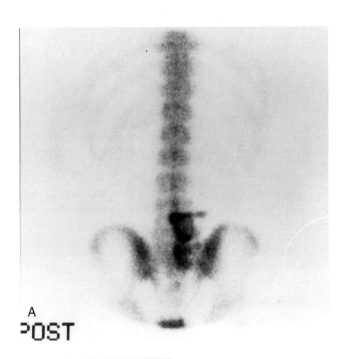

HEMANGIOMA

FIGURE 11–50   A.

Blood Pool Scan: There is irregular and incomplete filling of an antecubital mass on the 10 minute view.

FIGURE 11–50   B.

Delayed Bone Scan: The mass is well circumscribed and provokes no change in the nearby bones.

Cross References

Chapter 7: Hands and Feet—Bone and Soft Tissue Hemangioma of the Foot

Chapter 15: Solitary Liver Defects—Hemangioma

Chapter 17: Multiple Liver Defects—Multiple Hepatic Hemangiomas

Chapter 59: Venous Thrombosis—Leg Hemangioma on Tagged RBC Scan

Chapter 72: Tumors—Giant Hemangioma (Kasabach-Merritt Syndrome)

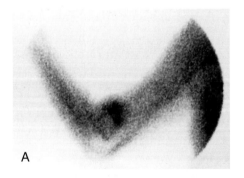

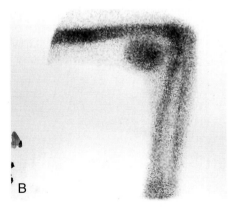

MÖNCKEBERG'S SCLEROSIS (VASCULAR OSSIFICATIONS)

FIGURE 11–51.
Delayed Bone Scintigraphy: The superficial femoral arteries are well seen bilaterally.

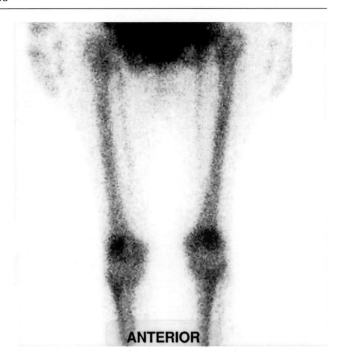

LYMPHEDEMA ON BONE SCAN

Patient 1: Prostate Cancer

FIGURE 11–52   A.
Bone Scan: There are marked soft tissue swelling and increased activity involving the right leg, especially in the subcutaneous tissue (dermal backflow) *(arrowheads)*.

Illustration continued on following page

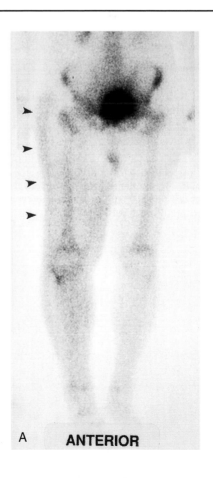

Patient 2: Testicular Cancer with Right Pelvic Mass

FIGURE 11–52   B.

Whole Body Anterior and Posterior Bone Scan: There is retained radioactivity in the soft tissues of the edematous right leg. The pelvic mass obstructs the lymphatics, displaces the bladder to the left, and obstructs the right kidney.

NOTE 1. Dermal backflow indicates lymphatic obstruction. This is best studied with intradermal injection of a radiocolloid in the extremity.

NOTE 2. Lymphedema can also be caused by patent but slow-flowing lymphatics. A swollen extremity may be present, but no dermal backflow will then be seen on lymphoscintigraphy.

Cross Reference

Chapter 61: Lymphatics—Lymphatic Obstruction

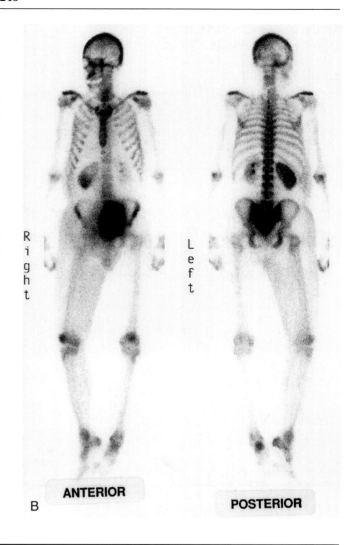

ANTERIOR   POSTERIOR

B

DEEP VENOUS THROMBOSIS ON BLOOD POOL IMAGING

FIGURE 11–53   A and B.

Anterior Lower Leg and Distal Thigh Blood Pool Scan: There are irregular vascular structures along the medial aspect of the larger right calf. The popliteal and distal femoral veins are not seen. The left calf has normal-appearing deep veins, including well-visualized popliteal and distal femoral veins.

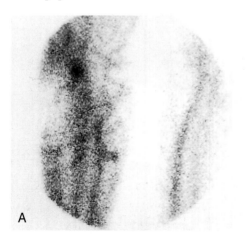

A

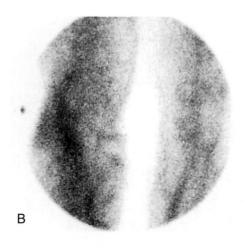

B

SCAR VISUALIZATION ON BONE SCAN

Patient 1

FIGURE 11–54   A.
Bone Scintigraphy: There is an inverted V accumulation of the MDP in two surgical incision scars.

Patient 2

FIGURE 11–54   B and C.
Anterior and Lateral Abdominal Bone Scans: An abdominal wall keloid has evidence of ossification.

Patient 3: Partial Scar Ossification

FIGURE 11–54   D.
Anterior Abdominal Bone Scan: The midline hot spot is partial ossification of a long abdominal surgical scar.

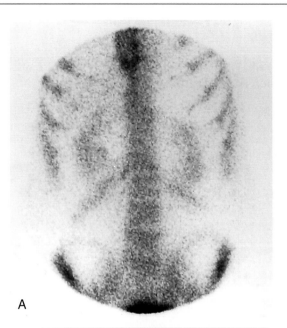

A

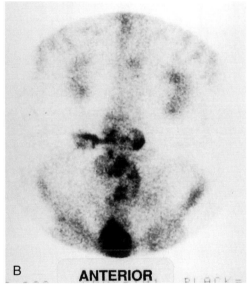

B   ANTERIOR

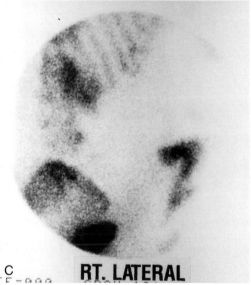

C   RT. LATERAL

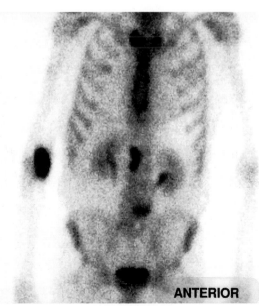

D   ANTERIOR

BONE SCAN OF FETUS AT 30 WEEKS' GESTATION

Patient: 28 Year Old Female with Giant Cell Tumor of the Right Tibia

FIGURE 11–55.

Anterior Whole Body Scan: There is uptake in the fetus *(arrow)*, persistent activity in the placenta *(arrowhead),* and marked uptake in the giant cell tumor in the right proximal tibial metaphysis. (From McKenzie A, Budd R, Yang C, et al: Technetium-99m-methylene diphosphonate uptake in the fetal skeleton at 30 weeks' gestation. J Nucl Med 35(8): 1338–1341, 1994.

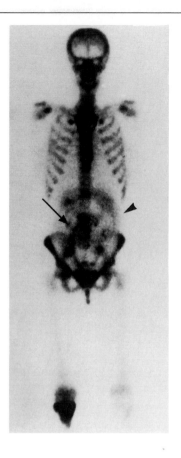

Chapter 12
Normal/Normal Variants

NORMAL PLANAR LIVER/SPLEEN SCAN

Patient 1

FIGURE 12–1   A to H.
Anterior, RAO, Right Lateral, RPO, Posterior, LPO, Left Lateral, and LAO Scans of the Liver and Spleen: The radiocolloid distribution should be homogeneous in both organs.

NOTE 1. The normal liver measures 10 to 15 cm in the right midclavicular line.

NOTE 2. The normal spleen should measure under 13 cm in its longest diameter.

NOTE 3. The splenic intensity should be less than the liver's radiocolloid accumulation. The bone marrow of the spine should be barely visible or nonvisualized.

NOTE 4. The number of views used for planar scans of the liver varies from laboratory to laboratory, but oblique views are definitely helpful in detecting masses and separating the left lobe from the spleen.

Illustration continued on following page

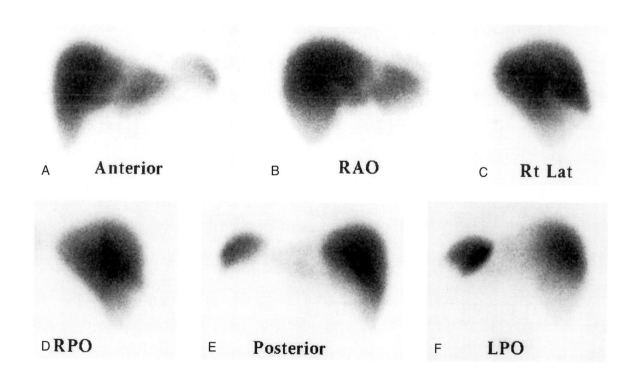

A   **Anterior**   B   **RAO**   C   **Rt Lat**

D **RPO**   E   **Posterior**   F   **LPO**

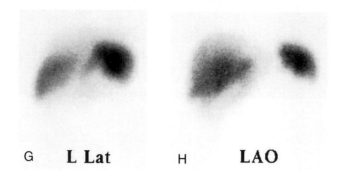

G   **L Lat**   H   **LAO**

NORMAL LIVER/SPLEEN SPECT SCAN

FIGURE 12–2   A to G.

Coronal, Transverse, and Sagittal ^{99m}Tc-Colloid SPECT Scans: There is homogeneous distribution of the radiocolloid within the liver, except for the intrinsic ducts and veins.(Portal venous and biliary structures = PB. Hepatic veins = HV. Porta hepatis = PH. Gallbladder fossa = G. Renal fossa = R.)

FIGURE 12–2   H.

Planar Posterior ^{99m}Tc-Colloid Liver and ^{99m}Tc-DTPA Renal Scans: The right kidney can be seen filling the renal fossa *(arrow).*

FIGURE 12–2   I to K.

Transverse, Coronal, and Sagittal ^{99m}Tc-Colloid SPECT Scan: The apparent mass in the posterior right lobe of the liver represents a prominent renal fossa.

NOTE. The spleen is almost always more intense than the liver on SPECT slices; therefore, one should evaluate radiocolloid distribution on the posterior SPECT raw data or on a planar scan.

Illustration continued on page 246

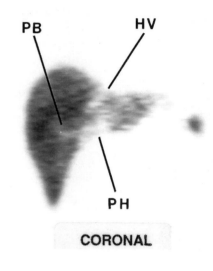

B   **CORONAL**

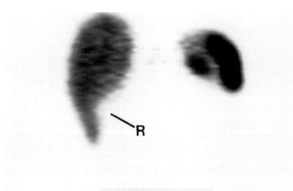

C   **CORONAL**

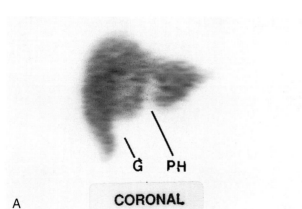

A   **CORONAL**

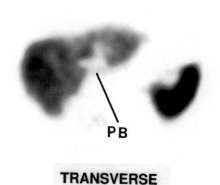

D   **TRANSVERSE**

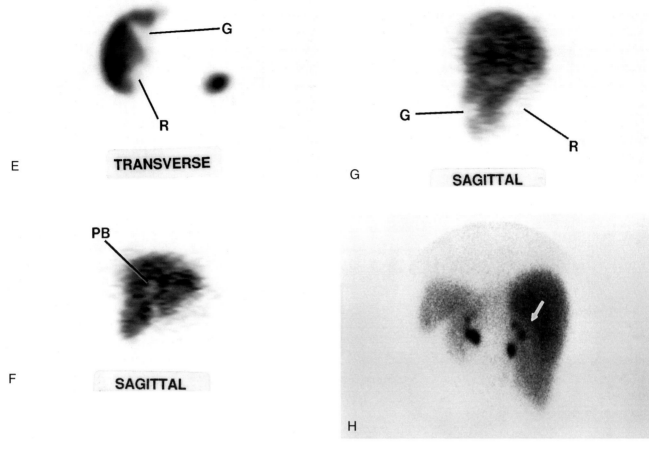

E   **TRANSVERSE**

G   **SAGITTAL**

F   **SAGITTAL**

H

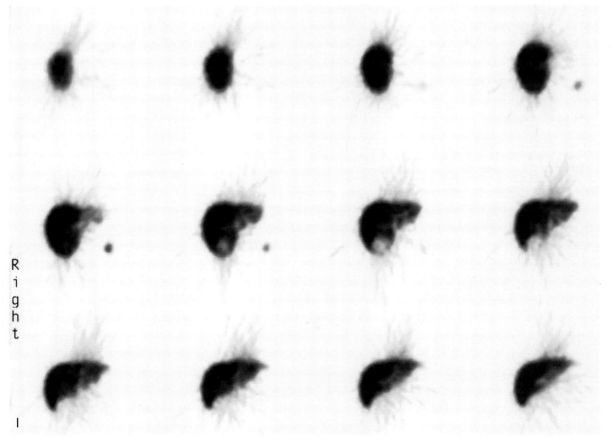

I

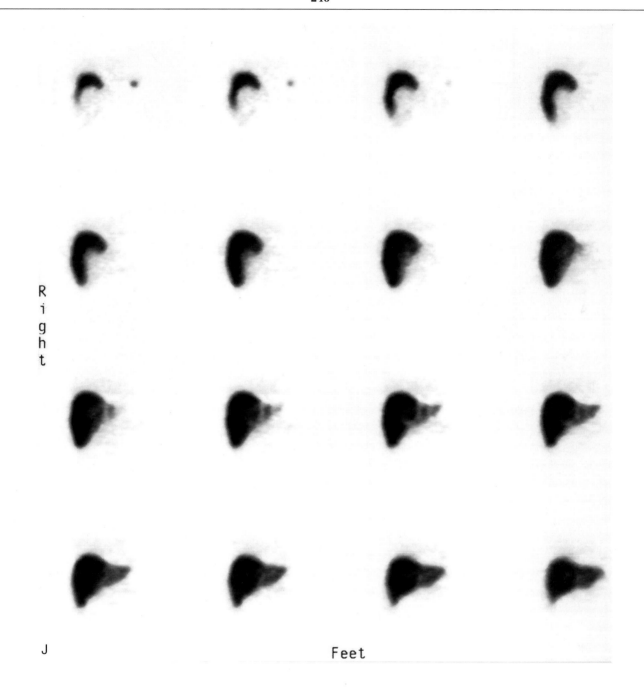

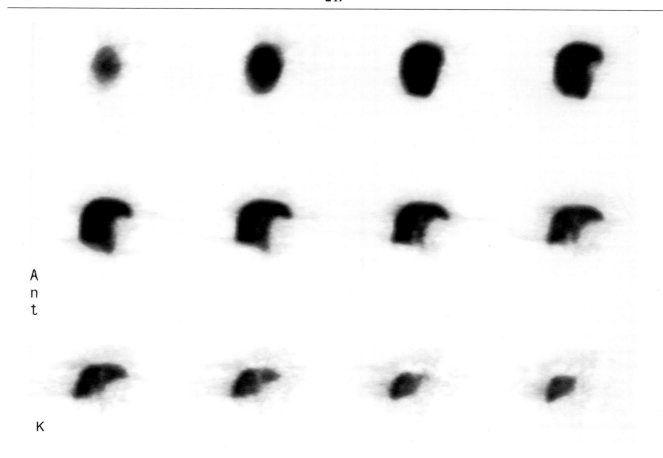

Chapter **13**

Hepatomegaly

ELONGATED LEFT LOBE OF THE LIVER

FIGURE 13–1   A to C.

Anterior, LAO, and Left Lateral Colloid Liver Scan: The left lobe of the liver *(curved arrow)* wraps around the abdomen to come in close proximity to the spleen.

Illustration continued on following page

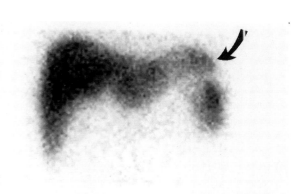

A   Rt. ANT. Lt.

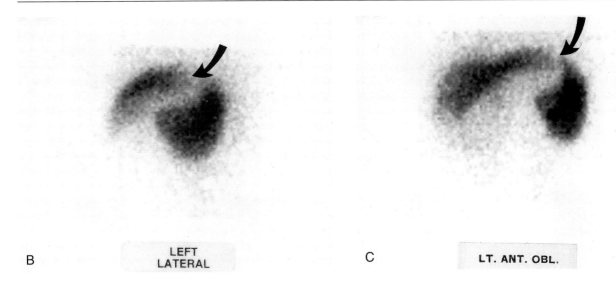

B — LEFT LATERAL

C — LT. ANT. OBL.

REIDEL'S LOBE

FIGURE 13–2   A to C.

Anterior, RAO, and Right Lateral Liver Scan: The extension of the right lobe inferiorly is a normal variant and does not represent hepatomegaly.

NOTE. The colloid accumulation in a Reidel lobe should be the same as in the rest of the liver.

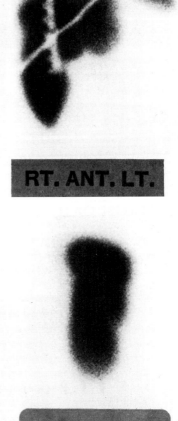

A — RT. ANT. LT.

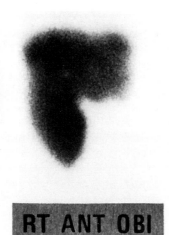

B — RT ANT OBI

C — Post. RT. LAT. Ant.

RIGHT ATRIAL REFLUX AND CONGESTIVE HEPATOMEGALY

Patient 1

FIGURE 13–3   A.

Blood Flow Scintigrams: The cardiac blood pool *(open arrow)* is separated from the liver by a pericardial effusion *(arrow)*.

FIGURE 13–3   B to C.

Liver Scan: The liver is enlarged (18 cm), the spleen has increased radiocolloid accumulation, but the bone marrow activity is normal.

Patient 2

FIGURE 13–3   D.

Anterior Blood Flow: There is reflux down the inferior vena cava *(arrow)* during right atrial systole.

Patient 3

FIGURE 13–3   E.

Posterior Blood Flow: The intermittent reflux down the inferior vena cava extends into the hepatic veins *(arrows)*, indicating right heart failure.

NOTE. The spleen in congestive hepatomegaly is usually normal in size if the patient has not developed cardiac cirrhosis. The bone marrow frequently has, at worst, mild radiocolloid accumulation.

Cross Reference

Section X Cardiac System, Chapter 56: Miscellaneous—Right Heart Failure

Illustration continued on following page

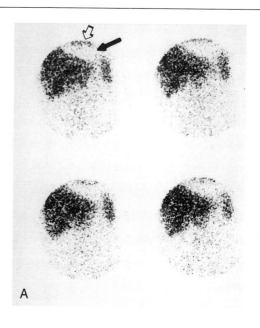

A

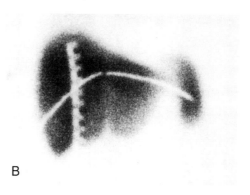

B

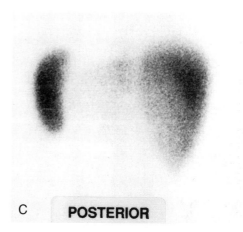

C   **POSTERIOR**

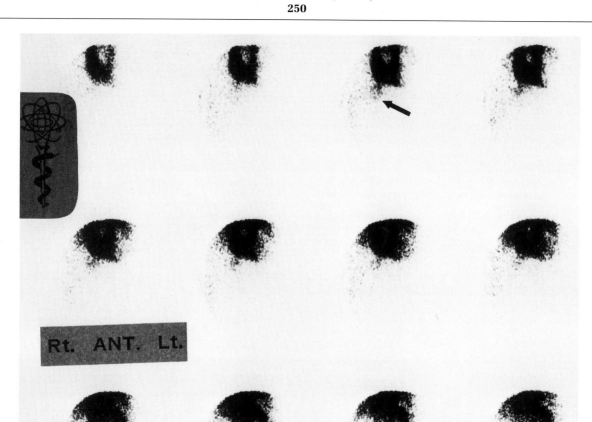

Rt. ANT. Lt.

D

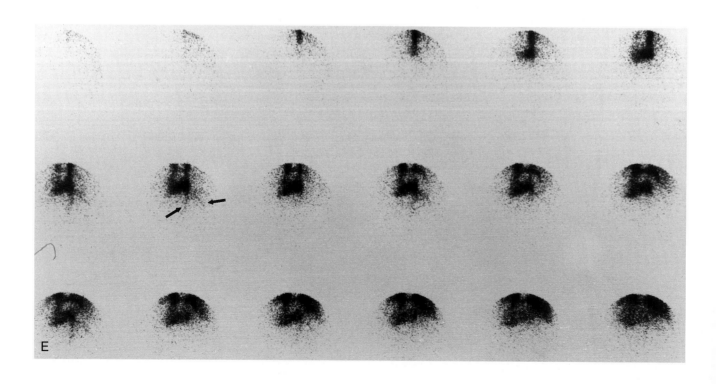

E

RENAL ACTIVITY WITH CARDIAC CIRRHOSIS

Patient 1

FIGURE 13–4   A.
Anterior Colloid Liver Scan: The liver is enlarged, and there is delayed clearance of the blood pool from the enlarged heart.

FIGURE 13–4   B.
Posterior Colloid Liver Scan: The left kidney has abnormal colloid accumulation, along with the bone marrow and spleen.

Patient 2

FIGURE 13–4   C and D.
Colloid Liver Scan: There is mottled colloid accumulation in the liver and increased kidney activity, along with a colloid shift to the enlarged spleen and bone marrow.

NOTE. Kidney visualization on colloid scintigraphy appears related to congestive heart failure.

Cross Reference

Chapter 20: Disorders of the Spleen—Splenomegaly

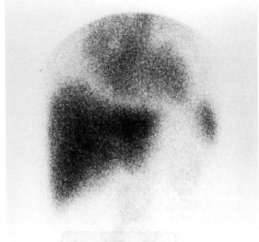

A   Rt. ANT. Lt.

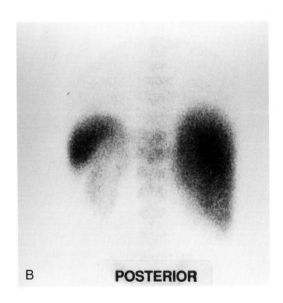

B   POSTERIOR

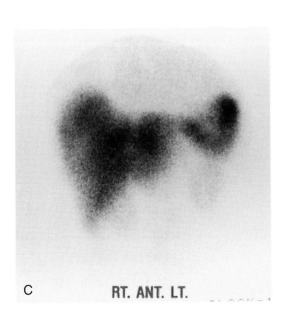

C   RT. ANT. LT.

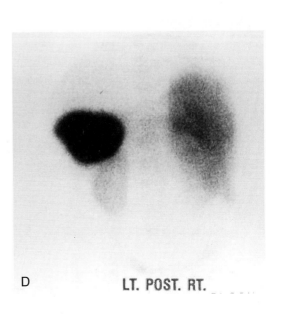

D   LT. POST. RT.

FATTY LIVER

FIGURE 13-5   A and B.

Colloid Liver Scan: The liver and spleen are enlarged with homogeneously decreased activity, although there is a mild colloid shift.

FIGURE 13-5   C and D.

Radioxenon Lung Scan: The accumulation of xenon in the liver *(arrow)* seen on the equilibrium scan is due to the fat solubility of xenon.

NOTE. Fatty livers may be acute and painful or chronic and asymptomatic. There usually is a mild hepatocellular colloid shift pattern.

Cross Reference

Chapter 15: Solitary Liver Defects—Fatty Liver Mass

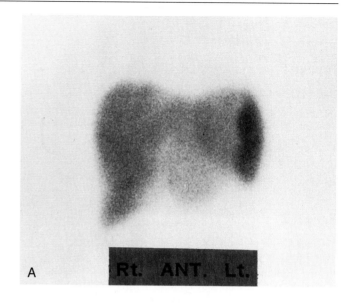

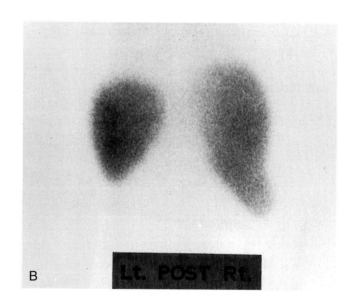

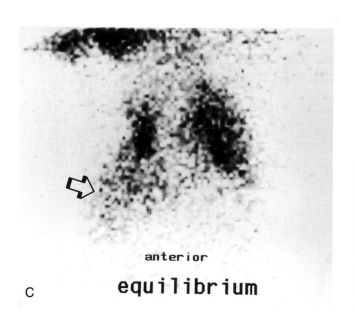

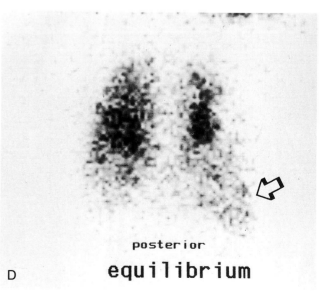

LEUKEMIC LIVER

FIGURE 13–6.
Colloid Liver Scan: The enlarged liver has diffusely decreased activity as compared with the markedly enlarged spleen.

NOTE. Infiltrative diseases, e.g., leukemia and lymphoma, usually do not have focal masses but rather have diffusely decreased colloid accumulation. Mass lesions are seen in less than 20 percent of cases.

Cross References

Chapter 18: Abnormal Liver Blood Flow—''Hot'' Spot in Liver

Chapter 20: Disorders of the Spleen—Tumors in the Spleen

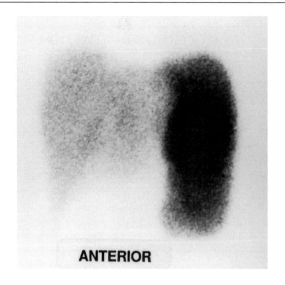

ANTERIOR

Chapter **14**
Liver Dysfunction

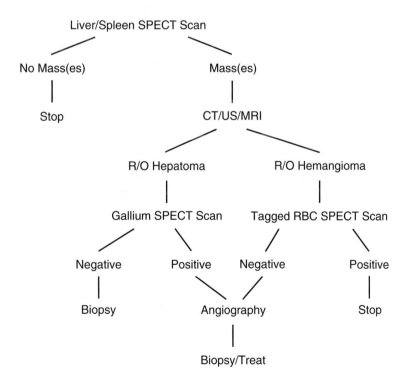

SUSPECT LIVER DYSFUNCTION

Liver/Spleen SPECT Scan

No Mass(es)   Mass(es)

Stop   CT/US/MRI

R/O Hepatoma   R/O Hemangioma

Gallium SPECT Scan   Tagged RBC SPECT Scan

Negative   Positive   Negative   Positive

Biopsy   Angiography   Stop

Biopsy/Treat

HEPATOCELLULAR DYSFUNCTION		
Figure	Degree of Dysfunction	Colloid Activity
14–1A	Normal	Liver > Spleen—no marrow
14–1B	Mild	Liver ≤ Spleen—no marrow
14–1C	Moderate	Liver < Spleen—slight ↑ marrow
14–1D	Marked	Liver < Spleen (↑ size)— ↑ ↑ marrow
14–1E	Severe	Ascites, ↓ liver size, ↑ spleen, ↑ ↑ ↑ Marrow, ↑ lung

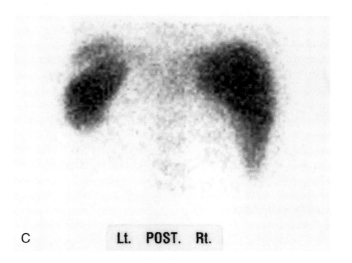

C   Lt. POST. Rt.

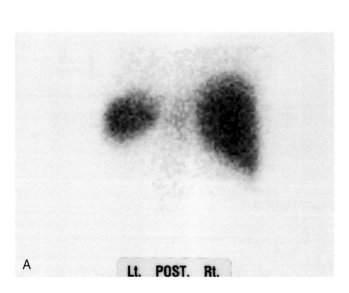

A   Lt. POST. Rt.

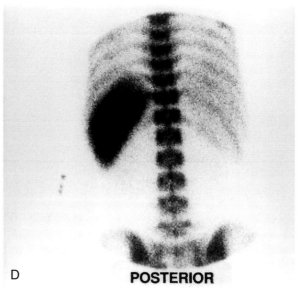

D   POSTERIOR

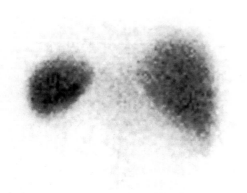

B   Lt. POST. Rt.

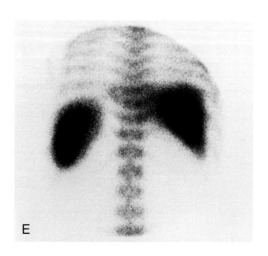

E

LIVER SIZE IN CIRRHOSIS

Patient 1: Hepatomegaly

FIGURE 14–2 A.
Anterior Liver Scan: The liver is enlarged, with irregular areas of decreased function.

Patient 2: Laennec's Cirrhosis

FIGURE 14–2 B.
Anterior Liver Scan: There is left lobe hypertrophy and right lobe atrophy. The spleen is enlarged.

Patient 3

FIGURE 14–2 C.
Anterior Liver Scan: The liver is barely visible, the spleen is intense, and the bone marrow has marked colloid accumulation.

Patient 4: Hepatic Atrophy

FIGURE 14–2 D.
Anterior Liver Scan: The liver is atrophic and is separated from the right abdominal wall by ascites. There is mild lung uptake.

NOTE 1. When the left hepatic lobe is hypertrophic, one might suspect alcoholic cirrhosis. This is because of the laminar flow of the portal veins, carrying the alcohol from the small bowel into the right portal vein. This can cause greater damage to the right lobe, with subsequent hypertrophy of the left lobe.

NOTE 2. The normal liver should abut the right abdominal wall, whereas the normal spleen may be separated from the left abdominal wall.

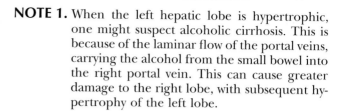

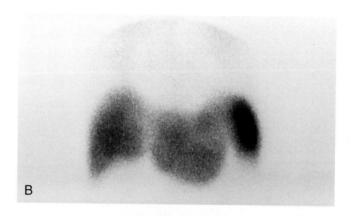

B

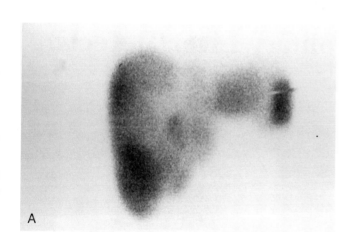

A

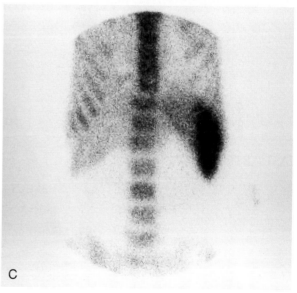

C

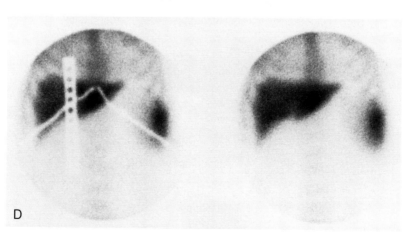

D

AMYLOID LIVER DISEASE

FIGURE 14–3.

[99mTc]-Pyrophosphate Myocardial Infarct Scan: There is diffuse accumulation of the radiopharmaceutical in the liver. Biopsy revealed amyloid deposits.

Cross References

Chapter 11: Soft Tissue Abnormalities—Diffuse Liver Activity on Bone Scan

Chapter 54: [99M]Tc-Pyrophosphate Scanning—Cardiac Amyloidosis

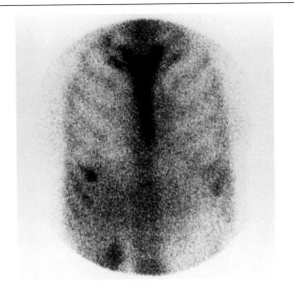

Chapter **15**

Solitary Liver Defects

BREAST ARTIFACT ON LIVER SCAN

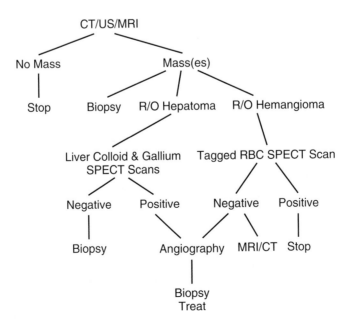

SOLITARY COLD LIVER DEFECTS	
1. Hemangioma	8. Adenoma
2. Primary neoplasm	9. Regenerating nodule
3. Metastatic neoplasm	10. Focal nodular hyperplasia
4. Abscess	11. Scar
5. Cyst	12. Artifacts, e.g., breast
6. Hematoma	13. Infarct
7. Fat	

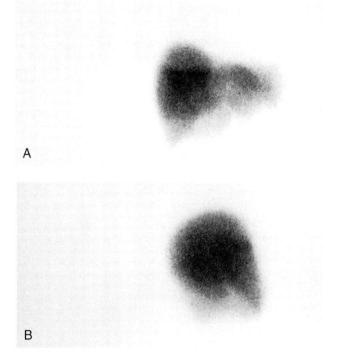

A

B

FIGURE 15–1 A.

Right Anterior Oblique Colloid Liver Scan: The decreased activity in the dome of the liver is due to breast attenuation.

FIGURE 15–1 B.

Lateral Colloid Liver Scan: The "defect" is no longer evident.

NOTE. When decreased activity is seen in the dome, especially with a curvilinear intense inferior border, and not seen on the lateral, breast artifact is likely. Raising the breast and repeating the study can confirm this.

FATTY LIVER MASS

Patient 1

FIGURE 15–2 A.

Colloid Liver Mass: The central liver has decreased activity that was of fat density on CT.

Patient 2

FIGURE 15–2 B.

CT Scan: The right lobe of the liver has focal areas of decreased density.

Cross References

Chapter 13: Hepatomegaly—Fatty Liver

Chapter 16: Hepatoma—Hepatoma in Suspected Fatty Liver

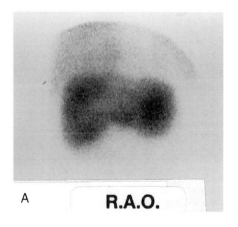

A **R.A.O.**

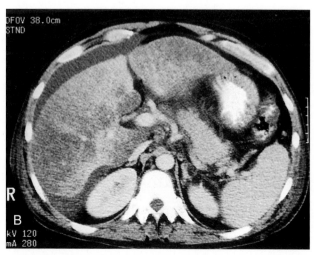

HEPATIC ABSCESS

Patient 1: *Bacteroides* Liver Abscess

FIGURE 15–3   A.
Colloid Liver Scan: The scan is normal.

FIGURE 15–3   B.
Gallium Scan: There is a "doughnut," or ringlike, gallium accumulation. There is a related pleural empyema.

Patient 2: *E. Coli* Abscess due to Retained Stones

FIGURE 15–3   C.
Colloid Liver Scan: There is a focal defect in the left lobe.

FIGURE 15–3   D.
WBC Scan: There is marked WBC accumulation in the left lobe.

Patient 3: Amoebic Abscess

FIGURE 15–3   E and F.
Blood Flow Scintigraphy: There is decreased flow to a huge right lobe mass.

FIGURE 15–3   G and H.
Right Anterior Oblique and Right Lateral Colloid Scan: The large multiloculated mass replaces most of the right lobe.

NOTE. A gallium scan may not distinguish between tumor or abscess, so if the clinical history is uncertain, a WBC scan should be done first.

Cross Reference

Chapter 16: Hepatoma—"Doughnut" Hepatoma

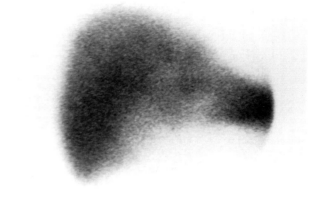

A   RT. ANT. OBL.

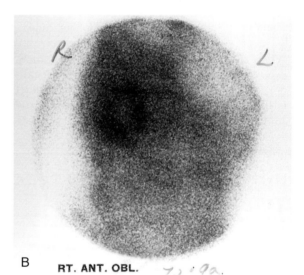

B   RT. ANT. OBL.

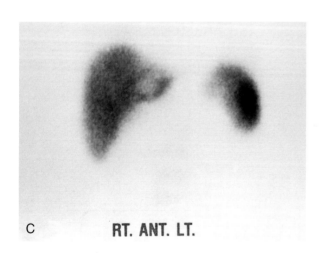

C   RT. ANT. LT.

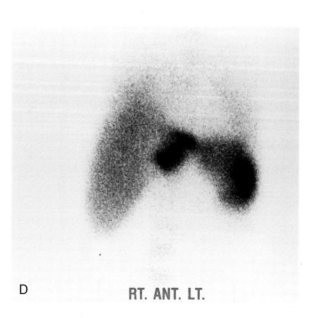

D   RT. ANT. LT.

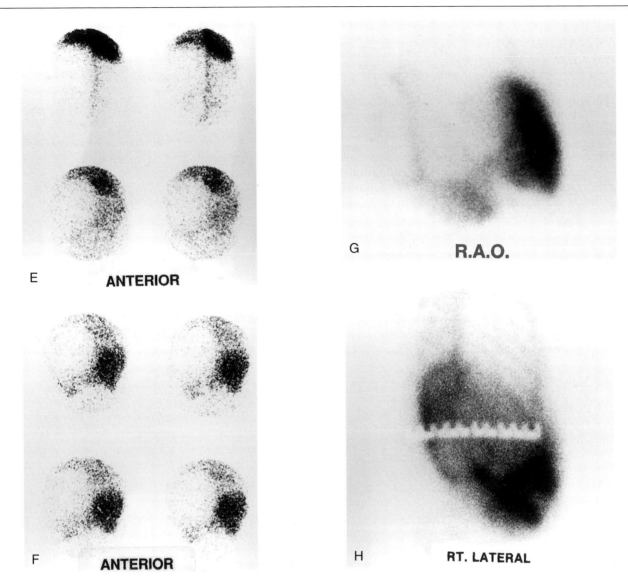

E   **ANTERIOR**

F   **ANTERIOR**

G   **R.A.O.**

H   **RT. LATERAL**

SUBHEPATIC ABSCESS

FIGURE 15–4   A.

Colloid Liver Scan: There is decreased colloid in the superior right lobe in a patient with a known hepatoma.

Illustration continued on following page

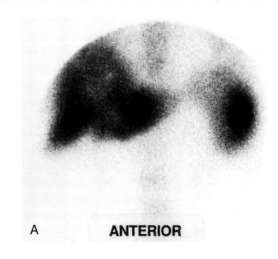

A   **ANTERIOR**

FIGURE 15–4   B.

WBC Scan: There is WBC accumulation below the liver *(arrow-heads)* but none within the liver mass.

NOTE 1. In about 3 percent of cancer patients, there is WBC accumulation in the tumor. The tumors need not be necrotic.

NOTE 2. Normal ^{111}In-WBC distribution to liver, spleen, and bone marrow may mask abnormal liver accumulation. Concomitant ^{99m}Tc-colloid liver scanning, with visual or computer subtraction, can be diagnostic.

Cross Reference

Chapter 71: Infectious Diseases—Metastases to the Liver on WBC Scan; WBCs in Tumor

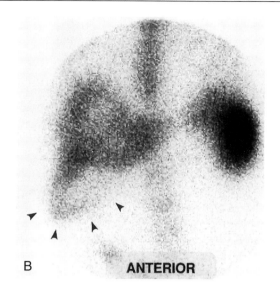

B   ANTERIOR

LACERATED LIVER

FIGURE 15–5   A to C.

Colloid Liver Scan: There is a linear defect representing a laceration cleaving the right lobe following an automobile accident.

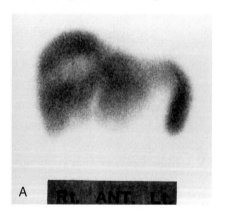
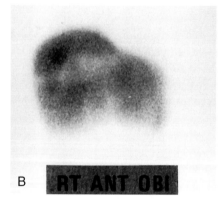
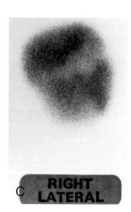

A RT. ANT. Lt.   B RT ANT OBl   C RIGHT LATERAL

BULLET IN LIVER

FIGURE 15–6.

Colloid Liver Scan: There is a focal defect representing the metallic bullet in the left lobe.

Cross References

Chapter 24: Bile Leaks—Bile Leaks

Chapter 39: Renal Defects—Bullet in Kidney

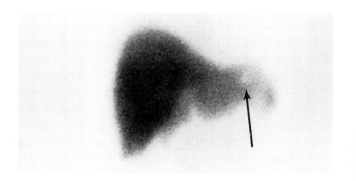

HEPATIC INFARCT

FIGURE 15–7.

Right Lateral Colloid Liver Scan: There is a wedge defect in the superior aspect of the right lobe *(arrow)*.

NOTE 1. Despite a dual blood supply, hepatic infarcts are more common than previously thought and are best detected on MR imaging.

NOTE 2. The liver is more susceptible to sudden portal vein damage than to hepatic arterial occlusion.

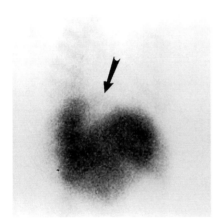

MASS LESIONS OF THE LIVER			
	Colloid	**Gallium**	**RBC**
Abscess	↓	↑	
Hepatoma	↓	↑	Normal or rarely ↑
Hemangioma	↓	Normal	↑
Adenoma	↓ *	Normal or ↑	
Regenerating nodule	↓	Normal	
Focal nodular hyperplasia	Normal, ↑, ↓	Normal	
Metastases	↓	Normal or occasionally ↑	

* May have normal colloid accumulation

HEMANGIOMA

FIGURE 15–8   A and B.

Colloid Liver Scan: There is a focal area of decreased colloid accumulation *(arrow)* in the inferior right lobe.

Illustration continued on following page

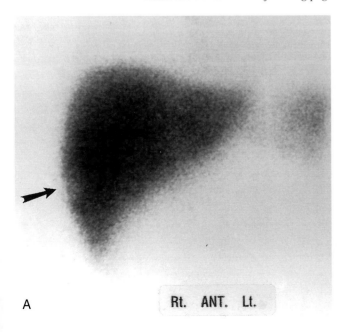

A   Rt. ANT. Lt.

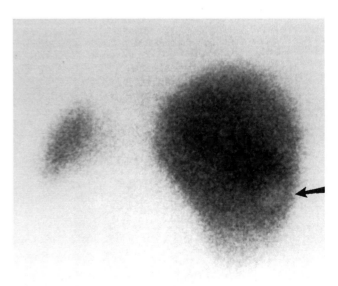

B   R.P.O.

FIGURE 15–8   C.

Tagged RBC Blood Flow: There is early blood flow to a focal area within the inferior right lobe *(arrow)*.

FIGURE 15–8   D.

Three Hour Delayed Tagged RBC Scan: There is persistent blood pooling in the right lobe abnormality.

FIGURE 15–8   E and F.

Gallium Scan: There is no abnormal gallium accumulation.

FIGURE 15–8   G.

Ultrasound: The mass is echogenic.

FIGURE 15–8   H.

Dynamic CT Scan: There is early opacification of the right lobe abnormality.

NOTE 1. Hemangiomas may be single but are often multiple. RBC scans may miss those smaller than 1.0 to 1.5 cm.

NOTE 2. Hemangiomas may have early or delayed blood flow but almost always have persistent tagged-RBC accumulation over hours.

NOTE 3. Hepatomas do not retain more RBCs as compared with normal liver.

Cross References

Chapter 7: Hands and Feet—Bone and Soft Tissue Hemangioma of the Foot

Chapter 11: Soft Tissue Abnormalities—Hemangioma

Chapter 16: Hepatoma—Well-Differentiated Hepatoma

Chapter 17: Multiple Liver Defects—Multiple Hepatic Hemangiomas

Chapter 18: Abnormal Liver Blood Flow—Hyperemia with Liver Metastases

Chapter 59: Venous Thrombosis—Leg Hemangioma in Tagged RBC Scan

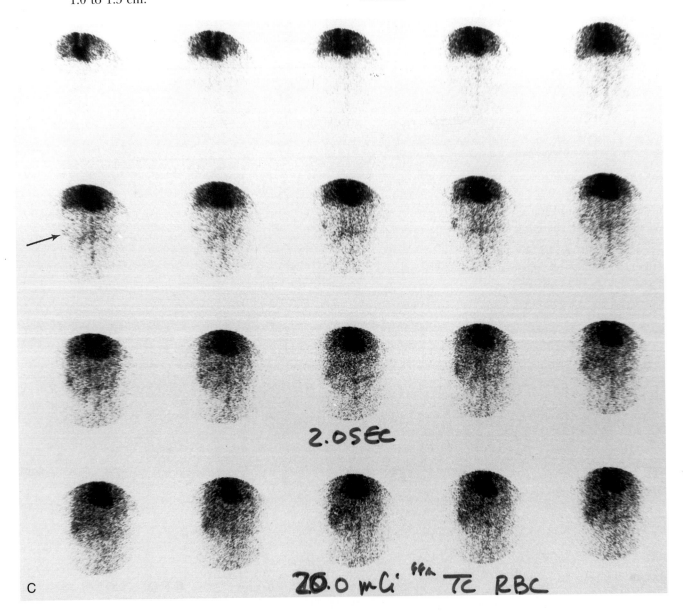

C

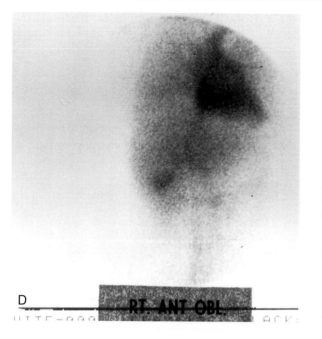

D   RT. ANT. OBL.

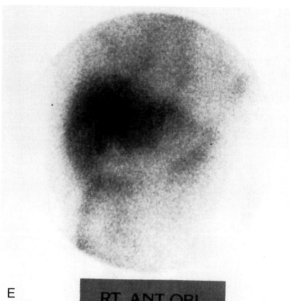

E   RT. ANT. OBL

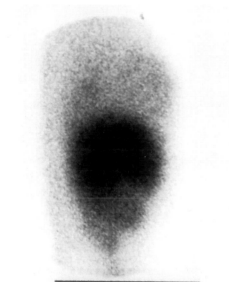

F   RIGHT LATERAL

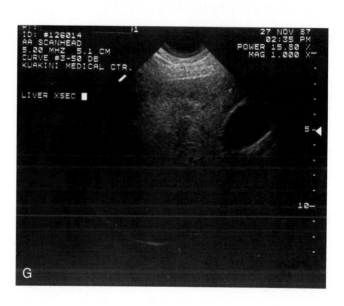

G

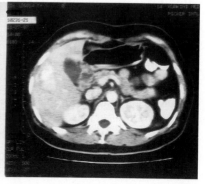

H

FOCAL NODULAR HYPERPLASIA

FIGURE 15–9   A.

Planar Anterior Radiocolloid Liver Scan: There is mildly increased activity along the inferior aspect of the right lobe.

FIGURE 15–9   B and C.

Coronal and Sagittal SPECT Scans: The increased colloid accumulation is better delineated as separate from the normal liver parenchyma.

NOTE 1. Radiocolloid accumulation in a focal liver mass should represent either focal nodular hyperplasia or a regenerating nodule.

NOTE 2. Hepatic adenomas do not retain radiocolloid because they have no reticuloendothelial cells.

NOTE 3. Focal nodular hyperplasia has normal hepatocytes and bile ducts and will excrete radiolabeled bile on hepatobiliary scanning.

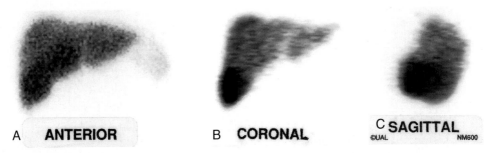

A **ANTERIOR**   B **CORONAL**   C **SAGITTAL**

REGENERATING NODULES

Patient 1: Alcoholic Liver Disease

FIGURE 15–10   A.

Right Anterior Oblique Colloid Liver Scan: The liver is inhomogeneous, with areas of decreased activity. The right lobe is separated from the ribs by ascites.

FIGURE 15–10   B.

Right Lateral Gallium Liver Scan: The central portion of the liver has decreased gallium accumulation, making a hepatoma unlikely.

Patient 2: Post-traumatic Hepatomegaly

FIGURE 15–10   C and D.

RAO and Right Lateral Colloid Liver Scan: The liver is enlarged but appears divided into three parts. There is concurrent splenomegaly.

FIGURE 15–10   E.

Transverse Liver SPECT Scan: The midline palpable abdominal mass was functioning hypertrophic liver tissue.

Patient 3: Post-traumatic Liver Mass

FIGURE 15–10   F.

Colloid Liver Scan: The palpated abdominal mass turned out to be functioning liver tissue. The spleen has been removed.

NOTE. Regenerating nodules occur following damage to the liver parenchyma. If they are mostly scar, there is no radiocolloid accumulation. If normal tissue hypertrophies (actually hyperplasia), there will be Kupffer cells, which can take up the radiocolloid.

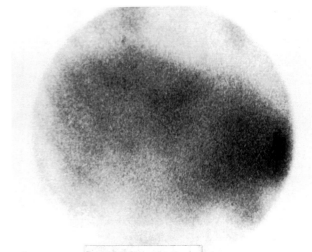

A **RT. ANT. OBL.**

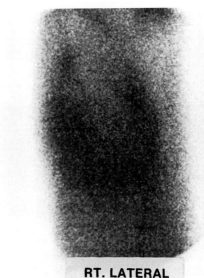

B **RT. LATERAL**

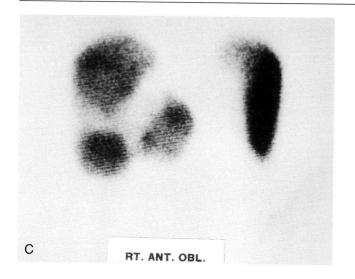

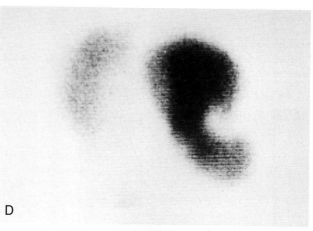

C RT. ANT. OBL.

D

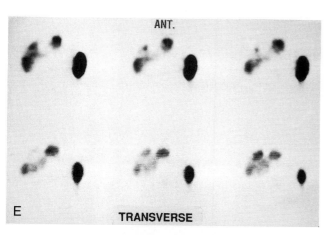

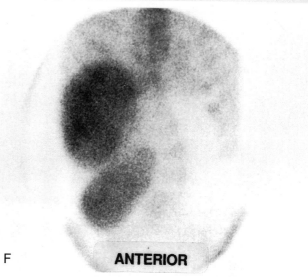

E ANT. TRANSVERSE

F ANTERIOR

SOLITARY HEPATIC MASS

Patient 1: Rapidly Growing Gastric Metastases

FIGURE 15–11   A.

Colloid Liver Scan: The scan is normal.

FIGURE 15–11   B. Liver Scan

3 Months Later: There is a large mass between the two lobes.

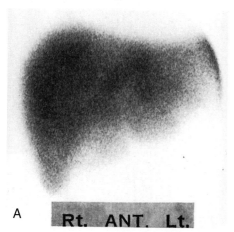

A Rt. ANT. Lt.

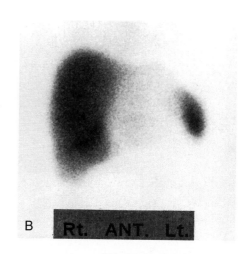

B Rt. ANT. Lt.

Illustration continued on following page

Patient 2: Hepatic Cyst

FIGURE 15–11 C.
Colloid Liver Scan: There is a large nonfunctioning mass between the right and left lobes of the liver.

NOTE. A colloid defect in the liver is totally nonspecific, requiring biopsy, ultrasound, CT, or MR scanning.

Cross Reference

Chapter 17: Multiple Liver Defects—Liver Metastases

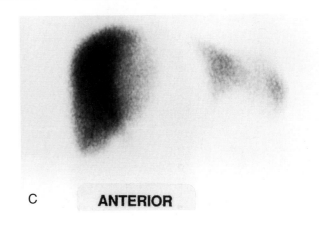

C **ANTERIOR**

EXTRINSIC LIVER MASS

Patient: Endodermal Sinus Tumor

FIGURE 15–12 A and B.
Colloid Liver Scan: There is an impression on the posterior aspect of the right lobe.

FIGURE 15–12 C and D.
Postoperative Colloid Liver Scan: The mass lesion is no longer present.

NOTE. Posterior masses impressing on the liver include neuroenteric masses, lung tumors, renal and adrenal tumors, retroperitoneal sarcomas, and metastases.

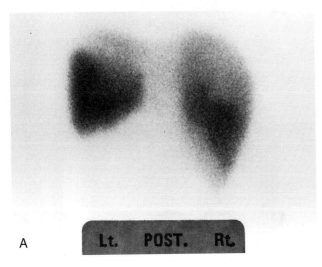

A **Lt. POST. Rt.**

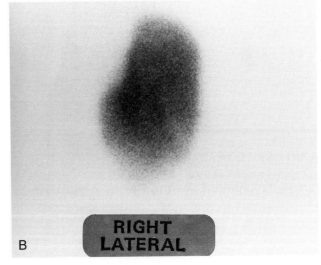

B **RIGHT LATERAL**

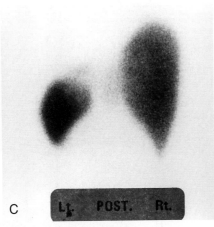

C **Lt. POST. Rt.**

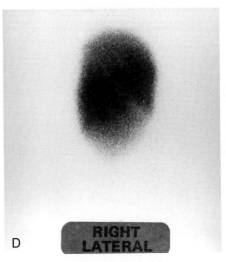

D **RIGHT LATERAL**

Chapter 16

Hepatoma

VASCULAR HEPATOMA WITH LUNG METASTASES

FIGURE 16–1 A.
Blood Flow Portion of Colloid Liver Scan: There is an early vascular blush in the liver, with early venous filling *(arrow)*.

FIGURE 16–1 B.
Colloid Liver Scan: The left lobe and the medial right lobe do not accumulate the radiocolloid (the black dots are markers).

FIGURE 16–1 C.
Gallium Scan: The left lobe has intense gallium accumulation along with the lung metastases.

Illustration continued on following page

NOTE 1. The liver should be the last abdominal organ to be seen on the blood flow study, since the majority of the blood supply comes via the portal venous system, not the hepatic arteries. Hepatomas derive 90 percent of their blood supply from the hepatic arteries, enlarging them and creating arteriovenous shunts.

NOTE 2. Gallium scanning is extremely sensitive in detecting hepatomas, although not specific.

Cross Reference

Chapter 18: Abnormal Liver Blood Flow—Hyperemia with Liver Metastases

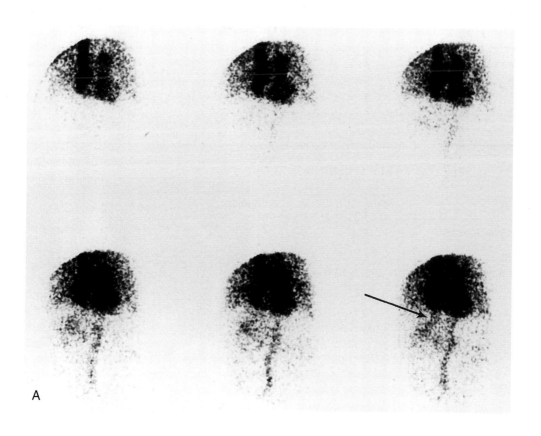

A

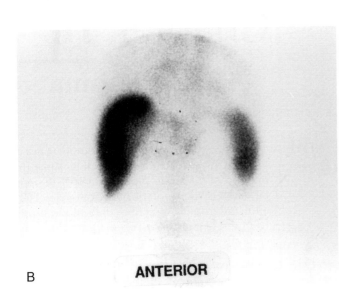

B   **ANTERIOR**

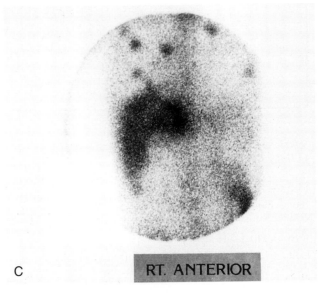

C   **RT. ANTERIOR**

"DOUGHNUT" HEPATOMA

Patient 1: Elevated Alpha-Fetoprotein

FIGURE 16–2.

Gallium Scan: This "doughnut" lesion is indistinguishable from an abscess. Clinical history is essential.

Cross Reference

CHAPTER 15: Solitary Liver Defects—Hepatic Abscess

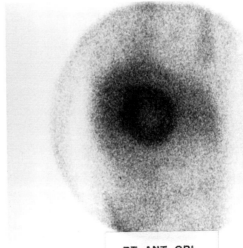

RT. ANT. OBL.

HEPATOMA IN SUSPECTED FATTY LIVER

FIGURE 16–3   A.

CT Scan of Liver: There is irregular low density within the liver believed to represent fat.

FIGURE 16–3   B.

Coronal Colloid Liver SPECT Scan: The right lobe has a large area of photon deficiency.

FIGURE 16–3   C.

Coronal Gallium SPECT Scan: Intense gallium accumulation fills in the right lobe defect.

Cross Reference

CHAPTER 15: Solitary Liver Defects—Fatty Liver Mass

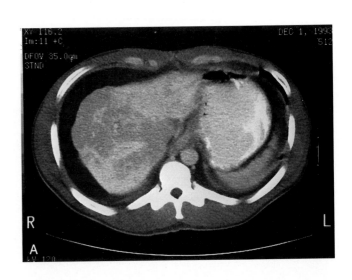

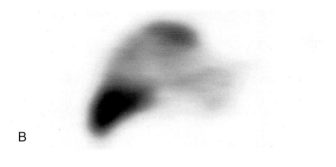

B

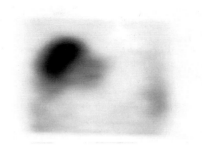

C

WELL-DIFFERENTIATED HEPATOMA

Patient 1

FIGURE 16–4   A.
Colloid Liver Scan: The inferior tip of the right lobe has decreased colloid.

FIGURE 16–4   B.
Gallium Scan: There is gallium accumulation within the defect.

FIGURE 16–4   C.
Coronal SPECT Tagged RBC Scan: The RBCs in the lesion are isointense with the "normal" liver.

FIGURE 16–4   D.
Hepatobiliary (HIDA) Scan: There is increased radiopharmaceutical accumulation in the region of the colloid liver scan defect. (This scan was done immediately after the tagged RBC scan.)

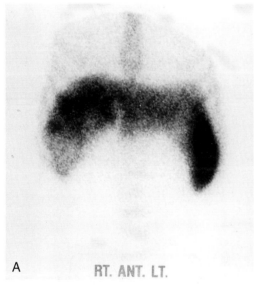

A   RT. ANT. LT.

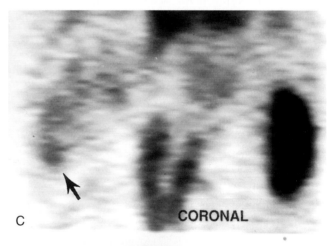

C   CORONAL

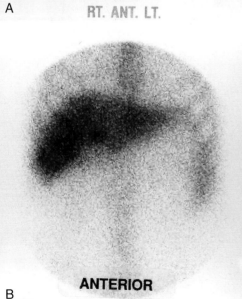

B   ANTERIOR

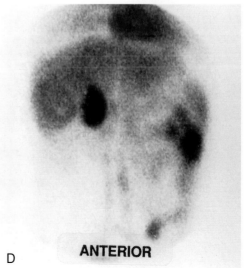

D   ANTERIOR

Illustration continued on following page

Patient 2

FIGURE 16–4 E.

Right Lateral Radiocolloid Scan: There is a large defect involving most of the right lobe of the liver.

FIGURE 16–4 F.

Right Lateral HIDA Scan: Much of the hepatoma takes up the hepatobiliary agent.

NOTE 1. Since the radioactivity in a hepatoma on a gallium scan may be isointense with the rest of the liver, a colloid liver scan should also be obtained.

NOTE 2. The hepatobiliary agents accumulate only in well-differentiated hepatocellular carcinomas.

NOTE 3. Biopsies may not be able to distinguish well-differentiated hepatomas from normal tissue. An abnormal gallium scan with normal histology necessitates further pathologic evaluation.

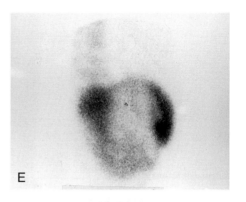
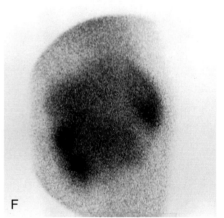

SUBTLE HEPATOMAS

Patient 1

FIGURE 16–5 A.

Blood Flow Portion of Colloid Liver Scan: There is early blood flow to the lateral aspect of the right lobe.

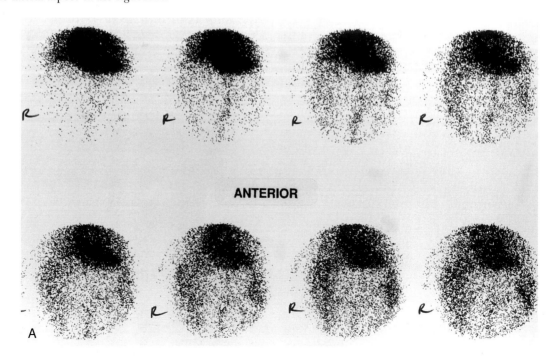

FIGURE 16–5 B.

Colloid Liver Scan: The liver is inhomogeneous, with no definite focal mass.

FIGURE 16–5 C.

Gallium Scan: There is homogeneous gallium accumulation, in both lobes, filling in the defects seen on the colloid scan.

Patient 2

FIGURE 16–5 D.

Colloid Liver Scan: There is a large right lobe liver defect. The patient is severely scoliotic.

FIGURE 16–5 E.

Gallium Scan: The defect has partially filled in.

Patient 3

FIGURE 16–5 F.

Gallium Scan: The marked gallium accumulation is so intense in the right lobe that the normal areas appear photon-deficient, e.g., the left lobe *(arrowheads)*.

Cross Reference

Chapter 17: Multiple Liver Defects—Multifocal Hepatoma

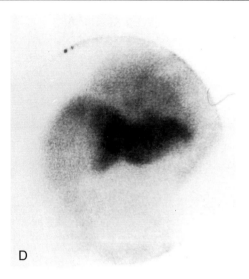

D

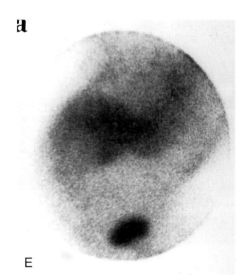

E

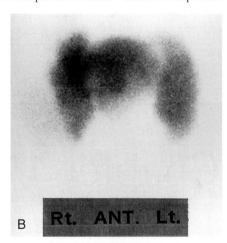

B   Rt. ANT. Lt.

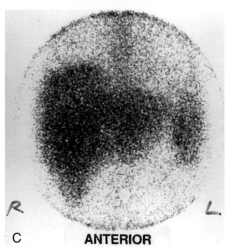

C   ANTERIOR

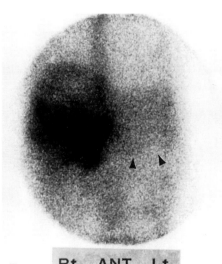

F   Rt. ANT. Lt.

GALLIUM-POSITIVE LIVER SCAN IN METASTATIC PANCREATIC CARCINOMA

FIGURE 16–6   A.

Colloid Liver Scan: The left lobe of the liver is not visualized.

FIGURE 16–6   B.

Gallium Scan: There is gallium accumulation in the left lobe.

NOTE. Gallium accumulation in pancreatic carcinoma is inconsistent and not usually valuable in evaluation of pancreatic masses or potential metastases to the liver.

Cross Reference

Chapter 71: Infectious Diseases—Infected Pseudocyst

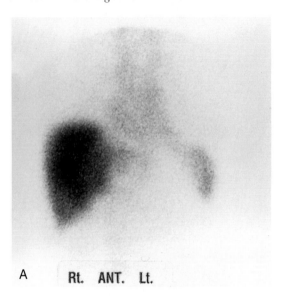

A   Rt. ANT. Lt.

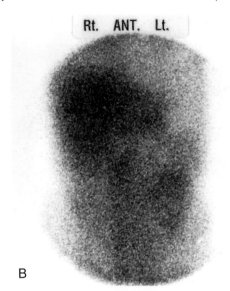

B

Rt. ANT. Lt.

Chapter 17
Multiple Liver Defects

MULTIPLE HEPATIC CYSTS

Patient 1: Polycystic Liver Disease

FIGURE 17–1   A to C.

Colloid Liver Scan: There are multiple focal defects within both lobes of the liver.

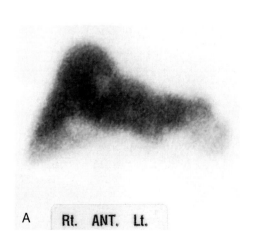

A   Rt. ANT. Lt.

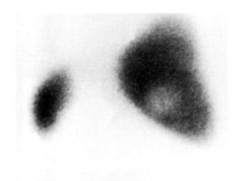

B Lt. POST. Rt.

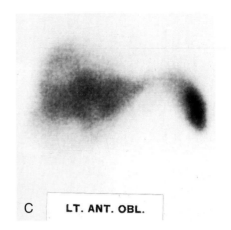

C LT. ANT. OBL.

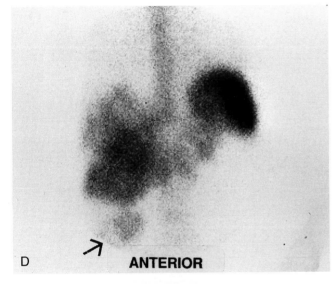

D ANTERIOR

Patient 2: Polycystic Liver Disease

FIGURE 17–1 D.

^{111}In-WBC Scan: There are numerous defects in the liver, none of which appears infected. The liver extends inferiorly *(arrow)* to the iliac crest.

Patient 3: Simple Cysts

FIGURE 17–1 E to G.

Colloid Liver Scan: There are at least two large masses within the right lobe. (Courtesy of Dr. Michael Kipper, Vista, CA.)

Cross Reference

Chapter 25: Choledochocysts—Caroli's Disease

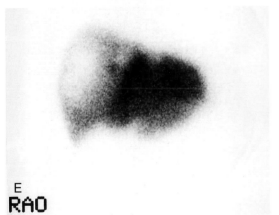

E
RAO

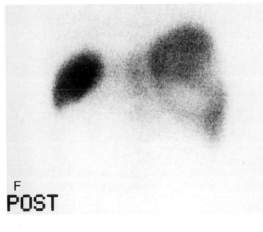

F
POST

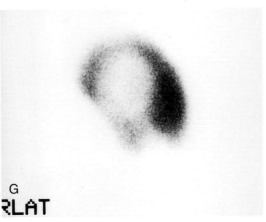

G
RLAT

MULTIPLE HEPATIC ABSCESSES

Patient 1

FIGURE 17–2 A.

Colloid Liver Scan: There are numerous focal defects in both lobes.

FIGURE 17–2 B.

Colloid Liver Scan 4 Months Later: After antibiotic therapy the abscesses have resolved. Hepatic function has improved.

Patient 2

FIGURE 17–2 C.

Colloid Liver Scan: There are two mass lesions in the dome of the right lobe, with overall diminished liver function.

FIGURE 17–2 D.

Colloid Liver Scan After 2 Weeks of Antibiotics: The masses are better defined owing to return of some hepatic function. Their sizes are unchanged.

FIGURE 17–2 E.

Colloid Liver Scan 2 Months After Initial Scan: The mass lesions have resolved, and the liver function has returned to near-normal. There is breast attenuation overlying the dome of the liver.

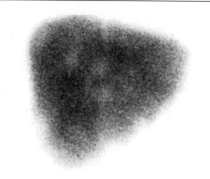

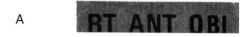

A

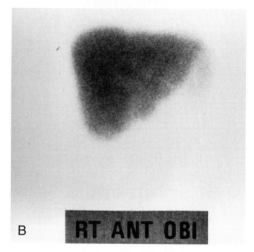

B **RT ANT OBI**

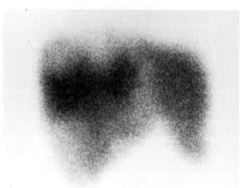

D **R.A.O.**

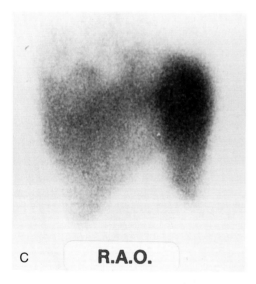

C **R.A.O.**

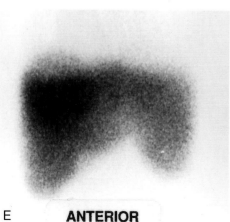

E **ANTERIOR**

NOTE 1. Multiple small abscesses in the liver are more commonly pyogenic rather than amoebic.

NOTE 2. Overall liver function may be reduced despite an apparent localized process.

NOTE 3. Liver abscesses are usually due to biliary obstruction (tumor, stone, stricture), ascending gastrointestinal infections, or penetrating trauma as well as to idiopathic causes.

MULTIPLE HEPATIC HEMANGIOMAS

Patient 1

FIGURE 17–3   A.

Planar Tagged RBC Scan: There are two and probably three hemangiomas in the liver, found incidentally on this GI hemorrhage study.

Patient 2

FIGURE 17–3   B.

Transverse Tagged RBC SPECT Scan: There are multiple areas of increased RBC accumulation, especially in the left lobe. (A = aorta. I = inferior vena cava.)

FIGURE 17–3   C.

CT Scan: There are several low-density masses in both lobes of the liver.

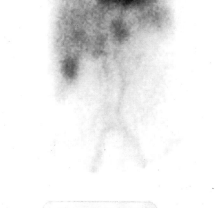

A   ANTERIOR   1ᵣ

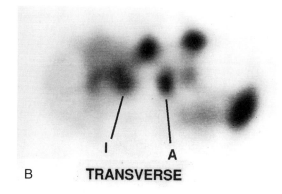

B   TRANSVERSE

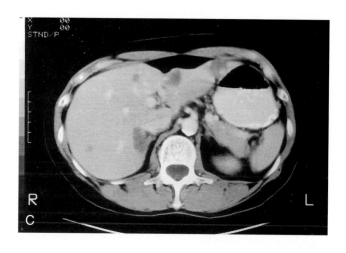

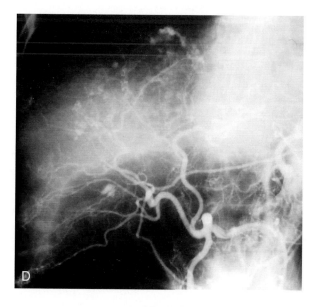

FIGURE 17–3   D.

Hepatic Arteriogram in Another Patient: There are numerous "puddles" of contrast medium, typical of hemangiomas.

Cross References

MULTIFOCAL HEPATOMA

Patient 1

FIGURE 17–4   A and B.
Colloid Liver Scan: There are multiple defects in each lobe of the liver.

FIGURE 17–4   C and D.
Gallium Scan: There are numerous foci of increased gallium accumulation, some of which are in areas that appear normal on the colloid liver scan.

Patient 2

FIGURE 17–4   E and F.
Anterior and Posterior Gallium Scan: There are three gallium collections in the right lobe.

NOTE. The presence of multiple foci of gallium accumulation in the liver requires clinical history to distinguish between abscesses and multifocal hepatoma.

Cross Reference

Chapter 16: Hepatoma—Subtle Hepatomas

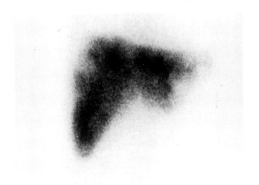

A   RT. ANT. LT.

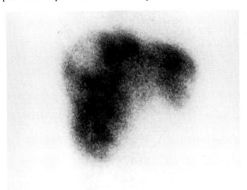

B   RT. ANT. OBL.

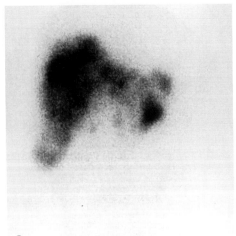

C   RT. ANT. LT.

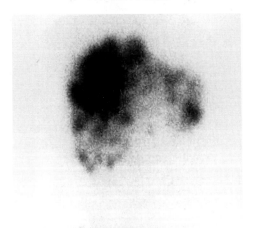

D   RT. ANT. OBL.

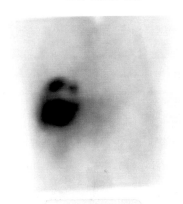

E   ANTERIOR

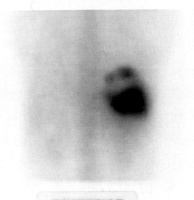

F   POSTERIOR

LIVER METASTASES

Patient 1: Rapidly Developing Metastases

FIGURE 17–5 A.
Colloid Liver Scan: The liver activity is homogeneous.

FIGURE 17–5 B.
Colloid Liver Scan 5 Months Later: The liver is virtually replaced by breast metastases.

Patient 2: Osteogenic Sarcoma

FIGURE 17–5 C to E.
Planar Colloid Liver Scan: There are multiple focal defects throughout both lobes of the liver.

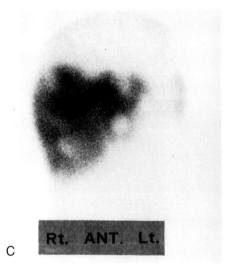

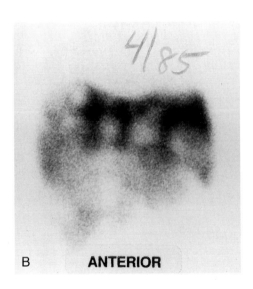

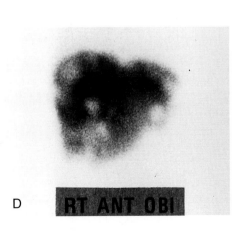

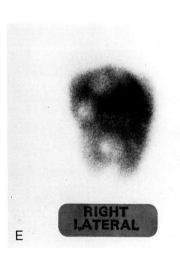

Illustration continued on following page

Patient 3: Breast Carcinoma

FIGURE 17–5 F to I.

Transverse and Selected Coronal and Sagittal SPECT Colloid Liver Scans: The number and distribution of the metastases can be clearly delineated.

Cross Reference

Chapter 15: Solitary Liver Defects—Solitary Hepatic Mass

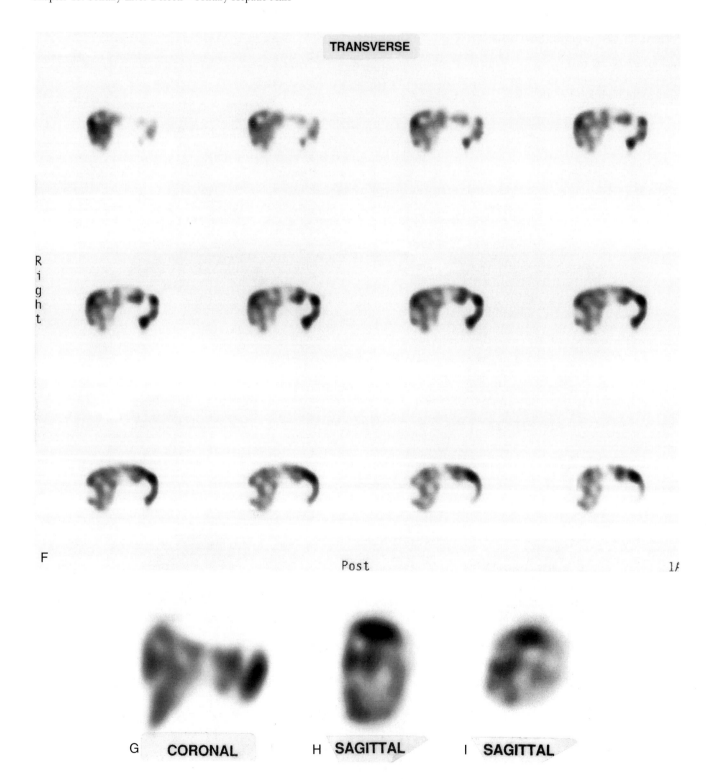

F Post 1*
G CORONAL   H SAGITTAL   I SAGITTAL

Chapter 18

Abnormal Liver Blood Flow

NORMAL HEPATIC BLOOD FLOW

FIGURE 18–1.

Blood Flow Scan with Colloid: In the normal order of flow the abdominal aorta fills first, the kidneys next, then the spleen, and last, the liver.

NOTE 1. The delay in normal hepatic visualization is due to the passage of the radionuclide bolus through the blood vessels of the bowel and spleen before reaching the liver via the portal vein.

NOTE 2. About 90 percent of blood flow to the liver is from the portal vein.

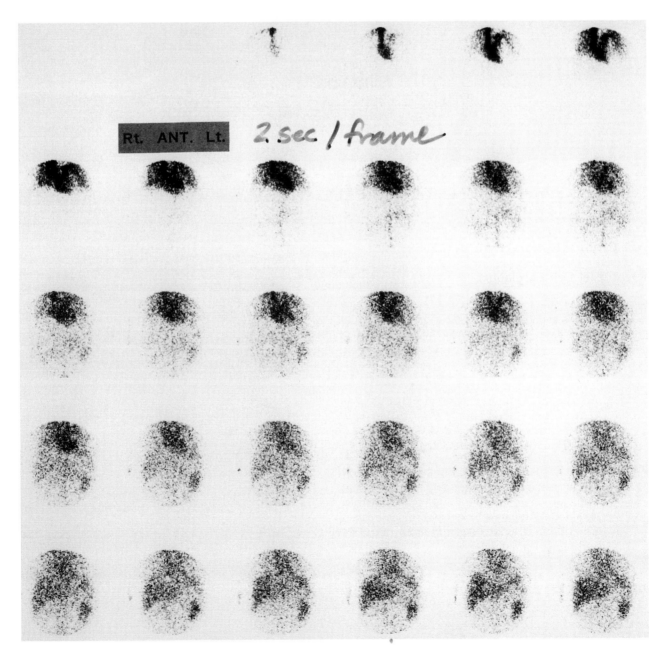

Rt. ANT. Lt. 2.sec/frame

EARLY ARTERIAL FLOW WITH PORTAL HYPERTENSION

FIGURE 18–2.

Blood Flow Scan: The liver is seen as soon as the aorta appears *(arrow)* owing to "arterialization": reduced portal venous flow and greater hepatic arterial flow.

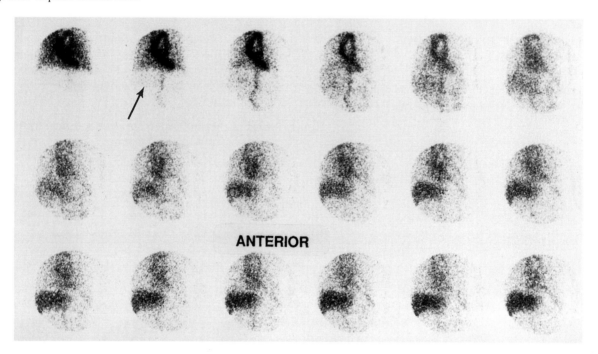

ANTERIOR

HYPEREMIA WITH LIVER METASTASES

Patient: Islet Cell Carcinoma

FIGURE 18–3.

Blood Flow Scan: There is early flow to a focal area in the right lobe of the liver. The static planar images revealed a solitary defect.

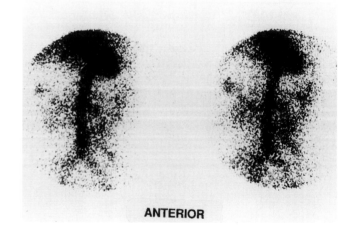

ANTERIOR

NOTE 1. All malignant lesions derive more than 90 percent of their blood supply from the hepatic arteries rather than the portal vein. However, not all tumors are hypervascular.

NOTE 2. Hypervascular metastases include renal cell carcinoma, islet cell carcinomas, melanoma, some sarcomas, breast carcinoma, and thyroid carcinoma. Hepatocellular carcinomas are also hypervascular, as are focal nodular hyperplasia and hepatic adenomas.

Cross References

Chapter 15: Solitary Liver Defects—Hemangioma

Chapter 16: Hepatoma—Vascular Hepatoma with Lung Metastases

"HOT" SPOT IN LIVER

FIGURE 18–4   A.

Blood Flow Study of Liver Scan: After injection of the colloid in an arm vein, the blood flow to the liver is rapid and has a normal pattern.

FIGURE 18–4   B and C.

Colloid Liver Scan: There is normal colloid accumulation in the right lobe. The left lobe has a defect from lymphoma.

Illustration continued on following page

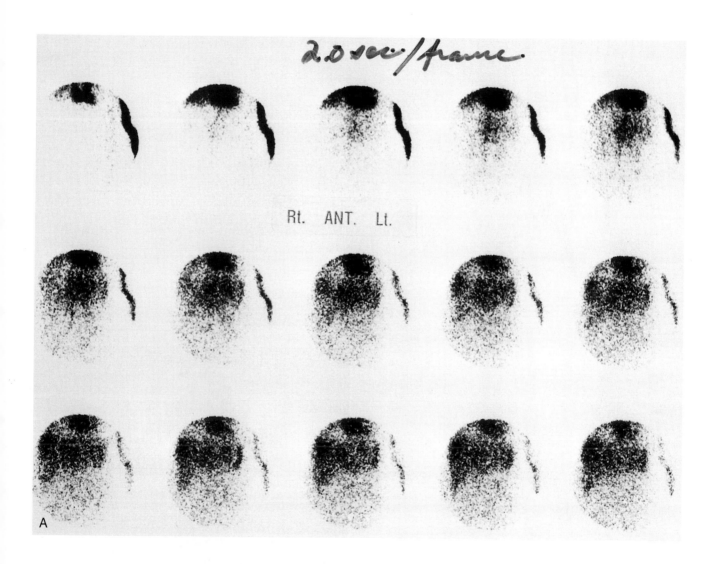

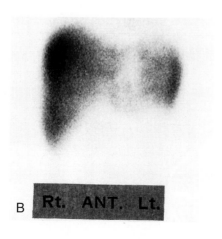

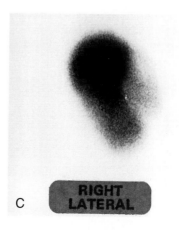

FIGURE 18–4 D.

Inferior Vena Cavagram: The IVC is obstructed. A collateral on the left side of the abdomen *(arrow)* leads to the umbilical vein *(arrowheads).*

FIGURE 18–4 E and F.

Repeat Colloid Liver Scan: There is a "hot" spot of colloid where the umbilical vein empties into the liver.

FIGURE 18–4 G.

CT Scan: The lymphoma has enveloped the IVC and abdominal aorta.

NOTE 1. "Hot" spots in the liver from collateral flow can be seen with either IVC or SVC obstruction.

NOTE 2. Vascular flow abnormalities should be considered as part of the differential diagnosis when a colloid scan "hot" spot is near the porta hepatis.

Cross Reference

Chapter 59: Venous Thrombosis—Liver Visualization with IVC Obstruction

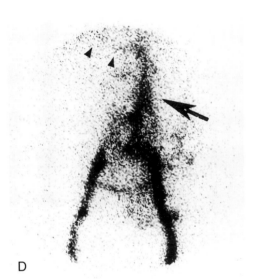

D

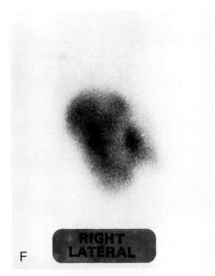

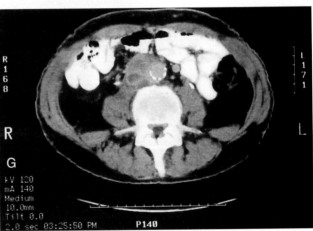

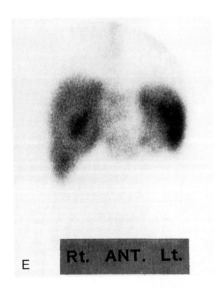

E

OBSTRUCTED ARTERIAL CHEMOTHERAPY CATHETER

FIGURE 18–5   A and B.
Anterior and Right Lateral ^{99m}Tc-Macroaggregated Albumin Catheter Flow and Albumin Colloid Liver Scans: The flow through the catheter accumulates only in the region surrounding the porta hepatis. The large mass in the posterosuperior right lobe of the liver receives none of the chemotherapeutic agents.

NOTE 1. The hepatic arterial catheter flow distribution should be checked by using the same flow rate as with the chemotherapy.

NOTE 2. A small amount of radiocolloid can be given after the arterial flow study to demonstrate the distribution of the catheter perfusion in terms of the liver anatomy and the tumor.

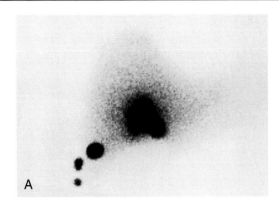

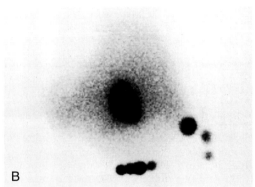

Chapter 19
LeVeen Shunts

PATENT LEVEEN SHUNT

FIGURE 19–1   A.
Anterior Abdomen Scan: The intra-abdominal injection of ^{99m}Tc-MAA can be seen in the right lower quadrant and in the LeVeen shunt tubing *(arrow)*.

Illustration continued on following page

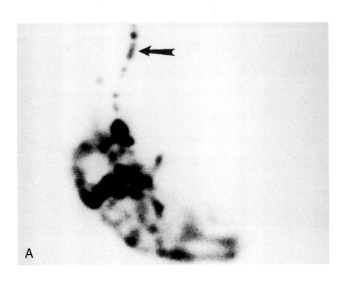

FIGURE 19–1 B.

Anterior Chest Scan: The lungs can be seen along with the shunt tubing, indicating patency of the LeVeen shunt. (Courtesy of Dr. Michael Kipper, Vista, CA.)

NOTE. A LeVeen shunt uses a one-way valve to drain ascitic fluid from the peritoneum into the central venous system, either the SVC or the subclavian vein.

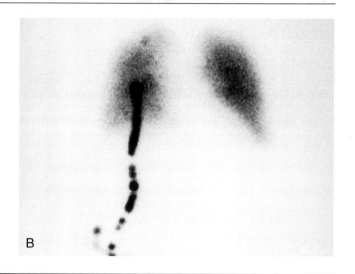

OBSTRUCTED LEVEEN SHUNT

FIGURE 19–2.

Radiocolloid and MAA Shunt Study: After injection into the LeVeen shunt tubing, there is no clearance by flow of fluid from the peritoneum. The minimal lung and liver activity is due to the injection volume's exceeding the capacity of the shunt tubing.

NOTE 1. LeVeen shunt obstruction is usually at the peritoneal end and is caused by fibrinous material.

NOTE 2. After intraperitoneal injection, an obstructed shunt will not be visualized. When the injection is made into the tubing, the lack of dynamic flow of the radiopharmaceutical indicates obstruction.

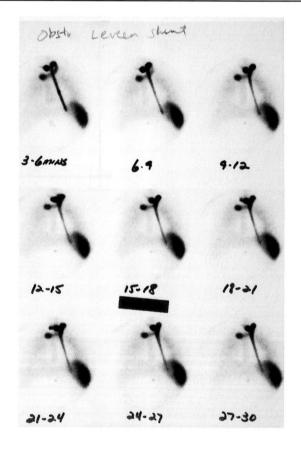

Chapter 20

Disorders of the Spleen

SPLENIC VARIANTS

Patient 1: Upside-down Spleen

FIGURE 20–1   A.

Colloid Scan: The spleen appears inverted.

Patient 2: Pelvic Spleen

FIGURE 20–1   B and C.

Colloid Scan: Although the patient has leukemia and the spleen is massive, its location in the pelvis is a normal variant.

Illustration continued on following page

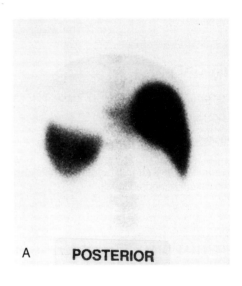

A   POSTERIOR

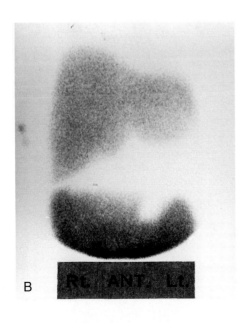

B   Rt. ANT. Lt.

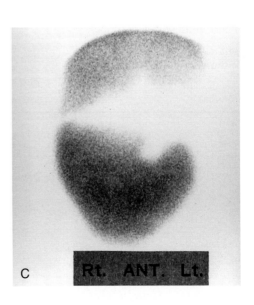

C   Rt. ANT. Lt.

Patient 3: Fetal Lobulation

FIGURE 20–1 D.

Colloid Scan: The round contours of the "defect" are more likely to be seen with fetal lobulation than with infarction or tumor.

NOTE 1. The splenic vascular pedicle can be long, allowing the spleen to move around in the abdomen. Rarely, torsion can occur.

NOTE 2. Although the liver should be against the lateral abdominal wall, the spleen need not be.

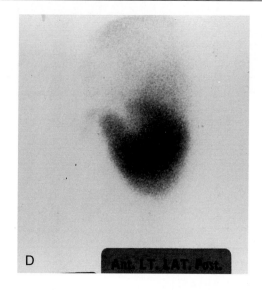

SPLENOMEGALY

Patient 1: Severe Chronic Congestive Splenomegaly

FIGURE 20–2 A and B.

Colloid Liver/Spleen Scan: The spleen is large, with markedly increased radiocolloid accumulation. The liver is atrophic, and the marrow has increased colloid.

DIFFERENTIAL DIAGNOSIS OF SPLENOMEGALY

1. Portal hypertension, including severe chronic congestive heart failure

2. Infections, especially viral and parasitic

3. Autoimmune disorders

4. Leukemias and lymphomas

5. Chronic anemias, hemolytic and megaloblastic

6. Storage diseases

7. Trauma

8. Cysts

9. Amyloidosis

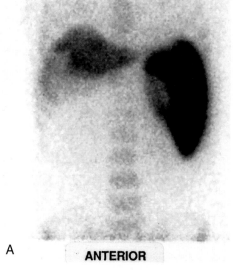

A   **ANTERIOR**

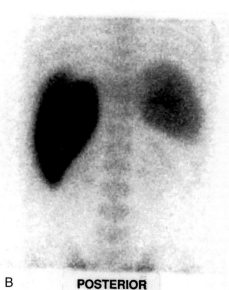

B   **POSTERIOR**

Patient 2: Polycythemia Vera

FIGURE 20–2   C and D.
The spleen is enlarged but has decreased activity, raising the question of leukemic infiltration.

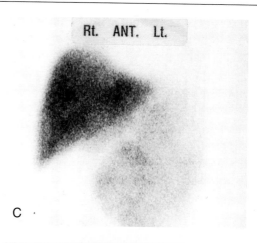

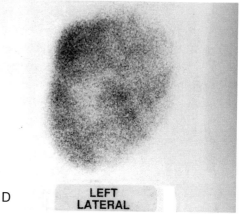

NOTE 1. The normal spleen should be less than 13 cm in its longest diameter.

NOTE 2. Congestive splenomegaly can be seen with cirrhosis, splenic vein occlusion, portal vein thrombosis, hepatic vein occlusion, and severe chronic congestive heart failure (cardiac cirrhosis).

NOTE 3. Banti's syndrome includes congestive splenomegaly, thrombocytopenia (hypersplenism), and gastrointestinal hemorrhage.

NOTE 4. In polycythemia vera there is splenomegaly, whereas in secondary polycythemia the spleen is usually normal in size.

Cross Reference

Chapter 13: Hepatomegaly—Renal Activity with Cardiac Cirrhosis

SUBPHRENIC ABSCESS SIMULATING SPLEEN

Patient 1: Post Splenectomy and Fever

FIGURE 20–3   A and B.
Posterior and Anterior ^{111}In-WBC Scan: The spleen has less activity than the liver.

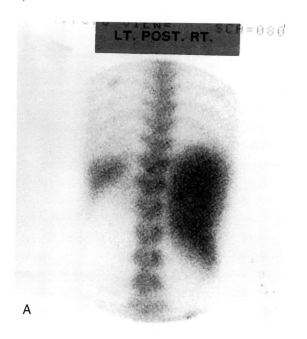

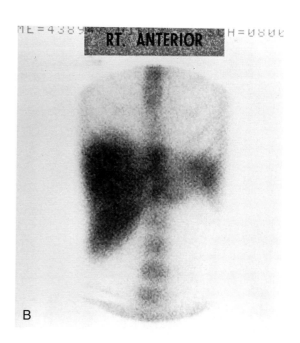

Illustration continued on following page

Patient 2: Fever in Patient with Remote History of Splenectomy

FIGURE 20–3   C and D.
Posterior and Left Lateral ^{111}In-WBC Scans: There is WBC accumulation under the diaphragm in the splenic bed.

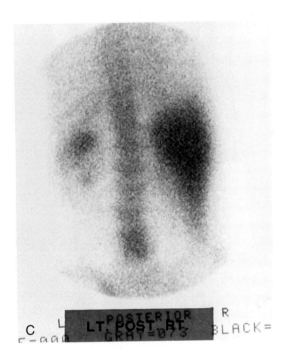

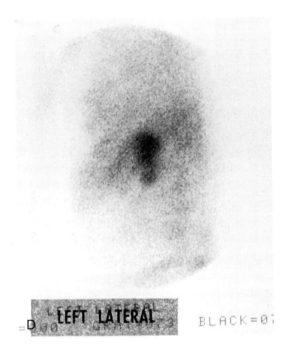

Patient 3: Normal Post Splenectomy

FIGURE 20–3   E and F.
Posterior and Anterior ^{111}In-WBC Scan: This is a normal appearance for a splenectomy patient.

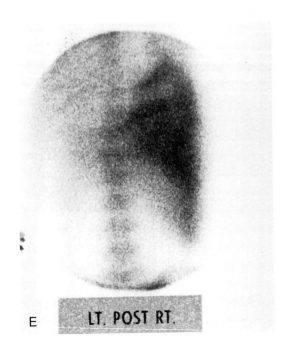

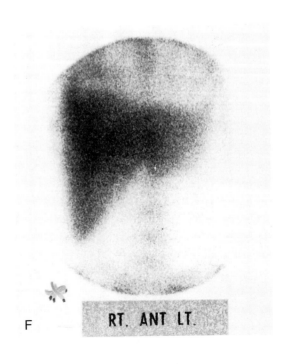

Patient 4: Normal Splenic Activity

FIGURE 20–3   G.

Posterior ^{111}In-WBC Scan: The accumulation of WBCs in the spleen is greater than in the liver and bone marrow.

NOTE 1. Knowing the history of splenectomy is critical in interpreting WBC scans.

NOTE 2. If the "splenic" activity is less intense than that of the liver, splenic infiltration with tumor, an error in the labeling process of the WBCs, and a subphrenic abscess in a postsplenectomy patient should be included in the differential diagnosis.

Cross Reference

Chapter 33: Gastrointestinal and Abdominal Infections—Pancreatitis

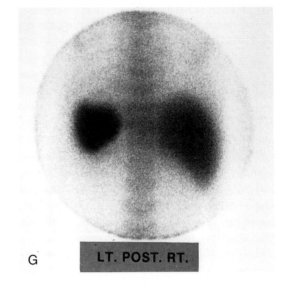

G   LT. POST. RT.

FRACTURED SPLEEN

Patient 1: Bicycle Accident

FIGURE 20–4   A and B.

Colloid Scan: There are at least three fragments of spleen after the traumatic event in this 9 year old boy.

Patient 2: Skateboard Accident

FIGURE 20–4   C to E.

Colloid Scan: The fracture extends partially through the splenic substance.

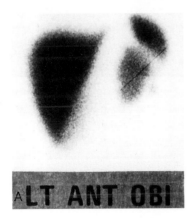

A LT ANT OBI

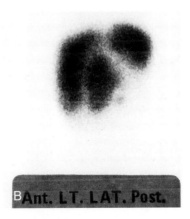

B Ant. LT. LAT. Post.

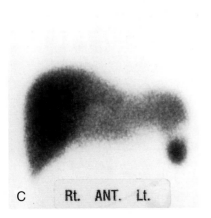

C   Rt. ANT. Lt.

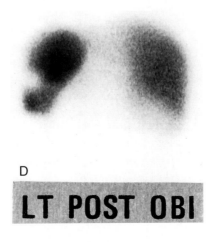

D   LT POST OBI

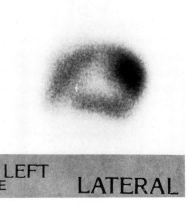

E LEFT   LATERAL

SPLENIC HEMATOMA

Patient 1: Automobile Accident

FIGURE 20–5 A.

Pretrauma Colloid Scan: There is mild hepatocellular dysfunction and hepatomegaly.

FIGURE 20–5 B.

Post-trauma Colloid Scan: There is now a mass in the upper pole of the spleen.

FIGURE 20–5 C.

Contrast-Enhanced CT Scan: The hematoma is well seen as lower density mass within the spleen.

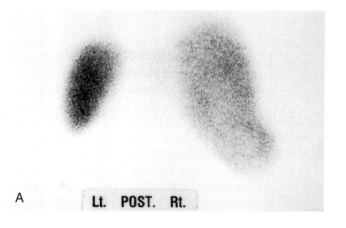

A Lt. POST. Rt.

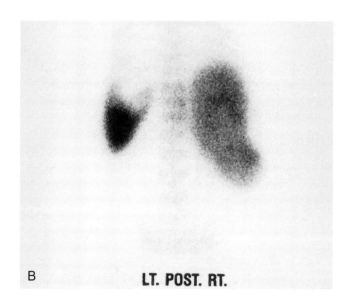

B LT. POST. RT.

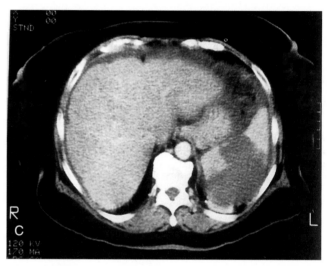

Patient 2: Bodysurfing Accident

FIGURE 20–5 D and E.

Colloid Scan: The pre-existing splenomegaly made this spleen more susceptible to trauma.

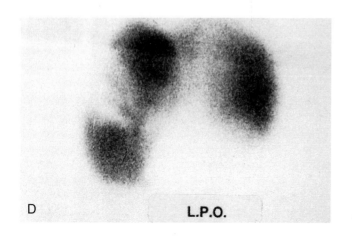

D L.P.O.

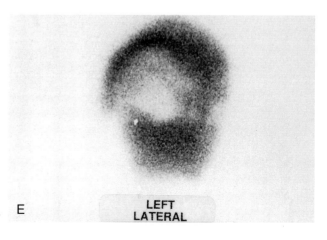

E LEFT LATERAL

ACCESSORY SPLEENS

Patient 1: Idiopathic Thrombocytopenia Purpura (ITP)

FIGURE 20–6   A and B.

Heat-Damaged Red Cell Study: There are two foci of RBC localization in the splenic bed. At surgery, these were splenic tissue.

Patient 2: ITP

FIGURE 20–6   C and D.

Heat-Damaged Red Cell Scan: A single accessory spleen was identified adjacent to the left kidney. A second accessory spleen *(arrow)* was not recognized at the time because of the relatively minor red cell accumulation.

Illustration continued on following page

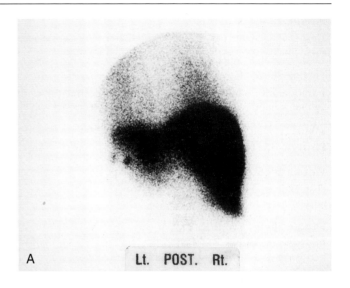

A   Lt. POST. Rt.

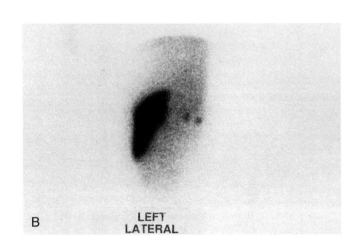

B   LEFT LATERAL

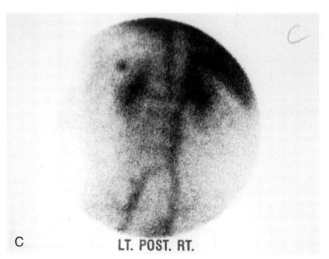

C   LT. POST. RT.

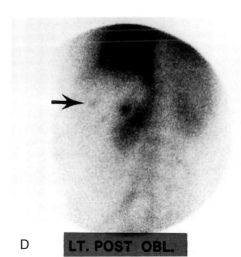

D   LT. POST OBL.

FIGURE 20–6   E and F.

Heat-Damaged Red Cell Scan 4 Months Later: The second accessory spleen now has enough function to be identified.

FIGURE 20–6   G.

Intraoperative Specimen Scan: Placing the specimen over the gamma camera confirms the removal of the accessory spleen.

Patient 3: ITP

FIGURE 20–6   H and I.

Heat-Damaged Red Cell Scan: Accessory splenic tissue is seen adjacent to the left kidney.

FIGURE 20–6   J and K.

Intraoperative Scans: The solitary focus is well seen, and moving it at surgery confirmed the specimen's activity (K).

FIGURE 20–6   L.

Heat-Damaged Red Cell Scan 10 Months Later: A second accessory spleen is now evident in the left midabdomen.

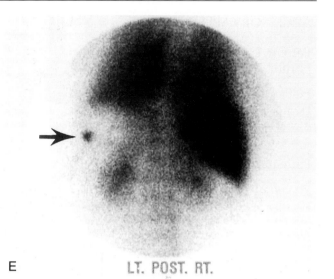

E   LT. POST. RT.

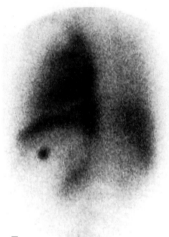

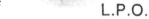

F   L.P.O.

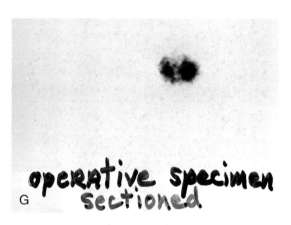

G   operative specimen sectioned

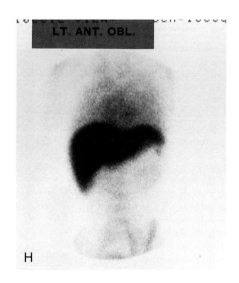

LT. ANT. OBL.

H

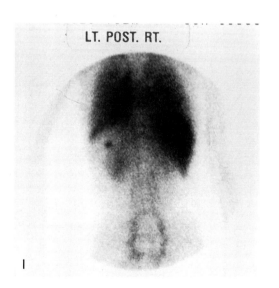

LT. POST. RT.

I

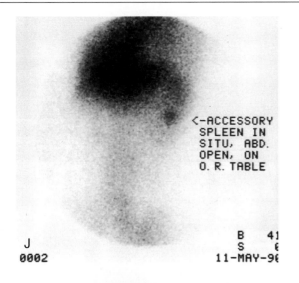

<-ACCESSORY
SPLEEN IN
SITU, ABD.
OPEN, ON
O. R. TABLE

J
0002

B   41
S   6
11-MAY-96

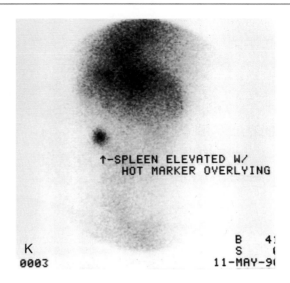

↑-SPLEEN ELEVATED W/
HOT MARKER OVERLYING

K
0003

B   4:
S   (
11-MAY-9(

L.A.O.

L
0004

B   7:
S   :
11-MAR-9

Patient 4: Status Post Splenectomy for Splenic Trauma During Gastric Surgery

FIGURE 20–6   M and N.

Coronal and Transverse ^{99m}Tc-Colloid Scan: There are two foci of colloid accumulation in the posterior left upper quadrant consistent with accessory splenic tissue.

NOTE 1. Accessory spleens can be found in the left upper quadrant, near the tail of the pancreas or the kidney, as well as in the mesentery or pelvis. There are rarely more than two, but one may not be functioning sufficiently at first relapse to be detected with scanning.

NOTE 2. Using a portable gamma camera in the operating room can help locate accessory spleens.

Illustration continued on following page

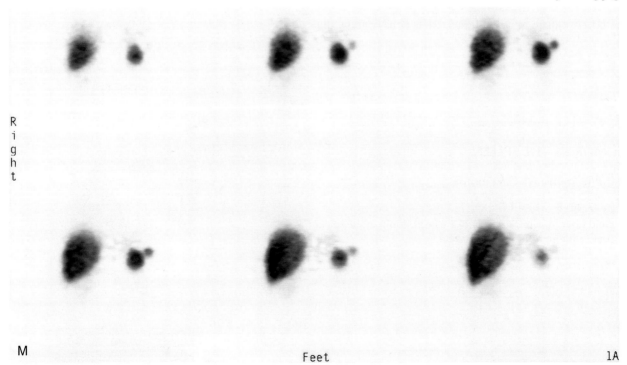

R
i
g
h
t

M

Feet

1A

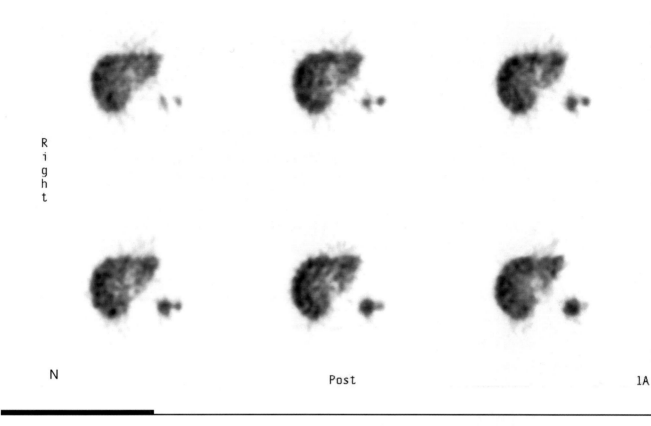

R
i
g
h
t

N   Post   1A

MESENTERIC IMPLANTS OF SPLENIC TISSUE

FIGURE 20–7.

Colloid Scan: Following splenectomy for a fractured spleen, splenic tissue became imbedded in the mesentery. The scan indicates an intact blood supply and presumed function.

NOTE. Surgical splenic implantation is no longer performed.

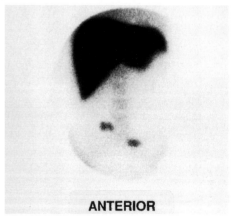

ANTERIOR

TUMOR IN THE SPLEEN

Patient 1: Breast Carcinoma

FIGURE 20–8 A and B.

Colloid Liver/Spleen Scan: There are focal lesions in the spleen *(arrows)*, although the liver is normal.

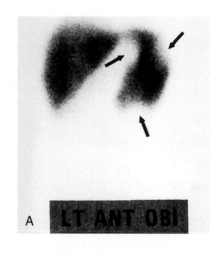

A   LT ANT OBl

Patient 2: Lymphocytic Leukemia

FIGURE 20–8   C and D.

Colloid Scan: There are focal masses in the spleen as well as the liver.

Patient 3: Leukemia

FIGURE 20–8   E and F.

Colloid Scan: The spleen has diffusely diminished activity, with an inhomogeneous pattern.

NOTE 1. Metastases to the spleen occur late in the course of disease and rarely cause symptoms or splenomegaly. Splenic involvement usually occurs when there is portal obstruction.

NOTE 2. Mass lesions from leukemia or lymphoma in the liver or spleen are distinctly unusual.

Cross References

Chapter 13: Hepatomegaly—Leukemic Liver

Chapter 18: Abnormal Liver Blood Flow—"Hot" Spot in Liver

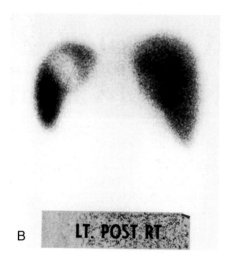

B   LT. POST RT.

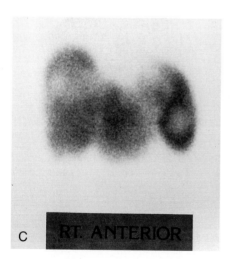

C   RT. ANTERIOR

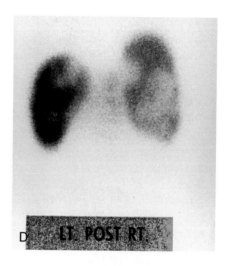

D   LT. POST RT.

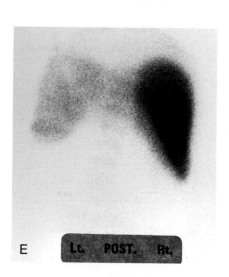

E   Lt. POST. Rt.

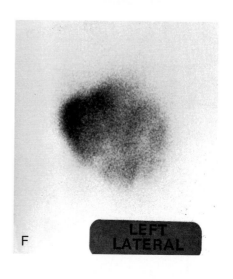

F   LEFT LATERAL

Chapter 21
Normal/Normal Variants

NORMAL HEPATOBILIARY SCINTIGRAPHY (HIDA)

FIGURE 21–1   A to D.

^{99M}Tc-Mebrofenin Scan (HIDA Scan): There is good extraction of the radiopharmaceutical by the liver parenchymal cells, with prompt conjugation and excretion of radiolabeled bile into the intrahepatic bile ducts. The gallbladder fills before the common duct empties into the duodenum. The liver has progressively diminished radioactivity over time.

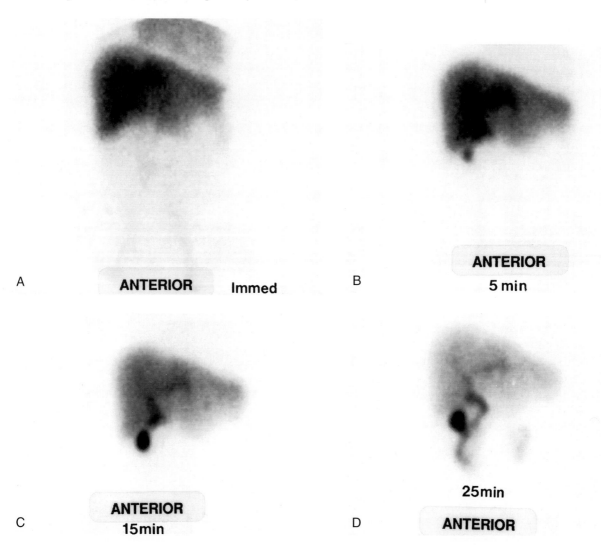

A   ANTERIOR   Immed

B   ANTERIOR   5 min

C   ANTERIOR   15min

D   25min   ANTERIOR

FIGURE 21–1   E.

Right Lateral HIDA Scan: The gallbladder (GB) is an anterior structure, distinguishing it from the more posterior duodenum (D).

Patient 2

FIGURE 21–1   F.

Anterior [99M]Tc-Mebrofenin Scan: The gallbladder can be seen filling the gallbladder fossa.

FIGURE 21–1   G.

Right Lateral Decubitus HIDA Scan: The gallbladder is not seen in its normal anterior location.

FIGURE 21–1   H.

Cross-table Lateral HIDA Scan: The gallbladder can be seen in its more usual position.

Patient 3

FIGURE 21–1   I.

Anterior [99M]Tc-Mebrofenin Scan: No gallbladder fossa is readily identifiable.

FIGURE 21–1   J.

Right Lateral HIDA Scan: A horizontal notch in the anterior liver can be seen.

FIGURE 21–1   K.

Delayed RAO HIDA Scan: The gallbladder fills and distends toward the left side, to overlie the gastric antrum and duodenal bulb.

FIGURE 21–1   L.

Delayed Right Lateral HIDA Scan: The gallbladder fills in the notch seen on the earlier right lateral scan.

NOTE 1. Although the correct term for this procedure is hepatobiliary scintigraphy, "HIDA" scan is commonly used for convenience.

NOTE 2. The normal gallbladder should fill within 40 minutes of injection and should distend to completely fill the gallbladder fossa. An incompletely filled gallbladder is abnormal, suggesting acalculous cholecystitis or "relieved" acute calculous cholecystitis.

NOTE 3. It is often preferable to do cross-table lateral scans, rather than right lateral decubitus scans, to confirm the filling of the gallbladder.

NOTE 4. Oblique views can be helpful when the gallbladder overlies the common bile duct, especially when there is bile in the duodenum.

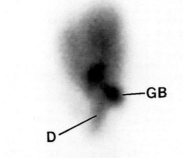

E

RT. LATERAL

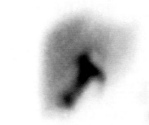

F

Anterior

G

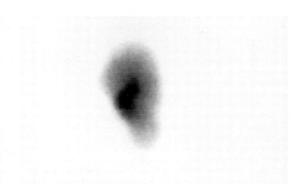

H

Cross-table Lateral

Illustration continued on following page

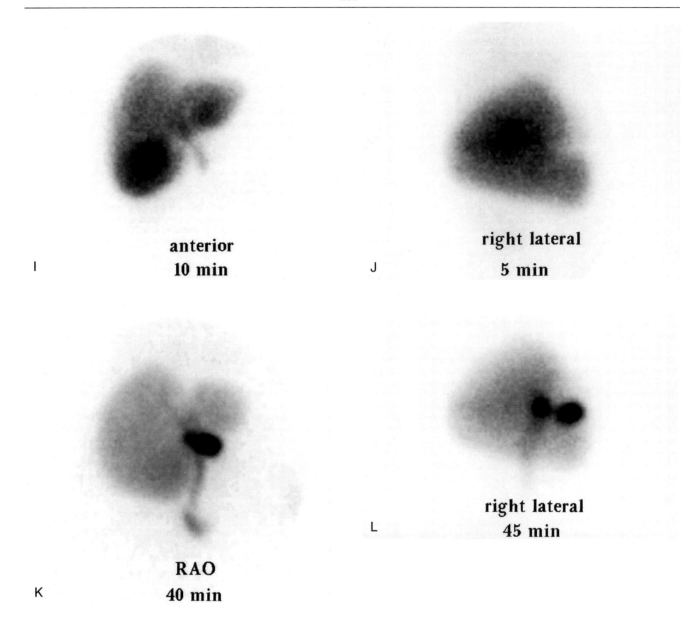

anterior
10 min

I

right lateral
5 min

J

RAO
40 min

K

right lateral
45 min

L

NORMAL MORPHINE-AUGMENTED HIDA SCAN

FIGURE 21–2 A and B.

HIDA Scan: After 4 mg of intravenous morphine at 50 minutes, the gallbladder filled and distended normally.

NOTE 1. Morphine will cause sphincter of Oddi contraction, increasing the pressure within the common bile duct, and allow bile to flow into the cystic duct if it is patent.

NOTE 2. With delayed distention to fill the gallbladder fossa, the differential diagnosis should include a sludge-filled gallbladder, chronic cholecystitis, or other nonobstructive gallbladder disease.

NOTE 3. With gallbladder visualization, acute calculous cholecystitis with cystic duct obstruction can be ruled out.

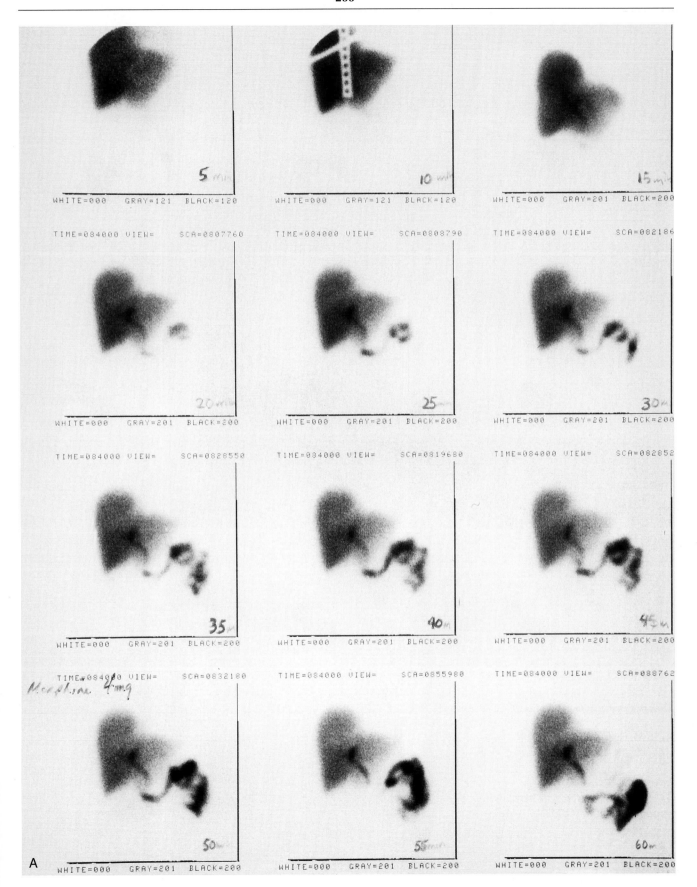

Illustration continued on following page

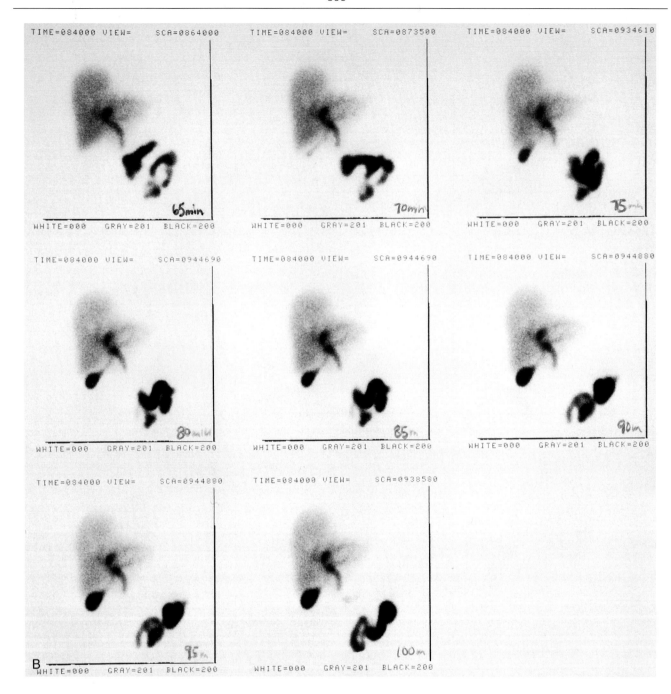

NORMAL GALLBLADDER EJECTION FRACTION

FIGURE 21–3   A.

Pre-Cholecystokinin (CCK) HIDA Scan: The gallbladder has distended to fill the gallbladder fossa.

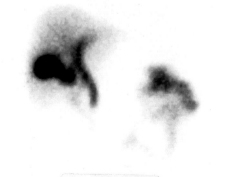

A

ANTERIOR

FIGURE 21–3   B.

Post-CCK HIDA Scan: There has been good contraction of the gallbladder.

FIGURE 21–3   C.

Gallbladder Ejection Fraction Graph: The time-activity curve demonstrates the reduction of the counts within the gallbladder following a CCK induced contraction. The gallbladder ejection fraction measures 80 percent.

NOTE 1. The normal gallbladder ejection fraction is greater than 50 percent.

NOTE 2. The loss of intensity within the gallbladder, more than the decrease in size, is indicative of the gallbladder ejection fraction.

NOTE 3. The synthetic CCK should be infused over 15 to 20 minutes to reduce cramping and nausea.

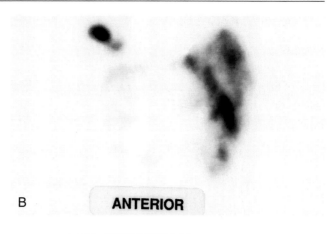

B   **ANTERIOR**

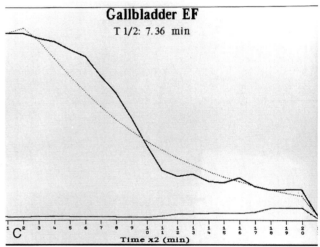

Gallbladder EF
T 1/2: 7.36 min

C   Time x2 (min)

HYPOPLASTIC GALLBLADDER

FIGURE 21-4   A and B.

HIDA Scan: The small gallbladder *(arrow)* was not inflamed at surgery.

NOTE 1. There is no appreciable gallbladder fossa on the early film.

NOTE 2. The differential diagnosis with this scan picture should include acalculous cholecystitis, severe chronic cholecystitis, and obstruction of the distal portion of a septate gallbladder.

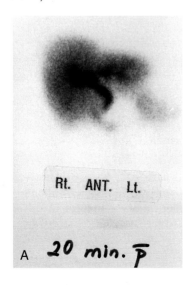

Rt. ANT. Lt.

A   20 min. $\bar{p}$

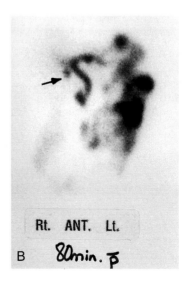

Rt. ANT. Lt.

B   80min. $\bar{p}$

INTRAHEPATIC GALLBLADDER

Patient 1

FIGURE 21–5   A and B.
Early Anterior and Right Lateral HIDA: There is no appreciable gallbladder fossa.

FIGURE 21–5   C and D.
Delayed Anterior and Lateral HIDA: The gallbladder sits high under the right lobe.

Patient 2

FIGURE 21–5   E and F.
Early Scan: The gallbladder fossa is seen only on the lateral scan *(arrow)* and is more posterior than usual.

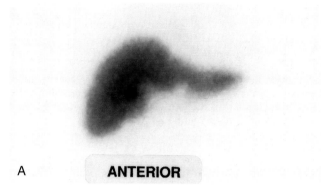

A   **ANTERIOR**

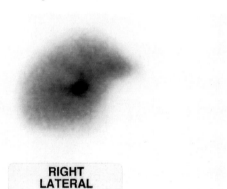

B   **RIGHT LATERAL**

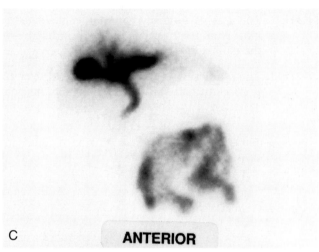

C   **ANTERIOR**

D **RT. LATERAL**

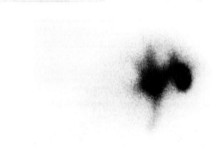

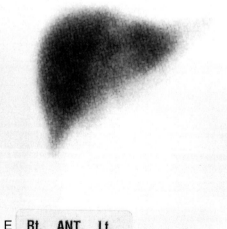

E **Rt.   ANT.   Lt.**

FIGURE 21–5   G and H.
Delayed HIDA Scan: The gallbladder fills and distends *(arrows)*. Poor concentration led to surgery and confirmation of the intrahepatic position.

NOTE. A right lateral view before and after the bile ducts are filled is often helpful in differentiating the gallbladder from bowel and liver.

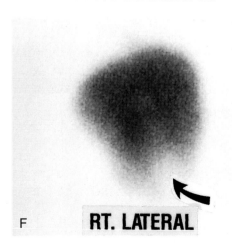

F   **RT. LATERAL**

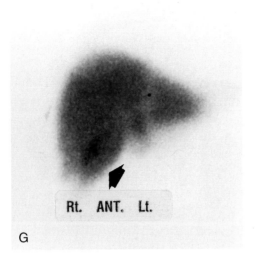

Rt. ANT. Lt.

G

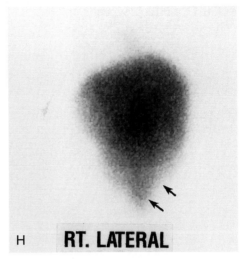

H   **RT. LATERAL**

SEPTATE GALLBLADDER

Patient 1

FIGURE 21–6   A.
HIDA Scan: There is a linear photon-deficient division of the gallbladder in the long axis.

Patient 2

FIGURE 21–6   B.
HIDA Scan: The distal end of the gallbladder is separated by a diaphragm.

NOTE. Septate gallbladders can have the dividing membrane in the long or short axis (gallbladder diaphragm). The septation may not be distinguishable from gallstones.

Cross Reference

Chapter 22: Cholecystitis—Incomplete Gallbladder Distention

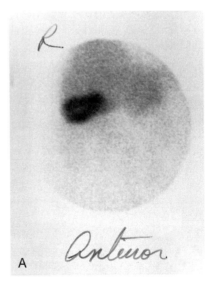

A

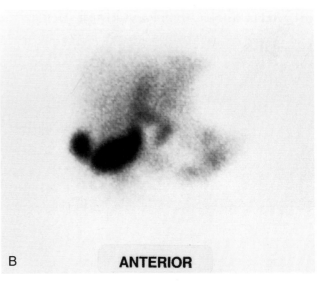

B   **ANTERIOR**

DUODENAL BULB ON HIDA SCAN

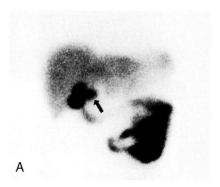

A

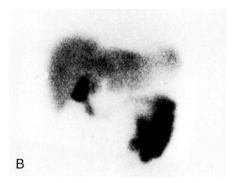

B

FIGURE 21–7 A.
HIDA Scan: The appearance of the duodenal bulb *(arrow)* can be confused with the gallbladder.

FIGURE 21–7 B.
Delayed HIDA Scan: Delayed imaging, especially after oral water, will show clearance of the duodenal bulb.

LOW ORIGIN OF CYSTIC DUCT

FIGURE 21–8.
HIDA Scan: The cystic duct arises from an unusually low position from the common hepatic duct.

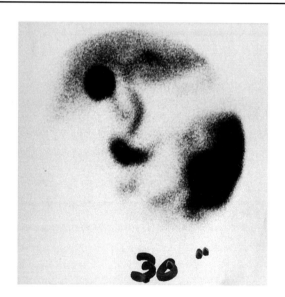

BILE REFLUX INTO THE PANCREATIC DUCT

FIGURE 21–9.
HIDA Scan: There is reflux of bile into a dilated pancreatic duct *(arrow)* as well as into the stomach.

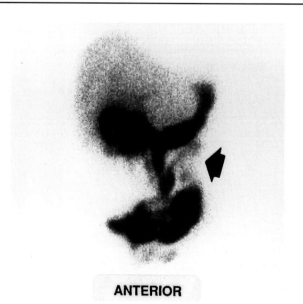

ANTERIOR

CLASSIC ACUTE CHOLECYSTITIS

FIGURE 22–1   A.

Blood Flow Scan: There is hyperemia along the inferior aspect of the liver.

FIGURE 22–1   B.

30 Minute HIDA Scan: The gallbladder is not visualized.

FIGURE 22–1   C.

Two Hour HIDA Scan: There is persistence of activity in the liver bordering the gallbladder fossa (the "rim sign").

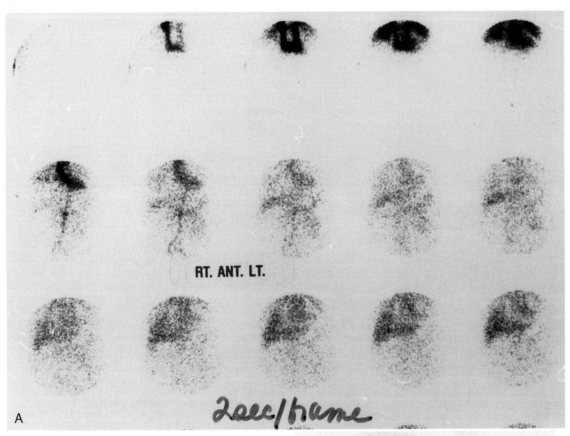

A

RT. ANT. LT.

2sec/frame

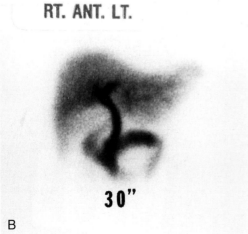

RT. ANT. LT.

B   30"

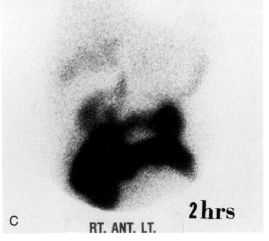

C   2hrs

RT. ANT. LT.

Illustration continued on following page

FIGURE 22–1   D.

Three Hour Computer-Enhanced HIDA Scan: There is entero-gastric reflux *(arrowhead)* and persistence of the rim sign *(arrow).*

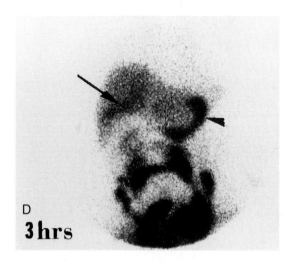

NOTE 1. Signs of acute cholecystitis include hyperemia, nonfilling of gallbladder despite morphine and/or long examination time, the rim sign, and incomplete gallbladder distention.

NOTE 2. Enterogastric reflux can be seen with many gallbladder conditions.

NOTE 3. The rim sign may be due to stasis of bile or increased delivery of the radiopharmaceutical because of the hyperemia.

ACUTE CHOLECYSTITIS ON MORPHINE-AUGMENTED HIDA SCAN

FIGURE 22–2   A.

Pre-Morphine HIDA Scan: The common duct and duodenum are well seen. No gallbladder can be seen.

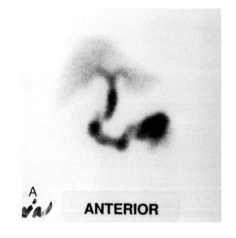

FIGURE 22–2   B.

Post-Morphine HIDA Scan: There is a good contraction of the sphincter of Oddi, without gallbladder visualization.

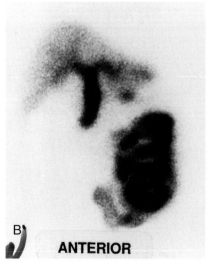

ACUTE ACALCULOUS CHOLECYSTITIS

FIGURE 22–3   A.

HIDA Scan: The gallbladder lumen is small *(arrow)*, and it filled only after morphine injection.

FIGURE 22–3   B.

CT Scan: The gallbladder wall is thickened. No stones are seen.

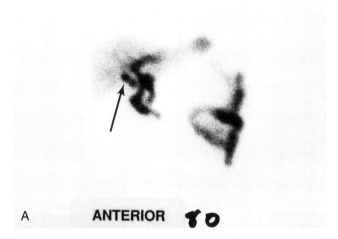

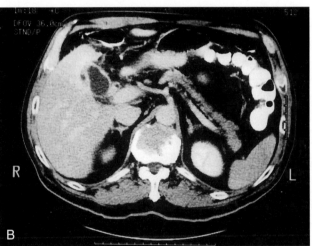

PERFORATED GANGRENOUS GALLBLADDER

FIGURE 22–4.

HIDA Scan: The common duct is faint and probably attenuated by the subhepatic abscess.

NOTE. The bowed, elongated, and poorly filled common bile duct is not a reliable sign of gallbladder perforation but, when seen, should lead to an ultrasound examination.

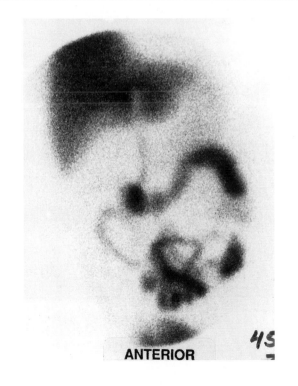

INCOMPLETE GALLBLADDER DISTENTION

Patient 1: Acalculous Cholecystitis

FIGURE 22–5 A.
HIDA Scan: A thin sliver of a gallbladder is seen *(arrowhead)*.

Patient 2: Relieved Acute Calculous Cholecystitis

FIGURE 22–5 B.
HIDA Scan: The gallbladder *(arrow)* has filling defects (stones) and does not distend fully. The patient's symptoms regressed soon after the examination.

Patient 3: Acute Cholecystitis

FIGURE 22–5 C.
HIDA Scan: The gallbladder fossa can be seen distal to the filled proximal gallbladder. There is also a rim sign.

FIGURE 22–5 D.
WBC Scan: There are WBCs accumulating in the distal portion of the gallbladder *(arrow)*.

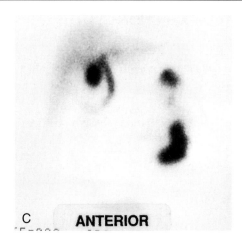

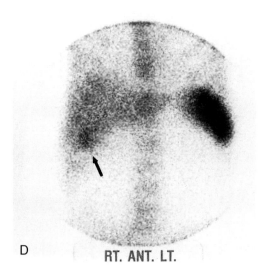

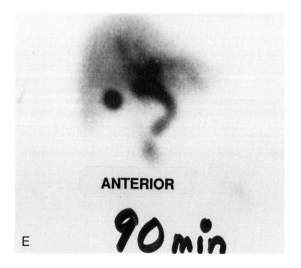

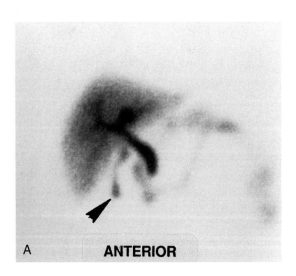

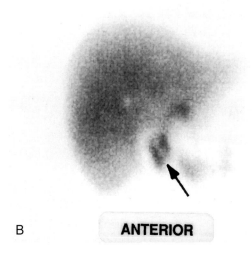

Patient 4: Stones Filling Proximal Portions of Septate Gallbladder

FIGURE 22–5 E.
HIDA Scan: The distal gallbladder fills but is separated from the bile ducts by a stone-filled proximal gallbladder.

Patient 5: Chronic Cholecystitis

FIGURE 22–5   F.

HIDA Scan: Filling defects (large stones) are seen within the proximal gallbladder. The distal gallbladder was completely occupied by stones and did not fill.

Patient 6: Hepatoma Invading Gallbladder Fossa

FIGURE 22–5   G.

HIDA Scan: The gallbladder does not distend to fill what appears to be the gallbladder fossa.

FIGURE 22–5   H.

Ultrasound: A mass is seen encasing the gallbladder.

NOTE 1. The normal gallbladder, even one with chronic cholecystitis, should always distend to fill the gallbladder fossa.

NOTE 2. Relieved acute cholecystitis occurs when the stone obstructing the cystic duct moves back into the gallbladder or is passed. Acute cholecystitis will recur frequently.

Cross References

Chapter 21: Normal/Normal Variants—Septate Gallbladder

Chapter 71: Infectious Diseases—Acute Cholecystitis on WBC Scan

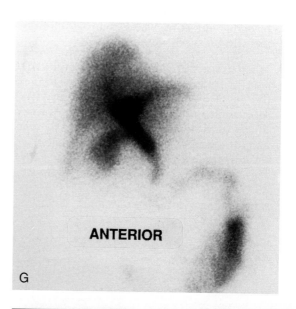

ANTERIOR

G

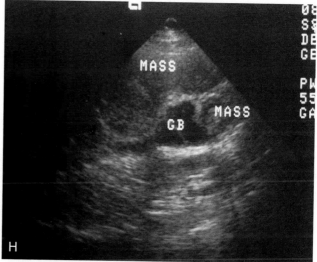

H

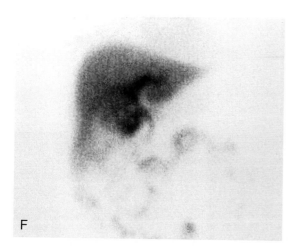

F

ABNORMAL GALLBLADDER CONTRACTILITY

Patient 1

FIGURE 22–6   A.

Pre-CCK HIDA Scan: The gallbladder distends to fill the gallbladder fossa.

FIGURE 22–6   B.

Thirty Minute Post-CCK Hida Scan: The gallbladder has not contracted significantly. The measured gallbladder ejection fraction was 10 percent.

Patient 2

FIGURE 22–6   C.

Gallbladder Time-Activity Curve: The contraction is poor, 32 percent before the curve turns upward during refilling.

NOTE 1. Visual analysis appears to work most of the time when using CCK. A measured gallbladder ejection fraction of less than 35 percent appears to be sufficiently below the normal range to have a high specificity for gallbladder disease.

Illustration continued on following page

NOTE 2. Symptoms need not be elicited when the CCK is given. The medium should be injected slowly over 15 to 20 minutes IV. We use 0.04 μgm/ kg over 15 to 20 minutes.

NOTE 3. The differential diagnosis of an abnormal gallbladder contractility includes chronic cholecystitis and biliary dyskinesia.

NOTE 4. When to Use CCK: (1) 3+ hours prior to HIDA scan in patient NPO for 48+ hours to clear the gallbladder of sludge; (2) during HIDA scan to measure gallbladder ejection fraction for chronic cholecystitis or biliary dyskinesia; and (3) to empty the gallbladder and bile ducts to study the bowel for obstruction.

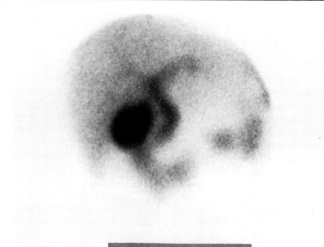

A   Rt. ANT. Lt.

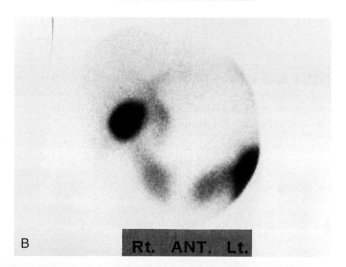

B   Rt. ANT. Lt.

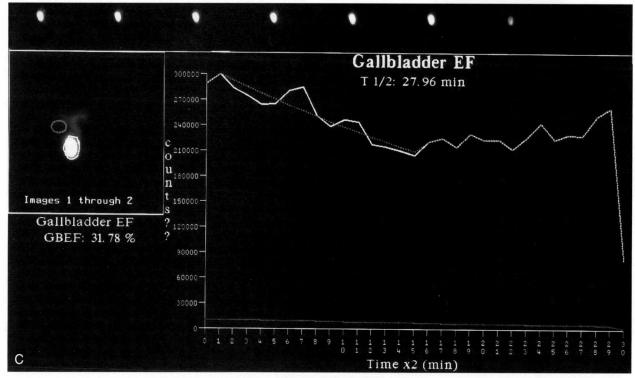

Chapter 23
Biliary Obstruction

TOTAL BILE DUCT OBSTRUCTION

Patient 1

FIGURE 23–1   A.
Twenty-four Hour HIDA Scan: The bile ducts and gallbladder never visualized over time.

Patient 2

FIGURE 23–1   B.
Twenty-four Hour HIDA Scan: There is an abrupt ending of the common bile duct *(arrow)*. There is also increased renal excretion of the radiopharmaceutical. The left kidney was hydronephrotic *(arrowheads)*. (Open arrow = right ureter.)

Patient 3: Biliary Atresia

FIGURE 23–1   C.
Four Hour HIDA Scan: There is no bowel seen at this time or on later scans. The kidneys and urinary bladder are seen as part of the extrahepatic excretory pathway.

NOTE 1. Ultrasound may not demonstrate biliary dilatation within 24 to 48 hours of total biliary obstruction.

NOTE 2. A newborn with jaundice should be placed on phenobarbital for 2 to 3 days prior to the scan to promote hepatic conjugation.

NOTE 3. False positive biliary atresia scans do occur.

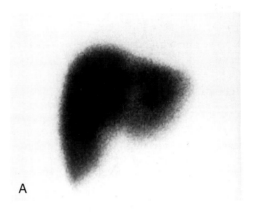

A

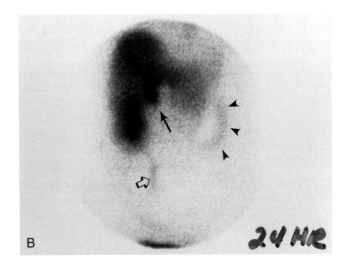

B   24 HR

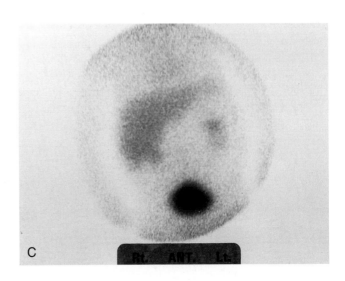

C   Rt.   ANT.   Lt.

PARTIAL COMMON DUCT OBSTRUCTION

Patient 1: Common Duct Stone

FIGURE 23–2   A.
Two Hour HIDA Scan: The extrahepatic duct is dilated and kinked, yet there is radiolabeled bile in the bowel.

Patient 2: Retained Common Duct Stone

FIGURE 23–2   B.
One Hour HIDA Scan: The left hepatic and the extrahepatic bile ducts are dilated.

Patient 3: Pancreatitis

FIGURE 23–2   C.
Ninety Minute HIDA Scan: There is delayed filling and emptying of the extrahepatic ducts, with compression by the enlarged pancreatic head. The second part of the duodenum is compressed as well.

Patient 4: Retained Common Duct Stone Without Obstruction

FIGURE 23–2   D.
Ninety Minute HIDA Scan: A stone in the distal common duct causes a filling defect *(arrow)*.

NOTE 1. A delayed scan is essential to confirm dilatation. Ultrasound can detect dilatation but cannot determine whether there is some bile passing into the bowel.

NOTE 2. Any patient on morphine or other opioids should have the medication stopped prior to beginning the HIDA scan. Morphine will markedly delay common duct visualization and emptying.

NOTE 3. Retained common duct stones can cause intermittent spasm and pain.

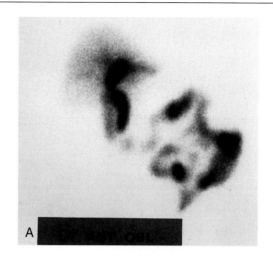

A

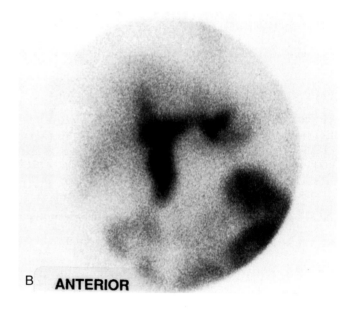

B   **ANTERIOR**

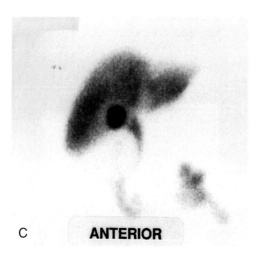

C   **ANTERIOR**

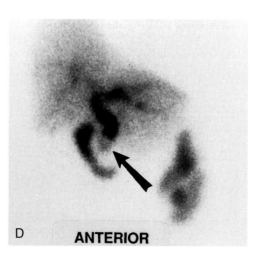

D   **ANTERIOR**

INTRAHEPATIC CHOLESTASIS

FIGURE 23–3 A.
Ninety Minute HIDA Scan: There is delayed filling and emptying of the normal-caliber common bile duct. The liver is enlarged.

FIGURE 23–3 B.
Seven Hour HIDA Scan: The bowel now has radiolabeled bile, indicating biliary tract patency.

NOTE 1. It may not be easy to distinguish intrahepatic from extrahepatic cholestasis, but at least partial patency of the bile ducts can be established when the bowel is seen.

NOTE 2. If the bilirubin is elevated, the bile ducts may not be seen, but bowel activity indicates biliary tract patency. Scans can be useful with serum bilirubins as high as 35 to 50 mg/dl.

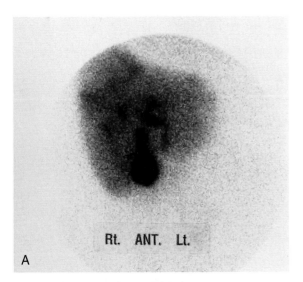

A

Rt. ANT. Lt.

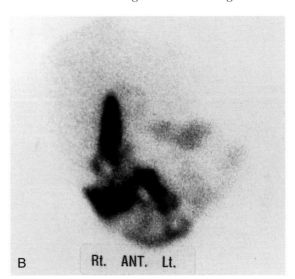

B

Rt. ANT. Lt.

Chapter 24
Bile Leaks

BILE LEAKS

Patient 1: Postoperative

FIGURE 24–1 A.
HIDA Scan: There is bile leaking into the peritoneum.

Patient 2: Auto Accident

FIGURE 24–1 B and C.
HIDA Scan: Bile collects anteroinferior to the liver in this post-cholecystectomy patient.

Patient 3: Trauma

FIGURE 24–1 D to F.
HIDA Scan: There is bile extravasation *(arrow)* from a fracture of the left lobe.

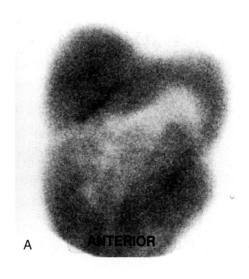

A ANTERIOR

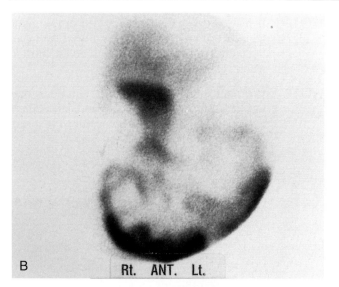

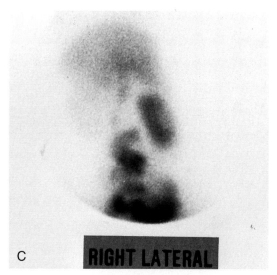

B   Rt. ANT. Lt.

C   **RIGHT LATERAL**

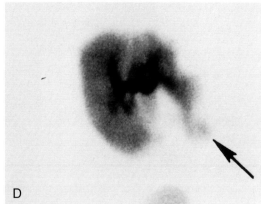

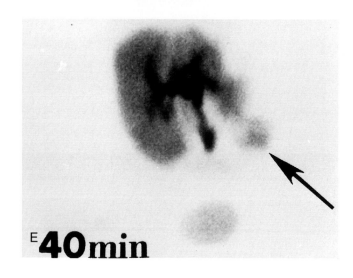

D

E **40min**

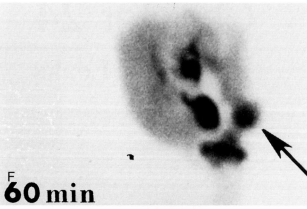

F
60 min

Patient 4: Postoperative

FIGURE 24–1   G to H.
HIDA Scan: There is a subcapsular collection of bile around the liver.

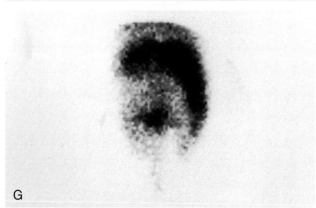

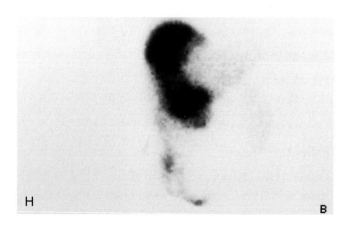

G

H   B

Patient 5: Skateboard Accident

FIGURE 24–1   I and J.

HIDA Scan: The liver is fractured *(arrow)*. There are focal collections of bile within the liver.

Patient 6: Postoperative

FIGURE 24–1   K.

HIDA Scan: Bile extravasation produced a collection overlying the left lobe of the liver.

Patient 7: Status Post Cholecystectomy

FIGURE 24–1   L and M.

HIDA Scan: The activity in the gallbladder fossa in this scan is extravasated bile from the cystic duct. It continues down into the peritoneum in the right paracolic gutter.

NOTE. Most bile leaks seal off spontaneously.

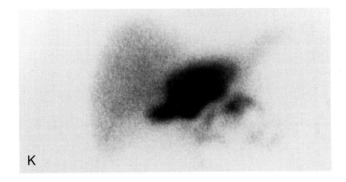

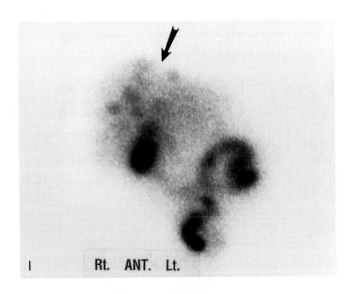

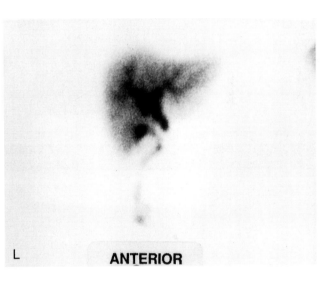

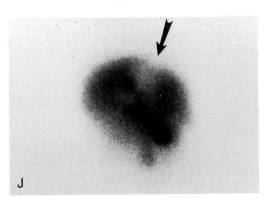

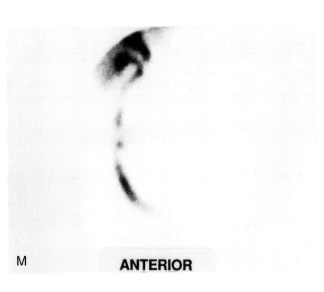

BOWEL PERFORATION

FIGURE 24–2.
HIDA Scan: There is extravasation of the radiolabeled bile into
the peritoneum. At surgery, a perforating ulcer was found in
the second part of the duodenum.

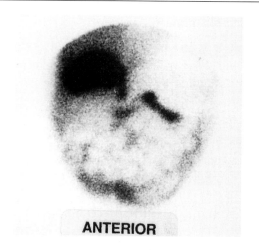

Chapter 25
Choledochocysts

CHOLEDOCHOCYST

FIGURE 25–1.
HIDA Scan: The common hepatic duct *(arrow)* is dilated but
does not obstruct bile flow.

NOTE 1. Choledochocysts are saccular or fusiform, most
commonly presenting with right upper quad-
rant pain and less often with jaundice or as
a mass.

NOTE 2. In early childhood, a choledochocyst may present with obstruction of the biliary tract,
whereas in adults and older children, pain is
more common.

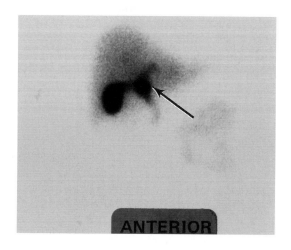

CAROLI'S DISEASE

FIGURE 25–2 A.
Thirty-five Minute HIDA Scan: There are focal areas of bile beginning to appear in the peripheral left lobe of the liver.

FIGURE 25–2 B.
Five Hour HIDA Scan: The left lobe is studded with focal bile collections.

FIGURE 25–2 C.
Colloid Liver Scan: There is diminished activity in the left lobe and medial right lobe.

FIGURE 25–2 D.
CT Scan: The dilated bile "cysts" are evident.

NOTE. Caroli's disease has focally dilated bile ducts ("cysts") that have a tendency to form stones and become infected. It is associated with congenital hepatic fibrosis.

Cross Reference

Chapter 17: Multiple Liver Defects—Multiple Hepatic Cysts

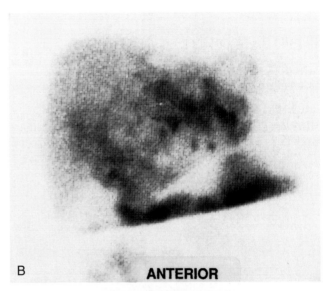

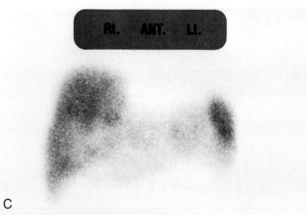

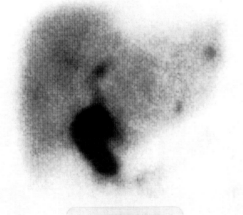

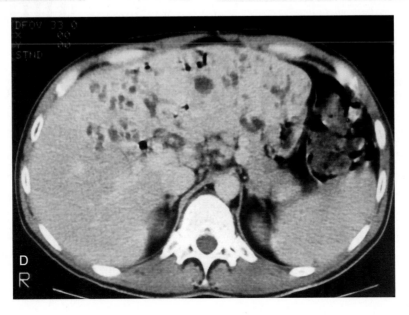

Chapter 26
Postsurgical Change

BILIARY DIVERSIONS

Patient 1: Cholecystojejunostomy for Pancreatic Carcinoma

FIGURE 26–1 A.
HIDA Scan: The diversion, done as part of a Whipple procedure, is patent.

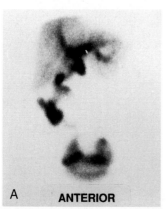

Patient 2: Choledochojejunostomy for Bile Duct Carcinoma

FIGURE 26–1 B.
HIDA Scan: Despite the diversion, there is biliary stasis in the dome of the right lobe, presumably from the intrahepatic tumor.

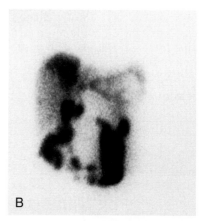

Chapter 27
Decreased Function on HIDA Scan

Patient 1: Chronic Liver Failure (Bilirubin = 23 mg/dl)

FIGURE 27–1 A.
HIDA Scan: There is residual parenchymal function and patent bile ducts. The activity below the liver is the kidney.

FIGURE 27–1 B.
Colloid Liver Scan: The liver has virtually no uptake of the radiocolloid.

DECREASED FUNCTION ON HIDA SCAN

1. Acquired Liver Parenchymal Disease

    a. Hepatitis, acute or chronic

    b. Cirrhosis

    c. Drugs

    d. Infections

    e. Neoplasms

2. Biliary Obstruction, Especially Chronic

3. Congenital Diseases of Bilirubin Metabolism

    a. Gilbert's disease

    b. Crigler-Najjar disease

    c. Dubin-Johnson syndrome

    d. Rotor's disease

4. Hemolysis

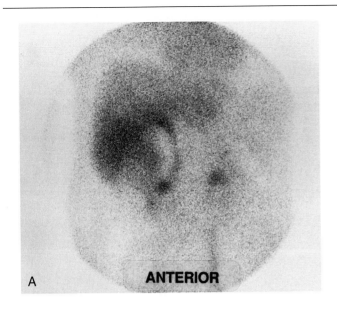

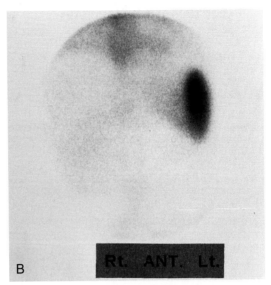

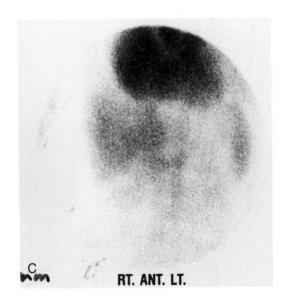

Patient 2: Cardiac Cirrhosis

FIGURE 27–1 C.

One Minute HIDA Scan: The cardiac blood pool is markedly enlarged.

FIGURE 27–1 D.

Forty Minute HIDA Scan: The liver has a mottled appearance, indicating areas of more severe hepatocellular dysfunction.

Patient 3: Hemolysis (Bilirubin = 32 mg/dl)

FIGURE 27–1 E.

HIDA Scan: Bilirubin, competing for binding sites, diminishes the concentration of the radiopharmaceutical in the liver and bile ducts *(arrow).*

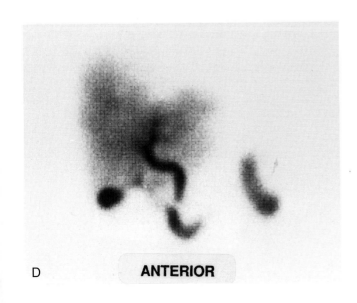

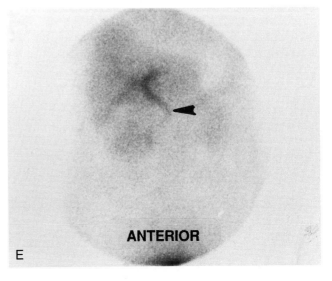

Patient 4: Jaundice (Bilirubin = 45 mg/dl)

FIGURE 27–1   F.

Sixty-five Minute HIDA Scan: The liver has decreased intensity, and no bile ducts can be seen.

FIGURE 27–1   G.

Twenty-four Hour HIDA Scan: With a longer scanning time and increased computer intensity, radiolabeled bile can be seen in the colon, indicating bile duct patency.

Patient 5: Acute Hepatitis

FIGURE 27–1   H.

HIDA Scan: The liver is barely discernible.

FIGURE 27–1   I.

Colloid Liver Scan: The liver has normal radiocolloid activity. (From Coel M, Denzer S: Disparate images in acute hepatitis using E-HIDA and sulfur colloid. Clin Nucl Med 7:315–317, 1982.)

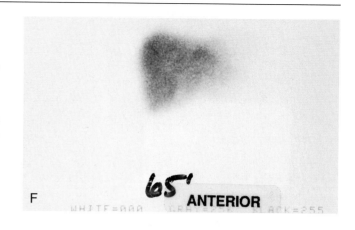

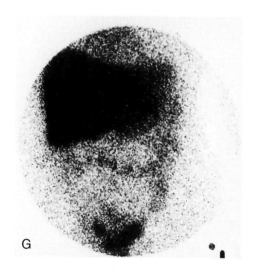

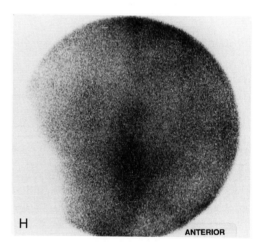

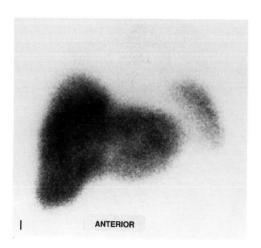

MASS LESIONS ON HIDA SCANS

Patient 1: Metastatic Disease to the Liver

FIGURE 27–2   A.
HIDA Scan: There are multiple foci of decreased activity.

Patient 2: Subhepatic Abscess

FIGURE 27–2   B.
HIDA Scan: A large "cold" area impressing upon the undersurface of the right lobe of the liver can be seen.

Cross Reference

Chapter 71: Infectious Diseases—Metastases to the Liver on WBC Scans

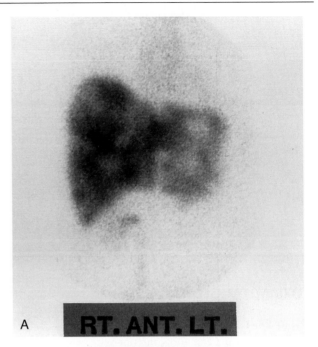

A   RT. ANT. LT.

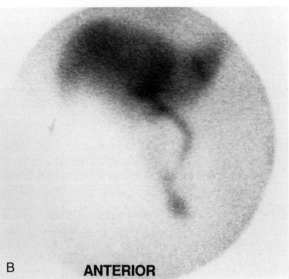

B   ANTERIOR

S E C T I O N   V

GASTROINTESTINAL SYSTEM

Chapter 28

Gastrointestinal Hemorrhage

NORMAL TAGGED RBC SCAN

FIGURE 28–1.

Tagged RBC Scan: The aorta, inferior vena cava, portal vein, splenic vein, and iliofemoral blood vessels are well seen. Some bladder activity occurs. The liver, spleen, kidneys, and penis will be seen because of their blood pools.

NOTE 1. Gastrointestinal hemorrhage is intermittent, with bleeding, then vasospasm, clot formation, and lysis followed by rebleeding.

NOTE 2. For GI bleeding studies, scanning should continue for 2 to 4 hours, unless the patient hemorrhages and the site of bleeding can be identified.

NOTE 3. Static images are taken every 5 minutes, with the computer acquisition at 30 sec/frame. A dynamic playback can be used to help identify which bowel segment is hemorrhaging.

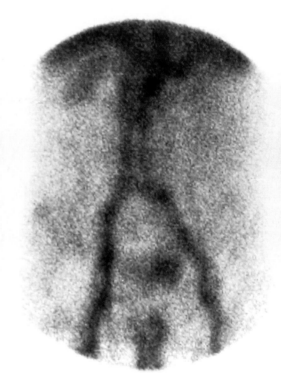

ANTERIOR

GI HEMORRHAGE ON BLOOD FLOW SCAN

Patient: Left Colonic Diverticular Hemorrhage

FIGURE 28–2   A.

Rapid Sequence Blood Flow Scans: Extravasation occurs immediately in the left lower quadrant.

FIGURE 28–2   B.

Three Minute Delayed Tagged RBC Scan: The left lower quadrant extravasation is beginning to spread out.

NOTE. Rapid-sequence scintiphotos can be obtained with either a tight radiocolloid bolus injection or the larger volume injection of tagged RBCs.

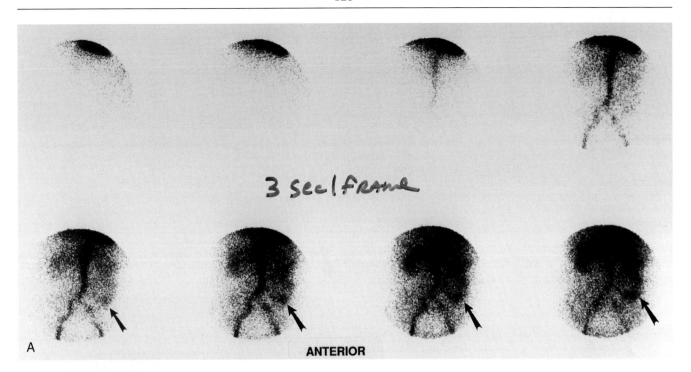

3 sec/frame

ANTERIOR

A

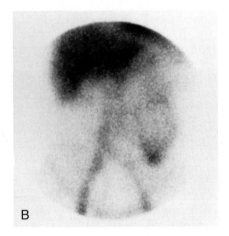

B

ACUTE GASTROINTESTINAL HEMORRHAGE

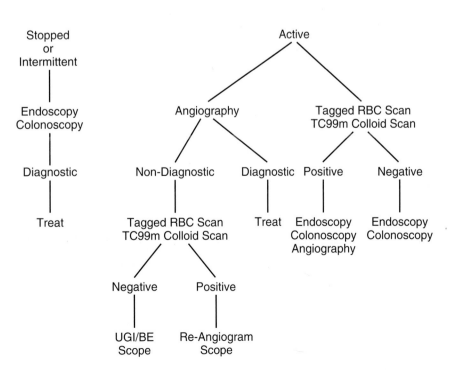

COLON DIVERTICULAR HEMORRHAGE

Patient 1

FIGURE 28–3   A.

Tagged RBC Scan: The extravasation of blood in the hepatic flexure *(arrow)* moved distally into the transverse colon.

FIGURE 28–3   B.

Superior Mesenteric Arteriogram: There is extravasation of contrast medium in the hepatic flexure *(arrow)*, best seen in the mucosal phase.

Patient 2

FIGURE 28–3   C.

Technetium Colloid Scan: There is extravasation in the ascending colon, which moved out of view over the liver.

NOTE 1. Arteriograms have approximately 4 seconds during which the contrast medium can detect extravasation. Radiocolloid scanning has approximately 5 to 15 minutes, whereas blood pool scans with tagged RBCs are capable of detecting the site of bleeding for several hours.

NOTE 2. The short effective scanning time and the inability to see over the liver make colloid scanning less useful for detecting intermittent bleeding.

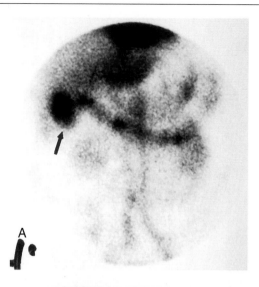

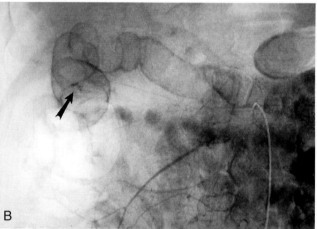

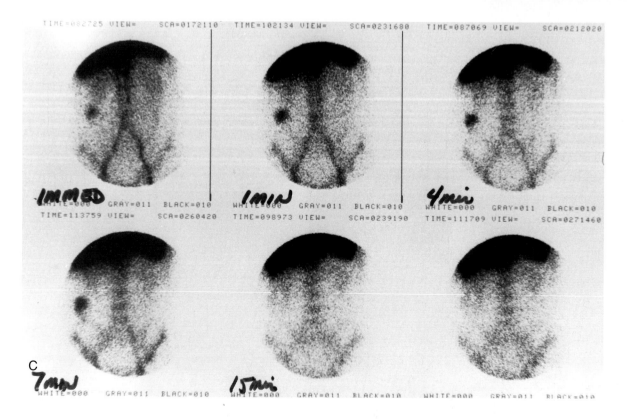

ANGIODYSPLASIAS

FIGURE 28–4.

Tc-99m Sulfur Colloid Scan: There is a "blush" in the right lower quadrant with a tortuous blood vessel draining cephalad.

NOTE. Angiodysplasias occur more frequently in the cecal region and more frequently in elderly patients.

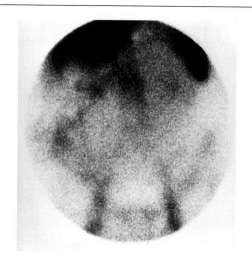

AORTOENTERIC FISTULA

Patient: 75 Year Old Male with Intermittent GI Hemorrhage

FIGURE 28–5.

Tagged RBC Scan: A saccular abdominal aortic aneursym is present just above the bifurcation. Extravasated blood can be seen in loops of jejunum.

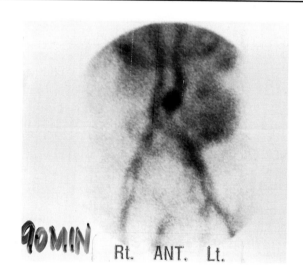

HEMORRHAGIC GASTRITIS

Patient 1

FIGURE 28–6   A.

Blood Flow Composite Scan: A summed image of the first seconds of the blood flow demonstrates stomach activity *(arrow)*.

FIGURE 28–6   B.

Tagged RBC Scanning: The stomach fills with extravasated blood. Endoscopy confirmed the bleeding.

Patient 2

FIGURE 28–6   C.

Sequential Tagged RBC Scintiphotos: There is immediate extravasation of blood in the left upper quadrant *(arrow)*. The filling of small bowel indicates that the hemorrhage is in the stomach rather than in the splenic flexure.

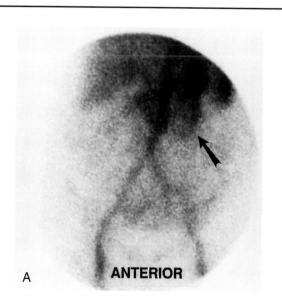

Illustration continued on following page

NOTE 1. Always scan the thyroid to check to see if there is free technetium, which would be excreted by the stomach.

NOTE 2. The stomach is not normally vascular and should not be seen on the blood flow study.

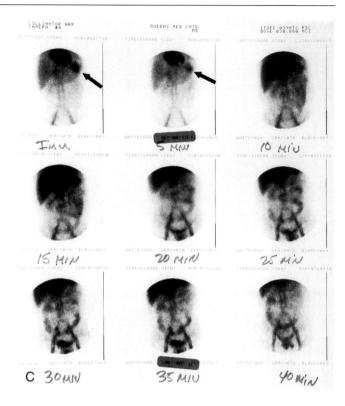

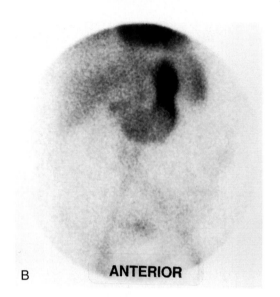

B   **ANTERIOR**

"CINE" OF GI BLEEDING

Patient 1

FIGURE 28–7   A.

Tagged RBC Scan: There is extravasation of blood in the central pelvis and in the small bowel, eventually reaching the colon at 35 minutes.

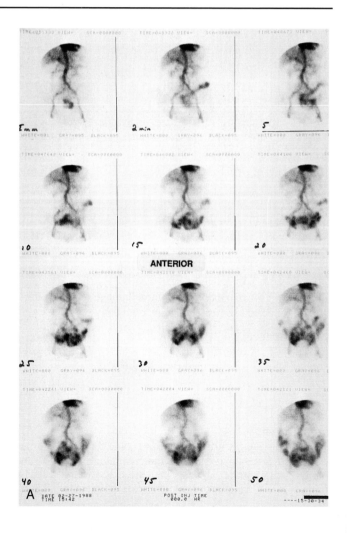

Patient 2: Bleeding Leiomyoma

Figure 28–7   B to F.

Sequential Tagged RBC Scans: There is extravasation of blood on the left side of the abdomen. Sequential scans establish the hemorrhage to be in the small bowel.

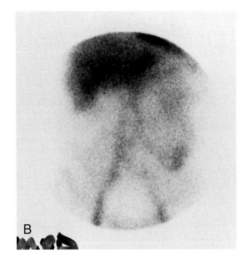

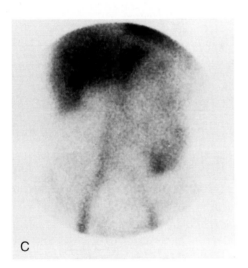

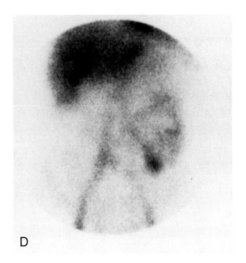

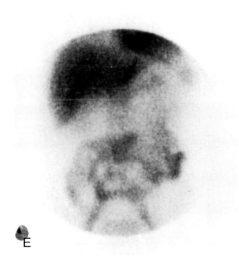

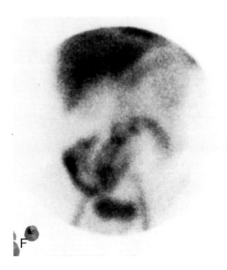

Illustration continued on following page

FIGURE 28–7   G.

Superior Mesenteric Angiogram: Extravasation of contrast medium *(arrowheads)* in the small bowel surrounds the tumor.

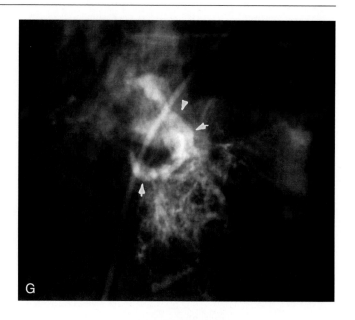

NOTE 1. Extravasated blood can move retrograde as well as antegrade.

NOTE 2. Acquiring the data on rapid computer acquisition and displaying as a cine loop can help identify the location of the hemorrhage more precisely, i.e., in separating small and large bowel hemorrhage.

Cross Reference

Chapter 33: Gastrointestinal and Abdominal Infections—GI Hemorrhage on WBC Scan

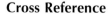

MULTIFOCAL GI HEMORRHAGE

FIGURE 28–8.

Tagged RBC Scan: There was simultaneous appearance of extravasated labeled RBCs along the transverse colon and small bowel in this patient with thrombocytopenia from leukemia.

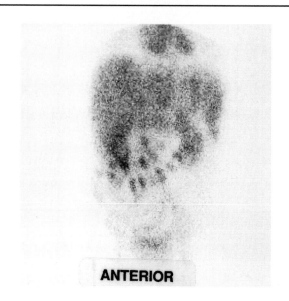

INFLAMMATION ON TAGGED RBC

FIGURE 28–9.

Tagged RBC Scan: There is hyperemia *(arrow)* in the RLQ that turned out to be a cecal infection secondary to appendicitis (typhlitis).

NOTE. Inflammation can cause hyperemia, which can be distinguished from GI hemorrhage by continued scanning. Over time, there is no transit of the radiopharmaceutical along the bowel.

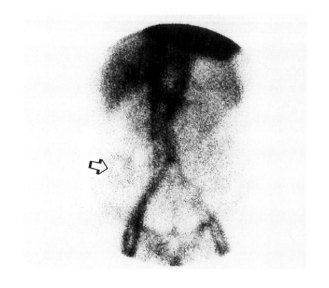

ASCITES ON TAGGED RBC SCAN

FIGURE 28–10.

Tagged RBC Scan: The mesenteric veins are straight but prominent. The small bowel is centrally located, with surrounding photopenic areas representing ascites.

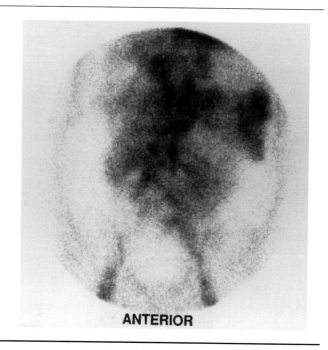

ANTERIOR

MESENTERIC VARICES

Patient 1: Portal Hypertension

FIGURE 28–11 A.

Tagged RBC Scan: There is a tangle of blood vessels in the mid-abdomen.

Patient 2: Pancreatic Carcinoma with Superior Mesenteric Venous Obstruction

FIGURE 28–11 B.

Tagged RBC Scan: The mesenteric varices can be seen in the left upper quadrant.

FIGURE 28–11 C to E.

Sequential RBC Scans: Jejunal hemorrhage *(arrow)* developed during the course of the scanning.

Patient 3

FIGURE 28–11 F.

HIDA Scan: There is a vascular loop *(arrow)* seen in the midabdomen in this patient with ascites.

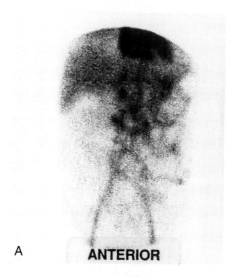

A   **ANTERIOR**

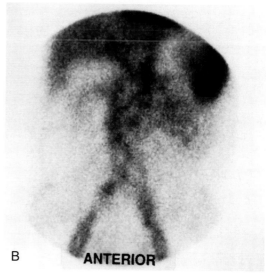

B   **ANTERIOR**

Illustration continued on following page

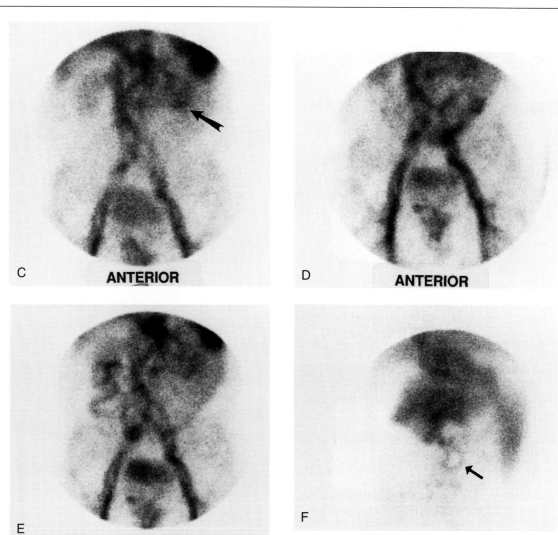

GALLBLADDER VISUALIZATION ON TAGGED RBC SCAN

FIGURE 28–12.
Tagged RBC Scan: The gallbladder can be seen on this tagged RBC scan.

NOTE 1. The gallbladder may be seen as a result of bleeding into the bile ducts (hematobilia) or blood breakdown products (hemolysis).

NOTE 2. Poor labeling can occur after multiple transfusions.

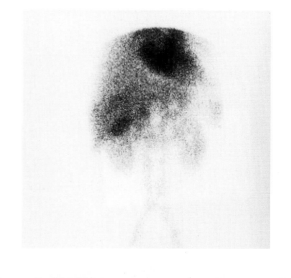

Chapter 29
Meckel's Diverticulum

NORMAL MECKEL'S DIVERTICULUM SCAN

FIGURE 29–1   A and B.

^{99m}Tc-Pertechnetate Scans: There is no focal accumulation of the ^{99m}Tc-pertechnetate over time.

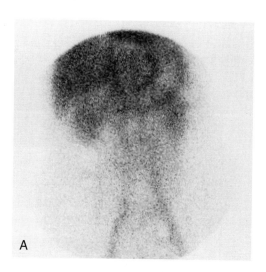

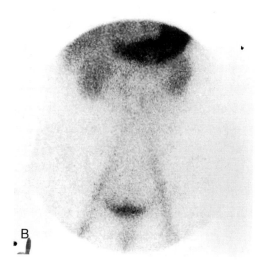

TECHNIQUE FOR SCANNING FOR MECKEL'S DIVERTICULUM

a. Glucagon, subcutaneous and IV, is an excellent way of delaying the gastric emptying, slowing intestinal motility, and preventing obscuration of the abdomen.

b. Subcutaneous pentagastrin stimulates gastric mucosa and may help in the detection of Meckel's diverticulum.

c. Oral cimetidine given 48 hours prior to the examination promotes retention of ^{99m}Tc-pertechnetate in gastric and ectopic gastric mucosa.

d. The patient should be fasting.

e. A bladder catheter is useful.

NOTE 1. This test will be positive only in those Meckel's diverticula that have gastric mucosa. These are the diverticula most likely to hemorrhage because of ulceration in the adjacent small bowel from the acid secretion.

NOTE 2. This test may have only a moderate sensitivity and specificity, but it is the best noninvasive diagnostic procedure. Reasons for negative examinations include Meckel's diverticulum with minimal or no gastric mucosa, ectopic gastric mucosal ulceration or necrosis, barium within the bowel, and poor patient preparation. About 50 percent of Meckel's diverticula do not have sufficient functioning gastric mucosa for detection on a technetium pertechnetate scan.

NOTE 3. Other conditions that can yield positive scans include intestinal neoplasms, ectopic gastric mucosa in enteric duplications, vascular malformations, and active bleeding sites.

MECKEL'S DIVERTICULUM

Patient: 57 Year Old Female

FIGURE 29–2 A and B.

Thirty Minute and 2 Hour ^{99m}Tc-Pertechnetate Scans: There is a small persistent focus of activity above the bladder in the RLQ *(arrow)*.

NOTE. Meckel's diverticula can be a cause of gastrointestinal hemorrhage in adults as well as in children.

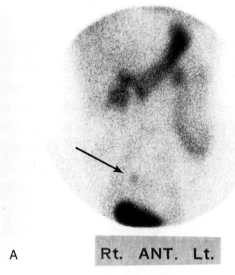

A   Rt. ANT. Lt.

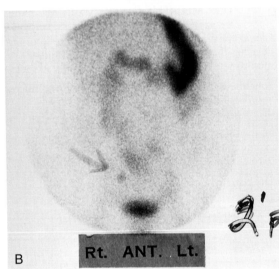

B   Rt. ANT. Lt.

UNUSUALLY LOCATED MECKEL'S DIVERTICULA

Patient 1: Three Year Old Female with Meckel's Diverticulum 2 Feet from Ileocecal Valve

FIGURE 29–3 A.

Four minute ^{99m}Tc-Pertechnetate Scan: There is a focal accumulation of the technetium pertechnetate in the left lower quadrant.

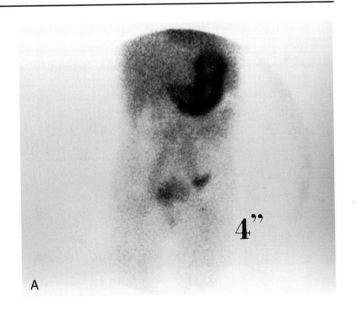

A

FIGURE 29–3   B.

Twelve Minute ⁹⁹ᵐTc-Pertechnetate Scan: There is radioactivity from acute bleeding in what proved to be a loop of small bowel.

Patient 2: Fourteen Year Old Male

FIGURE 29–3   C.

⁹⁹ᵐTc-Pertechnetate Scan: There is a focal accumulation of the radiopharmaceutical in the RUQ, lateral to a hydronephrotic kidney. At surgery a Meckel's diverticulum was found in the distal ileum. (Courtesy of Dr. Michael Kipper, Vista, CA.)

NOTE. Meckel's diverticula are most often in the RLQ or midline pelvis, but they can be elsewhere in the abdomen.

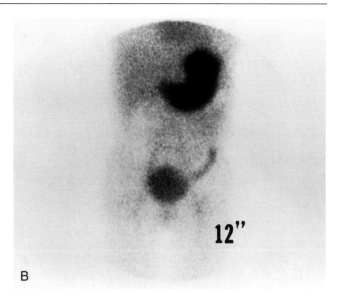

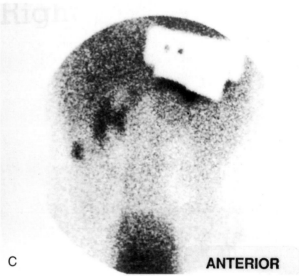

B

C

MECKEL'S DIVERTICULUM ON TAGGED RBC SCAN

Patient 1: Forty Year Old Male

FIGURE 29–4.

Tagged RBC Scan: There is RLQ extravasation of blood in what proved to be a Meckel's diverticulum.

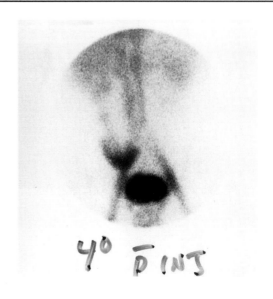

Chapter 30
Esophageal Studies

NORMAL ESOPHAGEAL SWALLOW

FIGURE 30–1.

Oral ^{99m}Tc-Colloid Scan: There is rapid clearance of the intact swallowed bolus within the normal 8- to 9-second transit time.

NOTE 1. Ten ml of water with 200 μCi of ^{99m}Tc-colloid is instilled in the mouth. The patient is asked to swallow once while standing or while lying supine.

NOTE 2. Rapid-sequence computer acquisition, 0.5 sec/frame, should be obtained as well as the rapid-sequence scintiphotos, at 2 sec./frame.

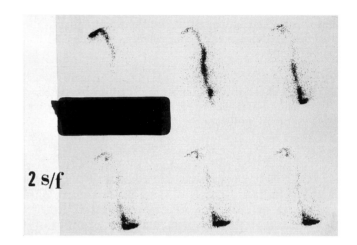

2 s/f

VALUE OF SUPINE ESOPHAGEAL MOTILITY STUDIES

Patient: Esophageal Dysmotility

FIGURE 30–2   A.

Upright Oral ^{99m}Tc-Colloid Scan: There is rapid clearance of the esophagus.

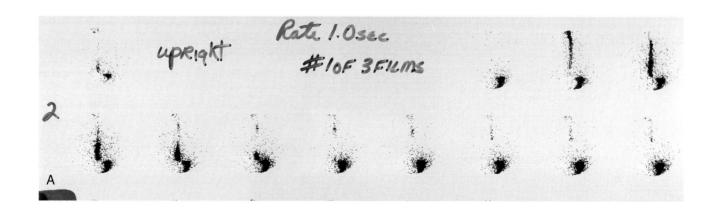

upright   Rate 1.0sec
#1 OF 3 FILMS

2

A

FIGURE 30–2 B.

Supine Oral ^{99m}Tc-Colloid Scan: There is splitting of the bolus, with to-and-fro movement, and delayed emptying into the stomach.

NOTE. Supine studies are more sensitive for esophageal dysmotility and gastroesophageal reflux.

SUSPECT ESOPHAGEAL DYSMOTILITY

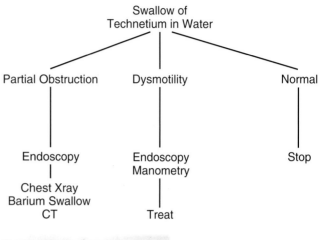

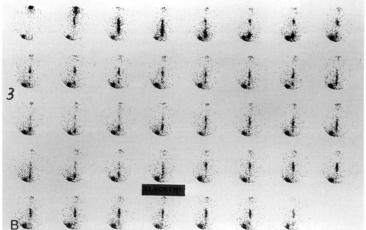

DISORDERED ESOPHAGEAL MOTILITY

Patient 1: Presbyesophagus

FIGURE 30–3 A.

^{99m}Tc-Colloid Scan: The poor emptying of the swallowed bolus at the esophagogastric junction is associated with retrograde movement.

Patient 2: Labial Insufficiency and Esophageal Dysmotility Following Stroke

FIGURE 30–3 B.

Oral ^{99m}Tc-Colloid Scan: The esophageal bolus divides in two, with retrograde and antegrade movement. There is a second column of activity on the skin *(arrow)* as a result of labial insufficiency.

Illustration continued on following page

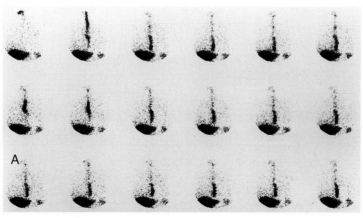

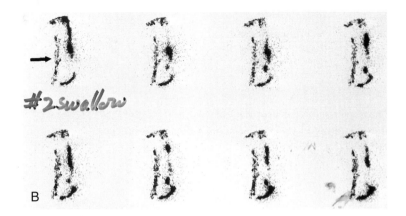

B

NOTE. Poor emptying at the esophagogastric junction can be due to esophageal spasm, stricture, hiatal hernia, neoplasm, achalasia, or foreign body.

ACHALASIA WITH ASPIRATION

FIGURE 30–4   A.

Oral ^{99m}Tc-Colloid Scan: There is distention and aperistalsis of the esophagus, with minimal emptying.

FIGURE 30–4   B.

Delayed Static Scan: The esophagus remains filled with the radiolabeled water, with activity in the lungs from aspiration.

NOTE. The use of ^{99m}Tc-colloid in 10 ml of water is a very sensitive technique for aspiration, more sensitive than Gastrografin, and causes less fluid shift in the lung.

Cross Reference

Chapter 48: Localized Infection—Aspiration Pneumonia from Achalasia

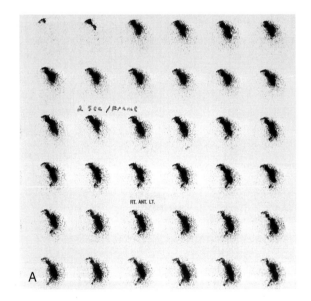

A

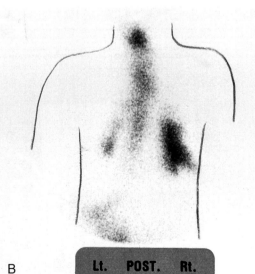

B

ESOPHAGEAL CARCINOMA

FIGURE 30–5.

Oral ^{99m}Tc-Colloid Scan: The swallowed bolus stops in mid-esophagus.

NOTE. Primary tumor, or invasion from lung carcinoma, should be considered in midesophageal obstructions. Occasionally, inflammatory strictures, especially from tuberculosis, can occur at this level.

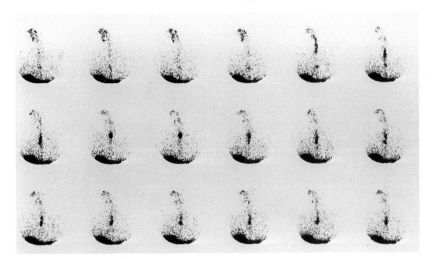

GASTROESOPHAGEAL REFLUX

FIGURE 30–6.

Sequential Supine Oral ^{99m}Tc-Colloid Scans: With the patient rolling over from supine to prone position, and back to supine, there is reflux *(arrow)*.

NOTE 1. Having the patient roll over to induce reflux is a more physiologic reproduction of symptomatic reflux than are compression techniques.

NOTE 2. A variation of this technique uses continuous computer acquisition with the patient remaining supine for 1 hour. Areas of interest are placed over the mid- and lower esophagus, and time/activity curves are drawn.

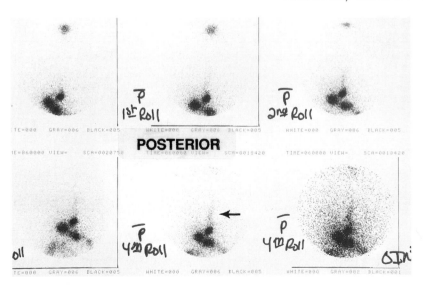

Chapter 31
Gastric Emptying

NORMAL GASTRIC EMPTYING

FIGURE 31–1   A and B.
Early and Late Gastric Emptying Scans: There is reduction of the size of the stomach over time. The intensity of the retained radioactivity also diminishes.

FIGURE 31–1   C.
Time-Activity Curve: The $T_{1/2}$ is 108 minutes (normal for our laboratory is 90 to 120 minutes).

NOTE 1. Gastric emptying is dependent on the caloric and protein content of the meal. Liquids always empty faster than solids.

NOTE 2. There are many choices for radioactive meals. We use a radiocolloid-labeled egg salad sandwich.

NOTE 3. Continuous scanning with computer acquisition over 2 hours should be done.

Illustration continued on following page

DELAYED GASTRIC EMPTYING

1. Physical Obstruction
   a. Congenital or acquired hypertrophic pyloric stenosis
   b. Peptic ulcer disease: edema, strictures
   c. Malignancy
   d. Bezoars
2. Diabetes
3. Drugs: anticholinergics, calcium channel blockers, opiates
4. Vagotomy
5. Collagen vascular diseases
6. Psychiatric disorders: depression, anorexia nervosa
7. Neuromuscular disorders
8. Hypothyroidism
9. Amyloidosis
10. Idiopathic

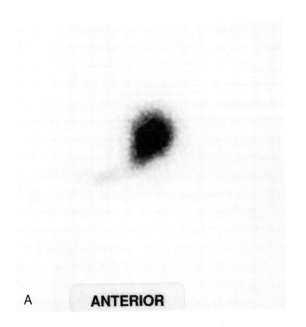

A   **ANTERIOR**

B   **ANTERIOR**

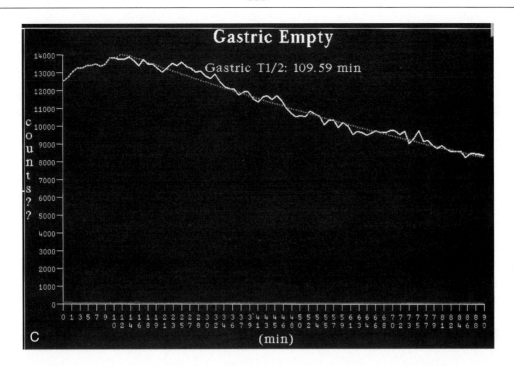

DELAYED GASTRIC EMPTYING

FIGURE 31–2   A and B.

Early and Late Gastric Emptying Scans: The small amount of material leaving the stomach was presumed to be in a liquid state. There is considerable retention of the radioactive meal within the stomach.

A   **ANTERIOR**

B   **ANTERIOR**

FIGURE 31-2 C.

Time-Activity Curve: The $T_{1/2}$ of 10 hours is far beyond the normal range.

NOTE. Even with the patient supine, the activity (food) in the more posterior fundus should be propelled anteriorly into the body and antrum.

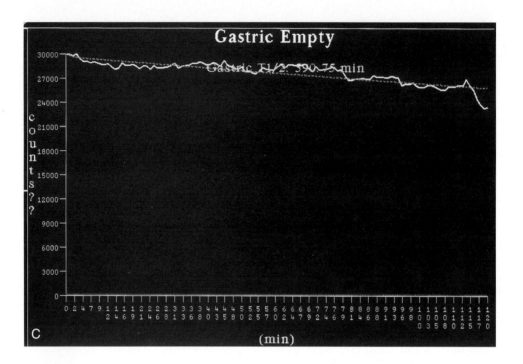

HIATAL HERNIA ON GASTRIC EMPTYING STUDY

FIGURE 31-3.

Gastric Emptying Scan: There is a separate collection of radioactivity superior to the normal location of the stomach. The gastric emptying time, including the hiatal hernia, was normal.

ANTERIOR

NORMAL SMALL
BOWEL FOLLOW-THROUGH

FIGURE 32–1   A to C.

Oral ⁹⁹ᵐTc-Colloid Scans: There is antegrade progression of the radiopharmaceutical through the bowel in this patient with Crohn's disease and suspected small bowel obstruction.

NOTE. The small bowel loops should be intertwined, adjacent to one another, and not dilated.

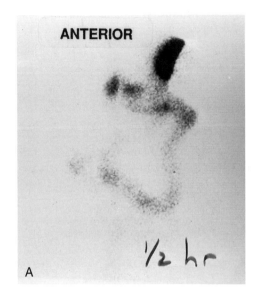

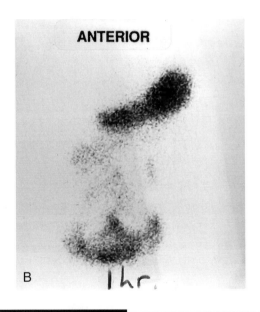

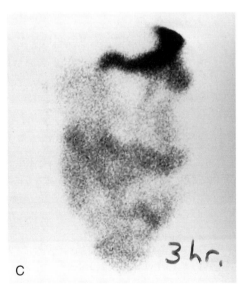

GASTROGRAFIN-AIDED SMALL
BOWEL FOLLOW-THROUGH IN
SMALL BOWEL ILEUS

FIGURE 32–2   A.

Oral ⁹⁹ᵐTc-Albumin Colloid Scan: At 8 hours the radiocolloid remained in the distal ileum with no further progression.

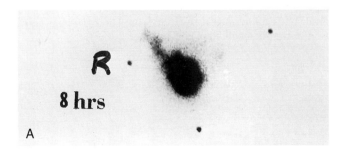

Illustration continued on following page

FIGURE 32–2   B and C.

[99mTc]-Albumin Colloid Scan soon after oral Gastrographin (1 tbs): Bowel peristalsis was stimulated, with the radiocolloid moving rapidly antegrade into the transverse and descending colon.

NOTE. This technique is useful in separating small bowel obstruction from "adynamic" ileus, and with less discomfort than intravenous CCK.

SUSPECT SMALL BOWEL OBSTRUCTION

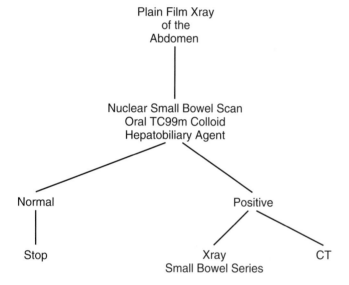

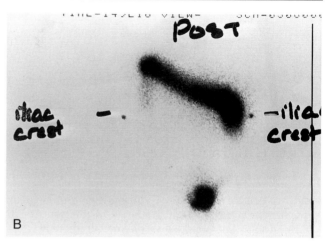

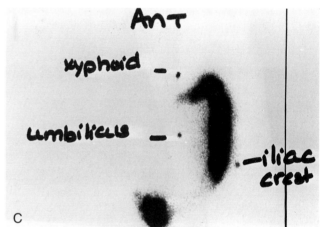

SMALL BOWEL OBSTRUCTION

Patient 1: Jejunal Leiomyoma

FIGURE 32–3   A.

Oral [99mTc]-Colloid and Gastrografin Scan: There was no progression of the radiocolloid over 4 hours.

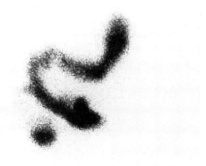

A

Patient 2: Adhesions

FIGURE 32–3   B and C.

Oral ^{99m}Tc-Colloid, Gastrografin, and HIDA Scans: The bowel is dilated and stacked. The radioactivity did not progress beyond the jejunum in the right abdomen *(arrow)* (gb = gallbladder; s = stomach).

NOTE 1. A small bowel follow-through examination can determine if there is an obstruction and where in the abdomen it is. The sensitivity of a gamma camera exceeds that of x-ray film using Gastrografin.

NOTE 2. This study can be performed with oral radiocolloid, oral macroaggregated albumin, and/or a hepatobiliary scanning agent.

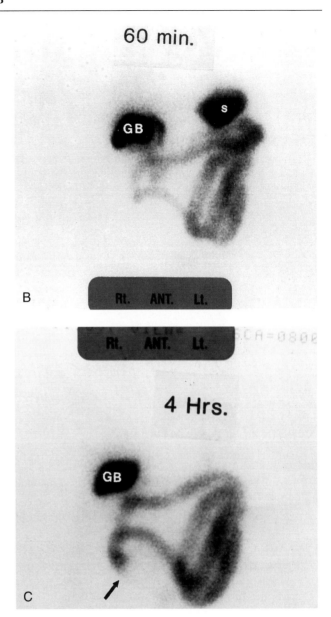

EFFERENT LOOP OBSTRUCTION AFTER BILLROTH II SURGERY

Patient 1

FIGURE 32–4   A.

Ninety Minute HIDA Scan: The bile refluxes into the stomach at the gastrojejunostomy *(arrow)*, but despite delayed imaging, there is little progression into the jejunum.

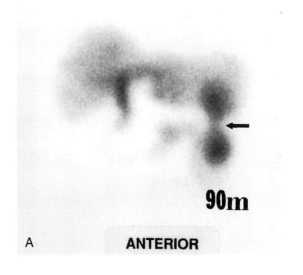

FIGURE 32–4   B.

Two Days Post Revision HIDA Scan: There is less reflux through the anastomosis *(arrow)* and more radiolabeled bile passing into the efferent loop *(open arrow)*.

Patient 2

FIGURE 32–4   C.

HIDA Scan: There is reflux across the stomach remnant into the esophagus *(open arrow)* but no significant flow into the efferent jejunal loop.

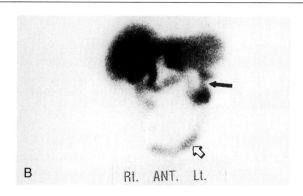

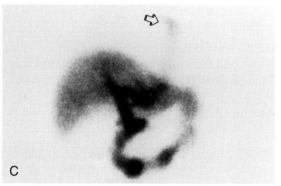

INTESTINAL NONROTATION

FIGURE 32–5   A and B.

HIDA Scan: The duodenum and the proximal small bowel are on the right side.

FIGURE 32–5   C.

Small Bowel Scan with Oral Radiocolloid: The stomach is on the left side, but the duodenum and jejunum are on the right, confirming the HIDA findings.

NOTE. Failure of the midgut to rotate after return to the fetal abdomen leaves the small bowel on the right and the stomach and colon on the left.

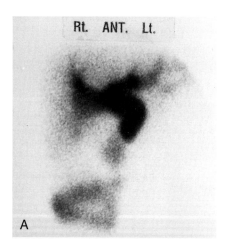

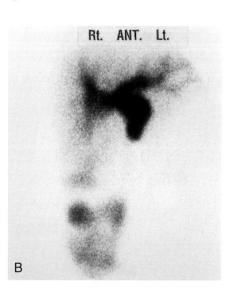

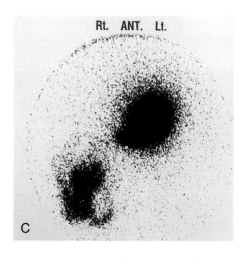

INTRAPERITONEAL SCINTIGRAPHY

Patient 1: Normal

FIGURE 32–6   A.

Anterior Intraperitoneal ^{99m}Tc-Colloid Scan: There is dispersion throughout the abdominal cavity.

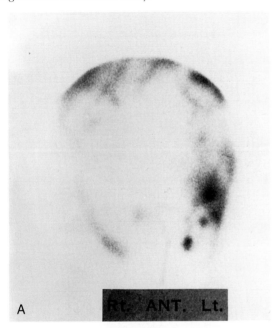

A

Patient 2: Loculation

FIGURE 32–6   B.

Anterior Intraperitoneal ^{99m}Tc-Colloid Scan: The radiocolloid remains concentrated in the midabdomen despite having the patient roll from side to side.

NOTE 1. Loculation of fluid within the abdomen is a contraindication for intraperitoneal chemotherapy or ^{32}P-colloid.

NOTE 2. This technique has been used to detect hernias of various forms.

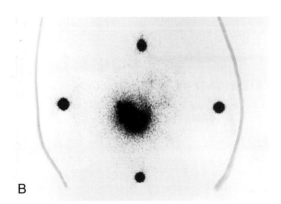

B

Chapter 33

Gastrointestinal and Abdominal Infections

NORMAL ABDOMINAL WBC SCAN

FIGURE 33–1   A and B.

^{111}In-WBC Scan: The spleen has greater activity than the liver, the bone marrow has mild activity, and there is no appreciable accumulation of the WBCs in the kidneys, bladder, or bowel.

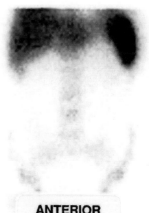

A

ANTERIOR

Illustration continued on following page

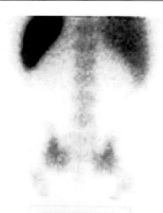

B   **POSTERIOR**

ENTERITIS AND COLITIS

Patient 1: Diffuse Enteritis

FIGURE 33–2 A.
WBC Scan: Virtually the entire small bowel has abnormal WBC accumulation.

Patient 2: Pseudomembranous Colitis

FIGURE 33–2 B.
WBC Scan: The WBCs are seen throughout the colon in this patient on long-term antibiotics.

Patient 3: HIV Colitis

FIGURE 33–2 C.
Gallium Scan: There is intense gallium accumulation in the colon.

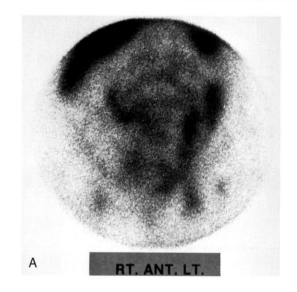

A   **RT. ANT. LT.**

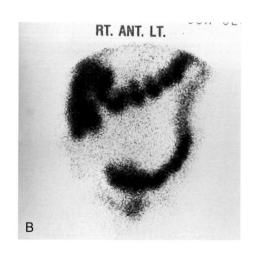

RT. ANT. LT.

B

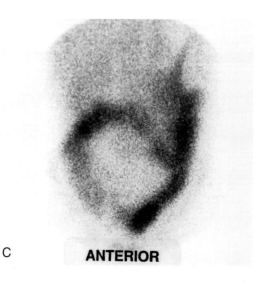

C   **ANTERIOR**

NOTE 1. There should be no WBC accumulation in the bowel on a normal scan.

NOTE 2. Unlike WBCs, gallium can normally be seen in the colon. However, intense gallium activity in the colon suggests active disease, which may or may not be symptomatic.

NOTE 3. Pseudomembranous colitis is caused by *Clostridium difficile* in patients on wide-spectrum antibiotics. Early on it may be silent, whereas later it presents as diarrhea and toxemia. A WBC scan will be positive before symptoms appear.

NOTE 4. HIV colitis is often caused by cryptosporidiosis or isosporidosis.

WHITE BLOOD CELLS IN BOWEL	
1. Diverticulitis	6. Ischemic colitis, bowel infarction
2. Ulcerative colitis	7. Behçet's vasculitis
3. Regional enteritis (Crohn's disease)	8. Swallowed WBCs from sinusitis and pneumonitis
4. Pseudomembranous colitis	9. GI bleeding
5. Bacterial and viral enterocolitis, including tuberculosis and arsine	10. Vigorous enemas

INFLAMMATORY BOWEL DISEASE

Patient 1: Crohn's Disease of Ileocecal Region

FIGURE 33–3 A.
WBC Scan: The most intense abnormality is in the right lower quadrant, in the ileocecal region. The ascending and transverse colon segments are also abnormal.

Patient 2: Crohn's Disease of Small and Large Bowel

FIGURE 33–3 B.
WBC Scan: The entire colon is abnormal. The central abdominal activity indicates involvement of the small bowel.

FIGURE 33–3 C.
WBC Scan 3 Months Later: The right colon is less active, but a dilated loop of small bowel is present in the midabdomen *(arrowheads)*.

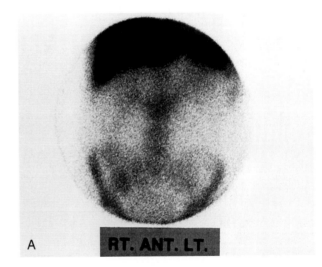

A   RT. ANT. LT.

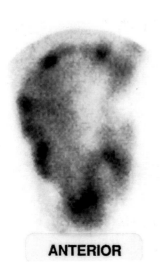

B   ANTERIOR

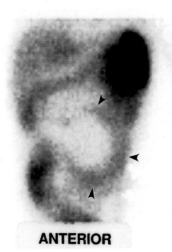

C   ANTERIOR

Illustration continued on following page

Patient 3: Crohn's Disease with Skip Lesions and Extramural Abscess

FIGURE 33–3 D.

WBC Scan: Short segments of small bowel and large bowel have WBC accumulation. The right lower quadrant has a large collection of white cells within an extramural abscess in the region of the terminal ileum and cecum.

Patient 4: Crohn's Disease Fistulas

FIGURE 33–3 E.

WBC Scan: The irregular pattern conforms to fistulas in the ileocecal region. The patient had a left flank infection as well.

Patient 5: Toxic Megacolon in Ulcerative Colitis

FIGURE 33–3 F and G.

Anterior and Posterior WBC Scans: There is intense WBC aggregation in the dilated, smooth transverse colon. Note the rectal activity.

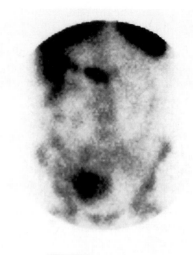

D **ANTERIOR**

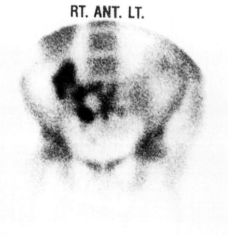

E

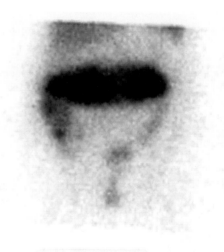

F **ANTERIOR**

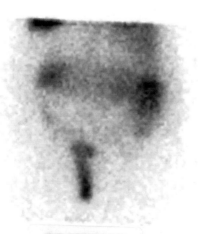

G **POSTERIOR**

FIGURE 33–3 H.

Abdominal Plain Film X-ray: The transverse colon is dilated, and there is a loss of haustral markings.

NOTE 1. WBC scanning is preferable to gallium scanning for abdominal inflammation or infections.

NOTE 2. The presence of labeled WBCs in bowel indicates active inflammatory disease.

NOTE 3. Right-sided colonic activity suggests Crohn's disease. Left-sided or diffuse disease, especially if the rectum is involved, suggests ulcerative colitis.

Cross References

Chapter 11: Soft Tissue Abnormalties—Enterovesical Fistula on Bone Scan

Chapter 71: Infectious Diseases—Pelvic Abscesses

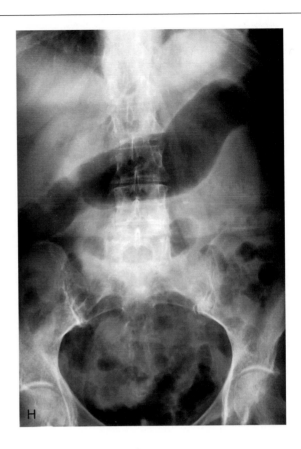

PANCREATITIS

Patient 1

FIGURE 33–4 A.

WBC Scan: The region of the head of the pancreas has intense WBC accumulation in a pancreatic abscess (phlegmon). The broad, ill-defined area of WBCs below represents extension of the inflammation into the adjacent peritoneum.

Patient 2

FIGURE 33–4 B.

Preoperative WBC Scan: The epigastric activity represents a lesser sac abscess from known pancreatitis.

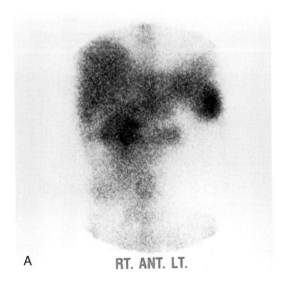

A RT. ANT. LT.

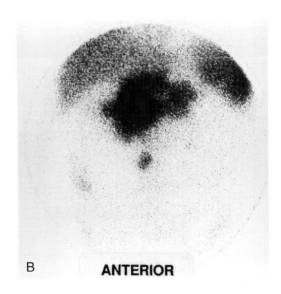

B **ANTERIOR**

Illustration continued on following page

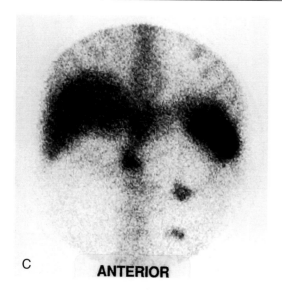

C   **ANTERIOR**

D   **ANTERIOR**

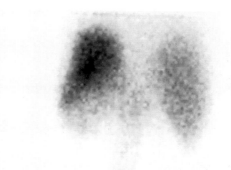

E   **POSTERIOR**

Patient 3: Stab Wound, Splenectomy, and Infected Pancreatic Pseudocyst

FIGURE 33–4   C.

Three Month Postoperative WBC Scan: There are three residual foci of infection.

FIGURE 33–4   D.

Anterior WBC Scan: The abnormal activity is in the epigastrium and left mid- and upper abdomen.

FIGURE 33–4   E.

Posterior WBC Scan: The activity in the left upper abdomen is infection, since the spleen had been removed.

Cross Reference

Chapter 20: Disorders of the Spleen—Subphrenic Abscess Simulating Spleen

PERITONITIS AND INFECTED ASCITES

Patient 1: 58 Year Old Male Alcoholic with Fever

FIGURE 33–5   A.

Gallium Scan: The U-shaped gallium accumulation along the pelvic floor *(arrowheads)*, below the colon, is indicative of peritonitis.

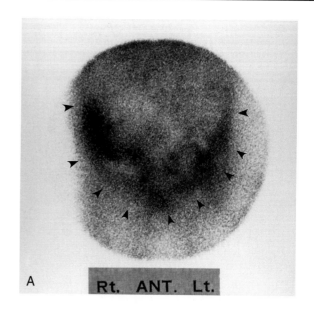

A   **Rt.   ANT.   Lt.**

Patient 2: 70 Year Old Male with Fever and Loculated Ascites

FIGURE 33–5 B and C.

RAO Abdomen and Anterior Pelvic WBC Scans: There is a broad area of abnormal WBC accumulation in the right abdomen that proved to be infected upon drainage.

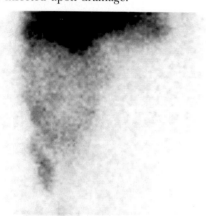

B

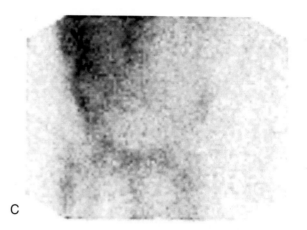

C

SWALLOWED WBCs

Patient 1

FIGURE 33–6 A.

Anterior Abdomen ^{111}In-WBC Scan: The ascending and transverse colon have intense WBC accumulation.

FIGURE 33–6 B.

Anterior ^{111}In-WBC Scan 6 Hours Later: The WBCs have moved out of the transverse colon.

FIGURE 33–6 C.

Anterior Chest ^{111}In-WBC Scan: There is an intense WBC accumulation in the right chest infection.

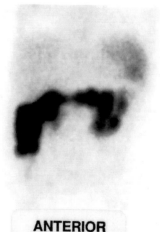

A

ANTERIOR

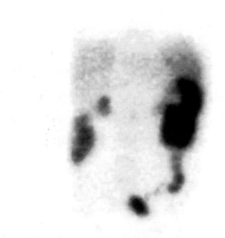

B

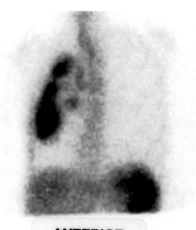

C

ANTERIOR

Illustration continued on following page

Patient 2: Active Parotitis, Ethmoiditis, and Pneumonitis

FIGURE 33–6   D and E.

WBC Scan: The focus of activity in the abdomen *(arrowhead)* was assumed to represent swallowed WBCs, since the patient was asymptomatic in the abdomen.

NOTE 1. All abdominal WBC scans should include the lungs and paranasal sinuses, since swallowed WBCs could be misinterpreted as an abdominal inflammatory focus.

NOTE 2. Delayed scans can document movement of swallowed WBCs, as opposed to inflammatory sites in the bowel and the abdomen, which would remain active in the same spot.

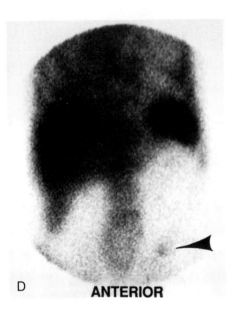

D   **ANTERIOR**

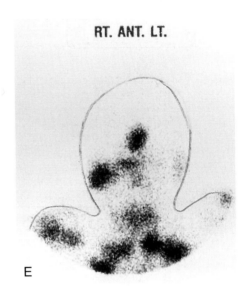

RT. ANT. LT.

E

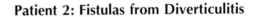

DIVERTICULAR AND APPENDICEAL ABSCESS

Patient 1: Diverticular Abscess (Diverticulitis)

FIGURE 33–7   A.

WBC Scan: The focal accumulation in the left lower quadrant *(arrow)* represents an abscess. The patient presented with left hip pain.

Patient 2: Fistulas from Diverticulitis

FIGURE 33–7   B.

Anterior WBC Scan: The large WBC accumulation has linear extensions *(arrow)*.

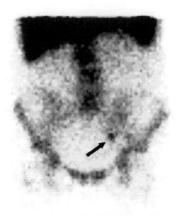

A   **ANTERIOR**

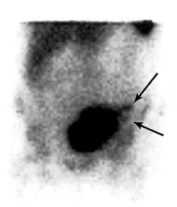

B   **ANTERIOR**

Patient 3: Appendiceal Abscess

FIGURE 33–7   C.
Three Hour Gallium Scan: The intense gallium collection in the RLQ is present before the rest of the bowel.

NOTE 1. Lower abdominal abscesses, especially near the sciatic nerve or obturator canal, can present with leg or hip pain.

NOTE 2. Acute infections can be scanned as early as 3 hours after injection with either labeled WBCs or gallium.

Cross Reference

Chapter 71: Infectious Diseases—Pelvic Abscesses; Unsuspected Abscesses

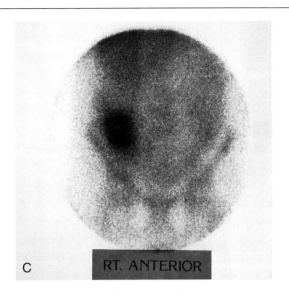

ABDOMINAL ABSCESS IN IMMUNOSUPPRESSION AND AFTER RADIATION THERAPY

Patient 1: Chemotherapy and Leukopenia

FIGURE 33–8   A.
Anterior Abdomen WBC Scan: The right gutter abscess accumulates WBCs despite the marrow suppression from chemotherapy.

FIGURE 33–8   B.
Posterior Chest WBC Scan: The bone marrow normally visualized on WBC scans is absent.

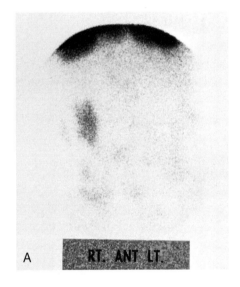

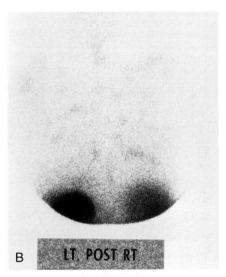

Illustration continued on following page

Patient 2: S/P Radiation Therapy

FIGURE 33–8 C.

WBC Scan: There is a RLQ abscess. The marrow activity is decreased below L4 from pelvic irradiation.

NOTE 1. Even in immunosuppressed patients, WBC scans or gallium scans will be effective.

NOTE 2. A white blood cell count minimum of 1500 WBC/mm^3 is necessary for effective labeling and scanning.

Cross Reference

Chapter 9: "Cold" Abnormalities—Radiation Change on Bone Scan

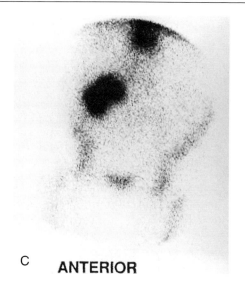

C **ANTERIOR**

GI HEMORRHAGE ON WBC SCAN

FIGURE 33–9 A and B.

Three- and 4-Hour WBC Scans: There are radiolabeled WBCs in the stomach that progress over time into the colon. This patient bled from a gastric ulcer.

NOTE. If the patient hemorrhages soon after the injection of WBCs, the extravasated blood with labeled WBCs will be seen in the bowel.

Cross Reference

Chapter 28: Gastrointestinal Hemorrhage

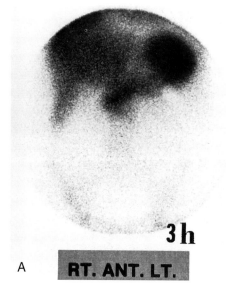

3 h

A **RT. ANT. LT.**

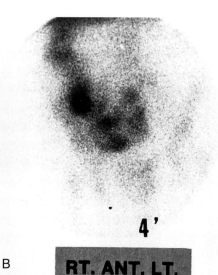

4'

B **RT. ANT. LT.**

Chapter 34

Disorders of the Salivary Glands

NORMAL SALIVARY GLANDS

FIGURE 34–1 A to D.

⁹⁹ᵐTc-Pertechnetate Salivary Gland Scan Pre- and Post-Lemon Administration: There is symmetric accumulation and excretion of the radiopharmaceutical from the parotid and submandibular glands. The parotid duct (Stensen's duct) is well seen.

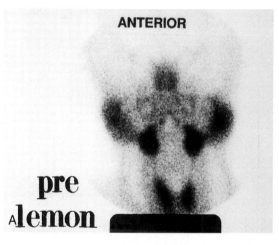

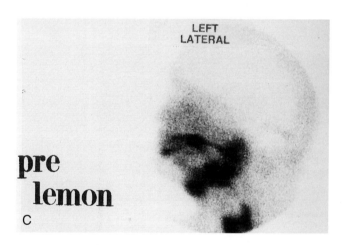

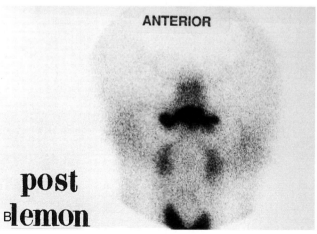

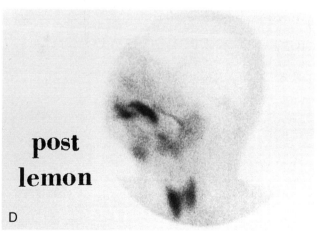

Illustration continued on following page

FIGURE 34–1 E to G.

Gallium Scan: The salivary gland activity is symmetric. The parotid activity is slighter greater than that of the submandibular glands.

NOTE. Any sour foods, such as lemon or pickles, can be used to stimulate salivary flow and excretion of the ^{99m}Tc-pertechnetate.

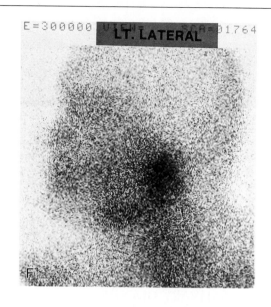

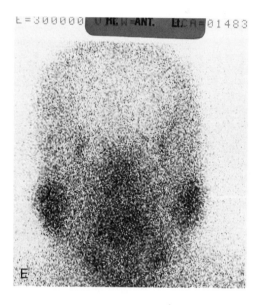

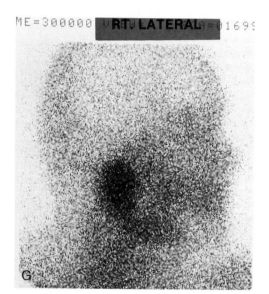

SJÖGREN'S SYNDROME (SICCA COMPLEX)

Patient 1

FIGURE 34–2 A.

^{99m}Tc-Pertechnetate Scan: There is nonvisualization of the salivary glands and no radiolabeled saliva in the oral cavity.

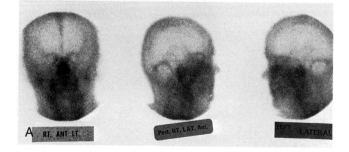

DIFFERENTIAL DIAGNOSIS OF SICCA COMPLEX	
Sjögren's syndrome	Systemic lupus erythematosus
Mikulicz syndrome	Other connective tissue diseases
Rheumatoid arthritis	

Patient 2: Inactive Sjögren's Syndrome

FIGURE 34–2   B and C.

Anterior and Left Lateral ⁹⁹ᵐTc-Pertechnetate Scans: There is some uptake of the radiopharmaceutical in the parotid and submandibular glands but no free saliva in the oral cavity.

FIGURE 34–2   D and E.

Anterior and Left Lateral Gallium Scans: None of the salivary glands has any gallium activity, although the lacrimal glands appear normal.

NOTE 1. Sicca complex involves a dry mouth (xerostomia) and dry eyes (xerophthalmia). The nose, pharynx, trachea, gastrointestinal tract, and vagina also have decreased glandular excretions.

NOTE 2. In the normal patient, there should be some uptake of gallium in the salivary glands, although it may be asymmetric and mild. An active process should have increased gallium accumulation.

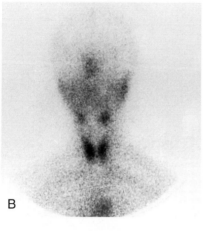

B

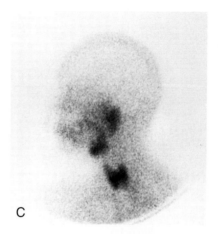

C

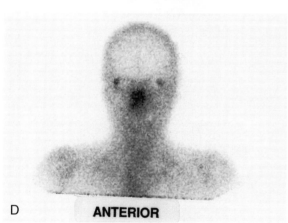

D   **ANTERIOR**

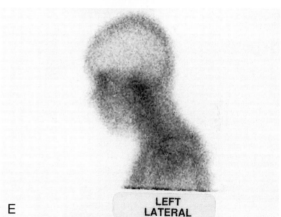

E   **LEFT LATERAL**

PAROTITIS

FIGURE 34–3   A to F.

⁹⁹ᵐTc-Pertechnetate Parotid Scans Pre- and Post-Lemon Administration: The parotid glands are irregular and small owing to recurrent infections.

FIGURE 34–3   G and H.

Gallium Scan: The left parotid gland has marked gallium accumulation from active infection.

Illustration continued on following page

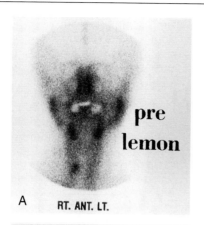

A   pre
     lemon
     RT. ANT. LT.

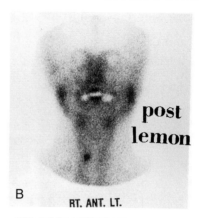

B   post
     lemon
     RT. ANT. LT.

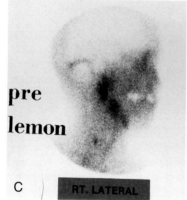

pre
lemon

C   RT. LATERAL

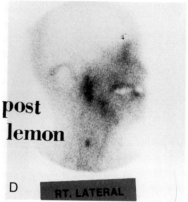

post
lemon

D   RT. LATERAL

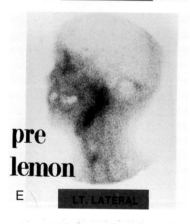

pre
lemon

E   LT. LATERAL

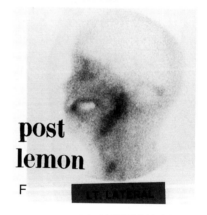

post
lemon

F   LT. LATERAL

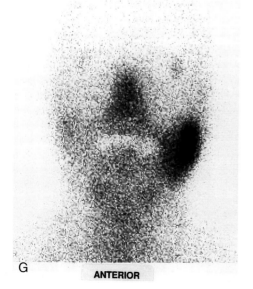

G   ANTERIOR

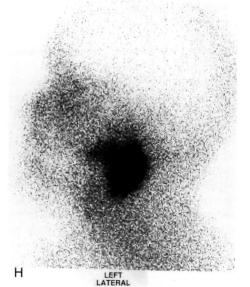

H   LEFT
     LATERAL

OBSTRUCTED PAROTID GLAND WITH INFECTION

Patient: Parotid Duct Stone

FIGURE 34–4 A to D.

Salivary Scans Pre- and Post-Lemon Administration: The parotid duct is not seen, and there is retention of the ^{99m}Tc-pertechnetate in the right parotid gland.

FIGURE 34–4 E to F.

Gallium Scan: The marked gallium accumulation indicates infection behind the blockage.

NOTE. Tumors and scarring as well as stones can cause salivary obstruction.

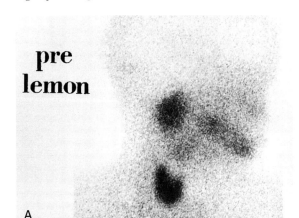

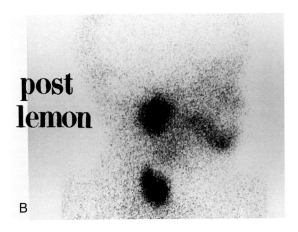

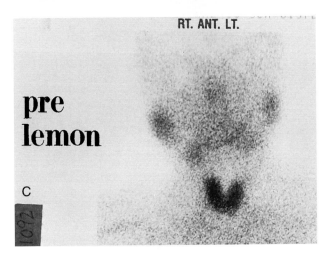

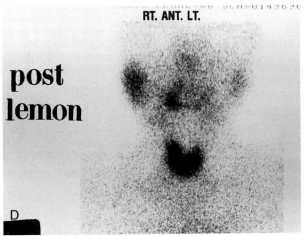

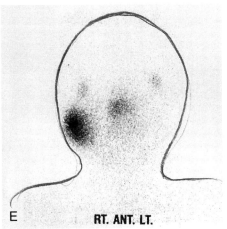

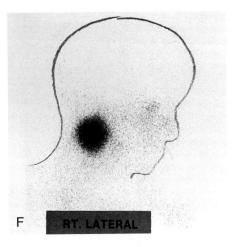

SALIVARY GLAND ABSCESSES

Patient 1: Parotid Abscess

FIGURE 34–5 A.

⁹⁹ᵐTc-Pertechnetate Salivary Scan: The inferior half of the left parotid gland is not visualized *(arrowheads)*.

FIGURE 34–5 B.

Gallium Scan: The palpable mass has intense gallium accumulation *(arrow)*.

Patient 2: Submandibular Gland Abscess

FIGURE 34–5 C.

WBC Scan: The right submandibular gland has increased WBC accumulation.

Patient 3: Cheek Abscess

FIGURE 34–5 D.

⁹⁹ᵐTc-Pertechnetate Salivary Scan: The parotid gland appears normal. The swelling is outlined by technetium markers.

FIGURE 34–5 E.

Gallium Scan: The abscess *(arrow)* anterior to the parotid gland did not obstruct the parotid duct.

NOTE 1. Normally there are no radiolabeled WBCs accumulating in the salivary glands.

NOTE 2. If abscess is suspected, a WBC scan is the most specific test. If a malignant tumor must be ruled out, a gallium scan is more definitive.

NOTE 3. Fine needle biopsy has replaced scintigraphy in the diagnosis of salivary gland tumors.

Cross Reference

Chapter 33: Gastrointestinal and Abdominal Infections—Swallowed WBCs

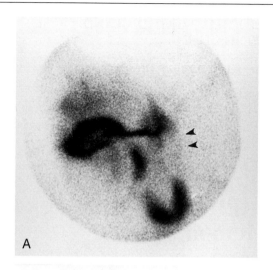

A

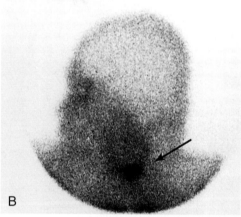

B

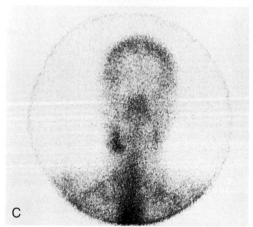

C

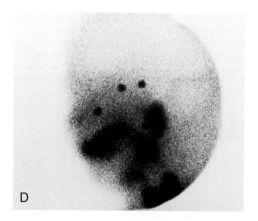

D

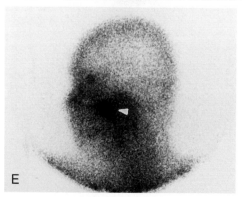

E

WARTHIN'S TUMOR

Patient: Bilateral Warthin's Tumor

FIGURE 34–6   A to F.

^{99m}Tc-Pertechnetate Scan Pre- and Post-Lemon Administration: After salivary stimulation there is retention of the ^{99m}Tc-pertechnetate in the functioning tumors.

FIGURE 34–6   G to I.

Gallium Scan: There is no abnormal accumulation of gallium in the neoplasms. The lack of activity in the left parotid gland is due to replacement of virtually the entire gland by tumor.

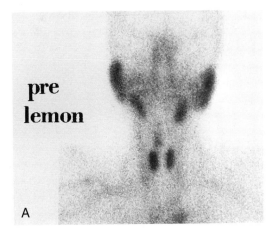

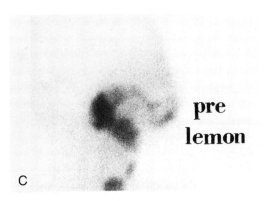

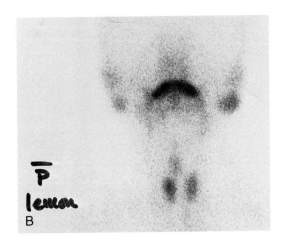

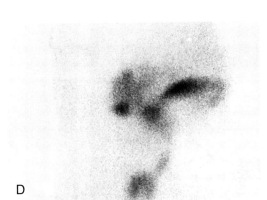

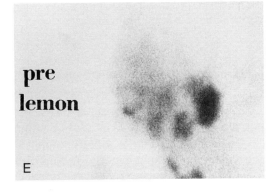

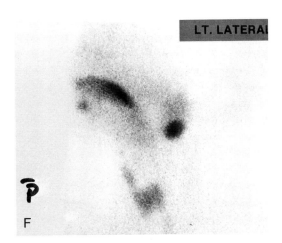

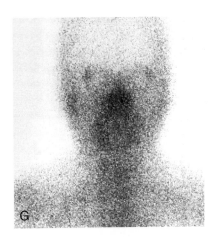

Illustration continued on following page

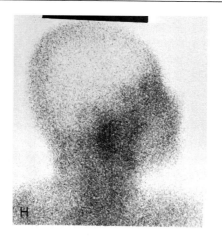

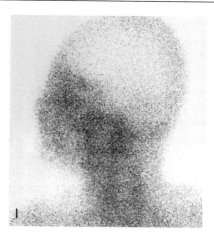

MIXED CELL SALIVARY TUMOR
WITH OBSTRUCTION

FIGURE 34–7 A and B.

^{99m}Tc-Pertechnetate Salivary Scan Post-Lemon Administration: The mass *(arrow)* in the inferior pole of the right parotid gland obstructs the outflow of saliva by invading the ducts.

NOTE 1. Except for Warthin's tumors, neoplasms of the salivary glands do not accumulate technetium pertechnetate.

NOTE 2. Salivary tumors include benign and malignant mixed cell, Warthin's (papillary cystadenoma lymphomatosum), neurofibroma, oncocytoma, squamous cell carcinoma, mucoepidermoid carcinoma, undifferentiated carcinoma, and lymphoma. The most common is the mixed cell type.

NOTE 3. A negative gallium scan virtually rules out a malignant salivary gland tumor. A positive scan can be seen with benign or malignant disease.

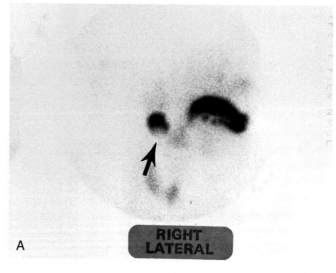

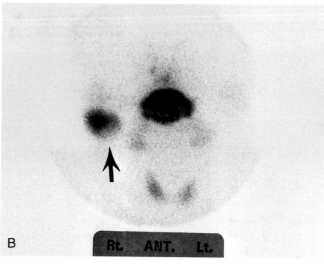

Chapter 35

Normal/Normal Variants

RENOGRAM CURVES

FIGURE 35–1   A.
Normal: $T_{1/2}$ <15 minutes.

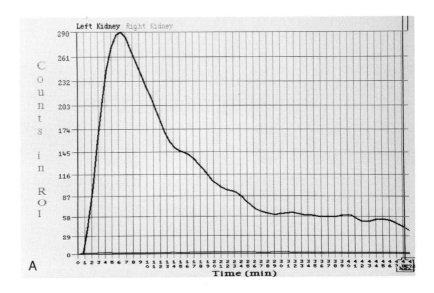

FIGURE 35–1   B.
Mild Renal Insufficiency: $T_{1/2}$ <30 minutes.

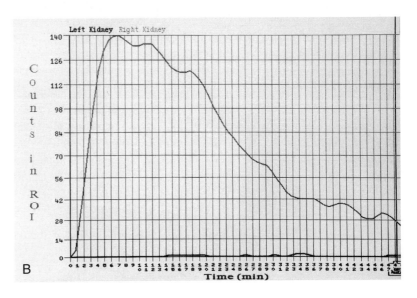

Illustration continued on following page

FIGURE 35–1   C.
Moderate Renal Insufficiency: $T_{1/2}$ >30 minutes.

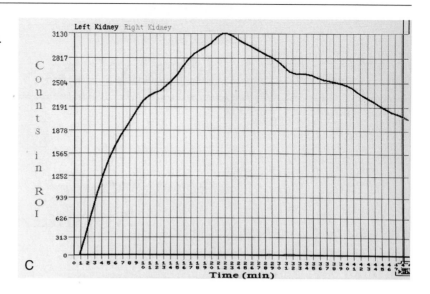

FIGURE 35–1   D.
Severe Renal Insufficiency.

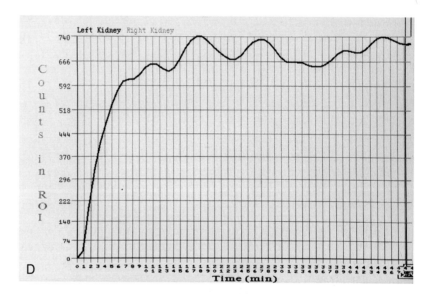

FIGURE 35–1   E.
Obstruction/ATN/Extrarenal Pelvis.

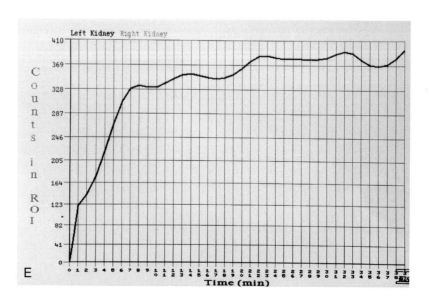

FIGURE 35–1   F.
Extrarenal Pelvis with Lasix.

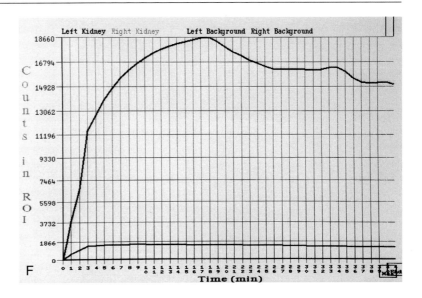

NORMAL RENAL SCAN

Patient 1

FIGURE 35–2   A and B.
Renal Blood Flow Scintigrams and Curves: The rapid sequence (0.5 sec/frame) study reveals aortic and renal appearance times. The curves demonstrate the bolus arrival in the aorta and kidneys. The spleen *(arrowhead)* also perfuses early.

FIGURE 35–2   C.
DTPA Renal Sequence: Sequential 30-second films allow for evaluation of glomerular filtration, the nephrogram phase, intrarenal and extrarenal collecting systems, and ureteral peristalsis.

Illustration continued on following page

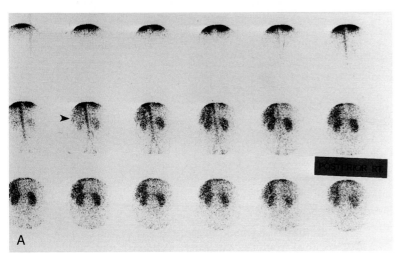

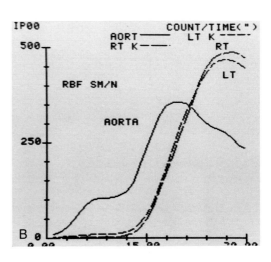

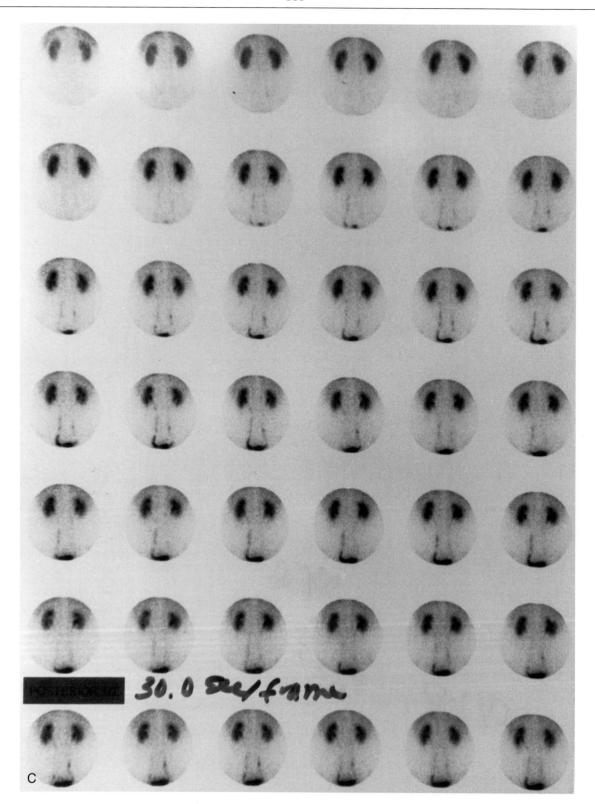

C

FIGURE 35–2   D.
DTPA Renal Curves: There is progressive loss of radioactivity from the kidneys.

FIGURE 35–2   E to I.
Delayed DTPA Static Images: The kidney sizes can be measured, kidney contours and cortex evaluated, and bladder voiding visually assessed. The normal adult kidney length is 9 to 14 cm.

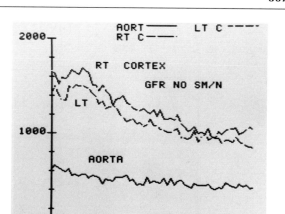

D

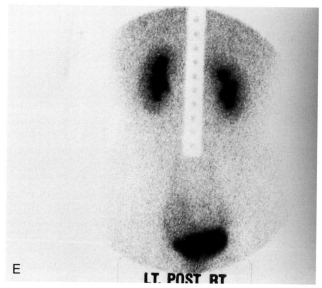

E

LT. POST. RT.

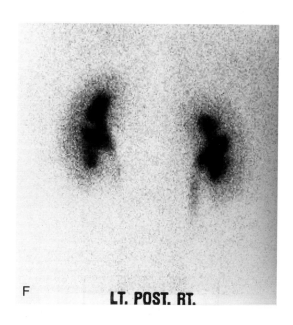

F   LT. POST. RT.

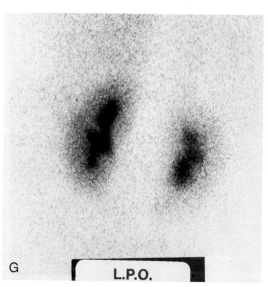

G   L.P.O.

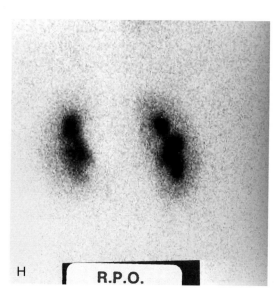

H   R.P.O.

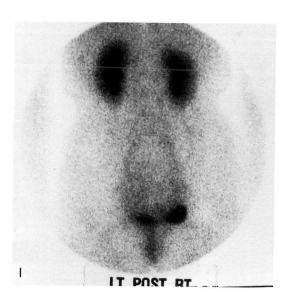

I   LT. POST. RT.

Illustration continued on following page

Patient 2

FIGURE 35–2   J and K.

Hippuran Renogram and Curves: Visual assessment is often as good as the computer-generated curves.

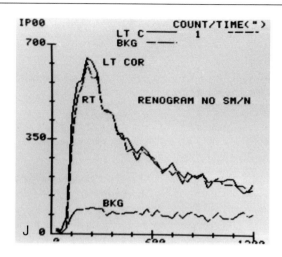

NOTE 1. Our "triple" renal scan is performed with 3 mCi ^{99m}Tc-DTPA for the blood flow and glomerular filtration rate (Gates technique). At the time of injection of 200 μCi ^{131}I-hippuran to assess tubular function, 12 mCi ^{99m}Tc-glucoheptonate is also given. The renogram is obtained, followed by the static images on the technetium window, using a medium-energy collimator.

NOTE 2. Regions of interest (ROIs) are drawn on a computer encompassing the cortex. Whole kidney ROIs can give an obstructive pattern when the calyces are dilated although not obstructed, e.g., postobstructive atrophy or extrarenal pelvis. This is due to stasis of urine in the aperistaltic collecting system.

NOTE 3. The early appearance of the spleen on the blood flow study should not be confused with the left kidney.

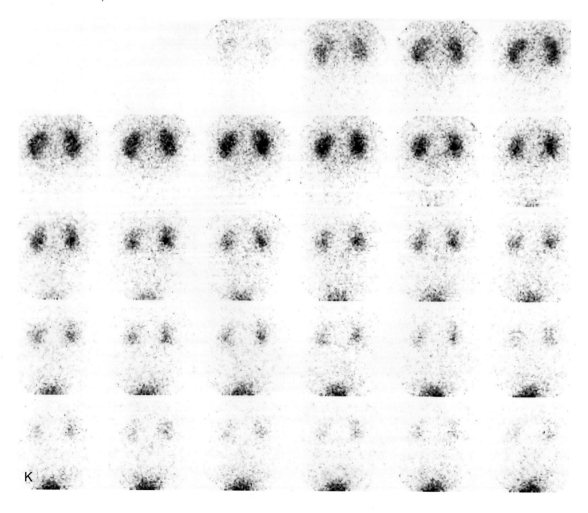

NORMAL NEWBORN RENAL SCAN

FIGURE 35–3.

^{99m}Tc-DTPA Scan: glomerular filtration is slower in newborns, and concentrating ability is less than older children and adults. Note the high activity in the body and soft tissues, with poor visualization of the collecting systems.

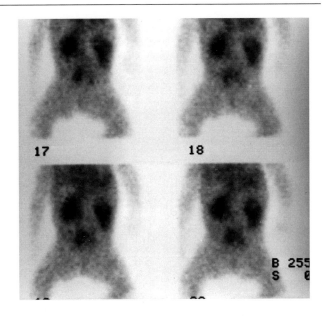

NORMAL UPPER POLE CALYCEAL DILATATION

FIGURE 35–4.

DTPA Renal Scan: The upper pole calices are often distended.

NOTE. Upper pole calyceal distention occurs when the scan is performed supine. The upper poles are more posterior (dependent) than the lower poles.

Cross Reference

Chapter 36: Unilateral Abnormalities—Lower Pole Calyceal Obstruction

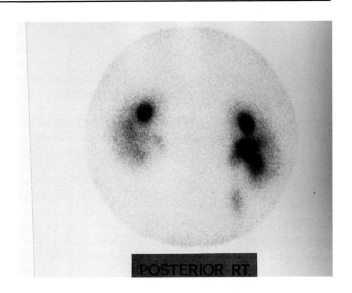

EXTRARENAL PELVIS

FIGURE 35–5   A and B.

Renal Scan: The right renal pelvis is markedly dilated. The sequential scan demonstrates good cortical clearance despite the distended renal pelvis.

Illustration continued on following page

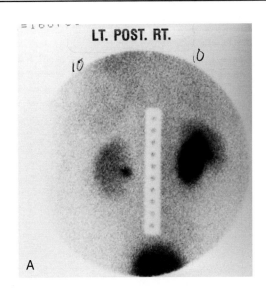

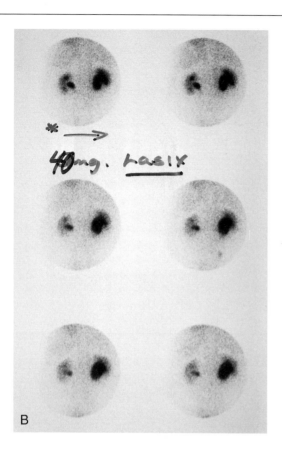

NOTE 1. The extrarenal pelvis has insufficient smooth muscle to generate and promote the peristaltic stripping wave, which begins at the renal calyx.

NOTE 2. A dilated extrarenal pelvis may not be distinguishable from ureteropelvic junction (UPJ) obstruction without a diuretic renal excretion scan.

NOTE 3. In UPJ obstruction, the renogram continues to show an obstructive pattern after administration of diuretic.

Cross Reference

Chapter 36: Unilateral Abnormalities—Ureteropelvic Junction Obstruction

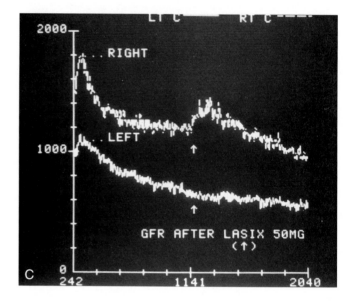

FIGURE 35–5 C.

DTPA Curves with Cortical Regions of Interest: Furosemide causes a momentary retention of the radiopharmaceutical in the cortex prior to the emptying of the extrarenal pelvis.

PELVIC KIDNEYS

FIGURE 35–6.

Bone Scan: The kidneys are more caudal than usual, with an extrarenal pelvis on the left. (Courtesy of Dr. Michael Kipper, Vista, CA.)

Cross Reference

Chapter 11: Soft Tissue Abnormalities—Pelvic Kidney

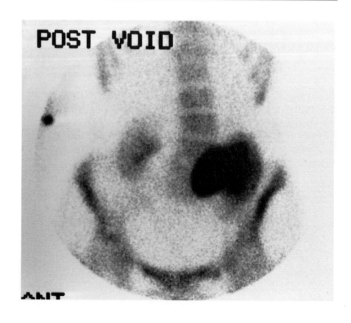

PTOTIC KIDNEY

Patient 1

FIGURE 35–7   A.
Supine DTPA Renal Scan: The kidneys are in a normal location.

FIGURE 35–7   B.
Upright Renal Scan: The right kidney drops inferiorly and rotates because of an incomplete Gerota's fascia.

Patient 2: Pseudomyxoma Peritonei

FIGURE 35–7   C.
DTPA Renal Scan: The left kidney is low-lying owing to a mass depressing and rotating the kidney. Both ureters are obstructed.

NOTE 1. Normal ptotic kidneys are most often seen in women and almost always are on the right side.

NOTE 2. With a low-lying kidney, a suprarenal mass should be considered, especially if there is distortion of the contour or if the left kidney is involved.

NOTE 3. Ptotic kidneys are asymptomatic, and there is an occasional association with renal arterial fibrodysplasia.

Cross Reference

Chapter 11: Soft Tissue Abnormalities—Ptotic Kidney on Bone Scan

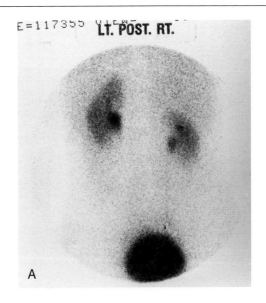

A

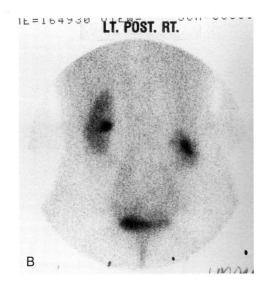

B

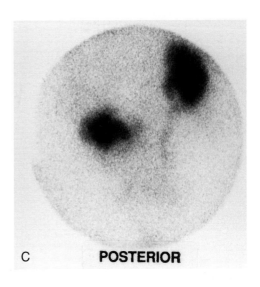

C   POSTERIOR

HORSESHOE KIDNEY

Patient 1

FIGURE 35–8   A.

DTPA Renal Scan: The renal pelves are anterolateral. The isthmus has minimal functioning tissue *(arrowheads)*.

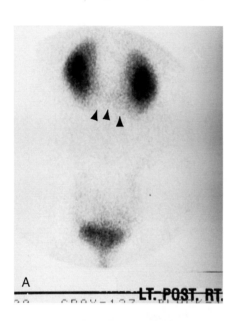

Patient 2

FIGURE 35–8   B.

Bone Scan: The isthmus on these horseshoe kidneys has considerable functioning tissue.

NOTE. Findings for horseshoe kidney include (1) medial lower poles, (2) anterior and anterolateral renal pelves with anterior ureters, (3) multiple renal arteries, and (4) more caudal location than normal.

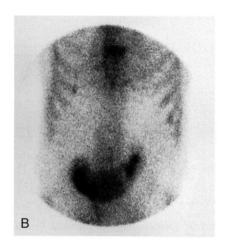

Chapter 36
Unilateral Abnormalities

DIFFERENTIAL DIAGNOSIS OF UNILATERAL ENLARGED KIDNEY	
1. Compensatory hypertrophy	7. Acute renal vein thrombosis
2. Duplicated collecting system	8. Polycystic kidney disease
3. Urinary obstruction	9. Unilateral cyst
4. Neoplasms, benign or malignant	10. Hematoma
5. Acute pyelonephritis	11. Arteriovenous malformation
6. Xanthogranulomatous pyelonephritis	

DIFFERENTIAL DIAGNOSIS OF SOLITARY VISUALIZED KIDNEY	
1. Nephrectomy	6. Neoplasm
2. Long-standing obstruction	7. Renal infarction, i.e., embolism
3. Trauma—torn renal pedicle, subcapsular hematoma	8. Transplant kidney
4. Congenital multicystic kidney	9. Acute pyelonephritis
5. Unilateral atrophic pyelonephritis	10. Xanthogranulomatous pyelonephritis

See also Chapter 11: Soft Tissue Abnormalities—Renal Cyst on Bone Scan.

SUSPECT NON-FUNCTION KIDNEY

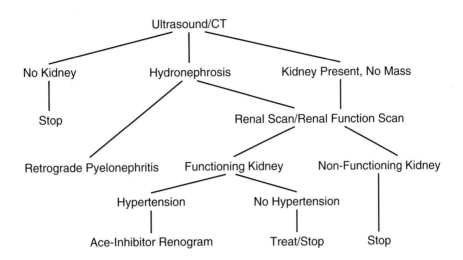

Ultrasound/CT

No Kidney — Hydronephrosis — Kidney Present, No Mass

Stop

Renal Scan/Renal Function Scan

Retrograde Pyelonephritis — Functioning Kidney — Non-Functioning Kidney

Hypertension — No Hypertension

Ace-Inhibitor Renogram — Treat/Stop — Stop

SOLITARY KIDNEY

Patient 1

FIGURE 36–1   A.
DTPA Renal Scan: The solitary right kidney is hypertrophic, measuring 16 cm (normal is 9 to 14 cm).

Patient 2

FIGURE 36–1   B.
DTPA Renal Scan: This kidney measures 11 cm in length, 2 years after the other kidney was removed for chronic obstruction with infection. There is also partial ureteral obstruction.

NOTE. The greatest hypertrophy will occur when one kidney is removed or is dysfunctional during childhood.

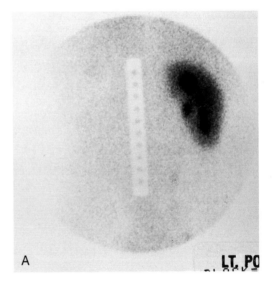

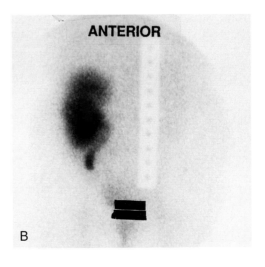

UNILATERAL POLYCYSTIC KIDNEY

FIGURE 36–2.

DTPA Renal Scan: The left kidney is markedly enlarged and distorted owing to intraparenchymal cysts. The right kidney is small and scarred.

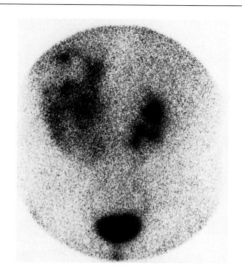

NOTE 1. The right kidney is probably small as the result of a more severe form of tubular dysplasia or atrophic pyelonephritis in utero or in early life.

NOTE 2. The continuum from normal, medullary sponge kidney, polycystic kidney, to multicystic kidney is one of tubular maldevelopment with variable obstruction of the tubules (Potter classification).

Cross References

Chapter 36: Unilateral Abnormalities—Urinoma

Chapter 37: Bilateral Abnormalities—Polycystic Kidney Disease

ACUTE PYELONEPHRITIS

Patient 1: Loss of Function

FIGURE 36–3 A.

DTPA Scan: Although the right kidney is barely visible, the presence of activity indicates an intact blood supply.

FIGURE 36–3 B.

Hippuran Renogram: The right kidney has no appreciable tubular function.

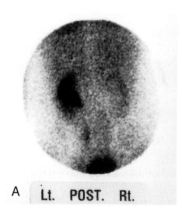

A   Lt. POST. Rt.

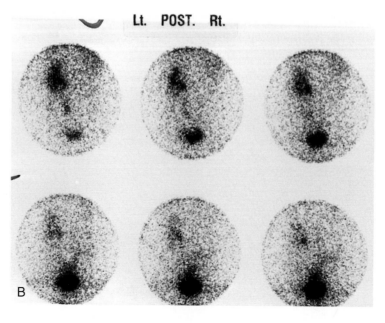

Lt. POST. Rt.

B

FIGURE 36–3   C.
Gallium Scan: The right kidney is enlarged and has intense gallium accumulation.

Patient 2: Pyuria

FIGURE 36–3   D and E.
WBC Scan: The right kidney (*arrow*) has abnormal WBC accumulation. The urinary bladder has WBCs as well, confirming the right renal WBC activity.

Patient 3: Infected Polycystic Kidney

FIGURE 36–3   F and G.
Posterior and Right Lateral WBC Scan: The right kidney is large and irregular and has marked WBC accumulation, especially in the right upper pole.

Illustration continued on following page

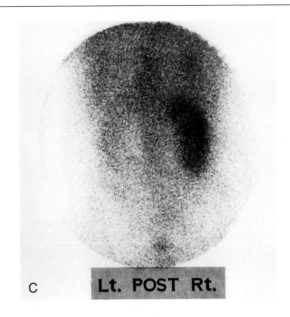

C   Lt. POST Rt.

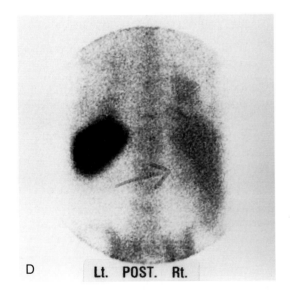

D   Lt. POST. Rt.

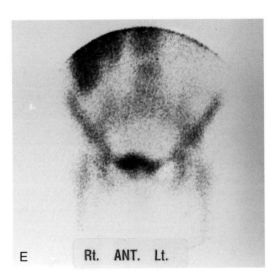

E   Rt. ANT. Lt.

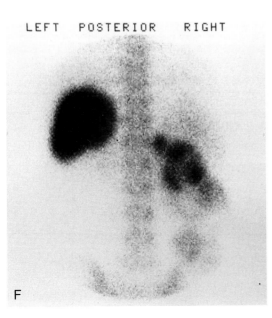

LEFT   POSTERIOR   RIGHT

F

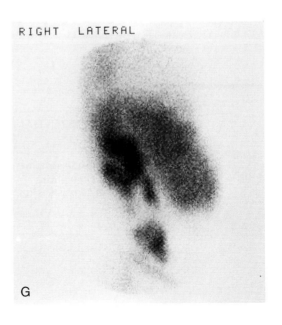

RIGHT   LATERAL

G

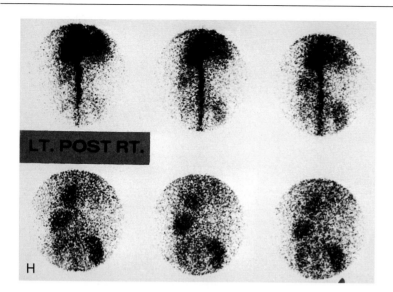

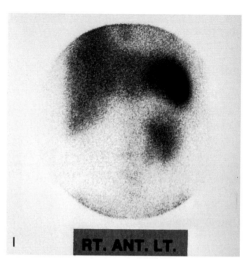

Patient 4: Reduced Blood Flow with Acute Pyelonephritis

FIGURE 36–3 H.

DTPA Renal Blood Flow: The left kidney has reduced blood flow.

FIGURE 36–3 I.

Anterior WBC Scan: The entire left kidney and renal pelvis have abnormal WBC accumulation.

NOTE 1. Renal blood flow may be reduced with acute pyelonephritis, probably owing to increased intracapsular pressure from renal edema.

NOTE 2. With acute pyelonephritis, the renal size increases while function decreases.

NOTE 3. Abnormal white cell accumulation in the right kidney may be subtle and may be confused with normal liver activity. Bladder activity is a confirmatory sign of renal infection.

WBC OR GALLIUM ACTIVITY			
	Acute Bacterial Pyelonephritis	Interstitial Pyelonephritis	Cystitis
Kidney activity	+	+	−
Bladder activity	+	−	+

Cross References

Chapter 37: Bilateral Abnormalities—Interstitial Pyelonephritis

Chapter 40: Bladder Abnormalities—Cystitis.

DIFFERENTIAL DIAGNOSIS OF UNILATERAL SMALL KIDNEY	
1. Chronic atrophic pyelonephritis (hypoplastic kidney)	6. Tuberculosis
2. Renal artery stenosis/ occlusion	7. Radiation therapy
3. Postobstructive atrophy	8. Chronic renal vein obstruction
4. Trauma	9. Extrarenal mass compressing and distorting kidney, including hematomas
5. Infarction	

CHRONIC PYELONEPHRITIS

Patient 1

FIGURE 36–4   A.
DTPA Renal Scan: The right renal calices are at the edge of the kidney owing to loss of cortex and scarring.

Patient 2

FIGURE 36–4   B to E.
⁹⁹ᵐTc-DMSA SPECT Scan: The left kidney has lost volume, particularly in the upper pole, and has an irregular cortex (B = axial; C = coronal; D = left sagittal; F = right sagittal; R = right.)

Cross Reference

Chapter 39: Renal Defects—Pyelonephritic Scarring

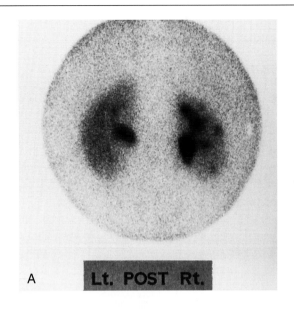

A   Lt. POST Rt.

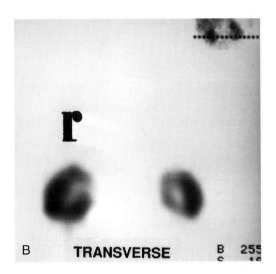

B   TRANSVERSE   B 255

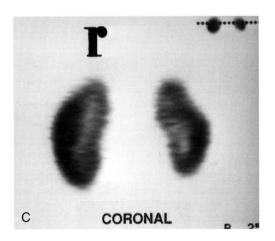

C   CORONAL   B 25

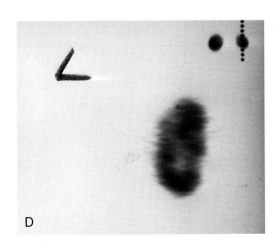

D

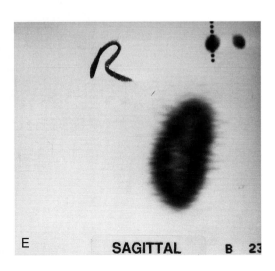

E   SAGITTAL   B 23

ATROPHY FROM REFLUX AND CHRONIC PYELONEPHRITIS

Patient 1

FIGURE 36–5 A.
DTPA Renal Scan: The right kidney has residual glomerular activity but is extremely small.

FIGURE 36–5 B.
Hippuran Renogram: Tubular function is virtually nonexistent in the right kidney.

FIGURE 36–5 C.
Retrograde Pyelogram: The ureter and intrarenal collecting system are dilated. Stones can be seen in the left kidney (*arrowheads*).

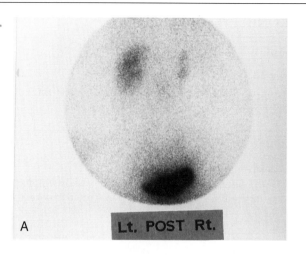

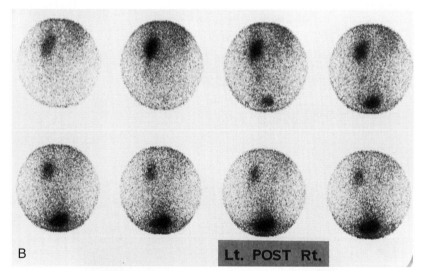

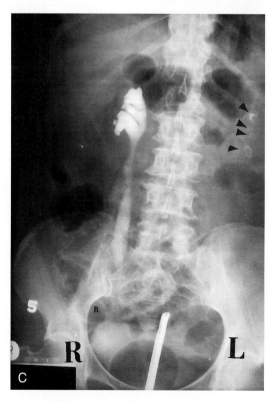

Patient 2

FIGURE 36–5   D and E.

DTPA and Hippuran Renograms: The left kidney is small but has considerable residual glomerular and tubular function.

FIGURE 36–5   F and G.

DTPA and Hippuran Renogram Curves: There is persistent, although diminished, function in the atrophic left kidney.

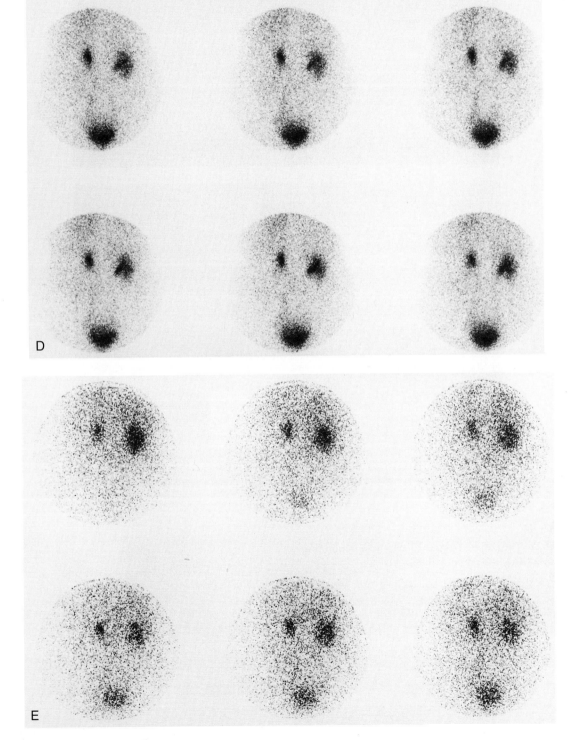

Illustration continued on following page

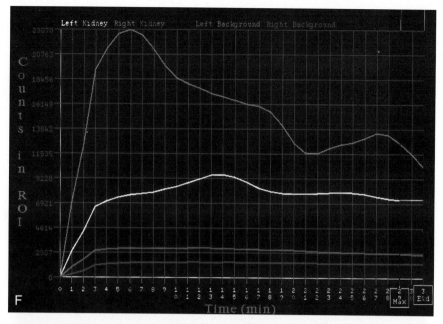

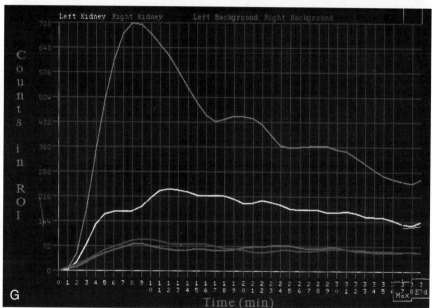

Patient 3

FIGURE 36–5 H.
DTPA Renal Scan: The patient has partial obstruction following reimplantation of the ureters for reflux.

FIGURE 36–5 I.
DTPA Renal Scan 5 Years Later: The right kidney has lost considerable parenchyma. The changes on the left are less pronounced, although function has been lost bilaterally.

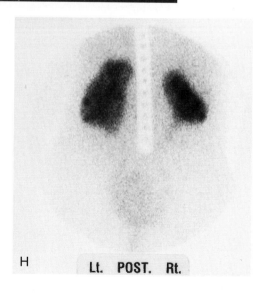

NOTE 1. Although long-standing reflux by itself may not damage the kidney, repeated infections together with reflux can cause scarring and atrophy.

NOTE 2. The unaffected kidney may appear to be mildly hydronephrotic owing to the increased urinary output.

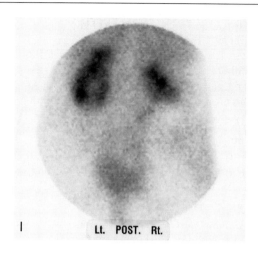

LOWER POLE CALYCEAL OBSTRUCTION

Patient: Transitional Cell Carcinoma

Figure 36–6.

DTPA Delayed Planar Scan: The right lower pole calyx is dilated in the supine position. This was due to an obstructing transitional cell carcinoma. An additional clue is the lack of dilatation of the midpole calyces.

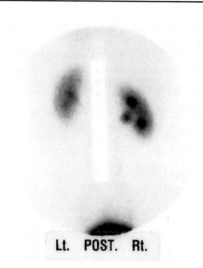

Cross References

Chapter 11: Soft Tissue Abnormalities—Obstructed Lower Pole Calyx

Chapter 35: Normal/Normal Variants—Normal Upper Pole Calyceal Dilatation

---

**DIFFERENTIAL DIAGNOSIS
OF URINARY OBSTRUCTION**

1. Calculus
2. Strictures—congenital, postinflammatory, post-traumatic, postoperative, radiation
3. Blood clot or sloughed papilla
4. Pus or fungus ball
5. Bladder outlet obstruction—prostatic hypertrophy or carcinoma
6. Carcinoma of the bladder
7. Ureterocoele
8. Retroperitoneal tumor—lymphoma, pseudomyxoma peritonei, sarcoma, metastatic disease
9. Pelvic tumor—carcinoma of the cervix
10. Retroperitoneal fibrosis
11. Urothelial tumor—transitional cell carcinoma
12. Trauma—torn ureter or clot
13. Crossing blood vessel, retrocaval ureter
14. Compression by aortic aneurysm
15. Ureteric valves
16. Horseshoe kidney
17. Endometriosis

URINARY OBSTRUCTION WITH "FLIP-FLOP" FUNCTION

FIGURE 36–7 A.

Early DTPA Renal Scan: The nephrogram phase demonstrates a faint rim of activity in the right renal cortex, with a relatively photopenic medulla ("rim sign").

FIGURE 36–7 B and C.

Lasix and DTPA Scan: The right kidney is enlarged, with little excretion despite the diuretic. The left kidney has faded after excreting its share of the radiopharmaceutical.

FIGURE 36–7 D.

DTPA Excretion Curves: There is clearance of the glomerular agent on the left after Lasix administration *(arrows)*. The right has a persistent upward slope, indicative of physical obstruction. There was no response to diuretic (L = Lasix).

Obstructed kidney scan findings in various patients include the following.

FIGURE 36–7 E.

Slow blood flow (bolus arrival curves).

FIGURE 36–7 F.

Delayed and prolonged visualization ("flip-flop" function).

FIGURE 36–7 G.

Rim of activity; enlarged kidney.

FIGURE 36–7 H.

Dilated collecting system; decreased activity distal to obstruction, e.g., ureter.

NOTE. The unaffected kidney may have a dilated collecting system owing to the increased load excreted (Fig. 36–7H) when the opposite kidney is functioning poorly.

Cross References

Chapter 3: Spinal Abnormalities—Spinal Osteomyelitis Associated with Hydronephrosis

Chapter 71: Infectious Diseases—Psoas Abscess

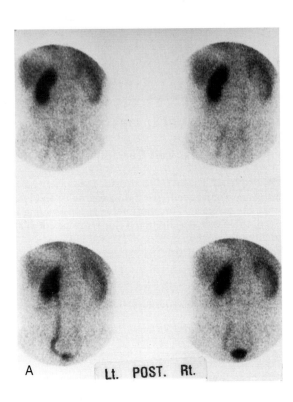

A   Lt. POST. Rt.

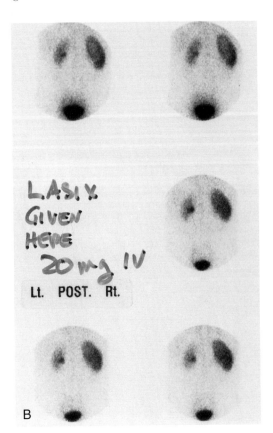

B

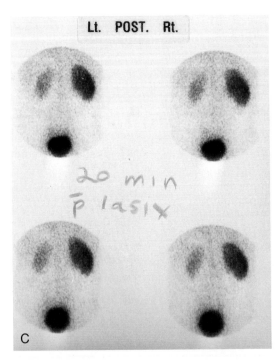

C

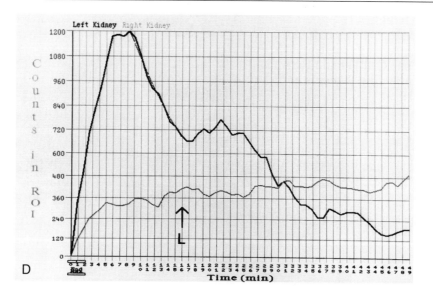

D

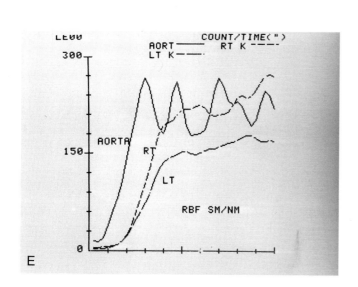

E

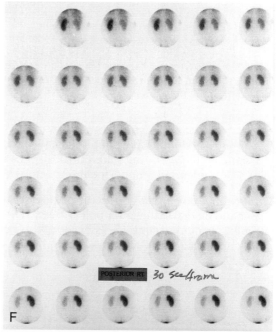

F

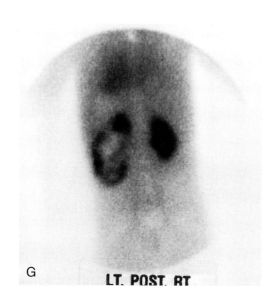

G   **LT. POST. RT.**

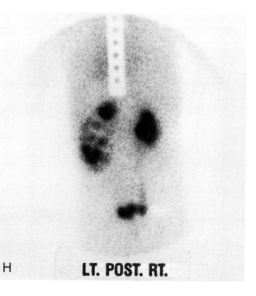

H   **LT. POST. RT.**

OBSTRUCTION OF DUPLICATE COLLECTING SYSTEM

Patient: Twenty-six Year Old Female with Bilateral Duplicate Collecting Systems and Recurrent Pyelonephritis

FIGURE 36–8   A to C.

DTPA Renal Blood Flow and Scan: The blood flow and glomerular filtration are markedly reduced in the upper pole of the right kidney. The renal pelves are both depressed and displaced away from the spine, the so-called drooping lily sign.

FIGURE 36–8   D.

Delayed Planar Glucoheptonate Scan: The upper pole of the right kidney has some viable tissue, although renal function proved to be minimal.

FIGURE 36–8   E.

Intravenous Urogram Reversed to Match the Renal Scan: The left upper collecting system has normal function and appearance. The left upper ureter is well seen, whereas the right upper pole duplicate system is only inferred by its mass effect.

FIGURE 36–8   F.

Bladder View from Intravenous Urogram: There is an ectopic ureterocoele on the right, low in the bladder, associated with partial obstruction of the upper pole ureter.

NOTE 1. An obstructed upper pole duplicate collecting system should be in the differential diagnosis of a nonfunctioning upper pole renal mass.

NOTE 2. The upper pole ureter enters the bladder inferior and medial to the lower pole's ureter. This finding is more frequently associated with reflux and obstruction and, in women, incontinence.

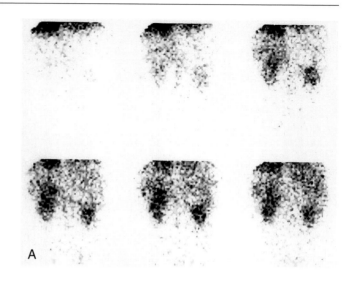

A

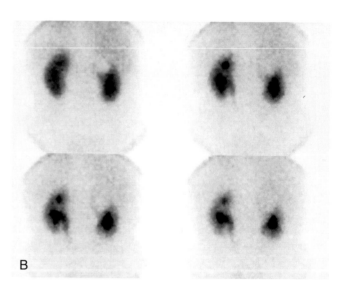

B

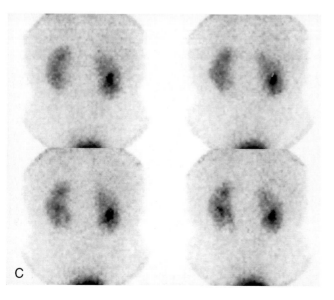

C

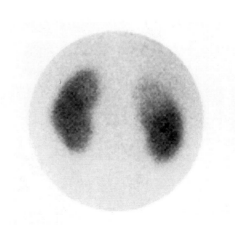

D

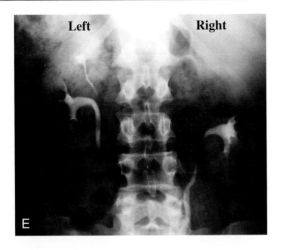
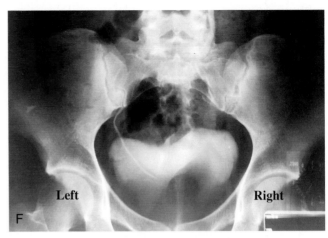

URETERAL OBSTRUCTION DUE TO RETROPERITONEAL TUMOR

FIGURE 36–9.
DTPA Renal Scan: The ureter is seen down to its middle third *(arrowhead)*; there is marked hydronephrosis.

NOTE. The lack of dilatation of the ureter suggests encasement rather than just luminal obstruction. (The obstruction in this case was due to carcinomatosis from stomach carcinoma.)

Cross Reference

Chapter 11: Soft Tissue Abnormalities—Urinary Obstruction on Bone Scan

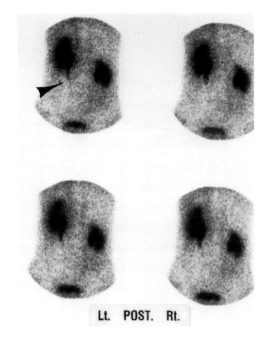

URETEROPELVIC JUNCTION (UPJ) OBSTRUCTION

Patient: Eight Month Old with Left UPJ Obstruction

FIGURE 36–10   A.
MAG₃ Renal Blood Flow Scan: The right kidney perfuses immediately, whereas the enlarged left kidney *(arrowheads)* takes longer. The spleen *(arrow)* fills early and should not be confused with kidney.

Illustration continued on following page

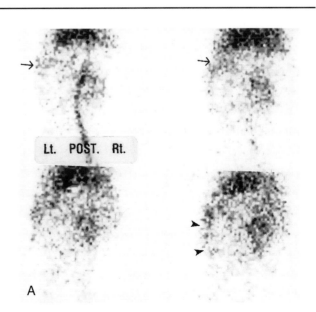

FIGURE 36–10   B.

Early Lasix MAG₃ Renal Scan: The left kidney is enlarged owing to the obstruction. The intrarenal collecting system is not filled yet (the rim sign).

FIGURE 36–10   C.

Delayed Lasix MAG₃ Renal Scan: There is massive dilatation of the left renal pelvis.

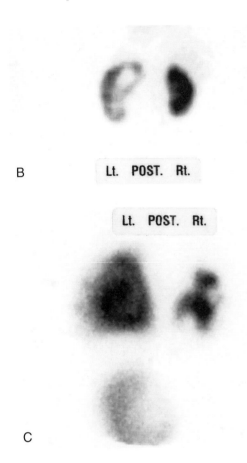

FIGURE 36–10   D.

Intravenous Urogram Film X-ray of the Abdomen: The left kidney is a large unopacified mass in the abdomen. The right kidney is normal.

NOTE. With children we use ⁹⁹ᵐTc-MAG₃, since the active process of tubular excretion allows for improved visualization and overall lower radiation.

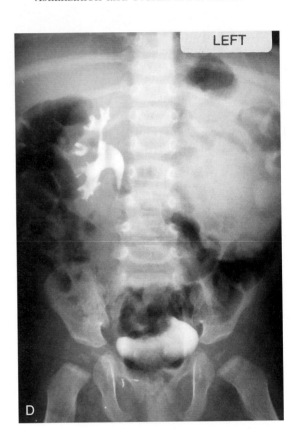

GALLBLADDER VISUALIZATION SIMULATING RENAL OBSTRUCTION

FIGURE 36–11   A and B.

⁹⁹ᵐTc-MAG₃ Renal Scan: The early scans demonstrate a small right kidney, whereas the later scans show an apparent obstruction of the kidney.

FIGURE 36–11   C and D.

Anterior and Right Lateral Renal Scans: There is a structure that has intense MAG₃ accumulation anterior to the right kidney that proves to be the gallbladder. There are small bowel loops filling as well (*arrow*).

FIGURE 36–11   E.

⁹⁹ᵐTc-MAG₃ Renogram Curve: The right renal function is poor, but there is no obstruction when cortical regions of interest are used. The second bump in the right excretion curve is due to filling of the gallbladder.

Cross References

Chapter 37: Bilateral Abnormalities—Extrarenal Hepatic Excretion

Chapter 38: Renal Transplant—Progressive Acute Renal Transplant Rejection

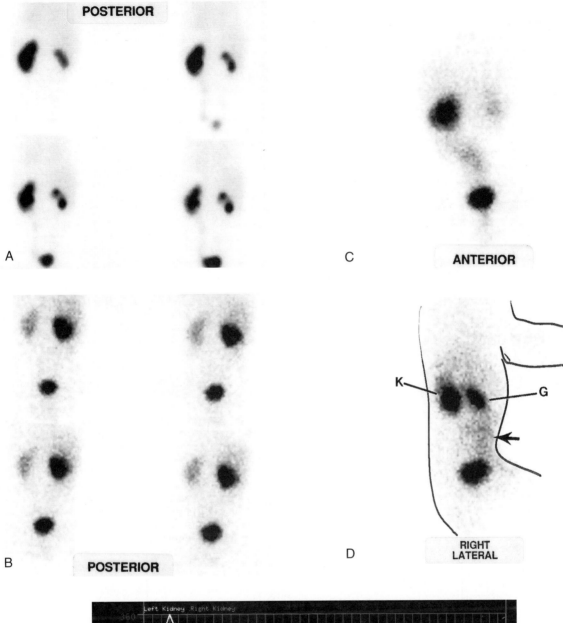

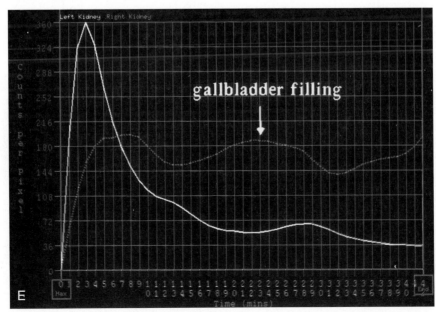

URETEROVESICAL JUNCTION OBSTRUCTION

FIGURE 36–12 A.

DTPA Renal Scan: There is hydronephrosis and hydroureter all the way down to the bladder.

FIGURE 36–12 B.

Post–bladder Catheterization Scan: The hydronephrosis and hydroureter remain.

NOTE. It may be important to catheterize the bladder, especially in children, to rule out urinary reflux as a cause of the collecting system dilatation.

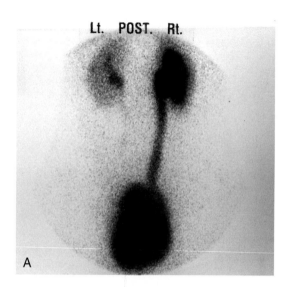

A

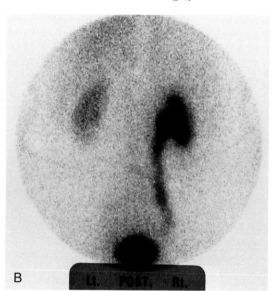

B

CAUSES OF URINARY EXTRAVASATION	
1. Trauma	5. Increased intra-abdominal pressure
2. Instrumentation	
3. Calculus	6. Polycystic kidneys
4. Urinary tract tumor	7. Surgery

URINOMA

Patient 1: Transected Left Ureter

FIGURE 36–13 A.

DTPA Renal Scan: There is extravasation of urine and hydronephrosis.

Patient 2: Polycystic Kidney Disease

FIGURE 36–13 B.

DTPA Renal Scan: There is an extrarenal collection of radiolabeled urine below the left kidney.

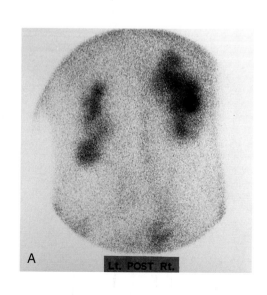

A

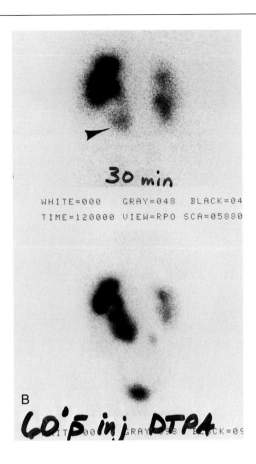

B

FIGURE 36–13 C.

Twenty-four Hour DTPA Renal Scan: The size of the urinoma has not expanded over time.

Cross References

Chapter 11: Soft Tissue Abnormalities—Urinoma on Bone Scan

Chapter 36: Unilateral Abnormalities—Unilateral Polycystic Kidney

Chapter 37: Bilateral Abnormalities—Polycystic Kidney Disease

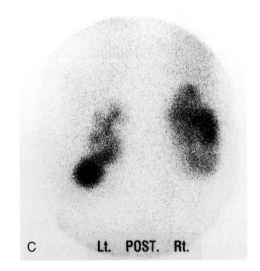

C   Lt. POST. Rt.

SUBCAPSULAR HEMATOMA OF THE KIDNEY

Patient 1: Bicycle Accident

FIGURE 36–14   A.

DTPA Renal Scan: There is minimal left renal glomerular function. A photon-deficient area *(arrow)* is seen just lateral to the kidney *(arrowhead).*

FIGURE 36–14   B.

CT Scan: The left kidney *(arrowhead)* is compressed by the large subcapsular hematoma.

Illustration continued on following page

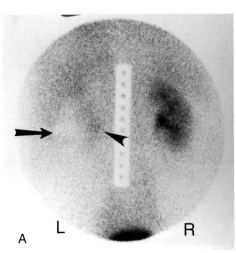

A   L   R

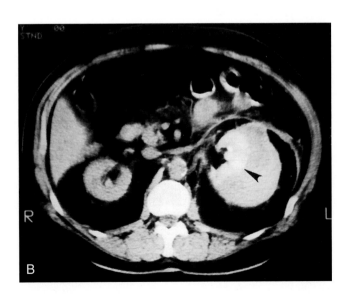

B

Patient 2: Jet Ski Accident

FIGURE 36–14   C and D.

DTPA Renal Scan: There is delayed function on the left. The left kidney has a crescentic rim of decreased activity *(arrowhead)* and an irregular cortical margin.

NOTE 1. Delayed function is presumably due to increased intracapsular pressure from a subcapsular hematoma.

NOTE 2. Subcapsular or perirenal hematomas can be a cause of hypertension (Page kidney).

NOTE 3. Tubular function probably persists because it is an active process, whereas glomerular filtration is passive and suffers owing to reduced perfusion.

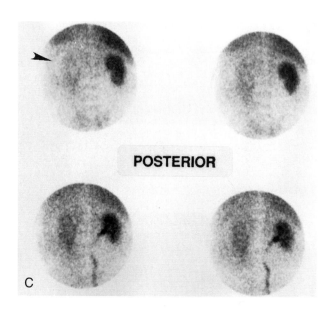

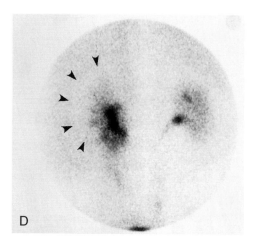

SUSPECTED RENAL ARTERY STENOSIS

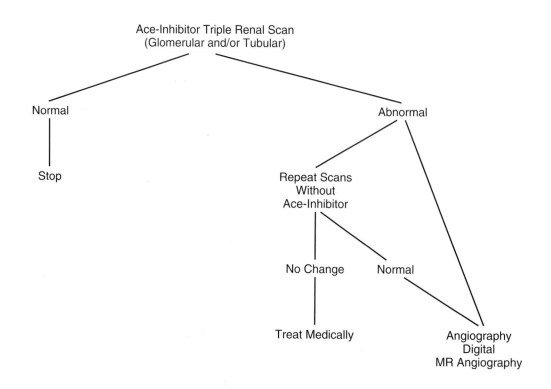

DIFFERENTIAL DIAGNOSIS
OF RENAL HYPERTENSION

1. Renal artery stenosis—
   atherosclerosis,
   fibrodysplasia

2. Renal artery aneurysm

3. Polycystic kidney disease

4. Collagen vascular disease

5. Renal infarcts with
   ischemic zones on
   periphery

6. Reninoma

7. End-stage renal disease

8. Giant renal cyst

9. Subcapsular or
   perirenal hematoma
   (Page kidney)

RENOVASCULAR HYPERTENSION

Patient 1: Main Renal Artery Stenosis and Renal Insufficiency

FIGURE 36–15 A.

Renal Blood Flow: The blood flow to the right kidney is not seen, and the flow to the left kidney is diminished *(arrow)*.

FIGURE 36–15 B.

Normalized Renal Blood Flow Curve: The right kidney has delayed flow with reduced slope.

FIGURE 36–15 C.

Captopril Hippuran Renogram: The right kidney retains the tubular agent. The left kidney has overall abnormal function.

Illustration continued on following page

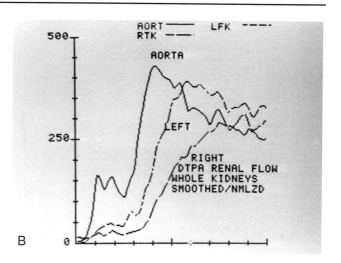

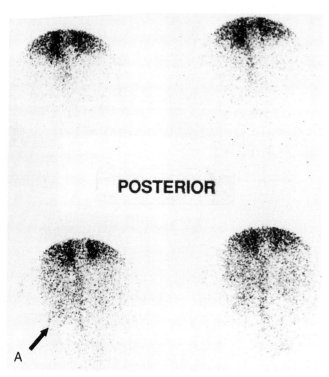

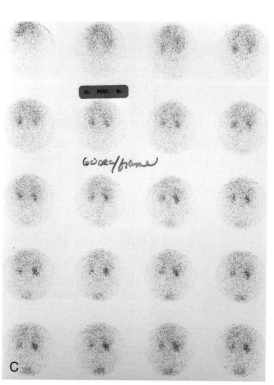

FIGURE 36–15   D.

Captopril Renogram Curve: The right kidney has an "obstructive" curve. The left kidney has diminished function but does excrete Hippuran.

FIGURE 36–15   E.

DTPA Renal Scan: The right kidney is small (7.5 cm); the left is normal (10 cm). (Normal = 9 to 14 cm.)

FIGURE 36–15   F.

Contrast Angiogram: The right renal artery is stenotic *(arrow)*. The aorta has moderate atherosclerosis.

Patient 2: Lower Pole Renal Artery Stenosis

FIGURE 36–15   G.

Pre–Captopril Hippuran Renogram: There is mildly delayed left renal function. The right kidney has almost no tubular function.

FIGURE 36–15   H.

Captopril Hippuran Renogram: The left kidney function is further delayed and has a progressive accumulation of the radiopharmaceutical.

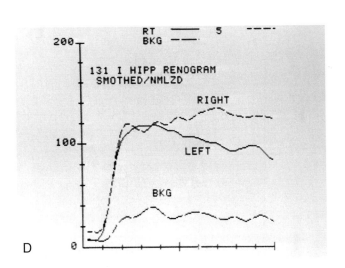

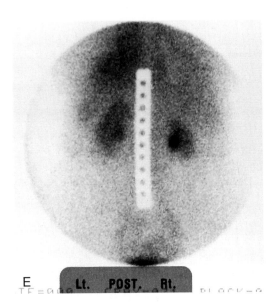

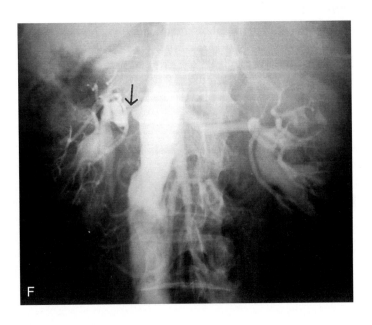

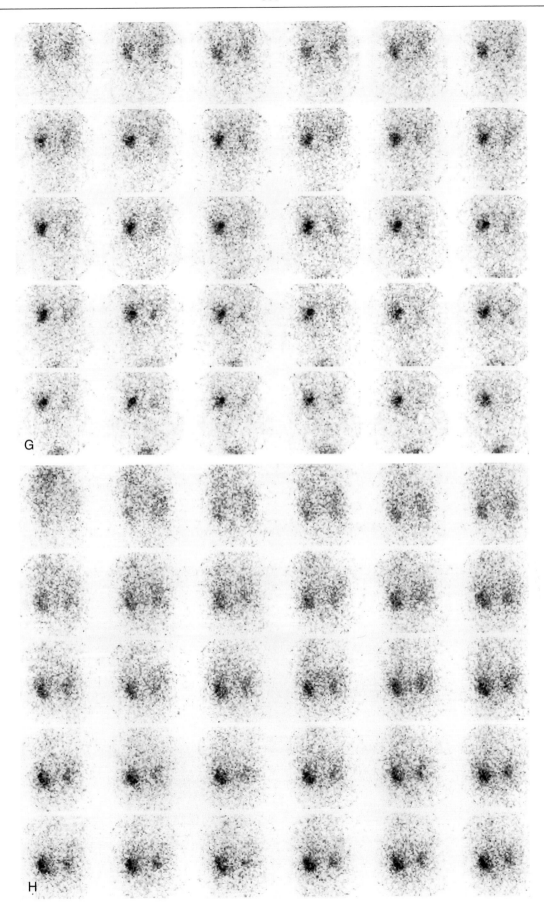

Illustration continued on following page

FIGURE 36–15   I and J.

Early and Late DTPA Renal Scans: The left lower pole retains the radiopharmaceutical while the rest of the left kidney and the right kidney wash out.

FIGURE 36–15   K.

Pre–Captopril Renogram Curve: Using left and right lower pole regions of interest, the poor function is evident.

FIGURE 36–15   L.

Captopril Renogram Curve: The left lower pole has progressive accumulation of the Hippuran.

FIGURE 36–15   M.

Digital Subtraction Angiogram: The left lower pole renal artery stenosis is well seen *(arrow)*. The upper pole artery was also stenotic. The right renal artery was patent.

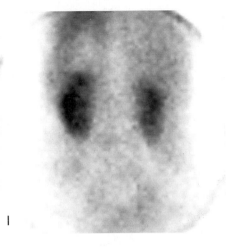

I

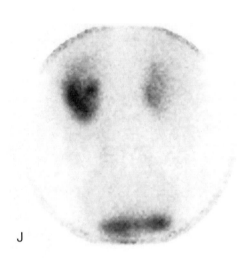

J

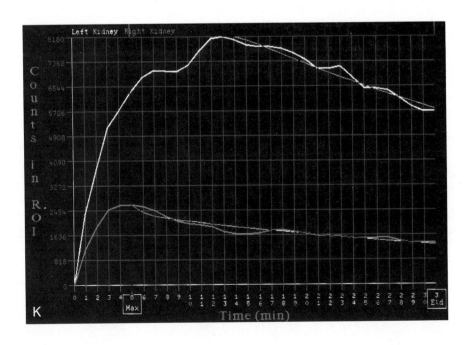

K

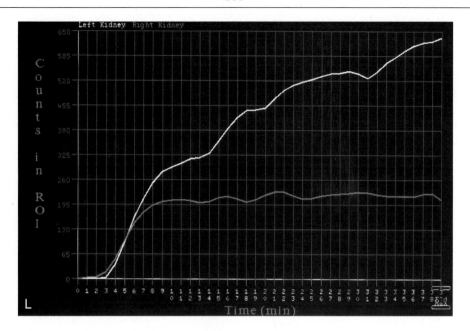

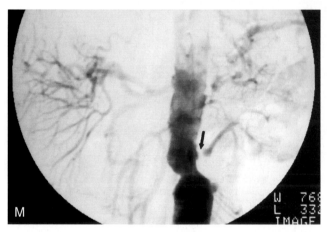

Patient 3: Fibrodysplasia

FIGURE 36–15 N.

Pre–Captopril ^{99m}Tc-MAG$_3$ Renogram: There is a mild delay of right renal washout.

Illustration continued on following page

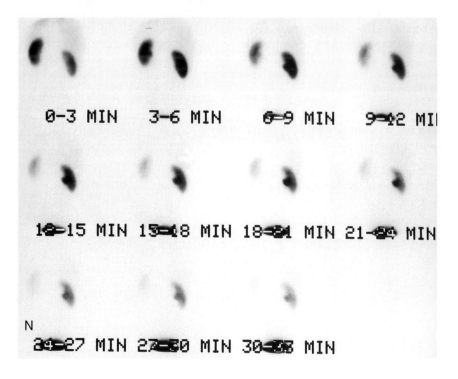

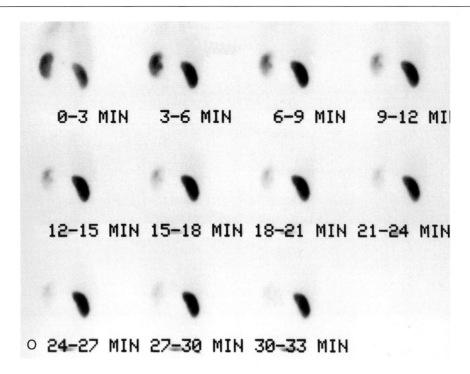

O 24-27 MIN 27-30 MIN 30-33 MIN

FIGURE 36–15   O.

Post–Captopril ^{99m}Tc-MAG$_3$ Renogram: The transit of the radio-pharmaceutical is so delayed in the right kidney that the renal pelvis has not filled by 30 minutes.

FIGURE 36–15   P.

Pre–and Post–Captopril ^{99m}Tc-MAG$_3$ Excretion Curves of the Right Kidney: The change due to the captopril is evident.

FIGURE 36–15   Q.

Digital Angiogram: There is a long irregular stenosis.

NOTE 1. A renogram with an ACE-inhibitor challenge is a good screening examination for renovascular hypertension, even with renal insufficiency. The sensitivity is almost 100% for stenosis >60%. Specificity is slightly lower.

NOTE 2. Segmental or ''accessory'' renal arteries can cause part of a kidney to be ischemic, also causing renovascular hypertension.

NOTE 3. A ''positive'' captopril renogram is a predictor of a kidney that will respond favorably after the renal artery is repaired.

NOTE 4. Fibrodysplasia includes medial fibromuscular dysplasia and intimal and adventitial fibrodysplasia.

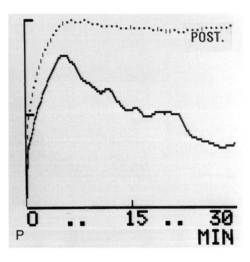

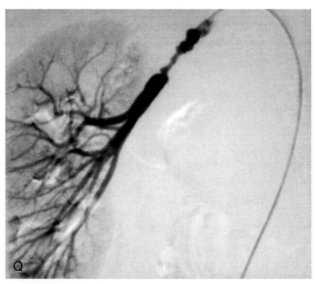

CAPTOPRIL "TRIPLE" RENAL SCAN TECHNIQUE

1. Stop ACE inhibitors for 48 hours

2. Stop diuretics for 48 hours

3. Only water by mouth for 4 hours

4. Captopril 50 mg PO with water

5. Normal saline 250 ml IV over 1 hour—optimal

6. Wait 1 hour; do ^{99m}Tc-DTPA study

7. ^{131}I-Hippuran renogram, with or without Lasix

8. Renal scan

NOTE 5. If the captopril renal scan is positive, a repeat scan without the ACE inhibitor can be obtained, or the patient can go directly to angiography. A negative examination is usually sufficient to forgo angiography.

Cross Reference

Chapter 37: Bilateral Abnormalities—Bilateral Renal Artery Stenosis

RENAL VEIN THROMBOSIS

Patient: A 46 Year Old Woman with Accidental Ligation of the Left Renal Vein During Surgery for Retroperitoneal Tumor

FIGURE 36–16 A.

^{99m}Tc-DTPA Scan: The left kidney has poor glomerular function but normal size.

Illustration continued on following page

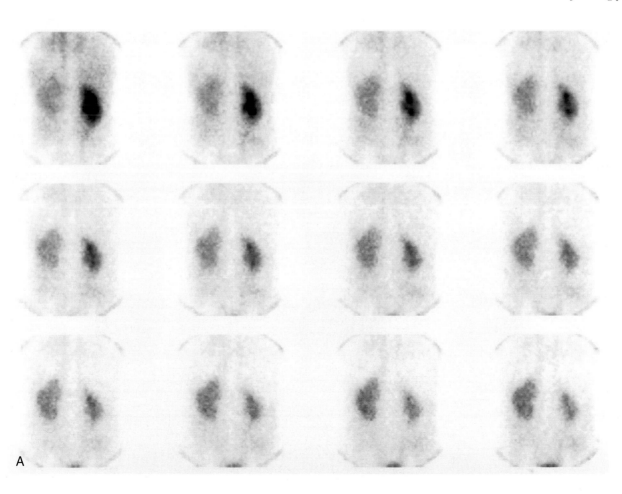

A

FIGURE 36–16   B.

⁹⁹ᵐTc-Glucoheptonate Scan for Kidney Size: The left kidney measures 12 cm in length; the right measures 11.5 cm. The difference is not significant.

FIGURE 36–16   C and D.

¹³¹I-Hippuran Lasix Renogram: The left kidney's tubular function is slow. There is no response to Lasix.

NOTE. Renal scanning is not diagnostic of renal vein thrombosis, but it can measure residual renal function. A tagged RBC scan with SPECT, spiral CT with bolused contrast, and MRI with MR angiography are noninvasive tests that can be used to diagnose renal vein thrombosis.

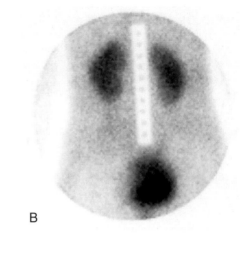

B

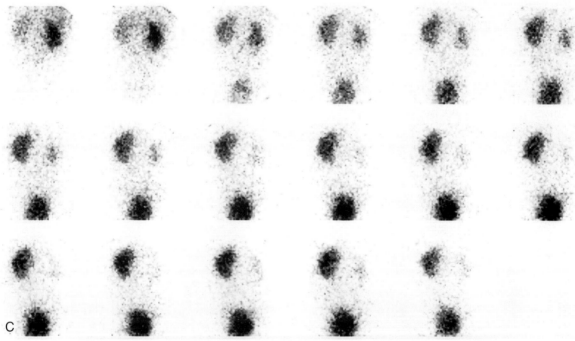

C

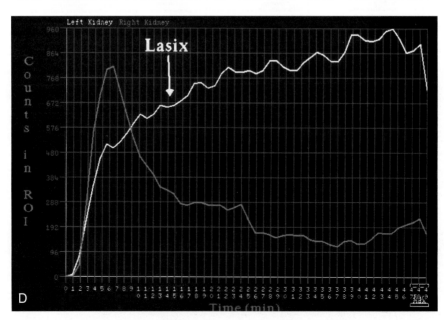

D

Chapter 37
Bilateral Abnormalities

RENAL ECTOPIA

FIGURE 37–1.

DTPA Renal Scan: The renal parenchyma is distorted, ectopic, malrotated, and difficult to objectively measure.

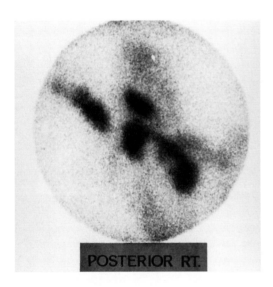

NOTE 1. Evaluation for renal function must be done visually in most cases.

NOTE 2. Renal ectopia is associated with other congenital abnormalities, especially of the spine.

POLYCYSTIC KIDNEY DISEASE

FIGURE 37–2.

DTPA Renal Scan: The kidneys are very large, with splayed collecting systems and numerous photon-deficient cysts surrounding the collecting systems.

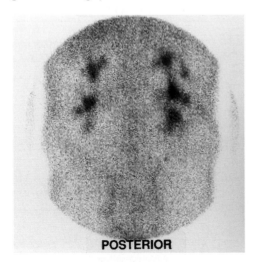

DIFFERENTIAL DIAGNOSIS OF BILATERAL ENLARGED KIDNEYS (>14 CM)

1. Diabetes mellitus, early
2. Polycystic kidney disease
3. Bilateral obstruction
4. Acute tubular necrosis
5. Acute bilateral pyelonephritis
6. Acute glomerulonephritis
7. Multiple myeloma
8. Lymphoma
9. Leukemia
10. Collagen vascular disease, i.e., systemic lupus erythematosus
11. Bilateral renal vein thrombosis
12. Amyloidosis
13. Medullary sponge kidneys
14. Congenital megacalices
15. Bilateral duplicated collecting system
16. Sickle cell anemia
17. Chemotherapy

See also Chapter 11: Soft Tissue Abnormalities—"Hot" Kidneys on Bone Scan.

NOTE 1. Adult polycystic kidney disease is associated with polycystic liver and berry aneurysms (up to 25 percent).

NOTE 2. These patients will all develop renal failure, hypertension, and possibly renal cell carcinoma.

NOTE 3. The disease is autosomal dominant with 100 percent penetrance if patients live long enough.

Cross Reference

Chapter 36: Unilateral Abnormalities—Unilateral Polycystic Kidney; Urinoma

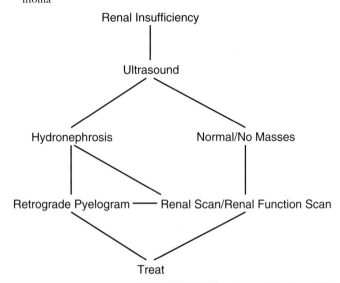

Renal Insufficiency

Ultrasound

Hydronephrosis   Normal/No Masses

Retrograde Pyelogram —— Renal Scan/Renal Function Scan

Treat

DIABETIC NEPHROPATHY (NEPHROSCLEROSIS)

FIGURE 37–3.

DTPA Renal Scan: Each kidney measures 7 cm in length (the normal is 9 to 14 cm), and both are grossly smooth.

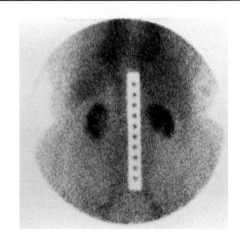

DIFFERENTIAL DIAGNOSIS OF SMALL KIDNEYS	
1. Diabetic nephropathy	5. Chronic atrophic pyelonephritis
2. Arteriolar nephrosclerosis secondary to chronic hypertension	6. Chronic glomerulonephritis
	7. Drug toxicity
3. Bilateral renal artery stenosis	8. Radiation
4. Generalized atherosclerosis	9. Hereditary nephropathy

TUBULOINTERSTITIAL NEPHROPATHY

Patient: Oxalate Nephropathy

FIGURE 37–4   A.

Initial DTPA Renal Scan: There is relatively normal glomerular function despite atrophy of the left kidney.

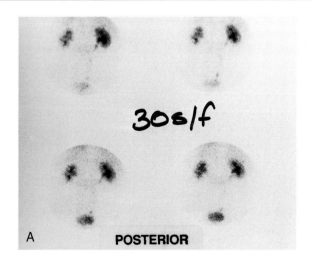

A   **POSTERIOR**

FIGURE 37–4   B.

DTPA Renal Scan 3 Years Later: Renal glomerular function has dramatically deteriorated.

FIGURE 37–4   C.

Hippuran Renogram: There is no discernible tubular function.

NOTE 1. Oxalate nephropathy can be seen with massive vitamin C intake, especially with gout. This may also be seen with inflammatory bowel disease (increased absorption).

NOTE 2. Hyperoxaluria is most often acquired, rarely genetic.

NOTE 3. This is one of several chronic tubulointerstitial nephropathies: analgesics, uric acid, hypercalcemia, heavy metals (e.g., lead), hemoglobinopathies, nephrosclerosis, radiation nephritis, granulomatous diseases, among others.

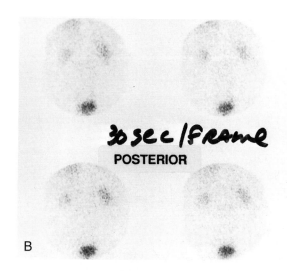

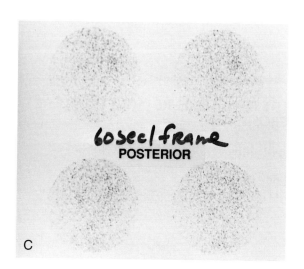

INTERSTITIAL PYELONEPHRITIS

FIGURE 37–5   A and B.

WBC Scan: There is abnormal WBC accumulation in both kidneys but none in the bladder.

NOTE. The lack of bladder activity indicates that there is no pyuria and, therefore, that the inflammation is interstitial.

Cross References

Chapter 36: Unilateral Abnormalities—Acute Pyelonephritis

Chapter 40: Bladder Abnormalities—Cystitis

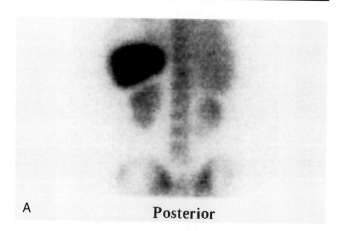

A   **Posterior**

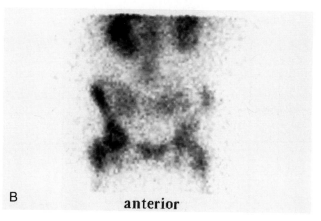

B   **anterior**

RENAL AMYLOIDOSIS

FIGURE 37–6.

Gallium Scan: There is increased gallium activity in both kidneys in this patient with recurrent septicemias from chronic paratyphoid. Biopsy revealed amyloid.

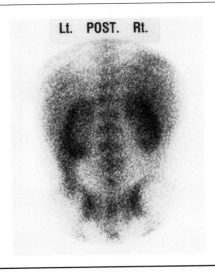

ACUTE RENAL FAILURE (ACUTE TUBULAR NECROSIS, ATN)

Patient: Intravenous Contrast Reaction

FIGURE 37–7   A.

Blood Flow Scan: There is symmetric perfusion of both kidneys.

FIGURE 37–7   B.

Blood Flow Time-Activity Curves: The right kidney has slightly slower blood flow.

FIGURE 37–7   C.

DTPA Renal Scan: The kidneys are well visualized, although neither the renal pelves nor the bladder has activity.

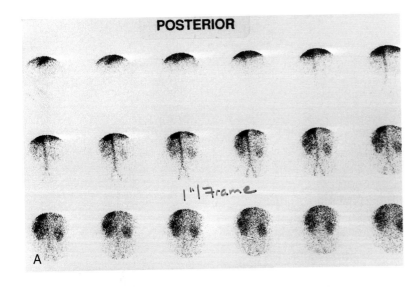

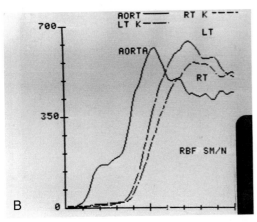

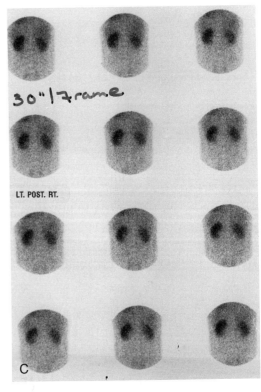

FIGURE 37–7 D.

DTPA Glomerular Time-Activity Curves: As the blood pool diminishes (aortic curve), the renal activity remains constant.

FIGURE 37–7 E.

DTPA Renal Scan: The kidneys are normal in size (10 cm, right; 11 cm, left).

FIGURE 37–7 F.

Hippuran Renogram: There is progressive accumulation of the tubular agent in both kidneys, with minimal bladder activity.

FIGURE 37–7 G.

Hippuran Tubular Time-Activity Curves: The curves have an "obstructive" pattern.

NOTE 1. ATN is suggested when the renal blood flow is near-normal, the glomerular curves are flat, there is no hydronephrosis, and the tubular agent has a rising curve.

NOTE 2. The combination of a glomerular filtered agent and a tubular excreted agent is often helpful in separating diseases affecting the individual components.

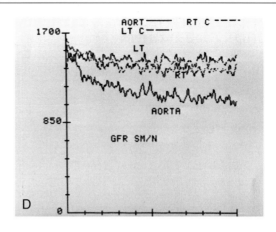

D

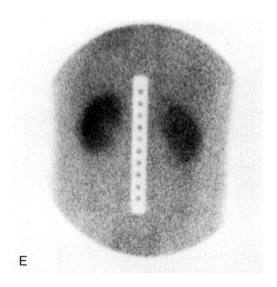

E

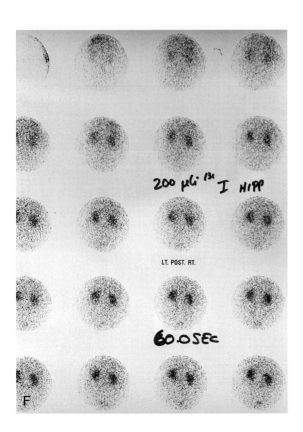

F

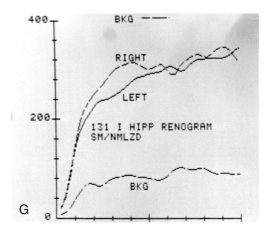

G

BILATERAL URETEROVESICAL JUNCTION OBSTRUCTION

Patient: S/P Bilateral Ureteral Reimplantations

FIGURE 37–8   A.
DTPA Renal Scan: There is bilateral hydronephrosis and hydro-ureter. The bladder is barely seen.

FIGURE 37–8   B.
Hippuran Renal Scan: There is slow accumulation of the radiopharmaceutical in each kidney.

FIGURE 37–8   C.
Hippuran Renogram Curves: Using cortical regions of interest, the data derived demonstrate high-grade obstruction on the left. The right kidney has a slow transit time of the radiopharmaceutical but does eventually excrete the material.

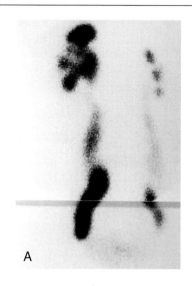

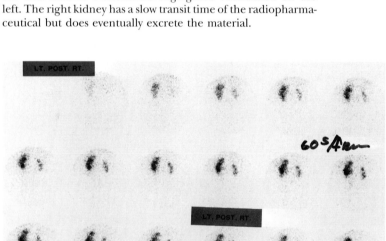

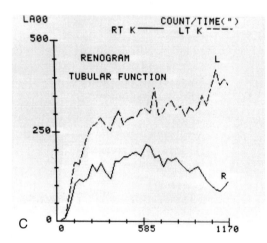

SEVERE BILATERAL RENAL FAILURE

Patient: Chronic Glomerulonephritis

FIGURE 37–9   A.
DTPA Renal Scan: There is very poor visualization of the kidneys and bladder.

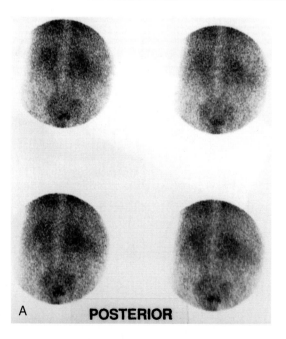

FIGURE 37–9 B.

FIGURE 37–9 B.

DTPA "Glomerular" Curves: The flat curves are only slightly above the blood pool as measured by the activity in the aorta. (The data are normalized.)

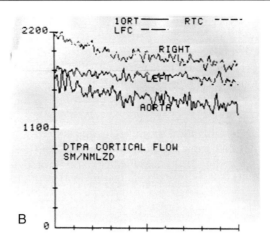

EXTRARENAL HEPATIC EXCRETION

Patient 1

FIGURE 37–10 A.

Anterior Abdominal ^{99m}Technetium DTPA Renal Scan: There is gallbladder and small bowel visualization in this patient with bilateral renal failure.

Patient 2

FIGURE 37–10 B.

Posterior ^{99m}Tc-MAG$_3$ Renal Scan: The liver can be seen above the obstructed right kidney.

Cross References

Chapter 36: Unilateral Abnormalities—Gallbladder Visualization Simulating Renal Obstruction

Chapter 38: Renal Transplant—Progressive Acute Renal Transplant Rejection

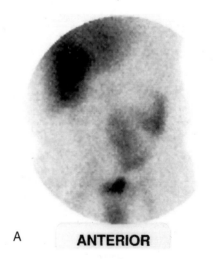

A **ANTERIOR**

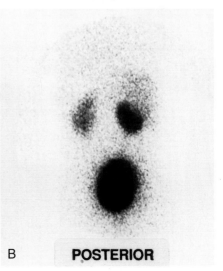

B **POSTERIOR**

ILEAL LOOP

FIGURE 37–11.

DTPA Renal Scan: There is renal collecting system dilatation with normal cortical thickness *(arrowheads).*

NOTE. The dilatation of the collecting systems is due to reflux from the ileal loop, which does not damage the cortex significantly and should not be interpreted as obstructive uropathy.

Cross Reference

Chapter 11: Soft Tissue Abnormalities—Ileal Loop on Bone Scan

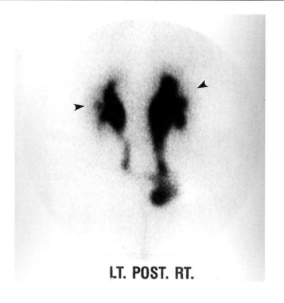

BILATERAL RENAL ARTERY STENOSIS

FIGURE 37–12   A.

Renal Blood Flow: There is late visualization of the kidneys.

FIGURE 37–12   B.

Renal Blood Flow Curves: Both renal blood flow curves have delayed bolus appearance times and flattened slopes.

FIGURE 37–12   C.

Captopril Hippuran Renogram: There is retention of the radiopharmaceutical in both kidneys.

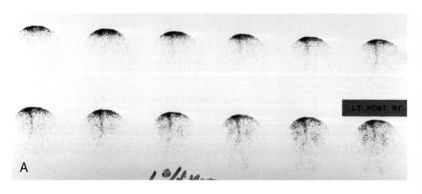

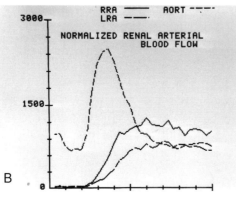

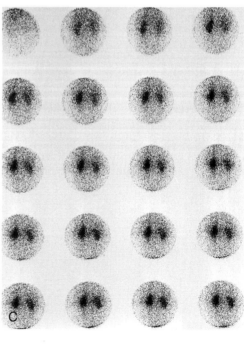

FIGURE 37–12   D.

Hippuran Renogram Curves: The bilateral "obstructive" curves suggest renal artery stenosis.

FIGURE 37–12   E.

Digital Subtraction Angiogram: The origins of both renal arteries have tight stenoses.

NOTE. Data suggest that those patients with an abnormal captopril renal study will improve with intervention by renal artery angioplasty or graft bypass.

Cross Reference

Chapter 36: Unilateral Abnormalities—Renovascular Hypertension

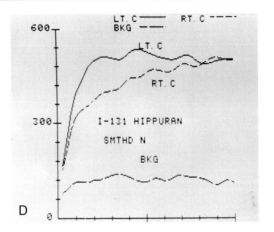

D

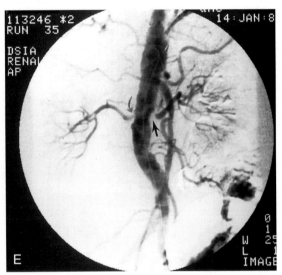

E

Chapter 38

Renal Transplant

NORMAL KIDNEY TRANSPLANT

FIGURE 38–1   A.

Blood Flow Scan: The perfusion is immediate and fills the entire graft.

FIGURE 38–1   B.

^{99m}Tc-MAG$_3$ Scan: The renal size and collecting system are normal. The appearance and drainage of the calyces are also normal. (Courtesy of Dr. Edward Hew, Honolulu, HI.)

Illustration continued on following page

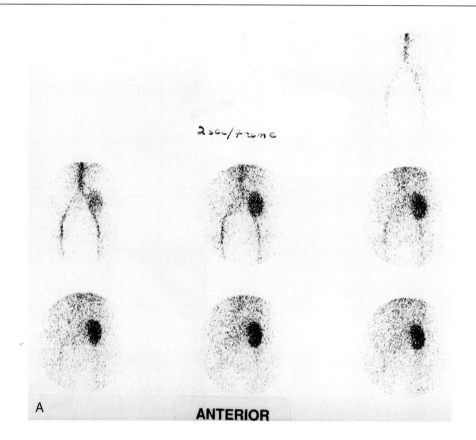

2sec/frame

A   **ANTERIOR**

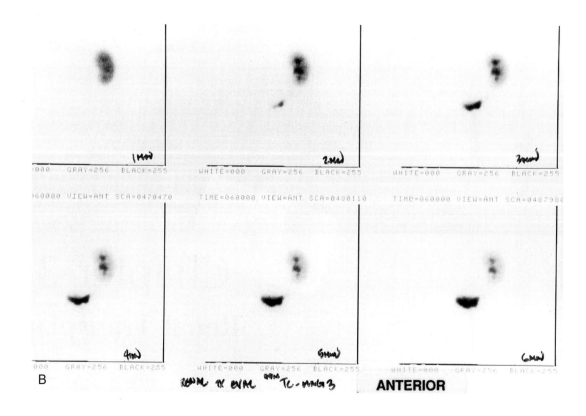

B   **ANTERIOR**

ACUTE REJECTION

FIGURE 38–2   A.

Initial Blood Flow Scan: There is slightly slow blood flow to
the transplant.

FIGURE 38–2   B.

Excretion Phase MAG₃ Scan: There is mildly reduced urinary
output (creatinine was 1.4 mg/dl).

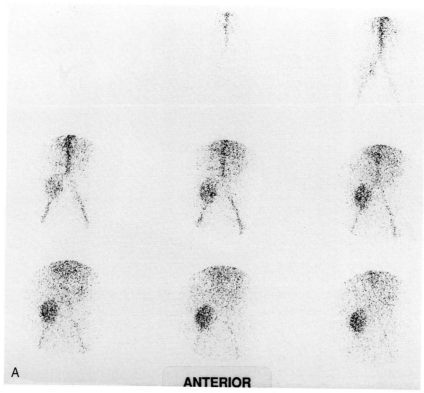

ANTERIOR

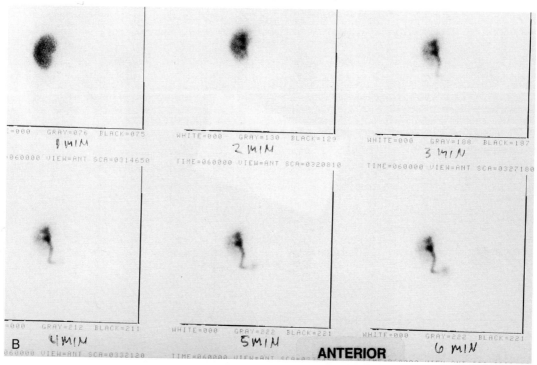

ANTERIOR

Illustration continued on following page

FIGURE 38–2   C.

Blood Flow Scan 5 Days Later: The blood flow is further diminished.

FIGURE 38–2   D.

Excretion Phase MAG_3 Scan: There is virtually no urinary output (creatinine = 1.5 mg/dl.) (Courtesy of Dr. Edward Hew, Honolulu, HI.)

NOTE. Hyperacute rejection occurs within minutes to hours after transplantation. Acute rejection may occur days to years after implantation. Acute rejection vasculitis usually develops within the first few months or when immunosuppression is stopped. Chronic rejection occurs after acute rejection is successfully treated.

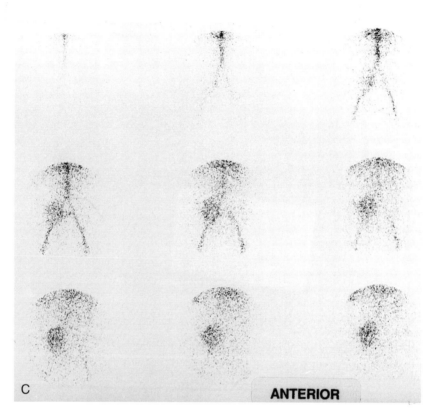

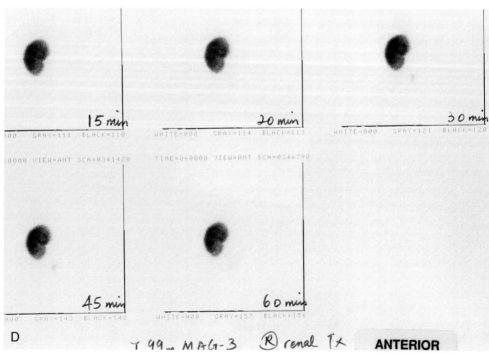

PROGRESSIVE ACUTE RENAL TRANSPLANT REJECTION

FIGURE 38–3   A.

Initial Blood Flow Scan: There are normal flow and perfusion to the transplant in the right pelvic fossa.

FIGURE 38–3   B.

One Hour MAG$_3$ Scan: The transplant retains the radiopharmaceutical, with no excretion into the bladder.

FIGURE 38–3   C.

Blood Flow Scan 4 Days Later: The blood flow has diminished significantly.

FIGURE 38–3   D.

MAG$_3$ Scan 4 Days Later: The transplant has less accumulation of the radiopharmaceutical and no excretion.

FIGURE 38–3   E.

Blood Flow Scan 17 Days After Initial Examination: There is further deterioration of the renal perfusion.

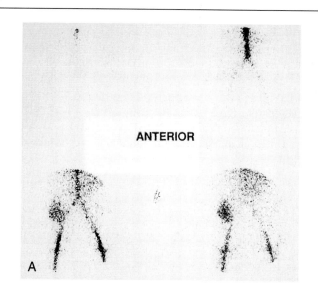

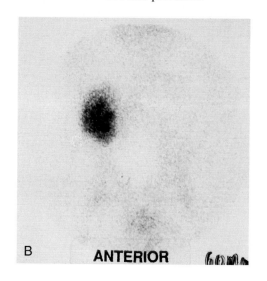

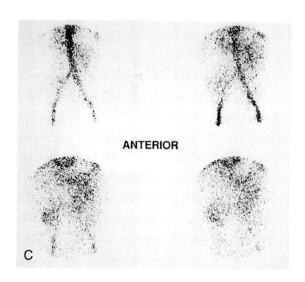

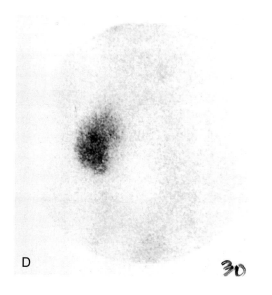

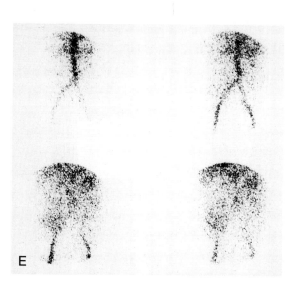

Illustration continued on following page

FIGURE 38–3 F.

MAG₃ Scan 17 Days After Initial Examination: With the film intensity turned up, the poorly functioning transplant can be seen as well as the gallbladder, common bile duct, and small bowel.

FIGURE 38–3 G.

Renal Ultrasound: The transplant kidney is swollen, with loss of the corticomedullary junction differentiation. (Courtesy of Dr. Edward Hew, Honolulu, HI.)

NOTE. With renal failure, biliary excretion of some waste products occurs.

Cross References

Chapter 36: Unilateral Abnormalities—Gallbladder Visualization Simulating Renal Obstruction

Chapter 37: Bilateral Abnormalities—Extrarenal Hepatic Excretion

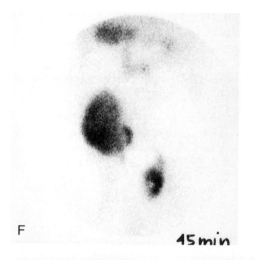

F   15 min

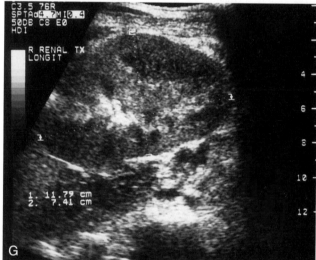

G

HYDRONEPHROTIC TRANSPLANT

Patient: Ureteric Kinking

FIGURE 38–4.

DTPA Scan: The transplant demonstrates a rim sign. The delayed DTPA and hippuran scans demonstrated no bladder activity. (Courtesy of Dr. Edward Hew, Honolulu, HI.)

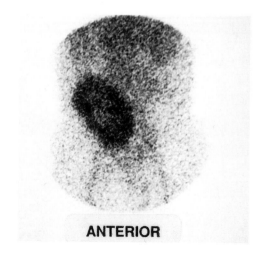

ANTERIOR

TRANSPLANT URINOMA SECONDARY TO NECROTIC URETER

FIGURE 38–5 A and B.

⁹⁹ᵐTc-DTPA Scan: There is extravasation of urine in the pelvis. The bladder is not seen.

FIGURE 38–5 C.

Postoperative Repair: The kidney retains normal function and excretes into the bladder. (Courtesy of Dr. Edward Hew, Honolulu, HI.)

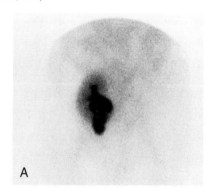

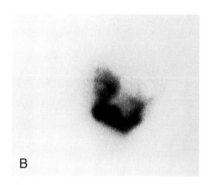

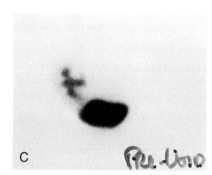

Chapter 39

Renal Defects

RENAL DEFECTS	
1. Simple cysts	7. Neoplasm, benign or malignant (primary or secondary)
2. Polycystic kidneys	
3. Abscesses	8. Foreign bodies
4. Infarcts	9. Staghorn calculus
5. Trauma	10. Vascular malformations
6. Pyelonephritic scars	

LUCENT RENAL PELVIS

FIGURE 39–1.

DTPA Scan: The renal pelvis does not appear to fill, although the kidney functions and the ureter displays peristaltic activity. The right kidney is nonfunctioning.

NOTE. The differential diagnosis of photopenic renal pelvis includes staghorn calculus, fibrolipomatosis (mostly seen in elderly patients), parapelvic cyst, and neoplasm.

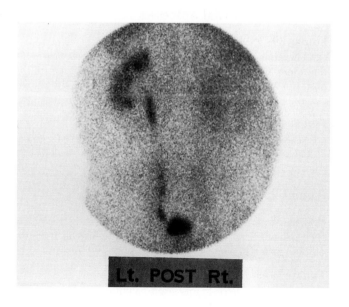

PYELONEPHRITIC SCARRING

FIGURE 39–2   A to C.
Renal Scan: The kidneys have irregular contours owing to focal scarring from recurrent infections.

NOTE 1. Pyelonephritis can cause focal scars, broad areas of cortical loss with calyceal dilatation, and overall loss of renal size and function.

NOTE 2. Small functioning kidneys are usually caused by chronic atrophic pyelonephritis.

Cross Reference

Chapter 36: Unilateral Abnormalities—Chronic Pyelonephritis

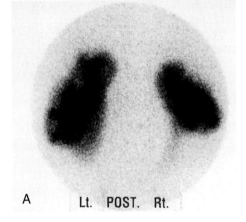

A   Lt. POST. Rt.

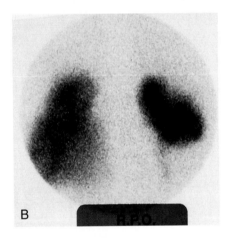

B   R.P.O.

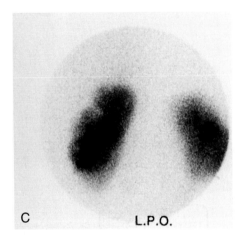

C   L.P.O.

RENAL ABSCESSES

Patient 1: Intrarenal Abscesses

FIGURE 39–3   A and B.
Glucoheptonate Renal Scan: There are focal defects *(arrows)* in the upper and lower poles of the left kidney, best seen on the posterior and LPO views. The renal parenchyma is inhomogeneous.

FIGURE 39–3   C.
CT Scan: A representative tomogram demonstrates one of several abscesses in the left kidney.

Patient 2: Pararenal Abscesses

FIGURE 39–3   D.
DTPA Renal Scan: The right renal contour has an irregular outline, with a greater defect in the upper pole *(arrow).*

FIGURE 39–3   E.
Gallium Scan: There is increased gallium accumulation surrounding the right kidney *(arrowheads),* with a more localized area in the upper pole *(arrow).*

NOTE 1. A pararenal abscess deforms the external contour of the kidney. The renal cortex may have diminished function.

NOTE 2. Intrarenal abscess—within the kidney parenchyma; pararenal abscess—within Gerota's fascia; perirenal abscess—outside Gerota's fascia.

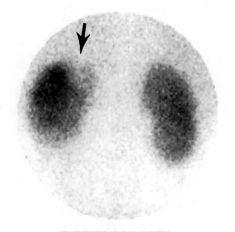

A   Lt. POST. Rt.

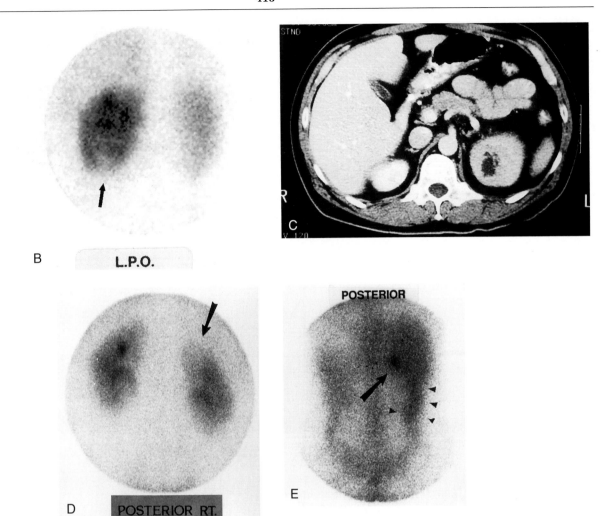

B L.P.O.

D POSTERIOR RT.

E POSTERIOR

FRACTURED KIDNEY

FIGURE 39–4   A.

DTPA Renal Scan: There is a peripheral photopenic defect *(arrow)*.

FIGURE 39–4   B.

Nephrogram Phase of Renal Arteriogram: The midpole of the kidney is less dense owing to the fracture and intrarenal hematoma. (The image is reversed to match the scan.)

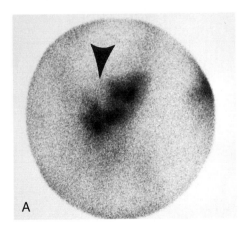

A

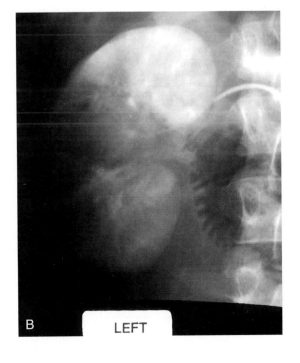

B LEFT

BULLET IN KIDNEY

FIGURE 39–5.
DTPA Renal Scan: There is a focal photon-deficient abnormality in the right kidney and loss of inferior pole parenchyma.

Cross Reference

Chapter 26: Bullet in Liver

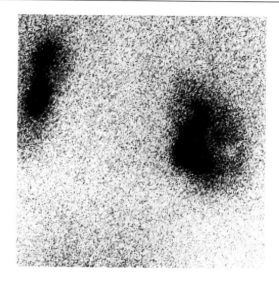

RENAL INFARCTS

FIGURE 39–6.
DTPA Renal Scan: There are large and small wedge defects *(arrowheads)* in this patient with atrial fibrillation.

NOTE. Sources of renal infarcts include thromboemboli from atrial fibrillation, intrarenal atherosclerosis, cholesterol emboli, periarteritis nodosa, and renal artery aneurysms.

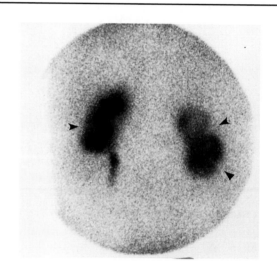

UNILATERAL SIMPLE CYSTS

Patient 1

FIGURE 39–7 A.
DTPA Renal Scan: In the early "nephrogram" phase, focal defects in the left kidney can be seen.

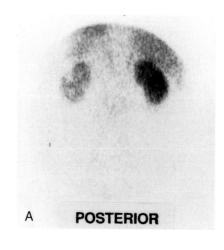

A   **POSTERIOR**

Patient 2

FIGURE 39–7 B.
DTPA Renal Scan: There are at least two round photon-deficient masses in the left kidney in a patient with renal failure.

NOTE 1. Only cysts larger than 1 to 1.5 cm will be detected with nuclear scanning, whereas ultrasound will detect smaller ones.

NOTE 2. Simple cysts may be single or multiple and generally have no clinical significance beyond recognition.

NOTE 3. Acquired cystic kidney disease is found in patients with chronic renal failure on long-term dialysis.

Cross Reference

Bone Chapter: Soft Tissue Abnormalities—Renal Cyst on Bone Scan

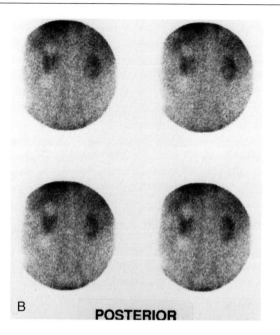

B

POSTERIOR

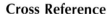

MULTIPLE ANGIOMYOLIPOMAS

FIGURE 39–8 A.
Blood Pool ⁹⁹ᵐTc-DTPA Scans: The left lower pole masses are hypervascular *(arrows)*.

FIGURE 39–8 B.
⁹⁹ᵐTc-Glucoheptonate Renal Scan: The kidneys each have several nonfunctioning masses, indistinguishable from cysts.

NOTE. Multiple angiomyolipomas are hamartomas, commonly, but not exclusively, found in patients with tuberous sclerosis.

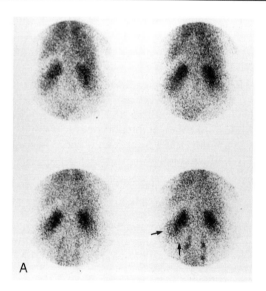

A

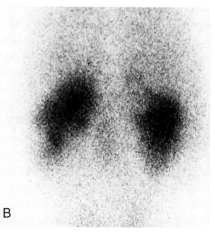

B

RENAL CELL CARCINOMA

Patient 1

FIGURE 39–9   A and B.

Glucoheptonate Renal Scans With and Without Computer Enhancement: There is a focal defect along the lateral margin of the right kidney *(arrow)*.

FIGURE 39–9   C.

Renal Ultrasound: There is a solid mass in the lateral right kidney.

FIGURE 39–9   D.

Contrast-Enhanced CT Scan: The mass *(arrow)* is solid and isodense with the kidney's parenchyma.

Patient 2: Hypervascular Tumor

FIGURE 39–9   E.

Renal Blood Flow: There is early blood flow to the left kidney *(arrows)*, which is markedly enlarged.

FIGURE 39–9   F.

Early DTPA Scan: The enlarged left kidney has an inhomogeneous nephrogram. Paravertebral venous collaterals *(arrowheads)* are evident owing to tumor invasion of the renal vein and inferior vena cava.

FIGURE 39–9   G.

Delayed DTPA Scan: The central portion of the left kidney is devoid of functioning renal tissue. Arrows show outline of kidney.

NOTE 1. A photon-deficient lesion on renal scan is nonspecific and requires CT or ultrasound to better define whether the defect is solid, cystic, scar, or other. If the photopenic lesion is hypervascular, it is a tumor, an abscess, or a vascular malformation.

NOTE 2. Changing display intensity can often make kidney defects more conspicuous.

NOTE 3. Renal cell carcinomas are usually hypervascular, often invading the renal vein and inferior vena cava, even growing into the right atrium.

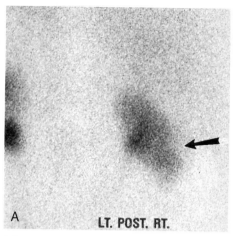

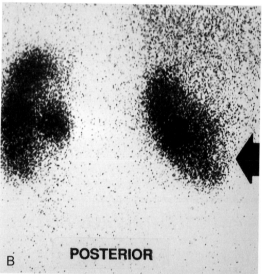

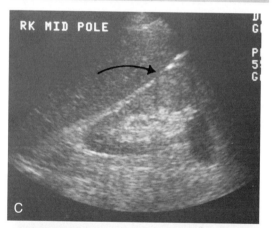

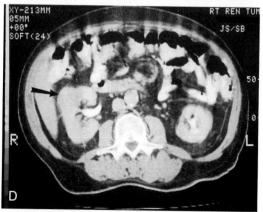

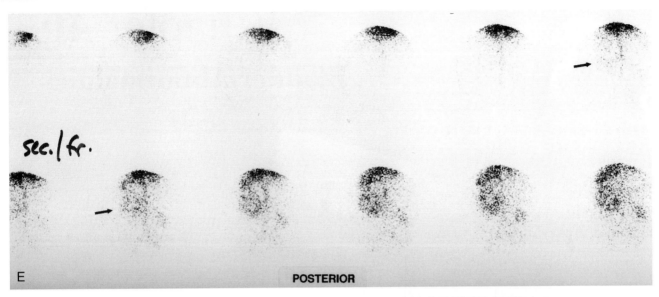

sec./fr.

E   **POSTERIOR**

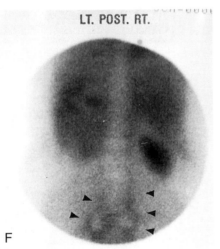

LT. POST. RT.

F

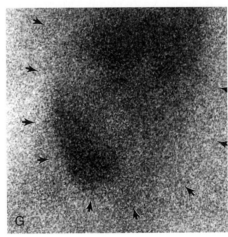

G

COLUMN OF BERTIN

Patient: Mass Found at Ultrasound

FIGURE 39–10   A.

Renal Ultrasound: There is a solid mass in the right kidney *(arrow)*.

FIGURE 39–10   B.

RPO ^{99m}Tc-DMSA Renal Scans: There is activity in the mass both early and late, indicating functioning renal tissue.

NOTE. A medullary mass on ultrasound or CT which functions on renal scan, can be left alone.

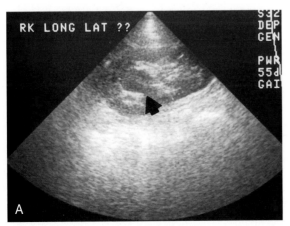

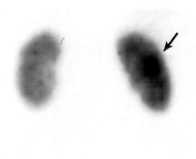

B   **POSTERIOR**

Chapter 40
Bladder Abnormalities

PASSIVE VESICOURETERAL REFLUX

FIGURE 40–1   A.

Radionuclide Cystogram: With the bladder filling, there is reflux up the right ureter.

FIGURE 40–1   B.

Static Radionuclide Cystogram Scan: The reflux fills the right renal pelvis.

NOTE 1. Active reflux occurs with voiding, whereas passive reflux will be seen as the bladder fills or is full.

NOTE 2. Sterile reflux may not cause renal parenchymal damage, whereas bacteriuria is associated with renal scarring.

NOTE 3. In general, one should have the patient upright on a bedpan with the back against the gamma camera during both the filling and the voiding phases of the cystogram.

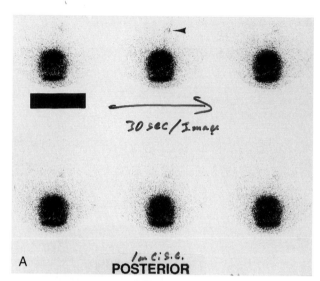

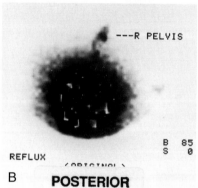

BLADDER DIVERTICULUM

FIGURE 40–2.

Anterior View of Bladder on DTPA Renal Scan: There is a diverticulum in the dome of the bladder.

NOTE. Bladder diverticula are associated with stasis, infection, stone formation, and ureteric obstruction and reflux (Hutch diverticulum).

Cross Reference

Chapter 11: Soft Tissue Abnormalities—Bladder Diverticulum on Bone Scan

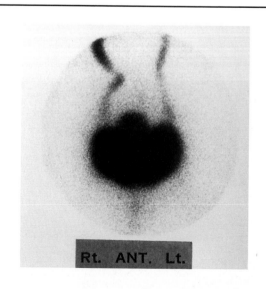

NEUROGENIC BLADDER WITH SECONDARY HYDRONEPHROSIS

FIGURE 40–3.
Bone Scan: There is a markedly enlarged urinary bladder and hydronephrosis.

NOTE. A neurogenic bladder can cause sufficient pressure on the pelvic and abdominal blood vessels that venous thrombosis, including IVC obstruction, can develop.

Cross References

Chapter 11: Soft Tissue Abnormalities on Bone Scan—Neurogenic Bladder.

Chapter 59: Pelvic Venous Thrombosis—Pelvic Venous Compression

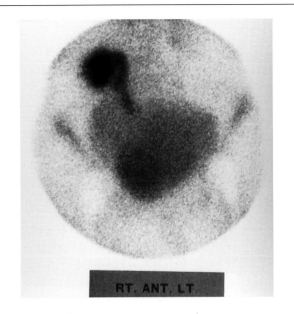

CYSTITIS

FIGURE 40–4   A and B.
Gallium Scan: Gallium can be seen in the urinary bladder. There was no renal accumulation (not shown), indicating that there is no pyelonephritis.

NOTE. The oblique view helps distinguish between rectal and bladder activity.

Cross References

Chapter 36: Unilateral Abnormalities—Acute Pyelonephritis

Chapter 37: Bilateral Abnormalities—Interstitial Pyelonephritis

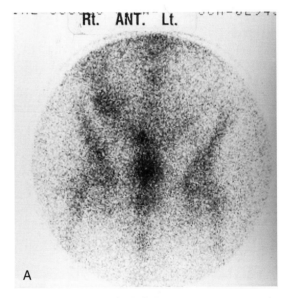

A

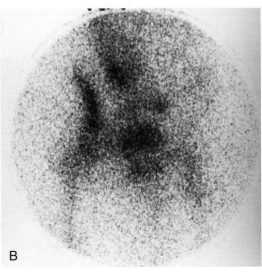

B

BLADDER HEMATOMA

FIGURE 40–5.

DTPA Renal Scan: The filling defect in the superior bladder was due to a large intramural hematoma.

FILLING DEFECTS IN THE BLADDER
1. Primary neoplasm
2. Blood clot
3. Foley catheter
4. Bladder stone
5. Ureterocele

See also Chapter 11: Soft Tissue Abnormalities— Impressions on the Bladder.

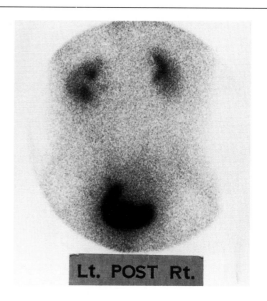

BLADDER PROLAPSE

FIGURE 40–6.

Posterior Pelvic and Lumbar Spine Bone Scan: The lower left figure demonstrates an hourglass-shaped bladder, extending down into the perineum. This, and not the degenerative disk disease, was thought to be the cause of the patient's incontinence.

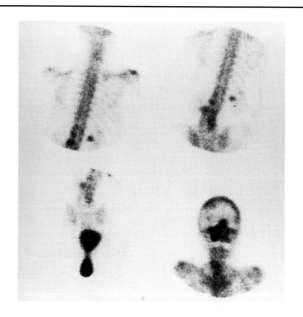

Chapter **41**

Disorders of the Testes

NORMAL TESTICULAR SCAN

FIGURE 41–1   A and B.

Composite of Blood Flow and Delayed Scans: The two sides of the scrotum have equal activity.

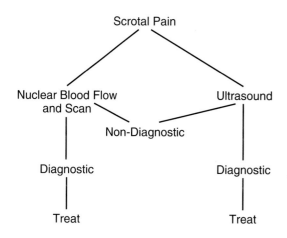

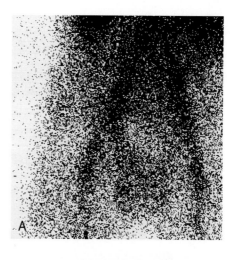

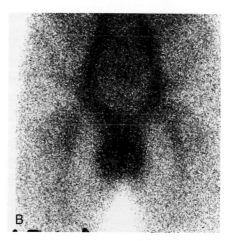

INCREASED SCROTAL BLOOD FLOW/POOL	
1. Epididymitis	4. Varicocele
2. Orchitis	5. Trauma
3. Missed testicular torsion	6. Tumor

EPIDIDYMO-ORCHITIS

Patient 1: Epididymo-orchitis

FIGURE 41–2   A.
Blood Flow Scan: The flow to the right scrotum is increased, especially to the right testis.

FIGURE 41–2   B.
Blood Pool Scan: The hyperemic right testis and epididymis are associated with a small reactive hydrocoele *(arrowhead)*.

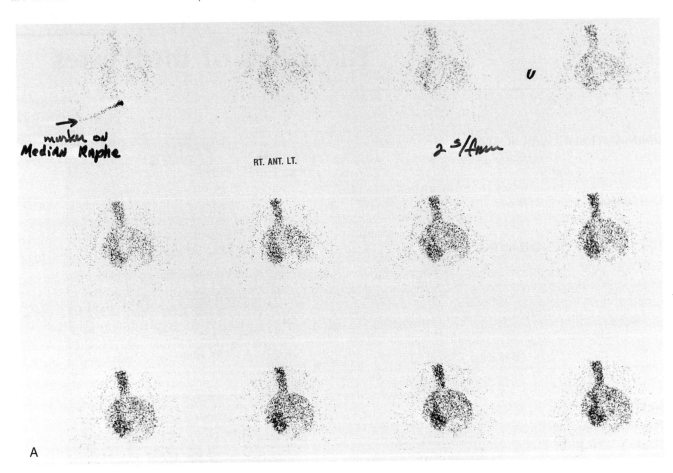

A

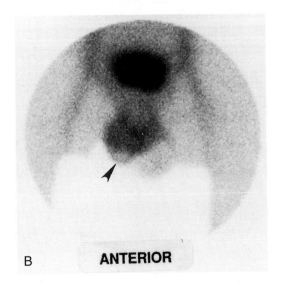

B   ANTERIOR

Patient 2: Epididymo-orchitis with Large Hydrocele

FIGURE 41–2   C.
Blood Flow Scan: Computer-generated images demonstrated increased flow to the left scrotum with a central photopenic area.

FIGURE 41–2   D.
Blood Pool Images: There is hyperemia above a round area of photopenia in the left scrotum.

NOTE. The differential diagnosis of a hyperemic testicular mass, with photopenic center (rim sign) includes epididymo-orchitis with hydrocele, testicular abscess, missed testicular torsion, epididymal cyst, hematoma, tumor, and hernia with intraperitoneal infection.

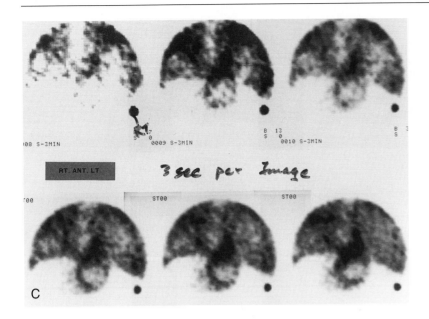

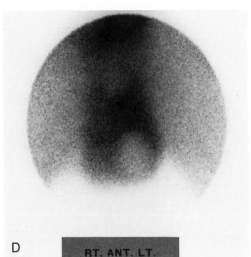

TESTICULAR ABSCESS WITH NECROSIS

FIGURE 41–3.

Blood Pool Scan: The enlarged right testis has a rim of hyperemia, although there is still some internal perfusion. After orchiectomy, the pathology demonstrated fibrosis, chronic inflammation, and necrosis.

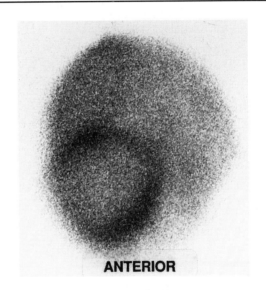

VARICOCELES

Patient 1: Varicocele

FIGURE 41–4 A and B.

Supine and Upright ^{99m}Tc-Labeled RBC Blood Pool Scan: There is a central area of blood pooling with a distended vein along the left side *(arrow)*.

Patient 2: Varicocele

FIGURE 41–4 C.

Blood Pool Scan: There is a dilated vein that does not end in a large venous plexus.

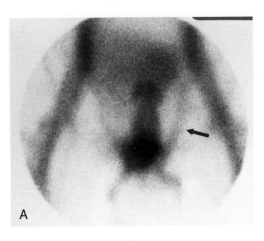

Illustration continued on following page

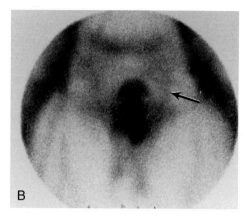

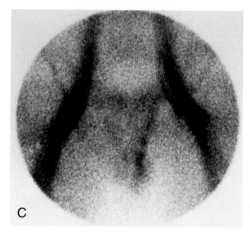

SCROTAL INFECTION

FIGURE 41–5.

WBC Scan: There is a scrotal infection associated with bilateral thigh and right abdominal wall cellulitis.

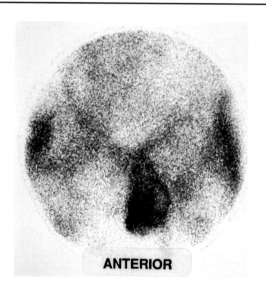

ANTERIOR

TESTICULAR TORSION

FIGURE 41–6.

Blood Pool Scan: There is decreased activity in the left scrotum *(arrow)*.

NOTE. The testicle may retract with torsion and should be looked for in a higher position than normal.

DECREASED SCROTAL BLOOD FLOW	
1. Acute torsion	5. Hernia
2. Hydrocele	6. Hematocele
3. Tumor	7. Spermatocele
4. Trauma	8. Testicular infarction

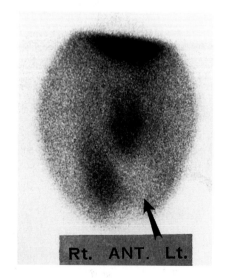

Rt. ANT. Lt.

HYDROCELE

FIGURE 41–7.

Blood Pool Scan: The right scrotum contains a photon-deficient ("cold") structure.

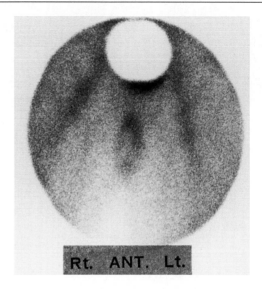

INTRASCROTAL HEMORRHAGE AND TESTICULAR INFARCTION

FIGURE 41–8.

Blood Pool Scan: The irregular photon-deficient area in the left scrotum is due to a post-traumatic hematoma. The testicle was infarcted.

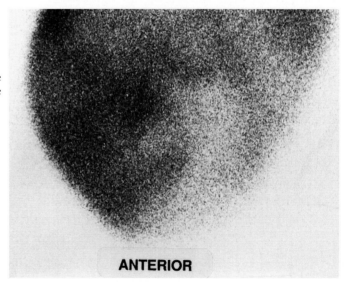

Chapter 42

Normal/Normal Variants

NORMAL LUNG SCAN

FIGURE 42–1   A to F.

Six View ^{99m}Tc-MAA Perfusion Lung Scans: The distribution of the radiopharmaceutical is homogeneous. The posterior aspects of the lungs have slightly greater activity owing to the supine position of the patient during injection.

NOTE. There is a gradient of activity depending on the position that the patient is in when injected. The distribution mirrors the blood flow changes owing to gravity. In the upright position the greatest activity is in the bases; the supine position has increased activity posteriorly.

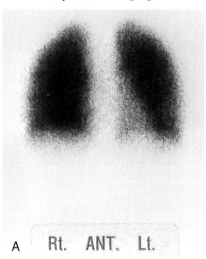

A   Rt. ANT. Lt.

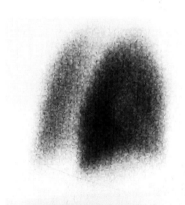

C   R.P.O.

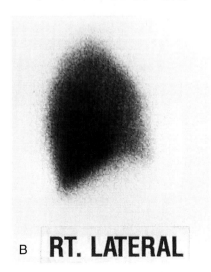

B   RT. LATERAL

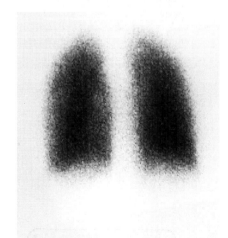

D   Lt. POST. Rt.

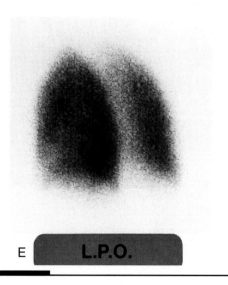

E **L.P.O.**

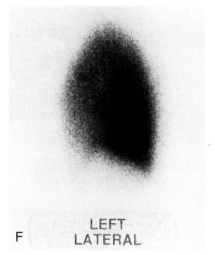

F LEFT LATERAL

NORMAL AEROSOL LUNG VENTILATION SCAN

Patient 1

FIGURE 42–2   A to F.

Six View Upright Aerosol Ventilation Scans: These views obtained before the perfusion lung scan demonstrate normal ventilation, with greater ventilation at the bases than at the apices.

Patient 2

FIGURE 42–2   G.

Anterior Aerosol Ventilation Scan: There is deposition of some of the Tc99m-DTPA along the tracheobronchial tree and the stomach in this patient with cardiomegaly.

NOTE 1. A xenon ventilation scan is best done in one position at a time. An aerosol ventilation scan can be done with multiple views.

NOTE 2. Tracheal and central bronchial deposition of the radioaerosol is common, as is stomach visualization from swallowed material.

NOTE 3. Intubated patients should be suctioned prior to administration of the aerosol to prevent "hot" spots from deposition on mucus.

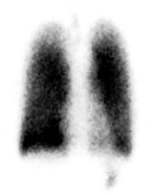

A **ANTERIOR**

B **RIGHT LATERAL**

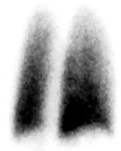

C **R.P.O.**

Illustration continued on following page

429

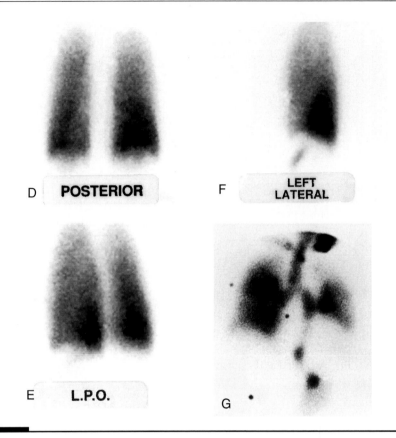

D **POSTERIOR**

F **LEFT LATERAL**

E **L.P.O.**

G

NORMAL RADIOXENON VENTILATION SCAN

FIGURE 42–3   A and B.

Posterior and RPO ¹³³Xe Ventilation Scans: There is homogeneous distribution of the radioxenon gas, with homogeneous washout throughout.

NOTE 1. Radioxenon ventilation scans can be performed after perfusion lung scans.

NOTE 2. Any position on the perfusion scan that demonstrates the defects best should be used with the ventilation scan.

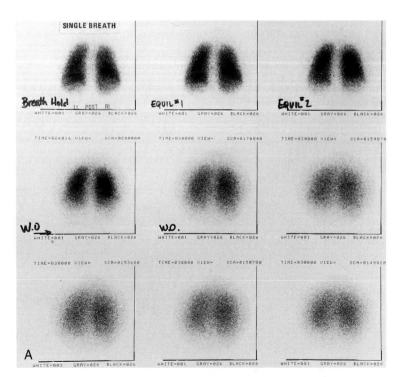

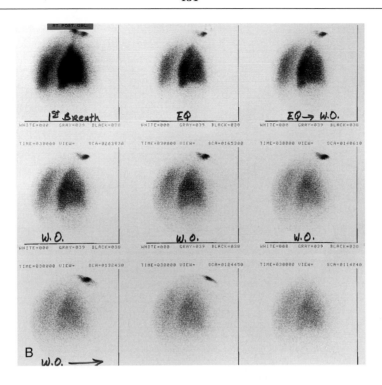

Chapter 43

Solitary Ventilation/Perfusion (V/Q) Mismatch

V/Q MISMATCHES

1. Pulmonary embolism, acute or chronic

2. Central bronchogenic carcinoma

3. Radiation therapy

4. Early pneumonia, especially tuberculosis

5. Emphysema

6. Bronchopleural fistula

7. Vasculitis, collagen vascular disease

8. Pulmonary artery compression or invasion by tumor (lymphoma, sarcoma)

9. Fibrotic sarcoid

10. Congenital pulmonary artery agenesis

11. Hilar adenopathy

12. Histoplasmosis, mediastinitis

PULMONARY EMBOLISM WITH SOLITARY V/Q MISMATCH

Patient 1: Solitary Segmental Abnormality

FIGURE 43–1 A to C.

Anterior, Posterior, and Right Posterior Oblique Perfusion Lung Scan: There is a solitary wedge abnormality in the superior segment of the right lower lobe, seen best on the RPO view.

FIGURE 43–1 D.

^{133}Xenon Ventilation Scan: There is normal ventilation in the region of the perfusion abnormality.

FIGURE 43–1 E.

Pulmonary Angiogram: Multiple filling defects and truncated pulmonary arteries indicate more diffuse emboli *(arrows)*.

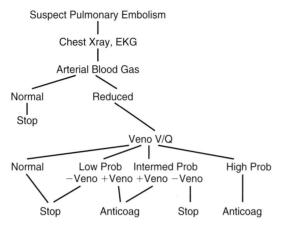

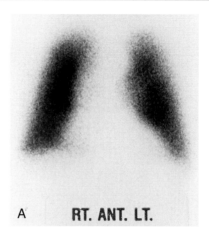

RT. ANT. LT.

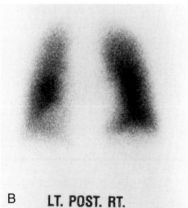

LT. POST. RT.

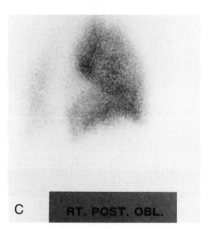

RT. POST. OBL.

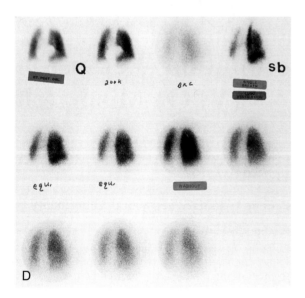

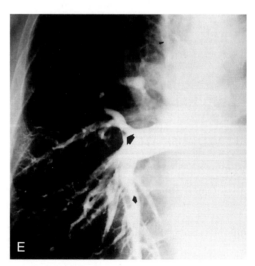

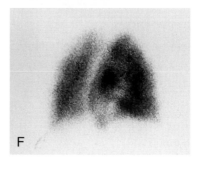

Patient 2

FIGURE 43–1 F.
RPO Perfusion Lung Scan: The segmental posterobasilar perfusion is reduced, along with several subsegmental defects.

FIGURE 43–1 G.
RPO ¹³³Xenon Ventilation Scan: The gas distribution is normal.

FIGURE 43–1 H.
Selective Right Lower Lobe Pulmonary Angiogram: Several thromboemboli are seen *(arrows)*.

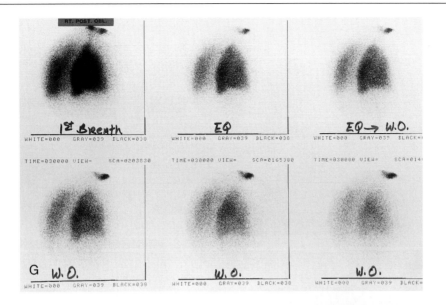

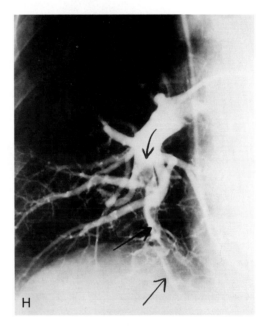

Patient 3

FIGURE 43–1   I to K.

Anterior, Posterior, and LPO Perfusion Scans: The solitary segmental perfusion deficit in the right lung is best seen on the LPO view *(arrow)*. The other abnormalities are subsegmental.

FIGURE 43–1   L.

LPO V/Q Scan: The right lower lobe superior segment *(arrow)* has normal ventilation.

FIGURE 43–1   M.

Right Pulmonary Artery Angiogram: Numerous large clots can be seen, and there is a paucity of blood vessels filling.

NOTE 1. These cases demonstrate the value of doing the perfusion scan first so that the optimal position for the ventilation scan can be chosen.

NOTE 2. There are many more emboli seen at pulmonary angiography than would be suspected by the number or size of lung perfusion abnormalities.

NOTE 3. Solitary segmental V/Q mismatches have a higher incidence of pulmonary embolism than one usually assigns to the intermediate probability category. These should be treated with anticoagulation.

NOTE 4. If the clinical suspicion is high or a pulmonary angiogram is not easily obtainable, the patient may be anticoagulated. An improved repeat perfusion scan in 1 week indicates that the solitary V/Q mismatch represents pulmonary embolism.

NOTE 5. Despite the low energy of radioxenon, an "opposite oblique" can be used to evaluate a segmental perfusion abnormality, i.e., an LPO position for a posterior right lung abnormality.

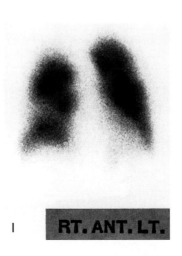

Illustration continued on following page

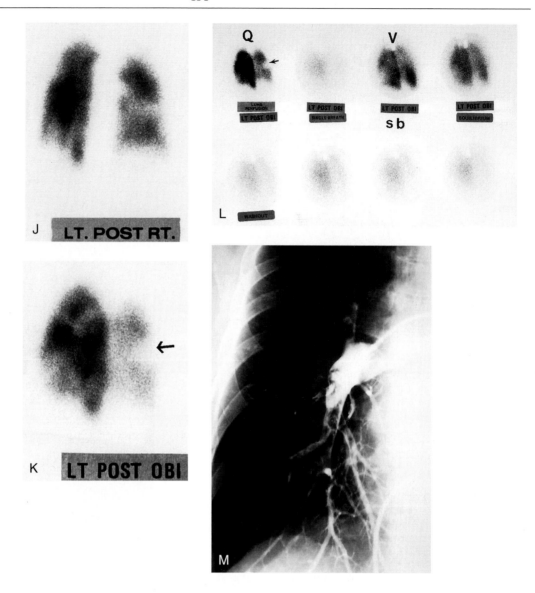

CHRONIC V/Q MISMATCH

FIGURE 43–2   A and B.

RPO V/Q Scan: The middle lobe has mismatched ventilation and perfusion (the right lower lobe is also abnormal).

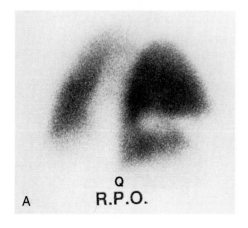

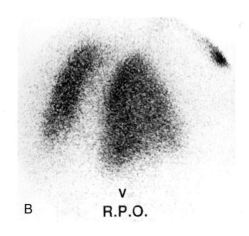

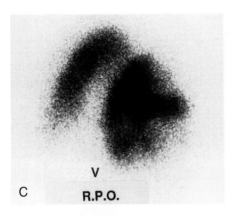

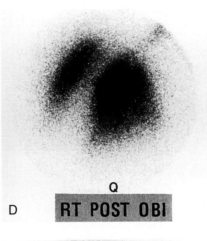

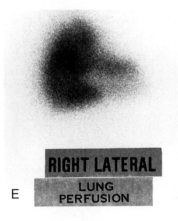

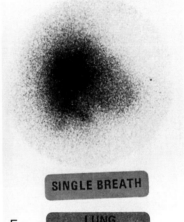

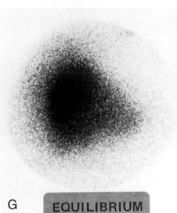

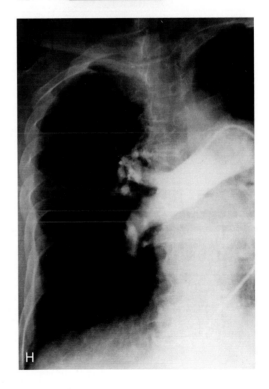

FIGURE 43–2   C and D.

RPO V/Q Scan 5 Years Later: The middle lobe has a persistent mismatch.

FIGURE 43–2   E to G.

6 Years Since Initial Scan, Right Lateral V/Q Scan: The first breath is abnormal in the middle lobe but normalizes on the equilibrium scan. Washout was normal.

FIGURE 43–2   H.

Pulmonary Arteriogram: The right interlobar pulmonary artery is occluded.

NOTE 1. Permanent occlusion of a pulmonary arterial segment usually causes a persistent V/Q mismatch or, occasionally, a single-breath abnormality.

NOTE 2. The lung usually remains viable owing to bronchial artery perfusion.

INACCURACY OF ROUTINE POSTERIOR VENTILATION SCANS

FIGURE 43–3 A and B.
Posterior Radioxenon Ventilation Scan: The equilibrium view has early washout in the left costophrenic angle.

FIGURE 43–3 C.
Posterior Perfusion Lung Scan: There is a matched perfusion abnormality in the left lower lobe.

FIGURE 43–3 D and E.
RPO V/Q Lung Scan: There is normal ventilation and multiple mismatched perfusion abnormalities in the middle lobe and right lower lobe.

NOTE. The radioxenon ventilation scan should be done with the patient in the position that best demonstrates the perfusion abnormalities.

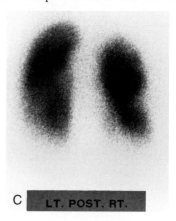

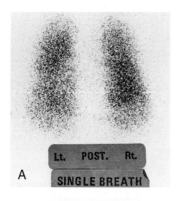

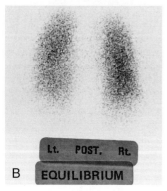

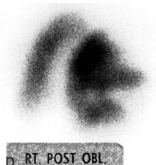

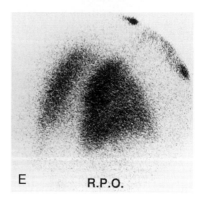

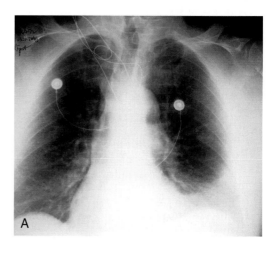

PLEURAL EFFUSION MASKING PULMONARY EMBOLISM

FIGURE 43–4 A.
Chest X-ray: There is increased density in the left lower lobe with a meniscus, indicating a pleural effusion.

FIGURE 43–4 B.
Posterior Perfusion Lung Scan: The lateral basal segment has decreased perfusion extending toward the midline.

FIGURE 43–4 C.
Single-Breath Portion of Ventilation Scan: There is a matched deficit in the lateral basal segment but a mismatch medially, raising the probability of pulmonary emboli. A pulmonary angiogram confirmed the presence of pulmonary embolism.

Cross Reference

Chapter 45: Solitary Matched Defects—Pulmonary Infarct and Pleural Effusion

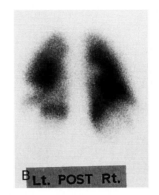

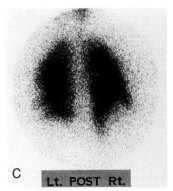

BRONCHOPLEURAL FISTULA

Patient 1

FIGURE 43–5 A.
Anterior Perfusion Lung Scan: There is no perfusion in the lateral right costophrenic angle *(arrow)*.

FIGURE 43–5 B.
Aerosol Ventilation Scan: The right costophrenic angle has accumulation of the radioaerosol *(arrow)*.

FIGURE 43–5 C.
Chest X-ray: The right lung *(arrowheads)* has pulled away from the right costophrenic angle.

Patient 2: Spontaneous Pneumothorax

FIGURE 43–5 D.
Anterior Aerosol and Perfusion Lung Scan: There is radioactivity in the right chest tube.

NOTE 1. Any pneumothorax that has a large enough leak can cause a V/Q mismatch, especially if the patient is on a ventilator.

NOTE 2. A radioxenon scan would demonstate delayed wash-in and delayed washout in the pneumothorax.

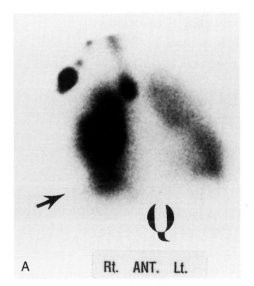

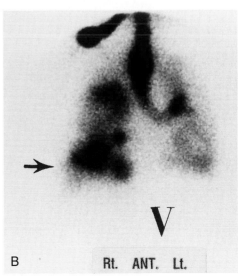

Illustration continued on following page

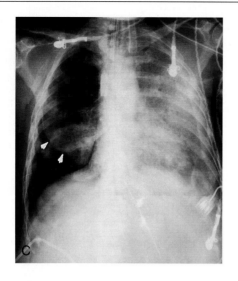

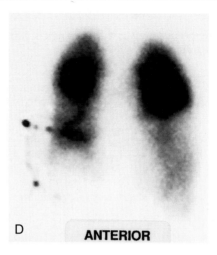

D **ANTERIOR**

FALSE POSITIVE V/Q SCAN

Patient: Fibrosing Mediastinitis

FIGURE 43–6   A.

Perfusion Lung Scan: The right lower and middle lobes have large perfusion deficits.

FIGURE 43–6   B.

Single-Breath and Equilibrium Xenon Ventilation Scans: The right lower lobe has good ventilation. There was no early or delayed washout. (Courtesy of Dr. Arnold Jacobson, Seattle, WA.)

NOTE. The pulmonary vasculature is more easily compressed than the cartilaginous bronchi.

Cross Reference

Chapter 45: Solitary Matched Abnormalities—Tumor on V/Q Scan

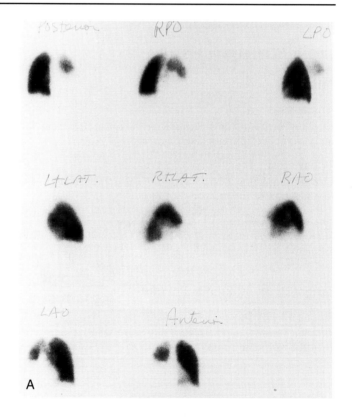

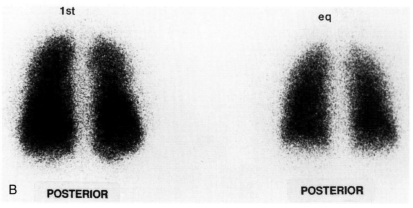

1st   eq

B **POSTERIOR**   **POSTERIOR**

PULMONARY EMBOLI LINES

FIGURE 44–1   A to F.
Perfusion Lung Scan: There are numerous linear and wedge defects.

FIGURE 44–1   G.
V/Q Scan: The ventilation scan is normal, although there is more rapid washout in the areas of severe perfusion deficiency (Q = perfusion; sb = single breath; eq = equilibrium; wo = washout).

NOTE. There are frequently linear nonsegmental perfusion abnormalities with pulmonary emboli.

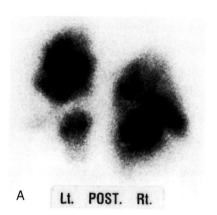

A   Lt. POST. Rt.

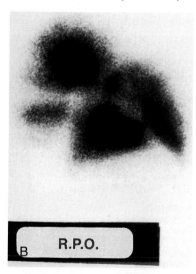

B   R.P.O.

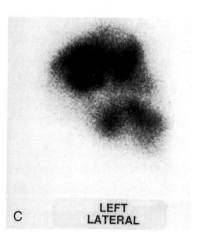

C   LEFT LATERAL

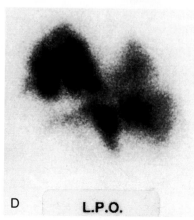

D   L.P.O.

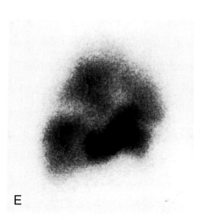

E

Illustration continued on following page

439

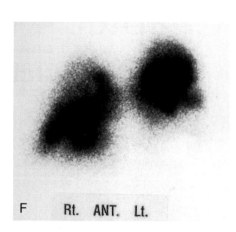

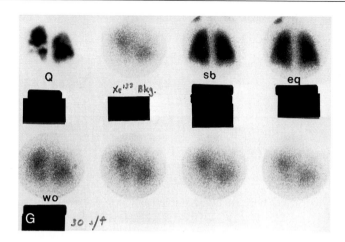

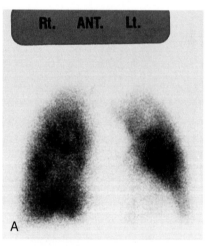

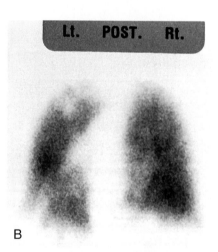

VALUE OF OBLIQUE VIEWS ON
V/Q SCANNING

FIGURE 44–2   A to D.
Perfusion Lung Scan: The best demonstration of the perfusion
abnormalities is on the LPO projection.

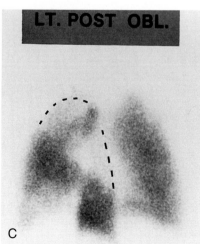

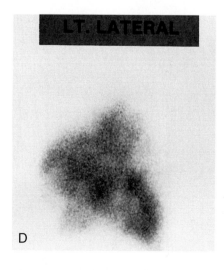

FIGURE 44–2 E.
LPO V/Q Scan: There is normal ventilation in areas of perfusion abnormality.

NOTE 1. A perfusion lung scan should have at least six views: anterior, posterior, both laterals, and both 45 degree posterior obliques.

NOTE 2. A radioxenon gas ventilation scan can be done *after* a ^{99m}technetium-macroaggregated albumin perfusion scan.

NOTE 3. The ventilation scan should be done in the projection that best demonstrates the abnormalities on the perfusion lung scan.

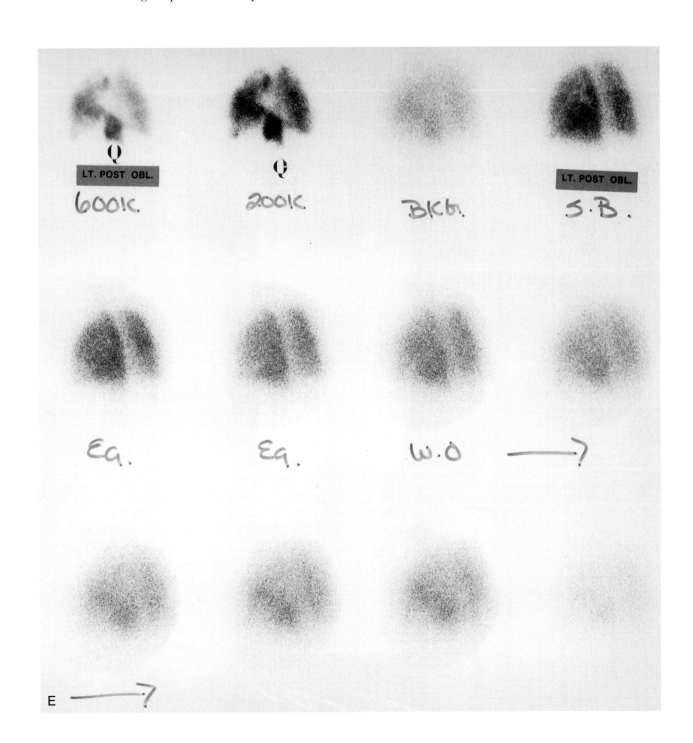

STREPTOKINASE FOR PULMONARY EMBOLISM

FIGURE 44–3   A and B.
Pre-Streptokinase Perfusion Lung Scan: There are multiple perfusion abnormalities.

FIGURE 44–3   C and D.
Post-Streptokinase Perfusion Lung Scan 1 Week Later: There is now normal perfusion throughout.

NOTE. Although streptokinase, urokinase, or thrombolytic agents can lyse thromboemboli, re-embolization may occur, probably more often than with anticoagulant therapy.

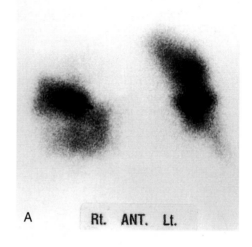

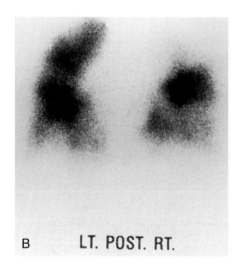

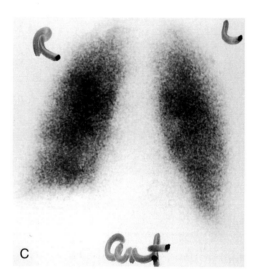

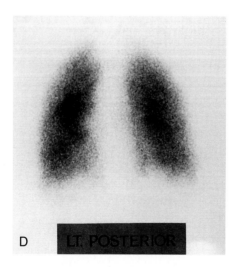

"CIGAR SIGN" IN PATIENT WITH PRE- AND POSTPULMONARY EMBOLECTOMY LUNG SCANS

FIGURE 44–4 A.
Chest X-ray: There is enlargement of the right pulmonary artery with a blunt end inferiorly *(arrow)*, the "cigar sign."

FIGURE 44–4 B and C.
Posterior V/Q Scan: There is normal ventilation as compared with the severely compromised right lung and left lower lobe perfusion.

FIGURE 44–4 D and E.
Pre– and Post–Right Lung Embolectomy Anterior Perfusion Lung Scans: There is improved perfusion to the right lung.

NOTE. The cigar sign is not common, but, when seen, it is fairly specific for pulmonary emboli.

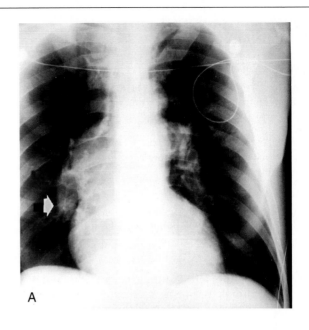

A

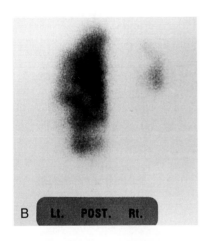

B Lt. POST. Rt.

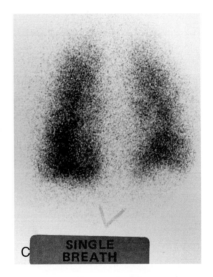

C SINGLE BREATH

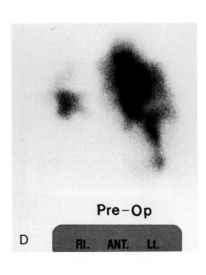

Pre-Op

D Rt. ANT. Lt.

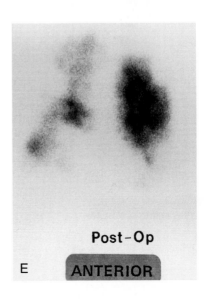

Post-Op

E ANTERIOR

RIGHT-TO-LEFT SHUNT WITH PULMONARY EMBOLISM

FIGURE 44–5   A.

Posterior V/Q Scan: Diffusely diminished right lung perfusion suggests central or saddle pulmonary emboli. The left lower lobe is also abnormal.

FIGURE 44–5   B.

Pelvic Nuclear Venogram: There is left iliofemoral thrombosis with multiple collateral veins.

FIGURE 44–5   C and D.

Scans of Brain and Kidneys: There is abnormal accumulation of the macroaggregated albumin particles in these organs.

NOTE 1. Right-to-left shunting occurs with pulmonary emboli owing to increased right heart pressures and opening of the foramen ovale.

NOTE 2. Less than 10 percent of injected MAA is normally found outside the lungs.

NOTE 3. This study demonstrates how paradoxical emboli may occur.

Cross Reference

Chapter 56: Miscellaneous—Right-to-Left Shunts

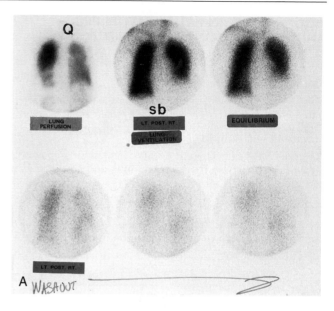

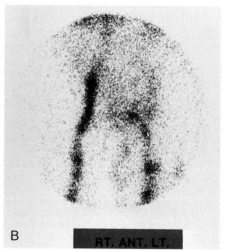

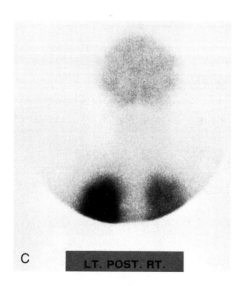

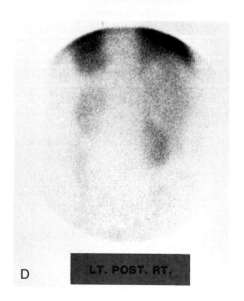

Chapter 45

Solitary Matched Defects

PULMONARY INFARCT AND PLEURAL EFFUSION

FIGURE 45–1   A.
Chest X-ray: There is a large left pleural effusion.

FIGURE 45–1   B and C.
Posterior V/Q Scan: There is a matched abnormality in the left base.

FIGURE 45–1   D.
Pulmonary Angiogram: A clot-filled lower lobe artery *(arrowheads)* is present. The pleural effusion compresses the lung, causing slow blood flow in shortened, irregular pulmonary arteries.

NOTE 1. Pulmonary infarcts are matched on V/Q scanning owing to parenchymal hemorrhage, edema, pleural effusion, and bronchospasm. The alveoli either are filled with fluid or are compressed.

NOTE 2. It can be difficult to diagnose pulmonary emboli in patients with pleural effusions without pulmonary angiograms, unless there are V/Q mismatches elsewhere.

NOTE 3. Less than 10 percent of pulmonary emboli result in infarction.

NOTE 4. The perfusion defect remains permanent in about 85 percent of pulmonary infarcts, albeit smaller.

Cross Reference

Chapter 43: Solitary V/Q Mismatches—Pleural Effusion Masking Pulmonary Embolism

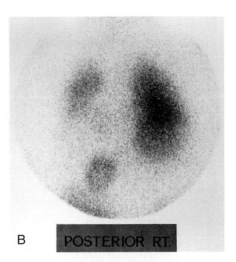

B   POSTERIOR RT.

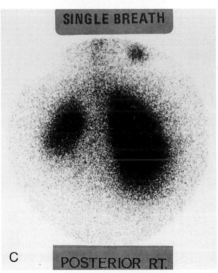

SINGLE BREATH

C   POSTERIOR RT.

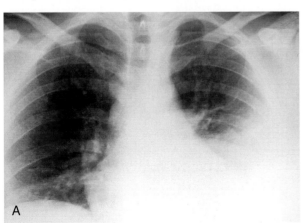

A

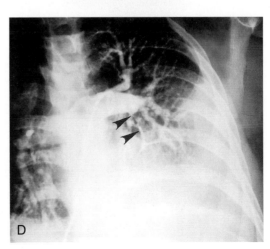

D

PLEURAL EFFUSIONS

Patient 1

FIGURE 45–2 A and B.
Left Lateral V/Q Scan: There is a matched V/Q abnormality coinciding with fluid in the major fissure.

Patient 2

FIGURE 45–2 C to E.
Anterior and Lateral Upright and Supine Liver/Lung Scans: In the upright position, the pleural effusion layers out between the lung and the diaphragm. In the spine position, the fluid is posterior.

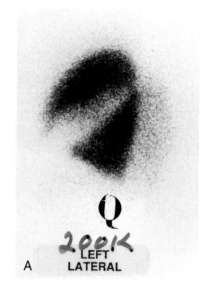

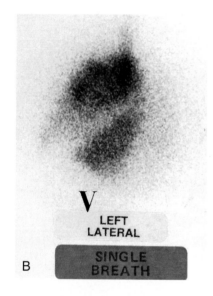

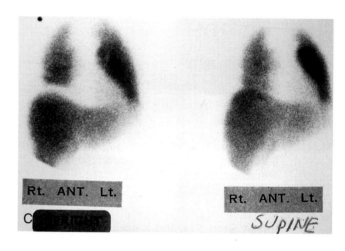

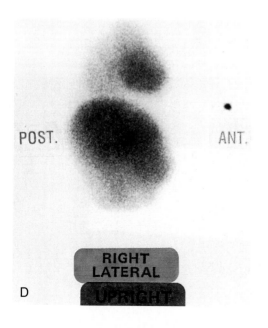

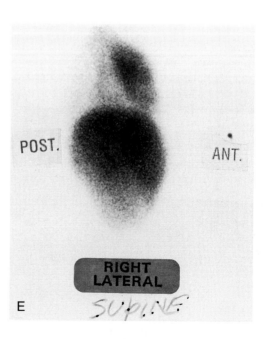

BULLOUS CYST

Patient 1: Active Tuberculosis

FIGURE 45–3   A and B.

Perfusion Lung Scan: There is virtually no perfusion in the left lung.

FIGURE 45–3   C.

Chest X-ray: There is a huge fluid-filled cyst occupying the left thorax, shifting the mediastinum to the right.

NOTE 1. Blebs and bullae characteristically have late wash-in and late washout.

NOTE 2. Bullae and blebs, which are air-filled, do not communicate with the bronchial tree. Rather, they get air via small pores in their walls connected to nearby alveoli.

NOTE 3. Blebs are peripheral; bullae are more central. Blebs are 1 to 2 cm in diameter; bullae are larger.

NOTE 4. Blebs may be congenital, whereas bullae are due to COPD and trauma, i.e., decompression disease. Pneumatocoeles are post-traumatic or postinflammatory.

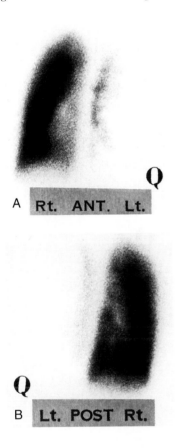

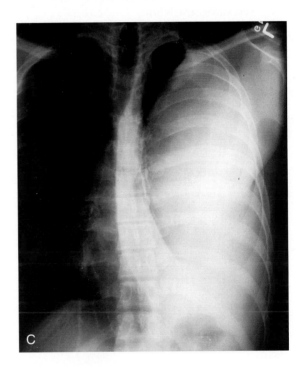

ATELECTASIS

FIGURE 45–4.

V/Q Scan: Both perfusion and ventilation are abnormal in the right lower and middle lobes (matched defects).

NOTE 1. In atelectasis, the airways are closed, but the chest x-ray may remain normal.

NOTE 2. Atelectasis may be due to retained secretions, pleural effusions, or loss of expiratory reserve volume. It is very common in the postoperative period and with ventilator patients.

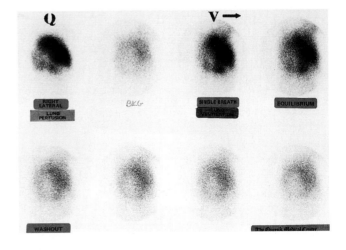

MUCUS PLUG

FIGURE 45–5   A to C.

Anterior and Posterior Perfusion and Posterior Aerosol Ventilation Scans: There is neither ventilation nor perfusion to the left lung.

FIGURE 45–5   D to F.

After Suctioning, and Reinjection, Anterior and Posterior Perfusion and Left Posterior Oblique Ventilation Scans: The perfusion and ventilation improved, although the huge heart still caused a considerable defect.

NOTE 1. The matched defect with mucus plugging is due to local hypoxia and local pulmonary arterial vasoconstriction.

NOTE 2. The mucus plug can be coughed up, causing a immediate return to normal perfusion.

Cross Reference

Chapter 47: Reverse V/Q Mismatch—Reverse Mismatch With Mucus Plug

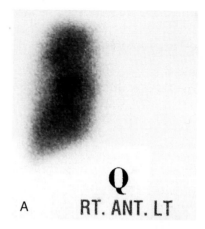

A   Q   RT. ANT. LT

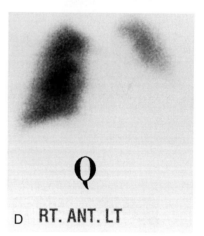

B Lt.   Q   POST.   Rt.

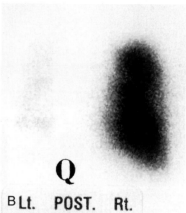

D   Q   RT. ANT. LT

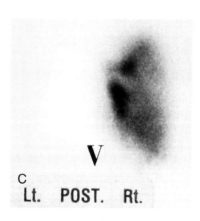

C   V   Lt. POST. Rt.

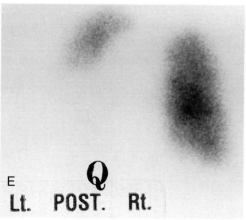

E   Q   Lt. POST. Rt.

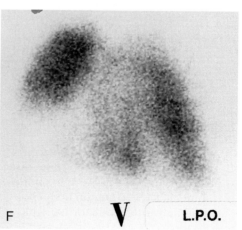

F   V   L.P.O.

TUMOR ON V/Q SCAN

Patient 1: Bronchogenic Carcinoma

FIGURE 45–6   A and B.

Right Posterior Oblique V/Q Scan: There are matching abnormalities in the middle lobe and the right lower lobe (Courtesy of Dr. Michael Kipper, Vista, CA.)

Patient 2: Mediastinal Leiomyosarcoma

FIGURE 45–6   C and D.

Posterior V/Q Scan: The entire left lung is devoid of ventilation and perfusion as the result of invasion of the left mainstem bronchus and pulmonary artery (Courtesy of Dr. Michael Kipper, Vista, CA.)

NOTE 1. Tumors replace, or fill, and compress normal alveoli, causing a reduction in pulmonary arterial perfusion and ventilation. This causes V/Q matched defects.

NOTE 2. Tumors of the hilum, particularly bronchogenic carcinoma, may decrease perfusion *without* invading or compressing the pulmonary artery. This can cause a false positive V/Q scan.

NOTE 3. Lymphomas and sarcomas can invade the mediastinal structures. All tumors can compress pulmonary vasculature and airways.

Cross Reference

Chapter 43: Solitary V/Q Mismatch—False Positive V/Q

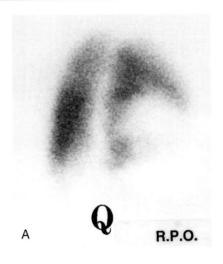

A   **Q**   R.P.O.

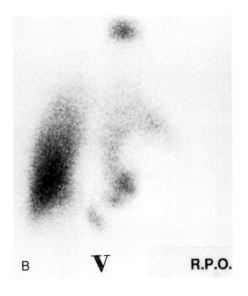

B   **V**   R.P.O.

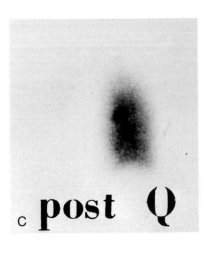

C **post Q**

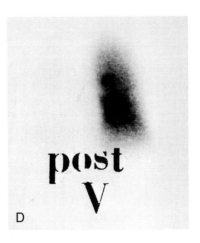

D **post V**

SCOLIOSIS AND AIR TRAPPING

Patient: 17 Year Old Female

FIGURE 45–7.

Posterior Radioxenon Ventilation Scan: There is slow washout of gas in the right lower lobe *(arrow)*.

NOTE. Scoliosis and pectus excavatum can be associated with lower lobe air trapping.

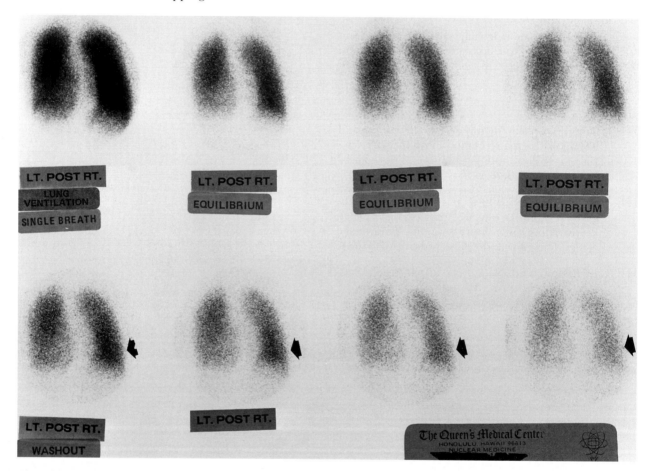

CONGESTIVE HEART FAILURE ON LUNG SCANNING

FIGURE 45–8 A to F.

Perfusion Lung Scan: There is diminished perfusion in the posterior lung fields, without pulmonary segmental distribution.

NOTE. With the patient injected supine, the redistribution of blood flow seen with congestive heart failure leaves a paucity of flow posteriorly. If the patient were injected upright, the bases would be hypoperfused.

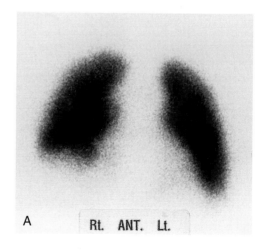

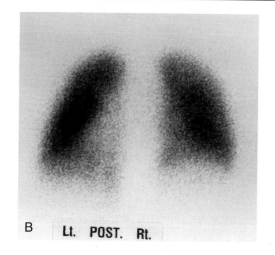

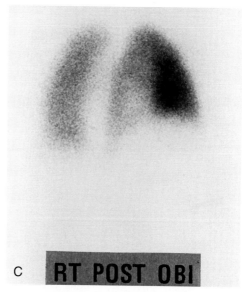

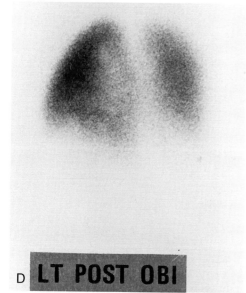

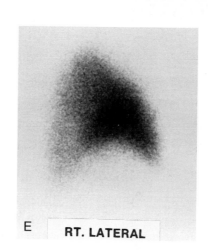

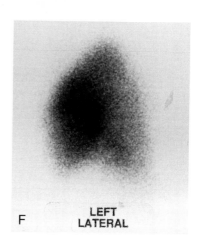

Chapter 46

Multiple Matched Defects

PULMONARY EMBOLISM (PE)
WITH BRONCHOSPASM

Patient 1: Unexplained Shortness of Breath

FIGURE 46–1   A.

LPO V/Q Scan: There are matching segmental defects in virtually all lung fields in this patient with high clinical suspicion for PE.

FIGURE 46–1   B and C.

Anterior and LPO Perfusion Scans: There are multiple perfusion abnormalities in both lungs.

FIGURE 46–1   D and E.

Anterior and LPO Perfusion Scans 8 Days Later: After anticoagulant therapy only, there is considerable improvement.

See illustration on following page

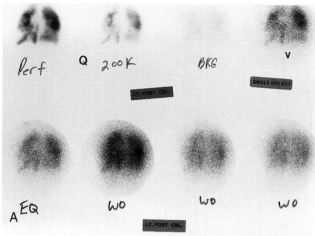

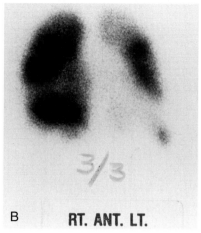

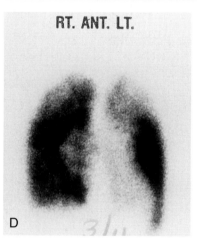

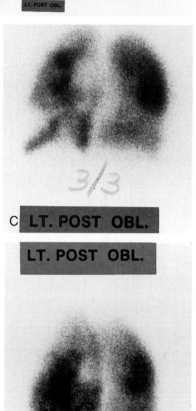

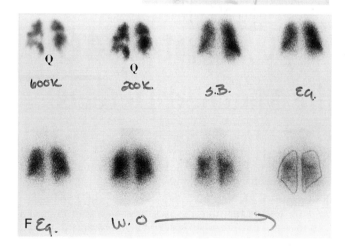

Patient 2

FIGURE 46–1 F.

V/Q Scan: The perfusion (Q) defects are matched by late wash-out on ventilation scanning. There is normal wash-in (single-breath equilibrium).

NOTE 1. Bronchospasm can be manifest as delayed wash-in and/or delayed washout.

NOTE 2. Pulmonary emboli can induce bronchospasm, presumably by release of a bronchoactive substance activated by ischemia.

NOTE 3. Bronchospasm occurring with acute PE usually lasts less than 24 hours.

NOTE 4. Pulmonary emboli with bronchospasm should be suspected in patients with multiple matching defects when there is no history of chronic lung disease.

NOTE 5. Pulmonary emboli should be considered, despite matching V/Q defects, when the perfusion scan demonstrates multiple wedgelike and linear perfusion abnormalities.

BRONCHIECTASIS IN A 5 YEAR OLD

FIGURE 46–2   A to D.
Perfusion Lung Scan: There is no perfusion to the apex and lower lung fields on the right.

FIGURE 46–2   E to H.
Aerosol Lung Scan: The only portion of the right lung that is ventilated is the anterior segment of the right upper lobe. The bronh4i here are markedly dilated *(arrows)*.

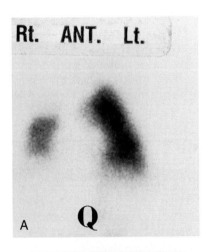

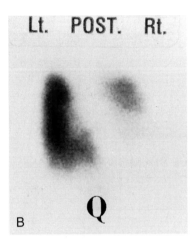

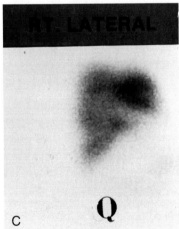

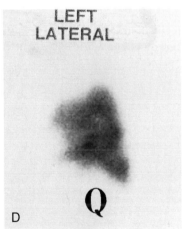

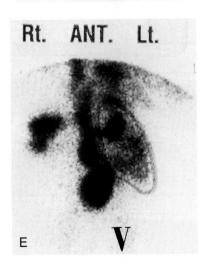

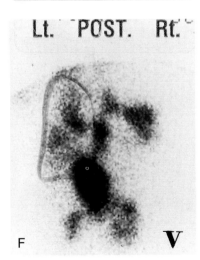

Illustration continued on following page

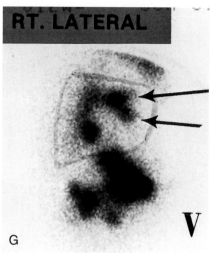

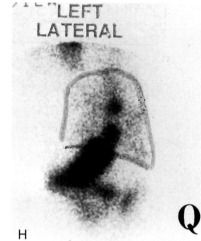

RESTRICTIVE PULMONARY DISEASE

Patient 1

FIGURE 46–3   A.

Posterior V/Q Scan: There is diminished apical perfusion with good early ventilation but early apical washout.

FIGURE 46–3   B.

Pulmonary Angiogram: The upper lobe vascularity is stretched and bowed.

NOTE. Restrictive pulmonary disease, or stiff lungs, has early wash-in and early washout because the bronchial connections are still intact.

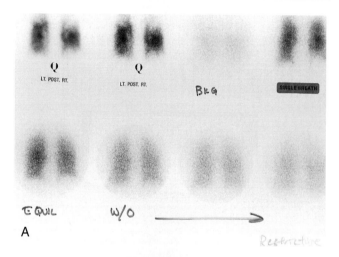

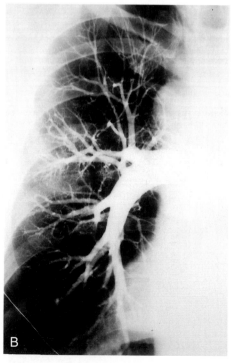

APICAL EMPHYSEMA

Patient 1

FIGURE 46–4   A.

Posterior Perfusion Lung Scan: There is markedly diminished perfusion to the right upper lobe as well as reduced perfusion to the left upper lobe.

FIGURE 46–4   B.

Posterior First-Breath Xenon Ventilation Scan: Neither upper lobe ventilates early.

FIGURE 46–4   C and D.

Posterior Equilibrium and Washout Ventilation Scans: The upper lobes have delayed ventilation.

Patient 2

FIGURE 46–4   E.

Posterior V/Q Scan: There is apical hypoperfusion that has delayed ventilatory wash-in. Washout of the right apex is delayed *(arrows)*. The left apex has diminished ventilation overall.

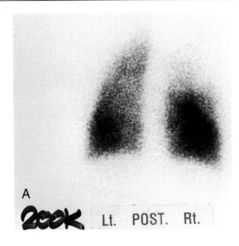

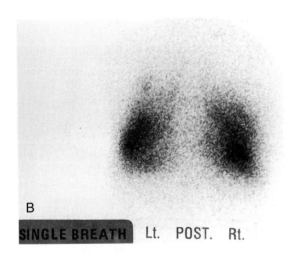

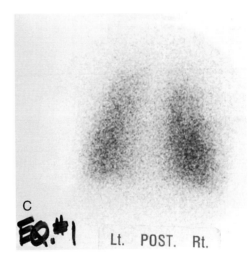

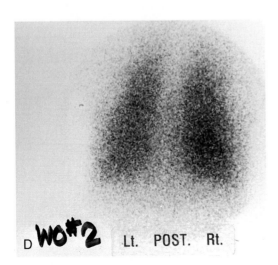

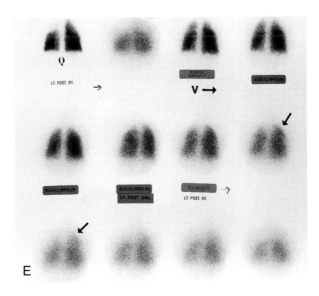

Illustration continued on following page

FIGURE 46–4 F.

Pulmonary Angiogram: The left lung vasculature is compressed from the bullae of the upper lobe.

NOTE. Emphysema, with blebs and bullae, classically has delayed ventilatory wash-in and washout.

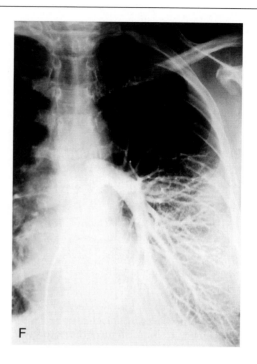

DIFFUSE EMPHYSEMA (COPD)

FIGURE 46–5 A to C.

Posterior, RPO, and LPO Perfusion Lung Scans: There are various-sized perfusion abnormalities in both lungs. There is a defect from an enlarged right pulmonary artery *(arrow)*.

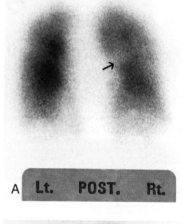

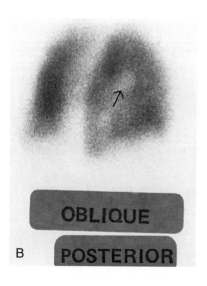

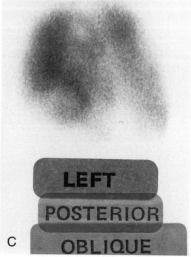

Illustration continued on following page

FIGURE 46–5   D to F.

RPO Ventilation Scan: There is delayed wash-in and washout in the area of the perfusion abnormalities, with significant retention of radioxenon even in late washout (Fig. 46–5F).

FIGURE 46–5   G.

Washout LPO Ventilation Scan: Apical and basilar air trapping can be seen.

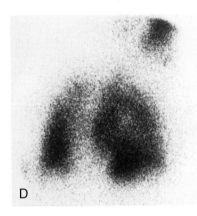

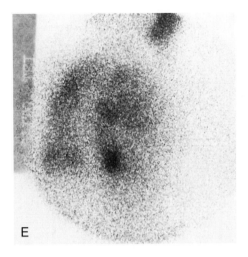

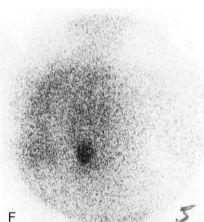

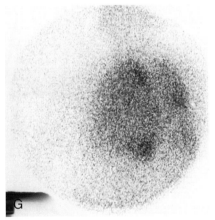

BULLOUS CYSTS

FIGURE 46–6   A and B.

Perfusion Lung Scan: There is very little perfusion to the right lung, which has round defects evident on the posterior view. (This scan was done after the aerosol ventilation scan.)

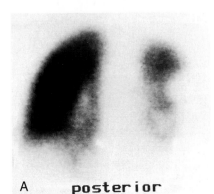

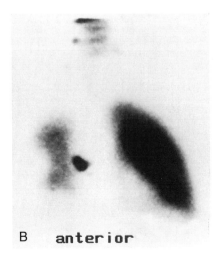

Illustration continued on following page

FIGURE 46–6   C to H.

Aerosol and Xenon Ventilation Lung Scans: There is no demonstrable ventilation to the cysts *(arrow)*. The liver, which was assumed to be fatty, takes up xenon at equilibrium *(arrowheads)*.

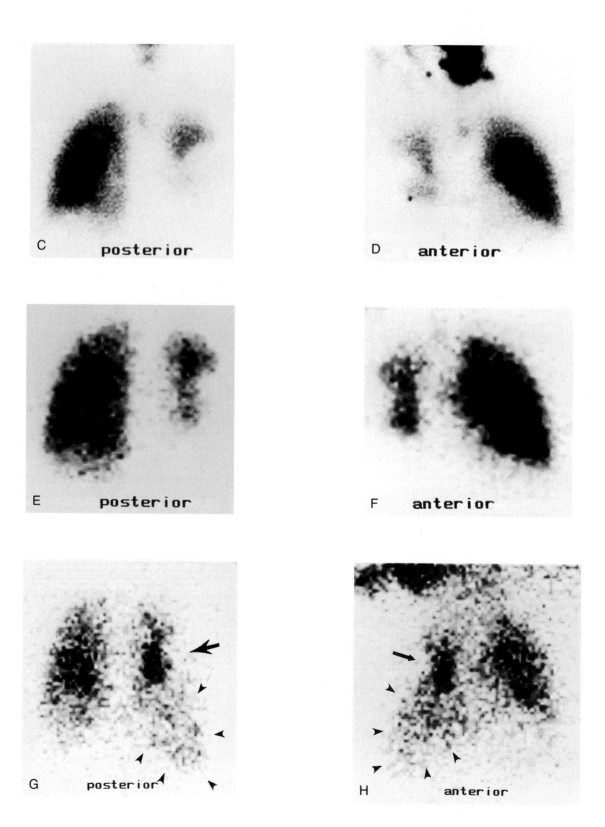

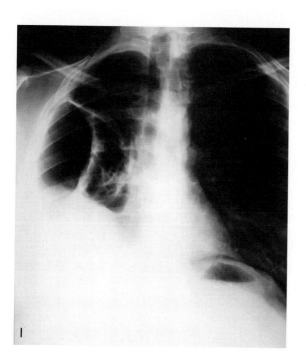

FIGURE 46–6   I.

PA Chest X-ray: There are several air-filled cysts evident, along with elevation of the right hemidiaphragm. There is no shift of the mediastinum to the left.

FIGURE 46–6   J.

CT Scan: The cystic changes of the right lung are evident.

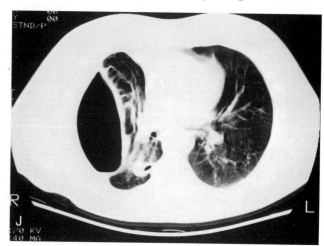

ALPHA-1-ANTITRYPSIN DEFICIENCY

FIGURE 46–7   A and B.

Anterior and Posterior Perfusion Lung Scans: There are multiple perfusion defects involving all lung fields, most marked at the base of the lungs.

FIGURE 46–7   C.

V/Q Scan: The ventilation scan is abnormal to the same degree as the perfusion lung scan, with basilar air trapping.

FIGURE 46–7   D.

CT Scan: There are numerous lower lobe bullae.

NOTE 1. Basilar V/Q matched abnormalities raise the possibility of an alpha-1-antitrypsin deficiency. Apical disease is more often seen with emphysema, especially from smoking.

NOTE 2. A theory suggests that the normal increased blood flow to the bases of the lungs brings more of the destructive proteases to these areas as opposed to the mid- and upper lung fields.

Cross Reference

Chapter 11: Soft Tissue Abnormalities—COPD on Bone Scan

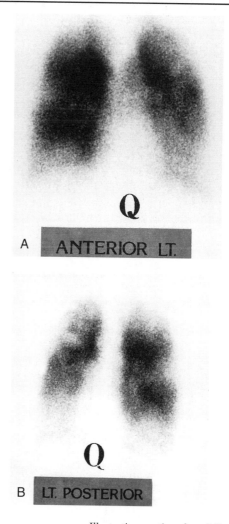

Illustration continued on following page

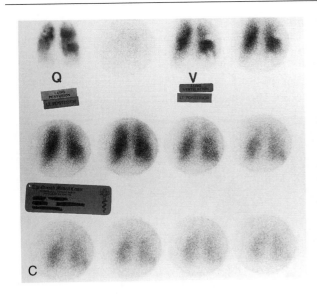

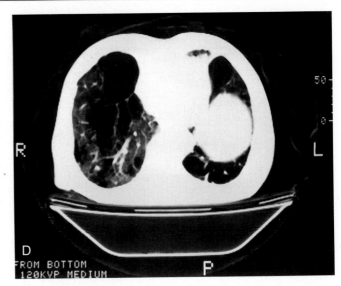

Chapter 47
Reverse V/Q Mismatch

REVERSE MISMATCH WITH MUCUS PLUG

FIGURE 47–1   A.
Posterior V/Q Scan: The radioxenon does not enter the left lung until very late. The perfusion to the left lung is mildly reduced.

FIGURE 47–1   B.
Posterior ^{99m}Tc-DTPA Aerosol Lung Scan After Suctioning, 24 Hours Later: There is now better ventilation to the left lung.

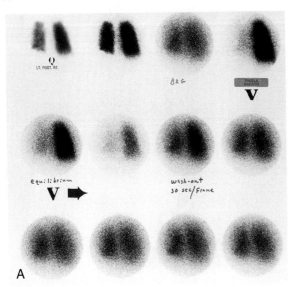

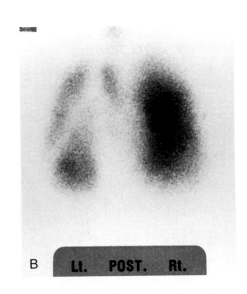

FIGURE 47–1   C.

Initial Chest X-ray: There is increased density to the left lung owing to loss of volume.

FIGURE 47–1   D.

Chest X-ray 24 Hours Later: There is now re-expansion of the left lung.

NOTE 1. Mucus plugs usually cause greater ventilation than perfusion abnormalities.

NOTE 2. The abnormalities, both on scan and on chest x-ray, can revert to normal immediately with movement of the plug after suctioning or coughing.

Cross Reference

Chapter 45: Solitary Matched Defects—Mucus Plug

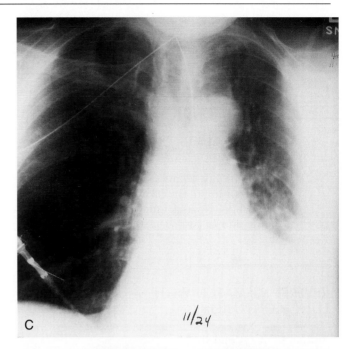

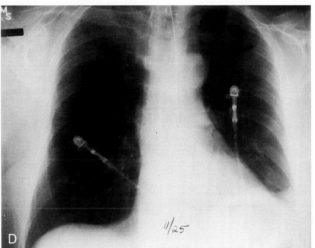

REVERSE MISMATCH WITH BRONCHIOLITIS OBLITERANS

FIGURE 47–2   A.

Anterior ^{99m}Tc-DTPA Aerosol Ventilation Scan: There is diminished ventilation in the periphery of both lung fields.

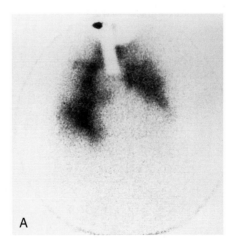

Illustration continued on following page

FIGURE 47–2   B.

Anterior ^{99m}Tc-MAA Perfusion Lung Scan: There is normal perfusion all the way out to the periphery of each lung.

NOTE 1. With severe reverse mismatches, the clinical and blood gas picture may suggest a right-to-left shunt. This is due to perfusion without ventilation.

NOTE 2. Bronchiolitis obliterans has marked narrowing or occlusion of the bronchioles caused by goblet cell metaplasia, mucus plugging, inflammation, and fibrosis.

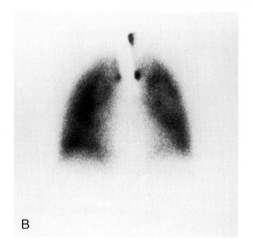

B

REVERSE MISMATCH WITH LUNG CONTUSION

FIGURE 47–3   A and B.

Posterior ^{99m}Tc-MAA Perfusion and ^{99m}Tc-DTPA Aerosol Lung Scans: The left lower lobe has normal perfusion but virtually no ventilation.

FIGURE 47–3   C and D.

Left Lateral Perfusion and Ventilation Scans: The left lower lobe has lost volume as well as ventilation. The major fissure is widened from fluid accumulation.

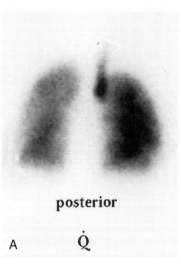

posterior

A $\dot{Q}$

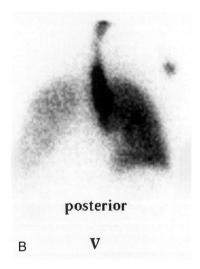

posterior

B   V

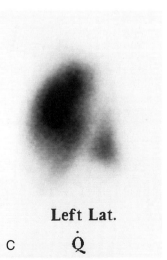

Left Lat.

C $\dot{Q}$

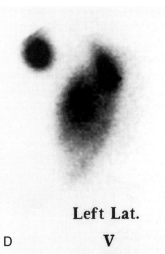

Left Lat.

D   V

FIGURE 47–3 E.

AP Chest X-ray: There is increased density behind the heart on the left owing to the collapsed left lower lobe.

NOTE. This case is unusual in that it has normal perfusion in an area of lung consolidation. The ventilation abnormality matches the left lower lobe collapse.

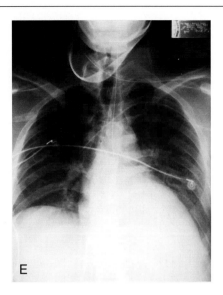

E

PERFORATION OF CENTRAL VENOUS LINE INTO PLEURAL SPACE

FIGURE 47–4 A.

Posterior Perfusion Scan: Injected through the central venous line, the ^{99m}Tc-MAA ended up in the left pleural fluid collection. The right lung is not seen.

FIGURE 47–4 B.

Posterior ^{133}Xenon Ventilation Scan: There is ventilation in the right lung and the left apex.

FIGURE 47–4 C.

Reversed Chest X-ray: There is a large left pleural fluid collection due to the intravenous fluids infused through the central venous catheter. (Courtesy of Dr. Alan Rothberg, Aurora, CO.)

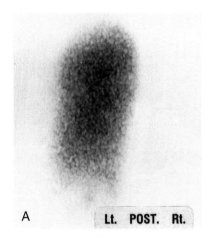

A **Lt. POST. Rt.**

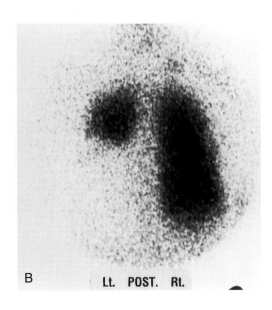

B **Lt. POST. Rt.**

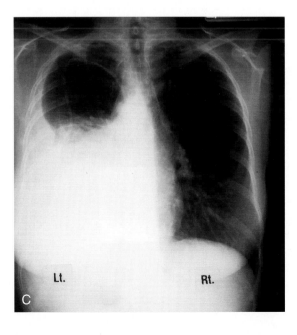

Lt. **Rt.**

C

PROGRESSION OF PNEUMONIA

FIGURE 48–1 A.
WBC Scan in Patient Following Partial Hepatectomy: There is localized right upper lobe WBC accumulation.

FIGURE 48–1 B.
WBC Scan 1 Month Later: There is now diffuse bilateral pulmonary infection. There is a small inflammatory focus at the site of the left chest tube *(arrow)*.

Cross Reference

Chapter 72: Tumors—Recurrent Tumor with Chest Infection

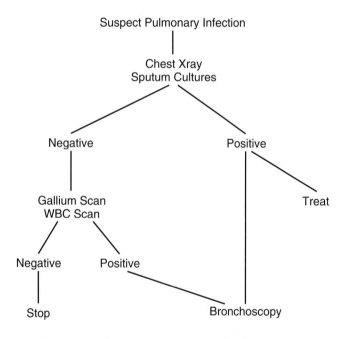

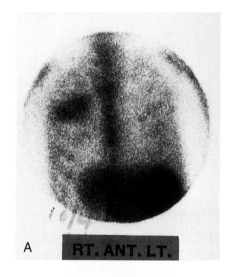

A   RT. ANT. LT.

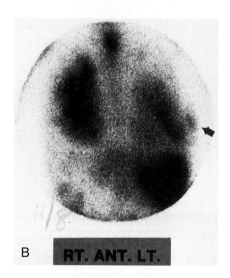

B   RT. ANT. LT.

ASPIRATION PNEUMONIA FROM ACHALASIA

FIGURE 48–2   A to C.

Gallium Scan: There are bilateral posterior pulmonary gallium accumulations.

FIGURE 48–2   D.

Technetium Colloid Esophageal Swallow: The esophagus is dilated, with an air-fluid level. (Courtesy of Dr. Michael Kipper, Vista, CA.)

NOTE 1. The most common segments involved in aspiration pneumonitis are the posterior aspects of the upper and lower lobes.

NOTE 2. Aspiration can occur with strokes, trauma, alcoholism, achalasia, various forms of tracheoesophageal diverticula, and spinal cord injuries and diseases.

Cross Reference

Chapter 30: Esophageal Studies—Achalasia with Aspiration

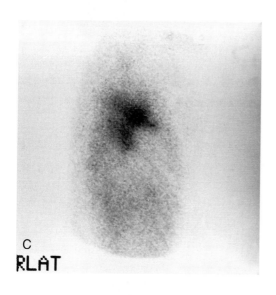

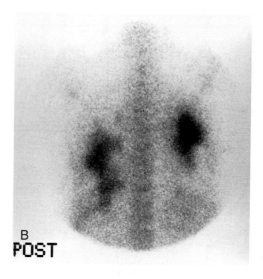

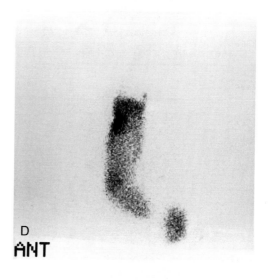

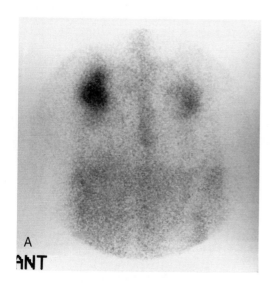

ACTIVE INTERSTITIAL PNEUMONITIS

Patient 1

FIGURE 48–3   A and B.

PA and Lateral Chest X-ray: There are prominent interstitial markings in a honeycomb pattern throughout the lungs.

FIGURE 48–3   C to F.

Gallium Scan: The abnormal gallium accumulation in the left lower lobe is best seen on the posterior and left lateral projections.

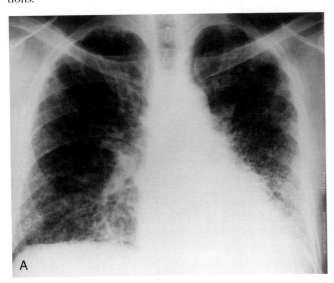

A

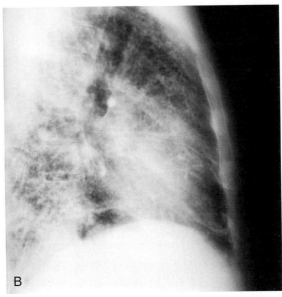

B

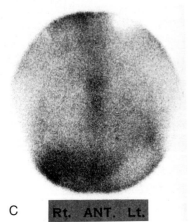

C   Rt. ANT. Lt.

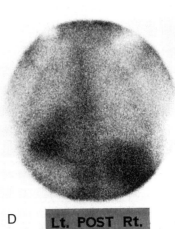

D   Lt. POST Rt.

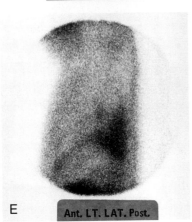

E   Ant. LT. LAT. Post.

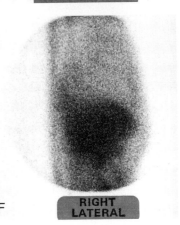

F   RIGHT LATERAL

Patient 2

FIGURE 48–3 G and H.

Right Lateral Gallium Scans Taken 2 Months Apart: There is clearing of the right lower and middle lobe inflammation following steroid therapy.

FIGURE 48–3 I.

Chest X-ray: There are increased linear markings in the lower halves of both lungs, unchanged over the 2 months.

Patient 3

FIGURE 48–3 J.

Chest X-ray: There is severe scarring and loss of volume of the right lung, with a large shift of the mediastinum to the right.

FIGURE 48–3 K and L.

Anterior and Lateral Gallium Scan: The lingula has increased gallium accumulation *(arrow)*, indicating the site of active inflammatory disease in this patient with an indeterminate chest x-ray.

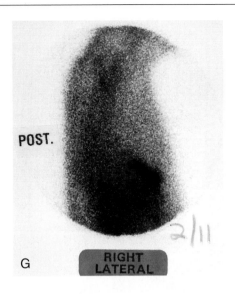

G

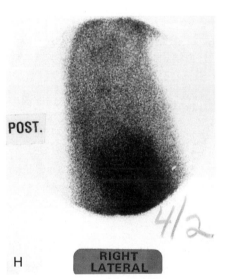

H

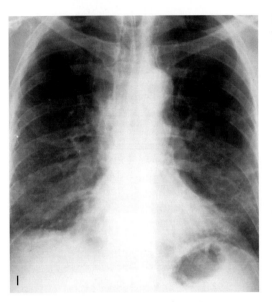

I

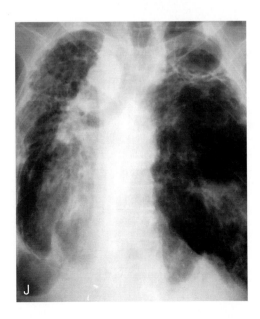

J

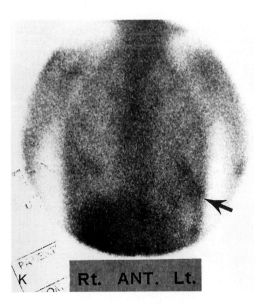

K

Illustration continued on following page

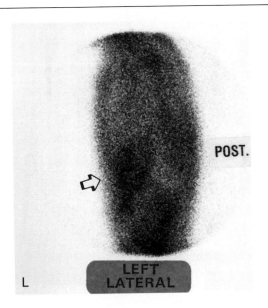

POST.

LEFT
LATERAL

L

NOTE. Although the chest x-ray may be diffusely abnormal, the gallium scan can determine the presence and extent of active disease.

Cross Reference

Chapter 71: Infectious Diseases—Inflammatory Lymph Nodes

ASPERGILLOSIS

FIGURE 48–4.

Gallium Scan: There is intense gallium accumulation in the right upper lobe.

NOTE. Aspergillosis is usually a unilateral upper lobe disease but is indistinguishable on gallium scan from bacterial pneumonia (especially *Klebsiella*, tuberculosis, sarcoid). A chest x-ray may be diagnostic for aspergillosis: a cavity with nodule.

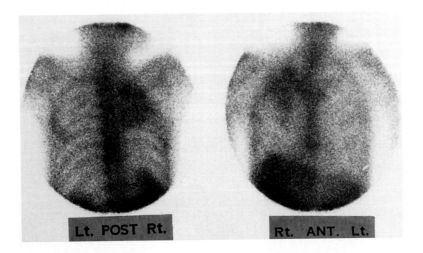

Lt. POST Rt.

Rt. ANT. Lt.

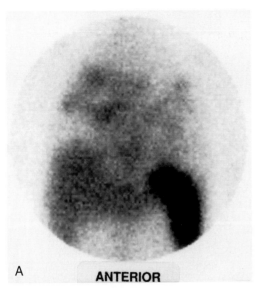

A **ANTERIOR**

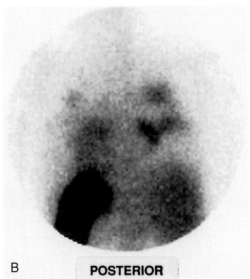

B **POSTERIOR**

LUNG ABSCESSES DUE TO INFECTED CENTRAL VENOUS CATHETER

FIGURE 48–5 A and B.
In-WBC Scan: Both lungs have multiple abscesses from septic emboli.

FIGURE 48–5 C.
AP Chest X-ray: There are multiple fluffy densities in the lungs, including right hilar adenopathy.

Cross Reference

Chapter 57: Infections—Septic Thrombus

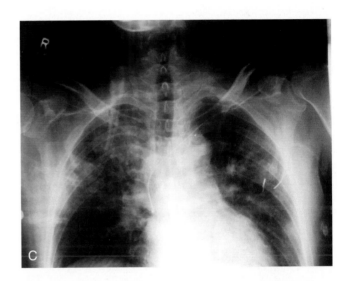

C

PERSISTENTLY ACTIVE LUNG ABSCESS ON GALLIUM SCAN

FIGURE 48–6 A to C.
Gallium Scan: There is a localized gallium accumulation in the posterior right lung.

RT. ANT. LT.

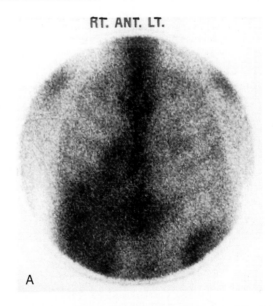

A

Illustration continued on following page

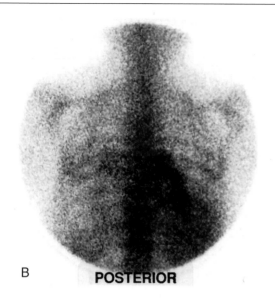

B   POSTERIOR

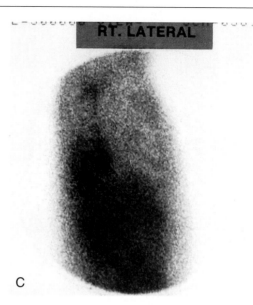

RT. LATERAL

C

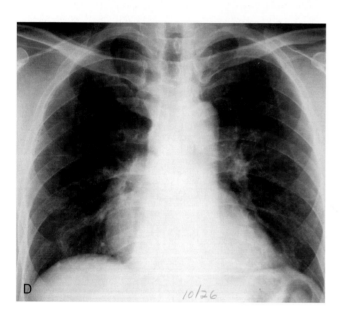

D   10/26

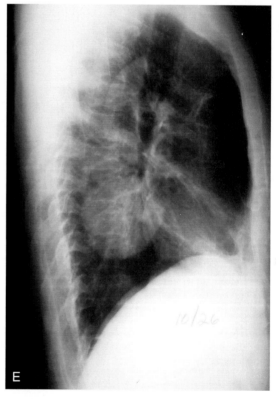

E   10/26

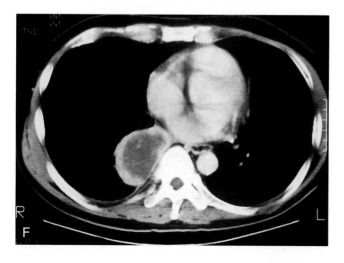

F

FIGURE 48–6   D and E.

PA and Lateral Chest X-rays: There is a smoothly marginated mass behind the heart on the right.

FIGURE 48–6   F.

CT Scan: There is a thick wall mass adjacent to the posteromedial pleura.

FIGURE 48–6   G and H.

Repeat Gallium Scan 2 Months Later: The abscess is larger and still accumulates significant amounts of gallium.

FIGURE 48–6   I.

Chest X-ray: The mass is larger.

NOTE. The chest x-ray cannot distinguish between pseudotumor and persistent abscess.

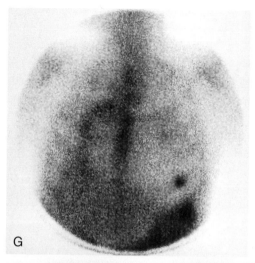

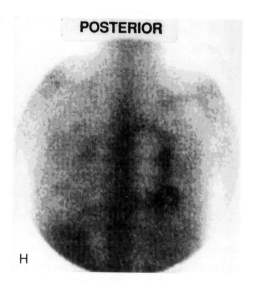

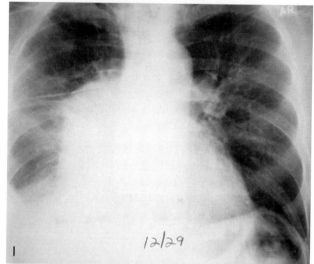

PLEURAL ABSCESS

Patient 1: Leukemia with Chronic Pleural Effusion and FUO

FIGURE 48–7   A.

Posterior Gallium Scan: There is a "doughnut" lesion in the right posterior costophrenic angle.

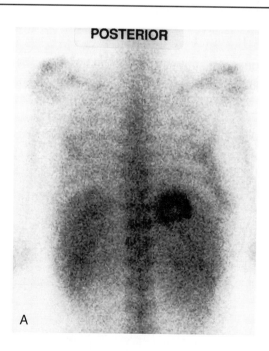

Illustration continued on following page

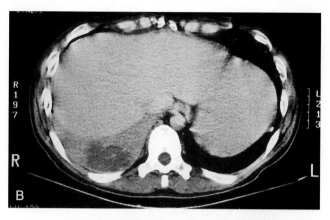

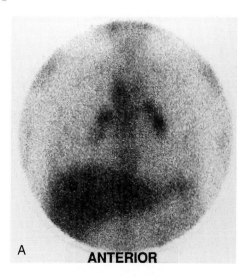

FIGURE 48–7   B.

CT Scan: There is a right pleural effusion surrounding an irregular low-density structure.

Patient 2

FIGURE 48–7   C.

^{111}In-WBC ^{99m}Tc-Colloid Subtraction Scan: There is a small, linear accumulation in the right posterior costophrenic angle. A subtraction of the technetium liver scan from the WBC scan demonstrates the infected pleural empyema.

FIGURE 48–7   D.

CT Scan: There is gas and fluid behind the liver in an abscess. Note the soft tissue swelling.

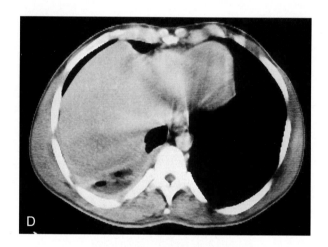

PULMONARY SARCOID

Patient 1: Type I Sarcoid

FIGURE 48–8   A and B.

Gallium Scan: There are active nodes in both hila and the right paratracheal region.

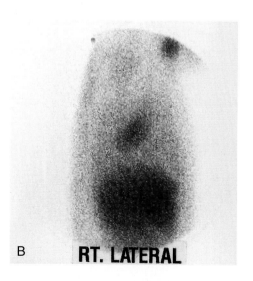

FIGURE 48–8   C.

Chest X-ray: The hilar nodes are enlarged, but there are no pulmonary parenchymal lesions.

Patient 2: Type II Sarcoid

FIGURE 48–8   D to F.

Gallium Scan: There is increased gallium activity in the peripheral lung parenchyma as well as probable right hilar adenopathy.

FIGURE 48–8   G.

Chest X-ray: There are fluffy densities in both lungs, with possible hilar lymphadenopathy.

NOTE 1. There may or may not be progression from one type to another.

NOTE 2. Blacks have a higher incidence of the disease and a worse prognosis than Caucasians.

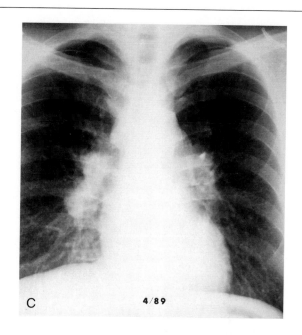

C   4/89

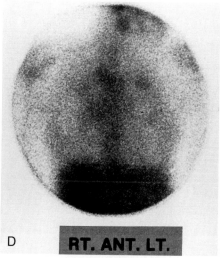

D   RT. ANT. LT.

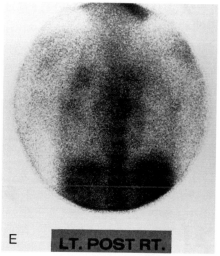

E   LT. POST RT.

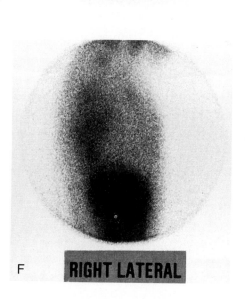

F   RIGHT LATERAL

STAGES OF THORACIC SARCOID	
I	Bilateral hilar adenopathy, normal lungs
II	Bilateral hilar adenopathy, pulmonary involvement
IIIA	Pulmonary lesions, no adenopathy, no lung fibrosis
IIIB	Pulmonary lesions, no adenopathy, pulmonary fibrosis

From Fraser RG, Paré JAP, Paré PD, Fraser RS, Genereux GP (eds): Diagnosis of Diseases of the Chest, ed. 3. Philadelphia: WB Saunders, 1995, p 2611.

Illustration continued on following page

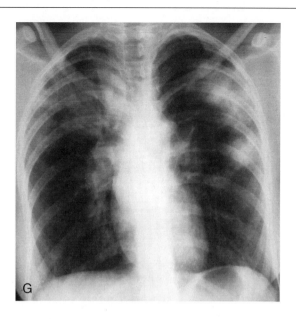

ABNORMAL GALLIUM BEFORE CHEST
X-RAY FINDINGS

FIGURE 48–9   A to C.

Gallium Scan: There is focal gallium accumulation in the superior segment of the right lower lobe.

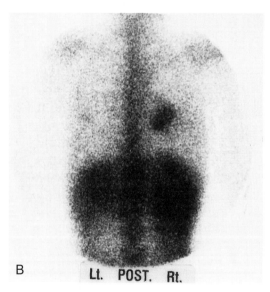

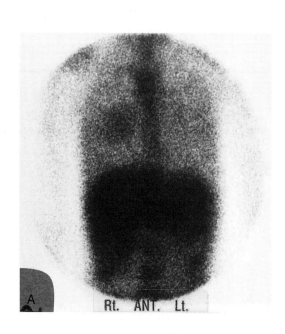

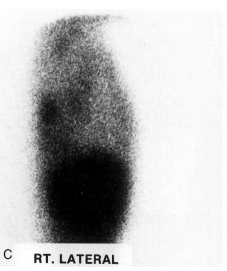

FIGURE 48–9 D.
Chest X-ray: normal.

FIGURE 48–9 E.
Repeat Chest X-ray (1 Week Later): There is now a pneumonitis evident in the superior segment of the right lower lobe.

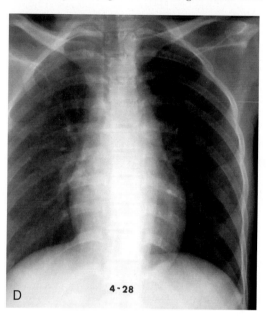

NOTE. The chest x-ray may be normal for 24+ hours even though there is a pneumonia. Hydrating a patient may help visualize the pneumonia on subsequent x-rays.

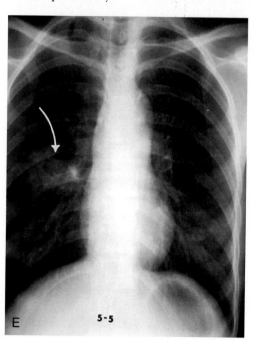

Chapter 49
Diffuse Infection

PNEUMOCYSTIS PNEUMONIA

Patient 1

FIGURE 49–1 A and B.
Gallium Scan: There is diffuse increased gallium accumulation in all lung fields.

FIGURE 49–1 C.
Chest X-ray: There are no findings suggesting infection.

Patient 2

FIGURE 49–1 D.
Gallium Scan: There is sparing of both apices.

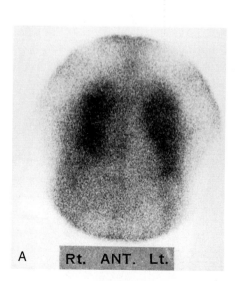

Rt. ANT. Lt.

Illustration continued on following page

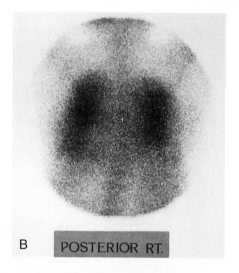

B   POSTERIOR RT.

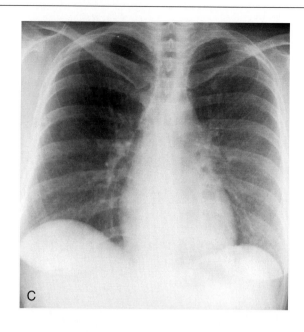

C

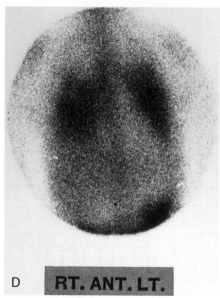

D   RT. ANT. LT.

Patient 3

FIGURE 49–1   E to H.

Anterior, Posterior, and Both Lateral Chest Gallium Scans: The gallium distribution is asymmetric, sparing the upper lobes and the superior segment of the right lower lobe and being less intense in the lingula.

Illustration continued on following page

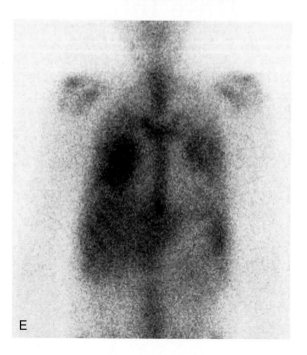

E

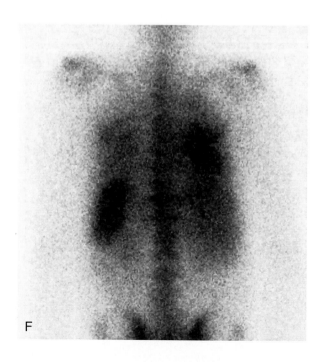

F

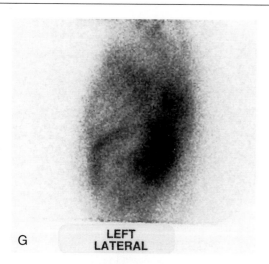

G **LEFT LATERAL**

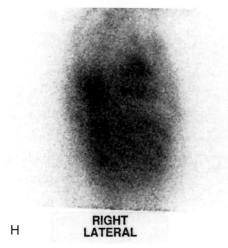

H **RIGHT LATERAL**

NOTE 2. Gallium and WBC scans are nonspecific and indicate only active inflammation. This can be miliary tuberculosis; bacterial or viral pneumonia (varicella, respiratory syncytial virus, CMV); protozoan, autoimmune, allergic, or idiopathic (e.g., sarcoid) pneumonitis; cytotoxic drug; or radiation pneumonitis.

NOTE 3. Although WBC scans can be effective with *Pneumocystis carinii* infections, and in other infections that have little or no WBC response, there can be false negative examinations. Gallium is better in infections that do not stimulate WBC response.

Cross Reference

Chapter 71: Infectious Diseases—WBC Scanning; Gallium Scanning (Tables 71–1 and 71–3)

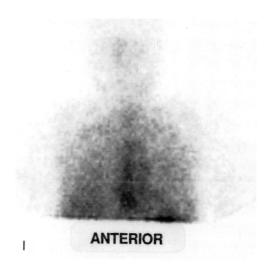

I **ANTERIOR**

Patient 4

FIGURE 49–1   I and J.

Anterior and Posterior ^{111}In-WBC Scan: There is no abnormal accumulation of white cells in the lungs

FIGURE 49–1   K and L.

Anterior and Posterior Gallium Scan 3 Days Later: There is intense focal activity in the right upper lobe and a milder abnormality in the superior segment of the right lower lobe.

FIGURE 49–1   M and N.

Sagittal and Coronal Gallium SPECT Scans: The focal abnormalities are better seen in the posterior segment of the right upper lobe and in the superior segment of the right lower lobe.

NOTE 1. Most *Pneumocystis carinii* infections are diffuse, but they may be focal. With prophylactic pentamidine aerosol inhalation, apical disease may develop, since upright inhalation delivers less drug to the apices.

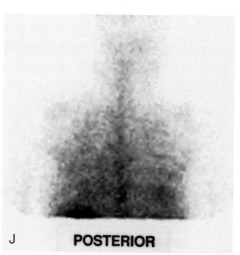

J **POSTERIOR**

Illustration continued on following page

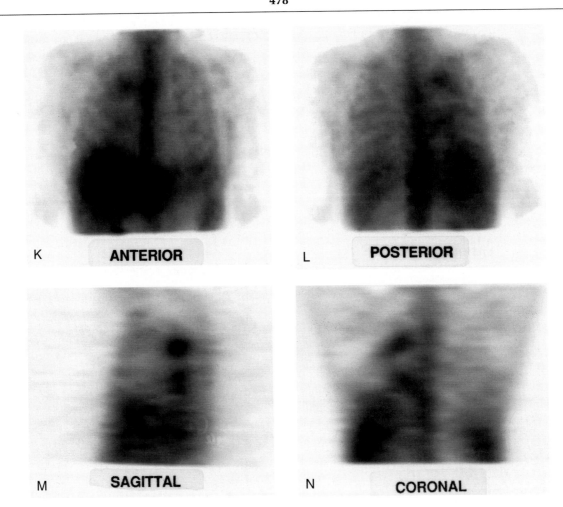

K **ANTERIOR**

L **POSTERIOR**

M **SAGITTAL**

N **CORONAL**

MILIARY TUBERCULOSIS

Patient 1

FIGURE 49–2   A and B.

WBC Scan: There is diffuse increased WBC accumulation in all lung fields.

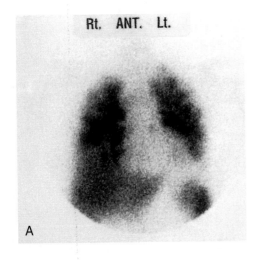

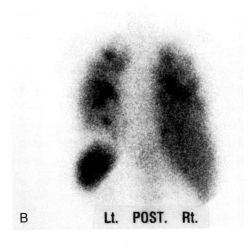

Patient 2: TB in Systemic Lupus Erythematosus with Steroid Therapy

FIGURE 49–2 C.

Anterior Gallium Scan: There is no gallium accumulation in the lungs.

FIGURE 49–2 D and E.

Anterior and Posterior Gallium Scan 3 Months Later: There is now diffuse gallium accumulation in all lung fields. Sputum samples were positive for acid-fast bacilli.

FIGURE 49–2 F and G.

Chest X-rays Taken 4 Days Apart: Increasing density and increased interstitial markings developed over 4 days. These x-rays were taken at the time that the gallium scan was positive.

NOTE 1. Repeat chest x-rays should be obtained if the initial one is normal and if the infection scan is positive.

NOTE 2. In interstitial pneumonitis from SLE, the arteritis involves the lower lung fields and should accumulate gallium when active.

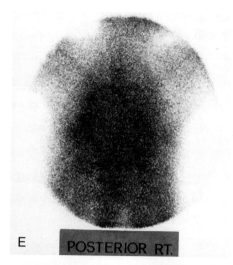

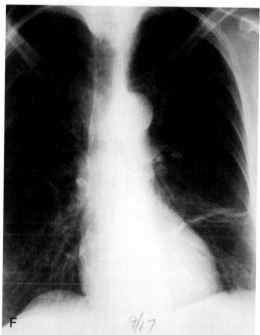

E   POSTERIOR RT.

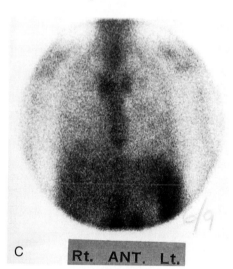

C   Rt. ANT. Lt.

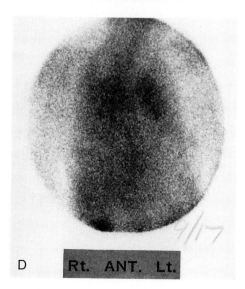

D   Rt. ANT. Lt.

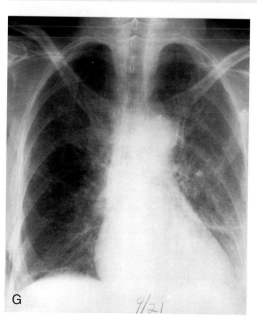

F   9/17

G   9/21

ADULT RESPIRATORY DISTRESS SYNDROME (ARDS)

Patient 1

FIGURE 49–3   A.
Gallium Scan: There is diffuse increased gallium throughout all lung fields.

Patient 2

FIGURE 49–3   B and C.
Anterior and Posterior Chest ^{111}In-WBC Scan: The WBCs have diffusely accumulated in both lungs.

FIGURE 49–3   D.
AP Chest X-ray: There is diffuse alveolar filling (''white-out'' lung).

FIGURE 49–3   E and F.
Anterior and Posterior Chest ^{111}In-WBC Scan 2 Weeks Later: There has been regression of the ARDS and a reduction of the WBC aggregation in the lungs.

NOTE 1. ARDS is an endotoxic pneumonitis, not necessarily caused by an infectious lung process.

NOTE 2. Pulmonary perfusion on V/Q scanning can be normal despite diffuse alveolar filling.

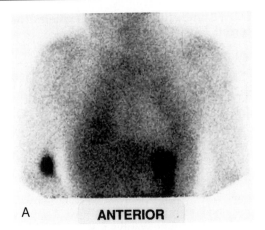

A   **ANTERIOR**

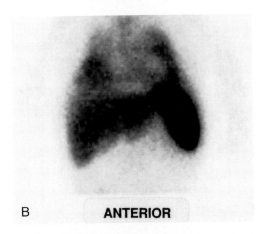

B   **ANTERIOR**

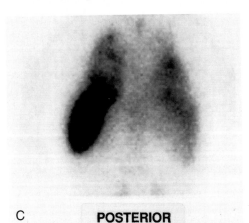

C   **POSTERIOR**

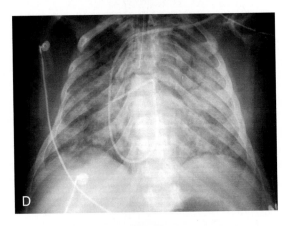

D

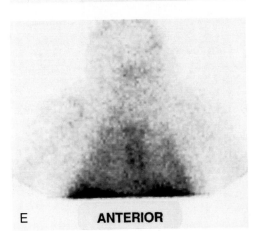

E   **ANTERIOR**

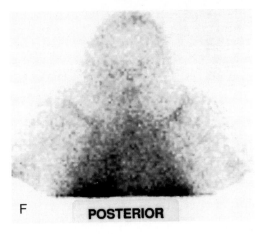

F   **POSTERIOR**

Chapter 50

Lung Tumors

BRONCHOGENIC CARCINOMA AND THALLIUM

Patient 1: Chest Mass

FIGURE 50–1 A.

PA Chest X-ray: There is a large mass in the left upper lobe at the level of the aortic arch, along with a large left pleural effusion.

FIGURE 50–1 B.

Anterior Thallium Scan: The mass in the left upper lobe takes up thallium. The pleural effusion has only minimal activity.

Patient 2: Lung Consolidation

FIGURE 50–1 C.

PA Chest X-ray: There is consolidation of the right upper lobe with loss of volume.

FIGURE 50–1 D and E.

Anterior and Posterior Thallium Planar Images: There is nodular right upper lobe thallium accumulation.

USES OF TUMOR SCANNING TO DETERMINE THE PROBABILITY OF MALIGNANCY	
1. In inoperable patients, or in patients at high risk for needle biopsy	4. To look for secondary sites of involvement
2. In patients who are reluctant to have biopsy or surgery	5. After therapy, to look for residual or recurrent neoplasm
3. When biopsies are negative or equivocal but suspicion remains	6. To differentiate malignant from benign processes

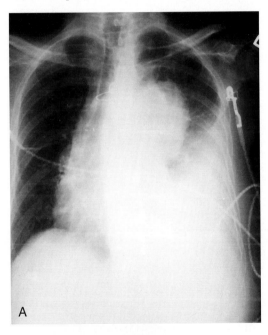

A

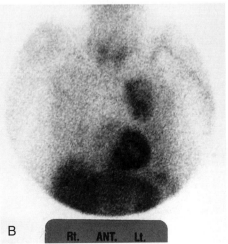

B Rt. ANT. Lt.

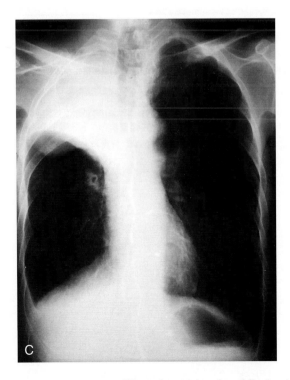

C

Illustration continued on following page

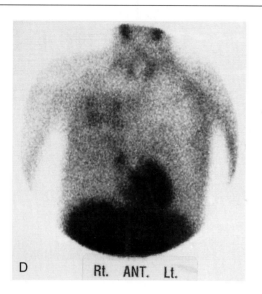

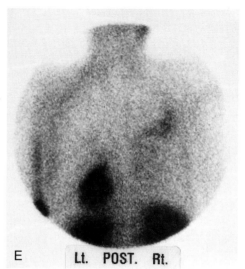

NOTE 1. Despite consolidation or pneumonitis, thallium goes to cells with high growth rates, such as malignant tumors.

Cross Reference

Chapter 72: Tumors—Lung Nodules

THALLIUM VS. SESTAMIBI

Patient: Bronchogenic Carcinoma

FIGURE 50–2   A to C.

Coronal, Sagittal, and Transverse Sestamibi SPECT Scans: The nodule in the superior segment of the left lower lobe accumulates sestamibi *(arrow)*.

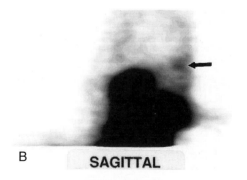

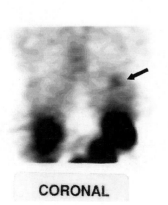

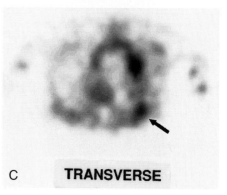

FIGURE 50–2   D and E.
Planar Sestamibi Chest Scans: There is no appreciable activity in the region of the tumor.

FIGURE 50–2   F to H.
Coronal, Sagittal, and Transverse Thallium SPECT Scans: There is mild thallium activity in the entire left lower lobe, with slightly greater activity in the region of the tumor *(arrows)*.

FIGURE 50–2   I and J.
Planar Thallium Chest Scans: The tumor nodule is faintly seen.

NOTE 1. No one tumor scanning agent will be accurate in all cases.

NOTE 2. SPECT scans usually are better in delineating activity in a mass and in detecting metastatic lymph nodes.

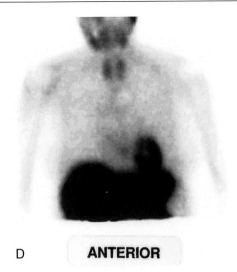

D   **ANTERIOR**

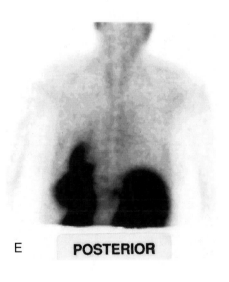

E   **POSTERIOR**

Suspect Active
Hilar/Mediastinal
Adenopathy

|

Chest Xray
(Compare to Old Xrays)

|

CT/MRI

|

<u>Spect Scan</u>
Gallium
Thallium
Sestamibi
Octreotide
FDG-Pet

Negative   Positive

| |

Stop   Biopsy/Treat

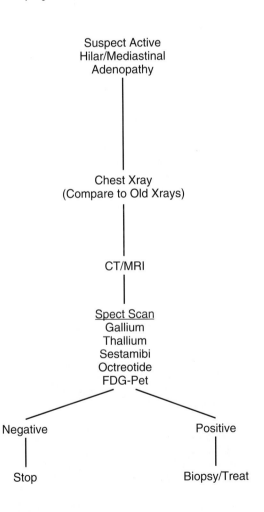

Cross Reference

Chapter 72: Tumors—Lung Nodule

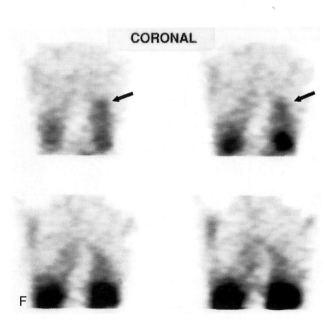

CORONAL

F

Illustration continued on following page

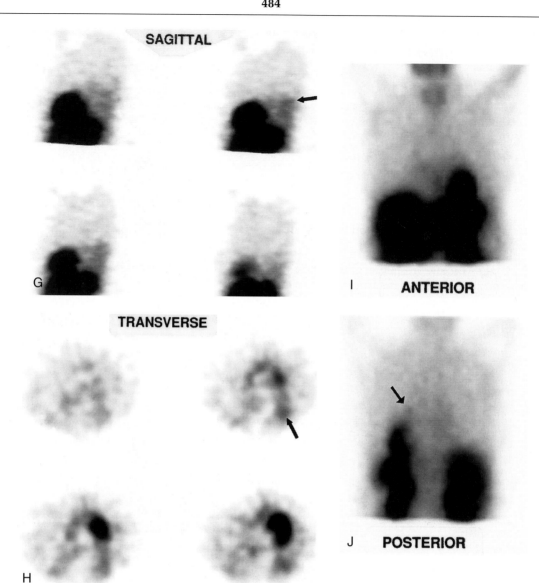

SAGITTAL

G

TRANSVERSE

H

I **ANTERIOR**

J **POSTERIOR**

TUMOR EXTENT ON GALLIUM SCAN VS. CHEST X-RAY

Patient 1: Leukemia

FIGURE 50–3 A and B.

PA and Lateral Chest X-rays: The middle lobe is partially opacified.

FIGURE 50–3 C.

Anterior Gallium Scan: There is greater lung and mediastinal involvement than the chest x-ray suggests, especially on the left.

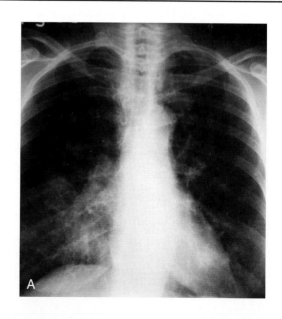

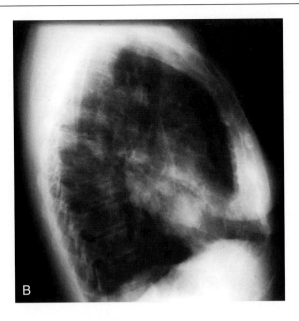

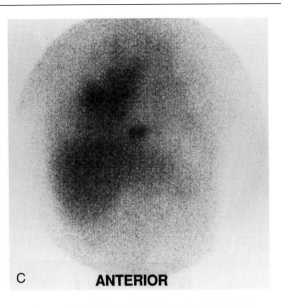

Patient 2: Lymphoma

FIGURE 50–3   D and E.

PA and Lateral Chest X-rays: There is a localized mass in the left hilum *(arrows)*.

FIGURE 50–3   F to H.

Anterior and Both Lateral Gallium Scans: There is marked gallium accumulation in the right superior mediastinum, middle mediastinum, and left hilum, findings less obvious on chest x-ray.

NOTE. CT is the mainstay for evaluating lymph node size. Gallium or another tumor scanning agent is better at evaluating for viable tumor, especially after therapy. Tumor involvement may be overestimated by size criterion alone.

Cross Reference

Chapter 72: Tumors—Gallium-Avid Lymphoma

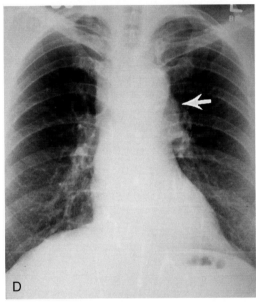

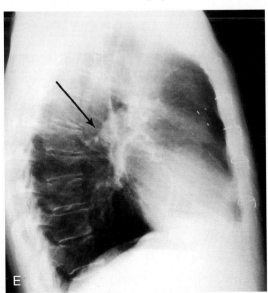

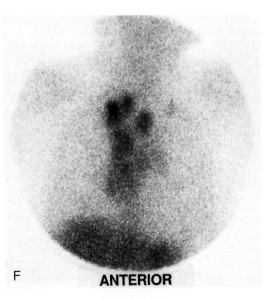

Illustration continued on following page

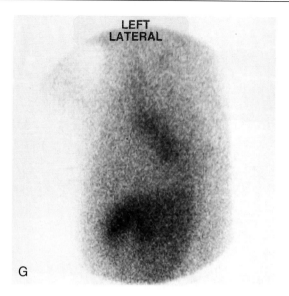

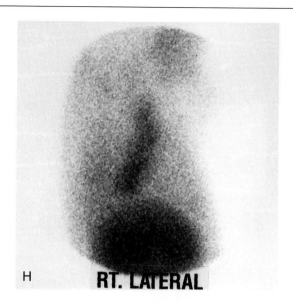

RESIDUAL MALIGNANT LYMPHOMA VS. SCAR

Patient: One Month After Chemotherapy

FIGURE 50–4   A and B.

PA and Lateral Chest X-rays: There is a mass at the level of the right hilum.

FIGURE 50–4   C.

CT Scan: The mass compresses or partially occludes the right mainstem bronchus.

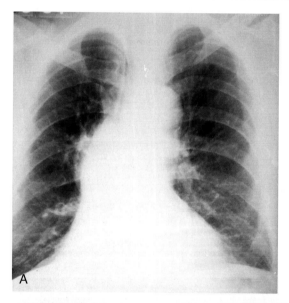

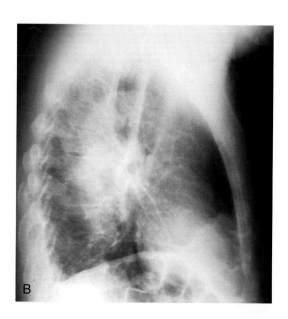

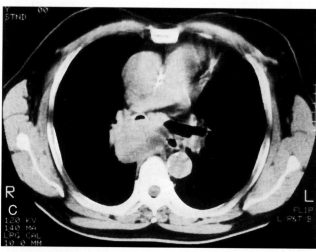

FIGURE 50–4   D.

Anterior Thallium Tumor Scan: There is active tumor along the periphery of the mass.

NOTE 1. Thallium, gallium, or sestamibi can distinguish residual or new tumor from scar or granulation tissue after surgery, radiation therapy, or chemotherapy.

NOTE 2. A residual mass on CT after therapy could be fibrotic tissue rather than persistent tumor.

Cross Reference

Chapter 72: Tumors—Lung Nodule

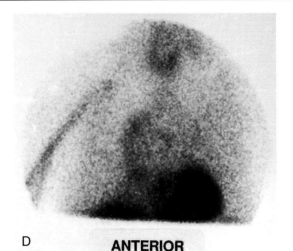

D   **ANTERIOR**

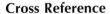

GLUCOHEPTONATE IN LUNG CANCER

FIGURE 50–5.

Anterior Chest ^{99m}Tc-Glucoheptonate Scan: The left lung nodule *(arrow)* demonstrated abnormal activity.

NOTE. The mediastinum is not as easy to evaluate soon after injection owing to persistent blood pool, making glucoheptonate a less desirable tumor scanning agent.

Cross Reference

Chapter 72: Tumors—Lung Nodule

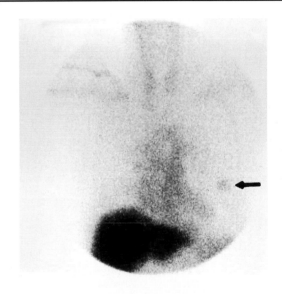

OCTREOTIDE: NON–SMALL CELL CARCINOMA OF THE LUNG

FIGURE 50–6   A to C.

Transverse, Sagittal, and Coronal [99m]Technetium Octreotide SPECT Scans of the Head: The solitary metastasis to the left deep parietal lobe accumulates the radiopharmaceutical. This was not visible on the planar scans.

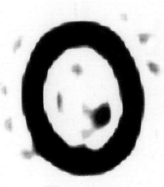

A   **Transverse**

Illustration continued on following page

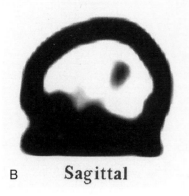

B   **Sagittal**

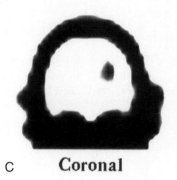

C   **Coronal**

FIGURE 50–6   D and E.

Anterior and Posterior ⁹⁹ᵐTechnetium Octreotide Planar Chest Scans: There is increased activity in a broad band across the right upper lobe. No activity is appreciable in the right hilum.

FIGURE 50–6   F to G.

Coronal ⁹⁹ᵐTechnetium Octreotide SPECT Chest Scans: Focal accumulation of the radiopeptide is seen in the right upper lobe and the right hilum *(arrows)*.

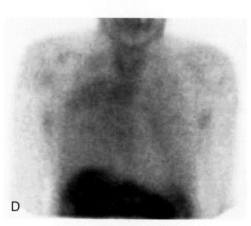

D

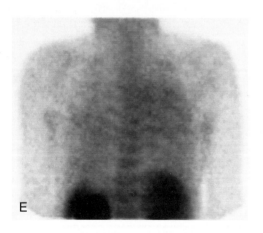

E

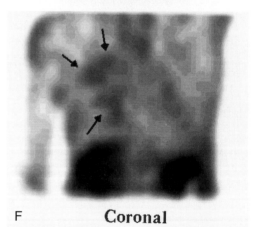

F   **Coronal**

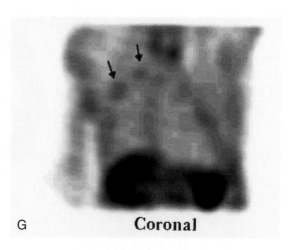

G   **Coronal**

FIGURE 50–6 H.

CT of the Thorax: The tumor in the right hilum is evident.

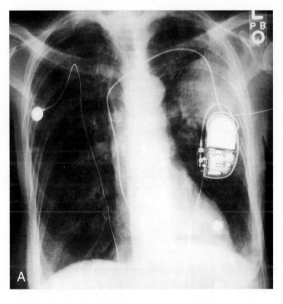

NOTE 1. SPECT scans are essential for most radiopeptide scans.

NOTE 2. The accumulation of the radio-octreotide in non–small cell carcinomas of the lung, and other non-neuroendocrine tumors, is due to surrounding activated lymphocytes, neuroendocrine cells, and venules as well as mild nonspecific binding within the tumor.

Cross Reference

Chapter 72: Octreotide—Carcinoid

WBC UPTAKE IN TUMOR

FIGURE 50–7 A.

PA Chest X-ray: There is a large density in the left upper lobe.

FIGURE 50–7 B.

WBC Scan (Anterior): There is a focal uptake of WBCs in the left upper lobe.

NOTE. WBCs can accumulate in tumors, probably owing to necrosis, or can accumulate distal to the neoplasm in an obstructive pneumonia.

Cross Reference

Chapter 71: Infectious Diseases—WBCs in Tumor

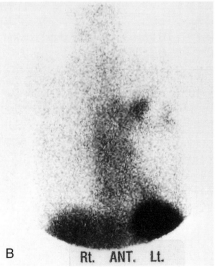

PULMONARY HEMORRHAGE ON RBC SCAN

Patient: Bronchiectasis

FIGURE 51–1 A.

Left Lateral Thorax on Tagged RBC Scan: There is abnormal accumulation of the radiolabeled RBCs in the left lower lobe *(arrow).*

FIGURE 51–1 B and C.

Anterior and Posterior Tagged RBC Scan: These views are normal. The left lower lobe activity is masked by the cardiac blood pool.

NOTE. It may be difficult to distinguish extravasation from hyperemia unless sequential scans are obtained.

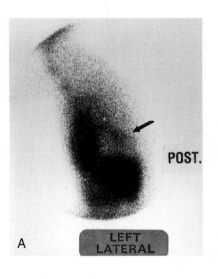
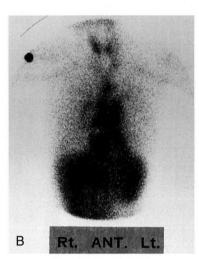
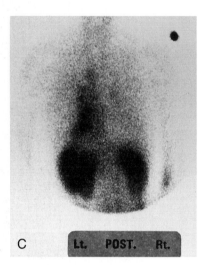

ABNORMAL DIFFUSION DUE TO SMOKING

FIGURE 51–2 A.

Posterior Supine ^{99m}Tc-DTPA Aerosol Scan: There is good filling of the upper lobe airways.

FIGURE 51–2 B.

RPO Aerosol Scan: This scan taken 10 minutes after the initial view demonstrates rapid absorption of the radioaerosol from the upper lobes with retention at the bases.

NOTE. Normal alveolar clearance should be approximately 1–1.5% min^{-1}. Smokers have a 2–5% min^{-1} clearance rate.

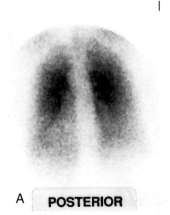
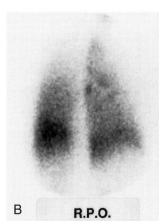

Chapter 52

Cardiac Ischemia

NORMAL MYOCARDIAL STRESS TESTS

Patient 1: SPECT Thallium Stress/Rest Scans

FIGURE 52–1   A.

Short Axis: The thallium is homogeneous in all walls until the septum becomes membranous *(arrow)* toward the base.

FIGURE 52–1   B.

Vertical Long Axis: The posteroinferior wall frequently has less thallium *(arrow)*, more evident after exercise. This is thought to be due to a partial volume effect with the diaphragm and attenuation.

FIGURE 52–1   C.

Horizontal Long Axis: There is homogeneous thallium distribution throughout the myocardium. The muscular septum is shorter than the lateral wall *(arrow)*. (Ap = Apex; A = anterior wall; S = septum; L = lateral wall; B = base or valve plane; I = inferior wall; RV = right ventricle.)

Illustration continued on following page

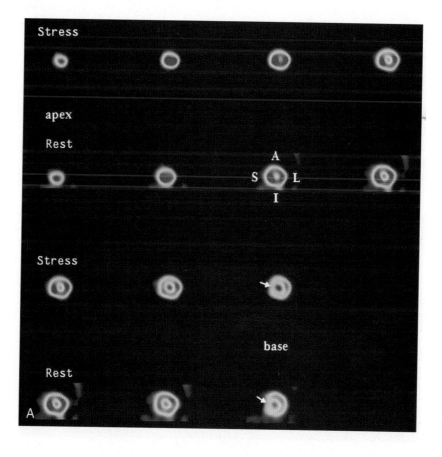

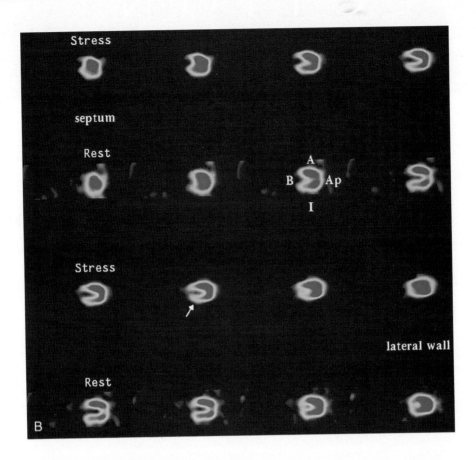

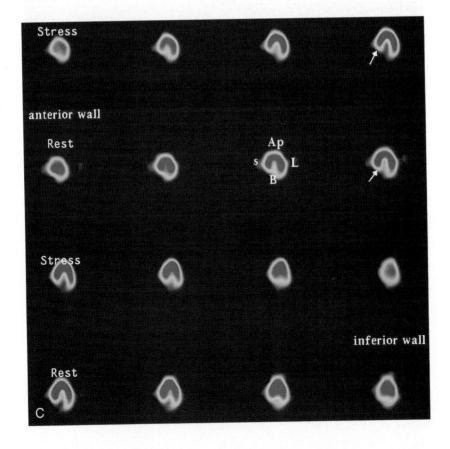

Patient 2: Planar Thallium Stress/Rest Scans

FIGURE 52-1   D and E.

Anterior Scan, 20 Degree Cranial Tilt: The cranial tilt allows for improved inferior wall evaluation.

FIGURE 52-1   F and G.

Forty-five Degree LAO, 15 Degree Caudal Tilt: The caudal tilt elongates the heart.

FIGURE 52-1   H and I.

Forty-five Degree LAO, 20 Degree Cranial Tilt

FIGURE 52-1   J and K.

Steep Lateral (≥LAO)

Illustration continued on following page

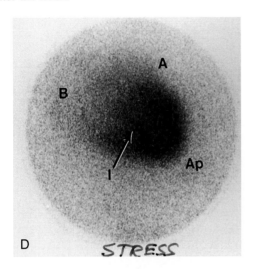

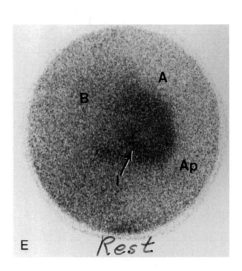

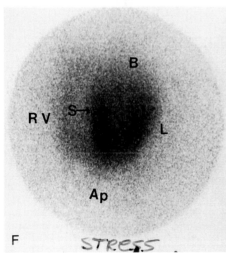

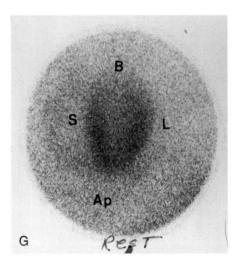

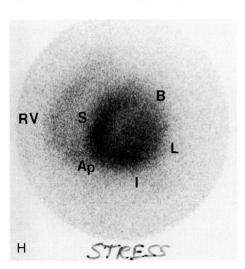

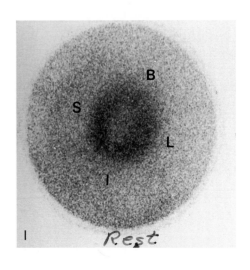

FIGURE 52–1 L and M.

Composite of Planar Thallium Stress/Rest Scans with Circumferential Curves: The washout should be at least 30 percent after 4 hours of rest for each myocardial segment.

NOTE 1. The base or valve plane should have little radiopharmaceutical, since there is virtually no muscle in the region.

NOTE 2. The stress left ventricular cavity size should be equal to, or smaller than, that on the resting scans. This is due to the shortened diastolic filling time.

NOTE 3. The proximal interventricular septum, the membranous septum, has very little of the radiopharmaceutical, since it has less muscle and more fibrous tissue.

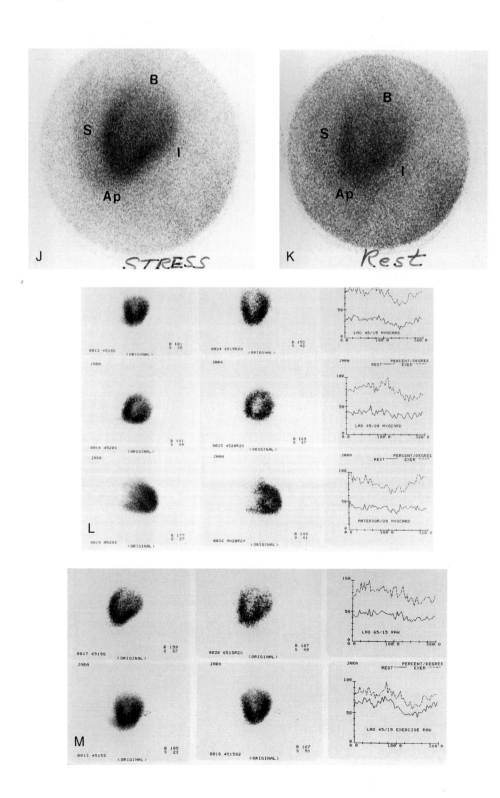

PAPILLARY MUSCLE HYPERTROPHY

FIGURE 52–2.

LAO Planar Rest Thallium Scans: The focal area of activity inside the ventricular cavity is presumed to represent hypertrophic papillary muscle.

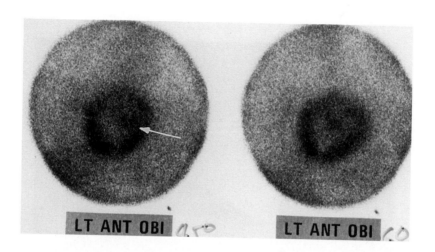

SINGLE VESSEL CORONARY DISEASE

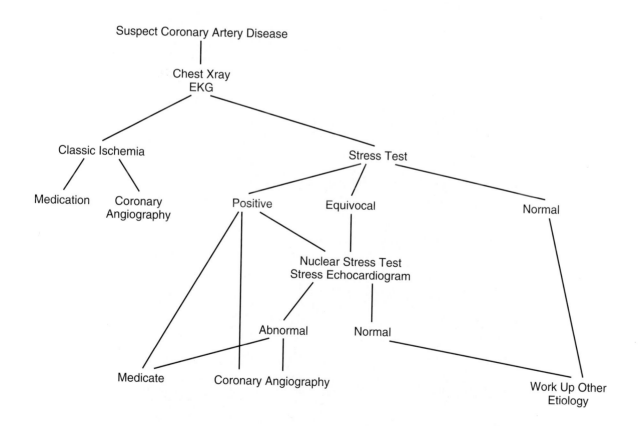

Patient 1: Anterolateral Ischemia, Disease of Diagonal Branch of LAD

FIGURE 52–3 A.

SPECT Thallium Stress/Rest Short Axis Scan: The anterior wall *(arrow)* has a transitory perfusion abnormality.

FIGURE 52–3 B.

Vertical Long Axis: The deficit extends from apex to base.

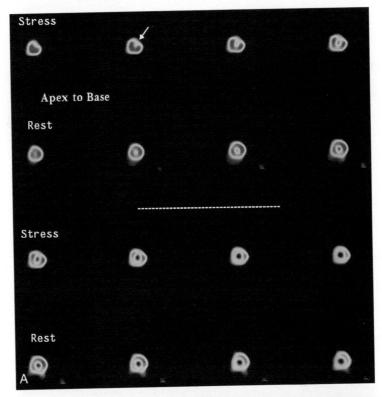

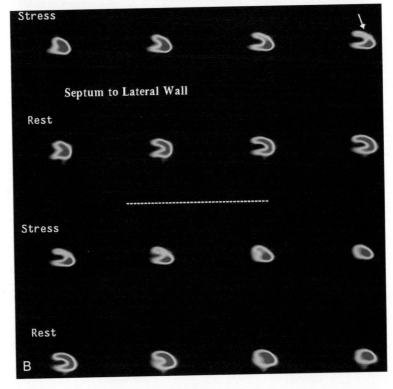

Patient 2: Lateral Wall Ischemia, Left Circumflex Disease

FIGURE 52–3   C.

SPECT Thallium Stress/Rest Short Axis: The lateral wall defect *(arrow)* extends into the inferior wall, sparing the anterolateral wall.

FIGURE 52–3   D.

Horizontal Long Axis

Illustration continued on following page

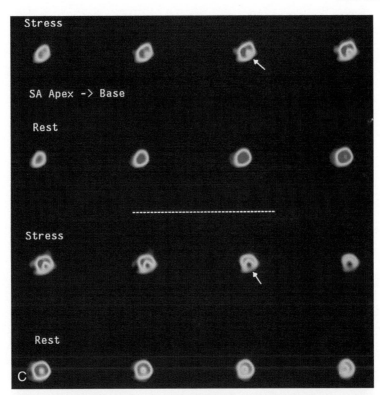

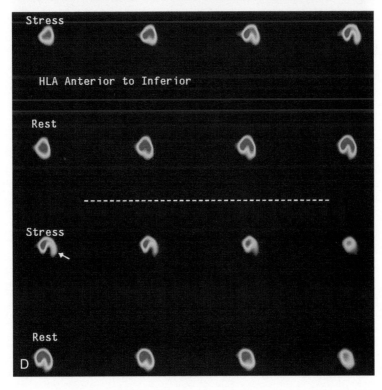

Patient 3: Inferior Wall Ischemia, Right Coronary Disease

FIGURE 52–3 E.
SPECT Thallium Stress/Rest Short Axis: The inferior wall defect does not fully recover after 4 hours of rest but definitely demonstrates an ischemic pattern.

FIGURE 52–3 F.
Vertical Long Axis

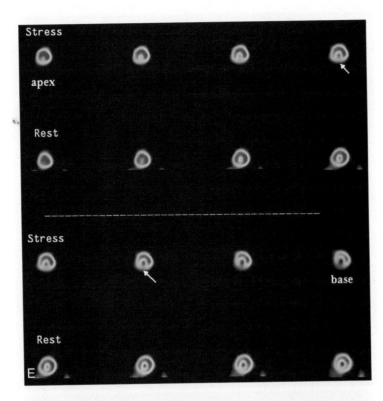

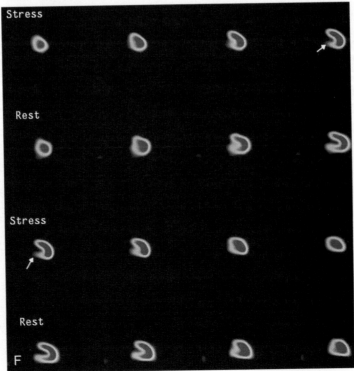

Patient 4: Inferior Wall Ischemia, Right Coronary Disease

FIGURE 52–3 G.

Forty-five Degree LAO Planar Thallium Stress (S)/Rest (R) Scan: The inferior wall has a reversible perfusion abnormality of the inferior wall.

NOTE. Although a perfusion abnormality may suggest disease of a specific coronary artery, because of numerous anatomic variations a coronary angiogram is necessary to identify the exact arterial branch involved.

VASCULAR DISTRIBUTION OF NORMAL CORONARY ANATOMY	
Anterior wall	Left anterior descending
Anterolateral wall	Diagonal branches of LAD
Lateral wall	Left circumflex
Posteroinferior wall	Obtuse marginal branch, left circumflex
Inferior wall	Right coronary
Apex	Distal LAD

INDICATIONS OF STRESS MYOCARDIAL IMAGING

1. Detection of ischemic coronary artery disease
   a. abnormal EKG during standard treadmill testing
   b. atypical chest pain
   c. in patients with other atherosclerotic disease
   d. in elderly patients undergoing major surgery
2. Detection of myocardium at risk after MI
3. Evaluation of extent of ischemia from stenoses seen on coronary arteriography
4. Any patient suspected of silent ischemia
5. Patients with strong family history of CAD at an early age

Thallium Stress Test

Normal — Abnormal

Abnormal: water only +/− nitrates

Normal → Stop

Normal → 4 hour redistribution scan with polar plots or washout curves

Abnormal → 4 hour reinjection scan

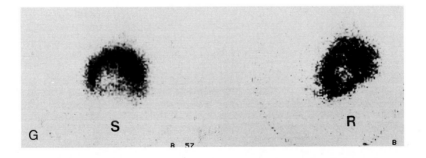

MULTIVESSEL CORONARY ARTERY DISEASE

Patient 1: Distal LAD and Left Circumflex Disease

FIGURE 52–4 A.

SPECT Thallium Stress/Rest Short Axis: The apex and the inferolateral walls have transitory perfusion abnormalities. The left ventricular cavity is mildly dilated after exercise, indicating left ventricular (LV) dysfunction.

FIGURE 52–4 B.

Horizontal Long Axis SPECT Scan: The basal lateral wall is foreshortened owing to a transmural myocardial infarct *(arrow)*. There is ischemia of the distal lateral wall.

Illustration continued on following page

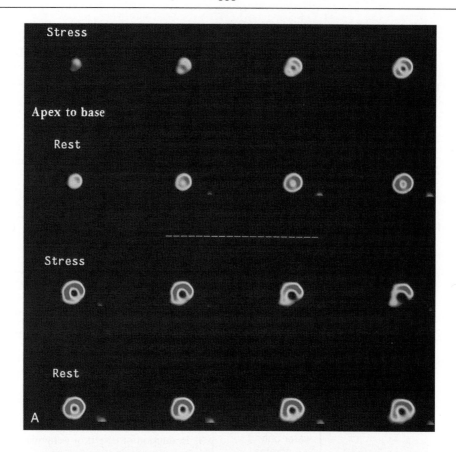

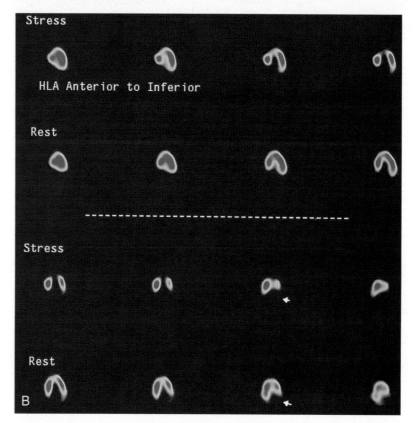

Patient 2: LAD and RCA Disease

FIGURE 52–4   C.

Forty-five Degree LAO Planar Thallium/Rest Scans: There are transitory perfusion abnormalities involving the anteroseptal and inferior walls.

NOTE. Multivessel ischemic disease will have at least two defects in separate vascular zones. It may also have a dilated ventricle, sometimes greater on the stress images than at rest, indicating LV dysfunction.

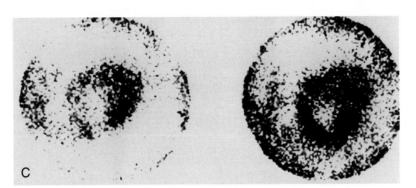

"BALANCED" ISCHEMIA

FIGURE 52–5   A to C.

Composite of Planar Thallium Stress (S)/Rest (R) Scans: There is a single discrete perfusion defect in the inferior wall near the apex, yet the left ventricle is dilated. The inferior wall also appears to have a reversed mismatch.

Illustration continued on following page

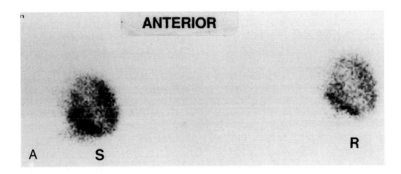

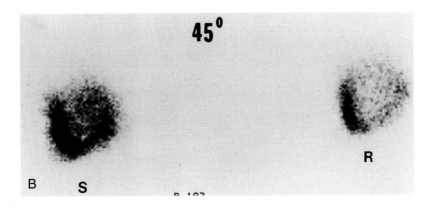

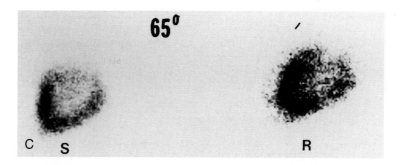

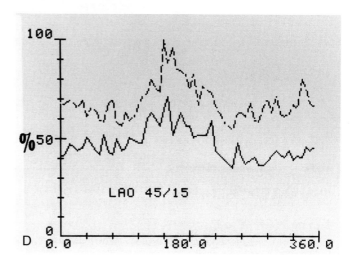

FIGURE 52–5 D.

Circumferential Curve: There is very little washout, <30 percent, in all parts of the myocardium.

NOTE 1. "Balanced" ischemia occurs with three-vessel disease, in which all walls are equally ischemic.

NOTE 2. A clue to "balanced" multivessel ischemic disease is ventricular dilatation and LV dysfunction with stress, with disproportionately small zones of ischemia.

LEFT VENTRICULAR DYSFUNCTION WITH STRESS

Patient 1

FIGURE 52–6 A.

SPECT Thallium Stress/Rest Short Axis Scans: The left ventricle is dilated after stress owing to the inferolateral infarct *(arrow)* combined with ischemic anterior, septal, and inferior walls.

Patient 2

FIGURE 52–6 B and C.

Pre-CABG Planar Thallium Stress/Rest Scan 45 Degree LAO: The left ventricular cavity is larger at stress than rest.

FIGURE 52–6 D and E.

Post-CABG Stress/Rest 45 Degree Scan: The mildly dilated ventricular cavity is now smaller after stress than at rest.

NOTE 1. The normal response with stress is for the ventricular cavity to be smaller because of the shortened end-diastolic filling time. In order to meet increased demand, the heart rate and ejection fraction increase, and the end-systolic volume decreases.

NOTE 2. LV dysfunction is diagnosed as dilatation of the ventricle with stress, which improves with rest. An increase in the pulmonary water is also present and is best seen as increased thallium in the lungs.

NOTE 3. Myocardial walls may appear thin on the stress tomograms owing to dilatation and ischemia.

NOTE 4. LV dysfunction may make perfusion abnormalities, especially infarcts, look larger on the stress tomograms when compared with the smaller heart at rest.

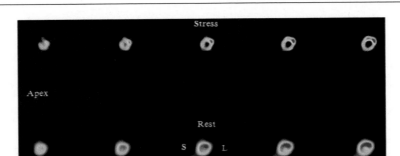

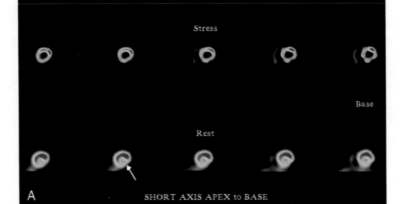

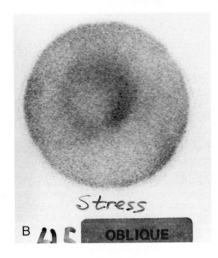

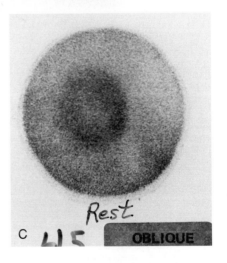

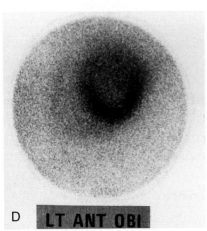

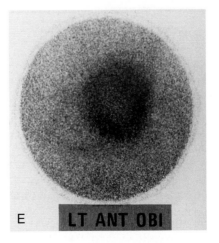

INCREASED PULMONARY WATER WITH STRESS

FIGURE 52–7   A and B.
Stress Planar Thallium Scans: The lungs have increased thallium.

FIGURE 52–7   C and D.
Four Hour Rest Thallium Scans: The lungs have cleared the thallium over the time between examinations.

NOTE 1. Increase in pulmonary thallium indicates increased pulmonary water, caused by LV dysfunction and congestive heart failure with stress.

NOTE 2. A ratio of lung:heart activity should be <0.5, although each laboratory should establish its own normal range.

NOTE 3. Increased pulmonary water is transient, "flash pulmonary edema," and rarely evident clinically as congestive heart failure.

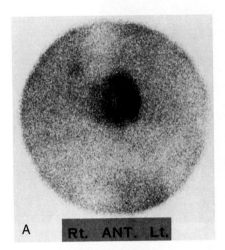

A   Rt. ANT. Lt.

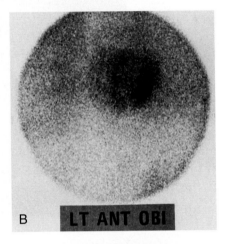

B   LT ANT OBI

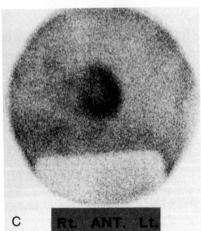

C   Rt. ANT. Lt.

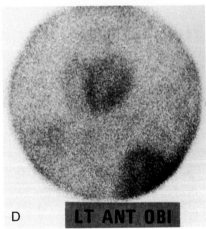

D   LT ANT OBI

INFARCT WITH ISCHEMIA

Patient 1: Anterior, Septal, and Right Ventricular Disease

FIGURE 52–8   A.
SPECT Thallium Stress/Rest Short Axis Scan: The ventricles are both dilated with viable, but ischemic, myocardium in the septum *(arrow)* as well as in the inferior and free walls of the hypertrophic right ventricle.

Patient 2: Cocaine Abuse in 17 Year Old

FIGURE 52–8   B.
SPECT Thallium Stress/Rest Short Axis: There is an inferolat-

eral nontransmural infarct with some ischemia *(arrow)*. There is also ischemia of the anteroseptal myocardium.

NOTE 1. When the right ventricle is well visualized on perfusion scanning, it is hypertrophic.

NOTE 2. Cocaine causes vasospasm and small vessel occlusions.

Cross Reference

Chapter 56: Miscellaneous—Cor Pulmonale with Severe Right Ventricular Hypertrophy

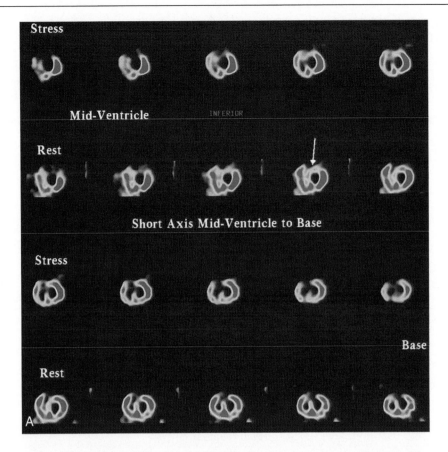

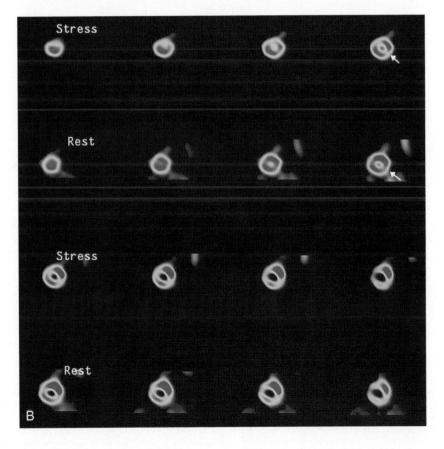

VALUE OF REINJECTION OF THALLIUM FOR HIBERNATING MYOCARDIUM

Patient 1

FIGURE 52–9   A.

SPECT Thallium Stress/Rest Scans: The presumed inferior and lateral wall infarcts have considerable viable myocardium, best seen with reinjection of thallium at rest.

Patient 2

FIGURE 52–9   B to I.

Short Axis and Vertical Long Axis ^{201}Tl Stress/Rest Scans: Even after 24 hours the inferior wall does not have significant amounts of thallium. After reinjection, the inferior myocardium can be determined to be viable (ex = exercise; ri = reinjection). (Courtesy of Dr. Derek Pang, Honolulu, HI.)

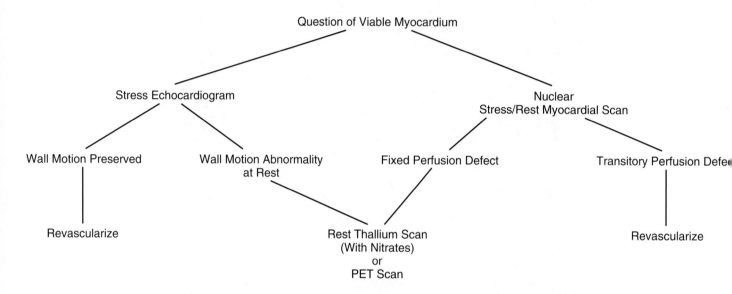

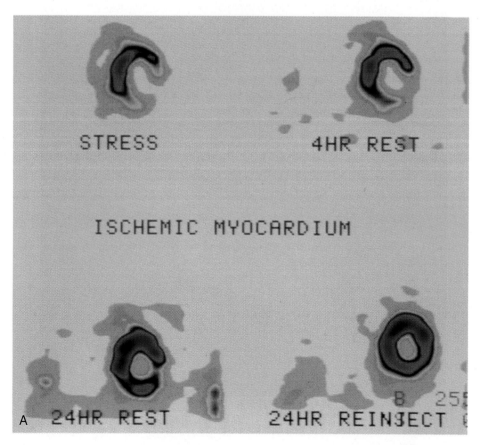

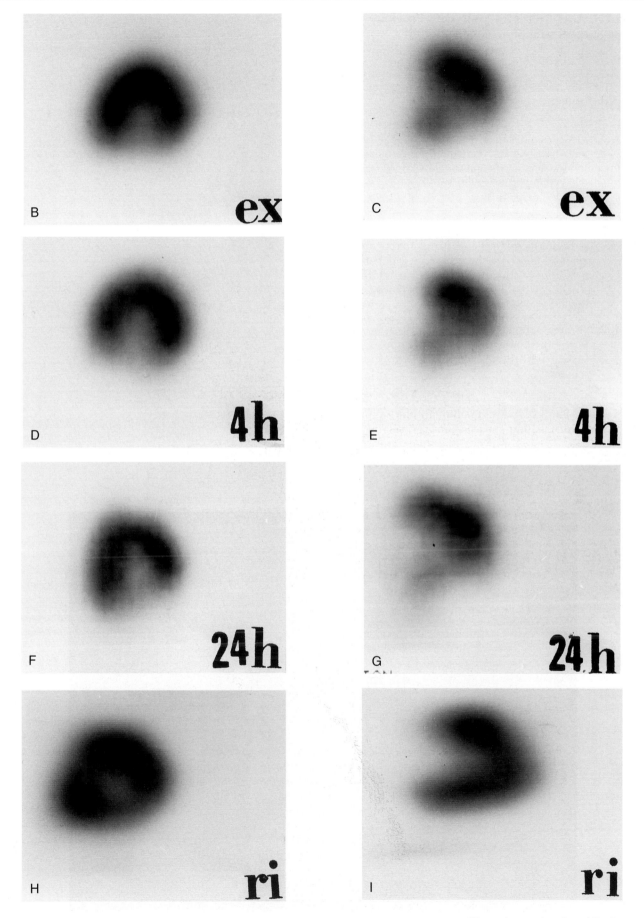

Illustration continued on following page

Patient 3: A 57 Year Old Male with Previous Bypass Surgery and Shortness of Breath

FIGURE 52–9   J and K.

Short Axis Stress and 4 Hour Rest/Reinjection/Nitrates [201]Tl Scans: The only "viable" myocardium appears to be the interventricular septum.

FIGURE 52–9   L.

Short-Axis 24 Hour Redistribution Thallium Scan: The inferior and lateral walls have viable, hibernating myocardium. The anterior and posterolateral walls appear infarcted but could be deeply ischemic and of low metabolic activity.

NOTE 1. There does not appear to be any need to wait 24 hours to reinject. All stress images can be reviewed immediately; a rest scan is performed in 4 hours with reinjection of an additional 1.5 mCi [201]thallium 20 minutes before scanning.

NOTE 2. Nitrates, either oral or topical, may be used during the 4 hour rest period to improve myocardial perfusion, relieving stress induced ischemia.

NOTE 3. ^{99m}Tc-sestamibi is purely a blood flow tracer and is not as good as thallium for the evaluation of hibernating myocardium. It will overestimate the size of myocardial infarctions.

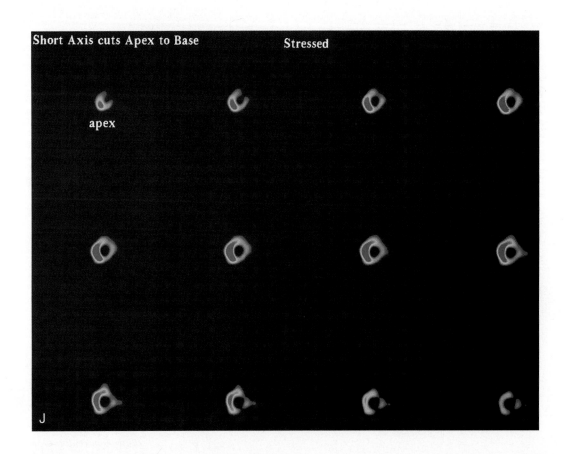

Short Axis cuts Apex to Base   Stressed

apex

J

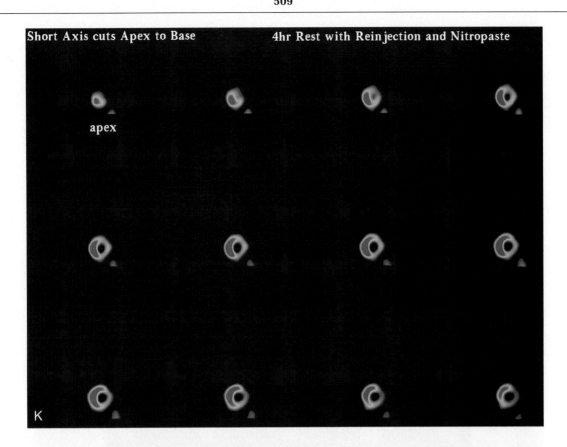

Short Axis cuts Apex to Base — 4hr Rest with Reinjection and Nitropaste

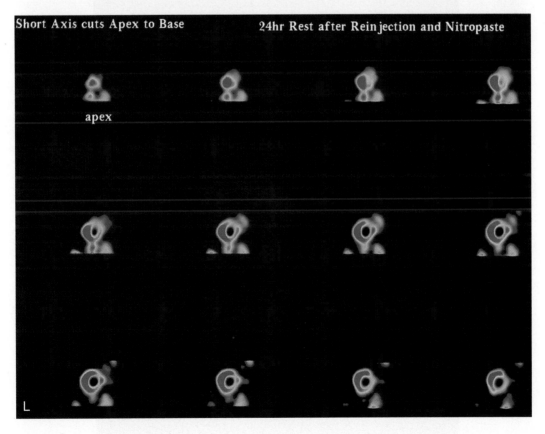

Short Axis cuts Apex to Base — 24hr Rest after Reinjection and Nitropaste

ISCHEMIA WITH INCOMPLETE REPERFUSION

FIGURE 52–10   A.

SPECT Thallium Stress/Rest Short Axis Scan: The anterior wall perfusion abnormality at stress incompletely normalizes, despite reinjection of thallium and oral 20 mg sorbitrate.

FIGURE 52–10   B.

SPECT Thallium Stress/Rest Vertical Long Axis: The anterior wall improves over time but does not become entirely normal.

NOTE. Any improvement in the size of the perfusion defect from stress to rest represents ischemia. Incomplete return to normal suggests profound ischemia rather than a coexisting nontransmural infarct.

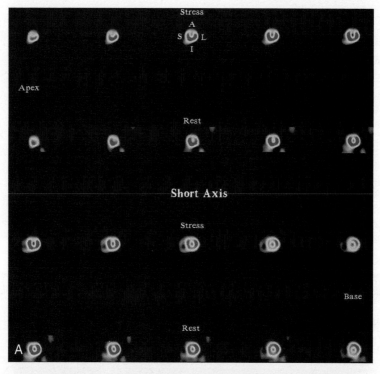

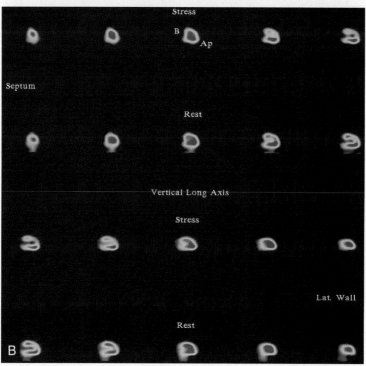

REVERSE REDISTRIBUTION

Patient 1

FIGURE 52–11   A and B.

SPECT Thallium Stress/Rest, Short Axis and Vertical Long Axis: The mild anterior wall perfusion deficit on the stress images is worse on the resting scans despite reinjection with an additional dose of thallium. The septum shows the more common pattern of improvement with rest and reinjection.

Patient 2

FIGURE 52–11   C.

Forty-five Degree LAO Stress/Rest Thallium Scans: The inferior wall has better perfusion after exercise than at rest.

Illustration continued on following page

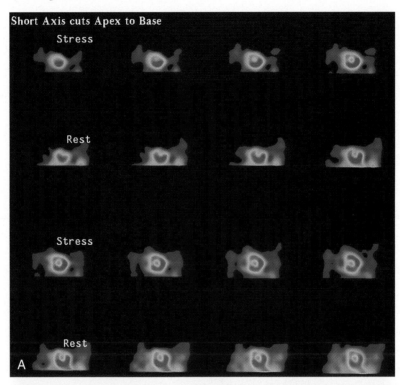

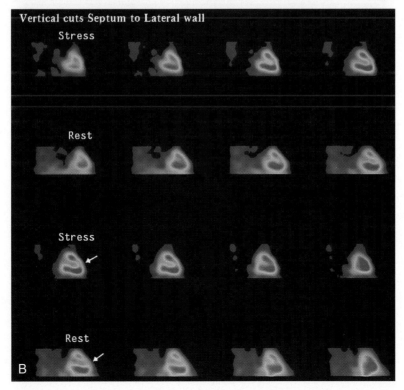

NOTE. Excessive washout or "reverse redistribution" is most often associated with ischemia.

Cross Reference

Chapter 52: Cardiac Ischemia—"Balanced" Ischemia

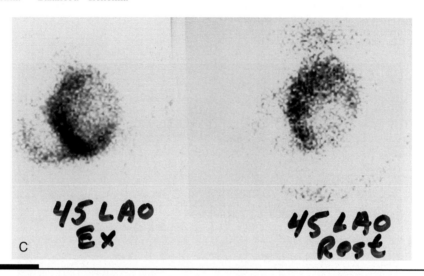

LEFT BUNDLE BRANCH BLOCK (LBBB) SIMULATING ISCHEMIA

Patient 1

FIGURE 52–12   A.

SPECT Thallium Stress/Rest Short Axis Scan: The septum has a transitory perfusion abnormality *(arrow)* in this patient with LBBB.

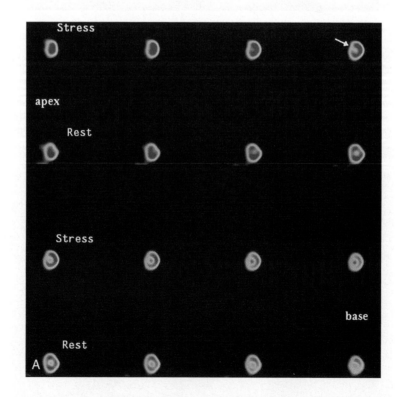

Patient 2

FIGURE 52–12   B and C.

Forty-five Degree LAO Planar Thallium Stress/Rest Scan: The septum *(arrow)* has a transitory perfusion abnormality.

FIGURE 52–12   D.

Circumferential Curves: The septal thallium accumulation is at 180 degrees *(arrow)* and has an abnormal (<30 percent) washout (difference between the two curves).

NOTE 1. LBBB, and occasionally RBBB, can cause a false positive scan for ischemia of the septum, possibly as a result of asynchronous septal contraction and/or septal perforating artery compression.

NOTE 2. One should suspect a bundle branch block rather than ischemia when only the septum is abnormal.

Chapter 53
Myocardial Infarction

NONTRANSMURAL INFARCTS ON STRESS/REST THALLIUM SCANS

Patient 1: Nontransmural Anteroseptal Infarct

FIGURE 53–1   A.

Stress and Rest Short Axis SPECT Scans: The diminished activity at the anteroseptal junction is seen on both examinations involving the same amount of muscle—a "fixed" perfusion defect (s = septum; l = lateral wall).

FIGURE 53–1   B.

Stress and Rest Horizontal Long Axis SPECT Scans (s = septum; l = lateral wall).

FIGURE 53–1   C.

Stress and Rest Vertical Long Axis SPECT Scans.

Illustration continued on following page

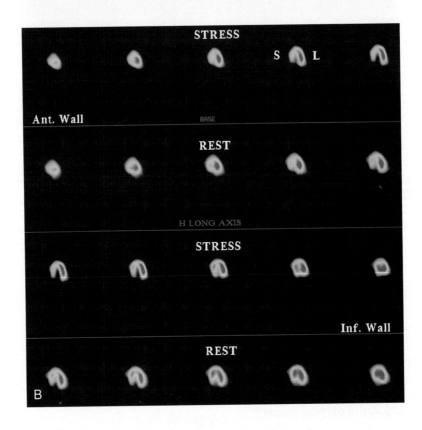

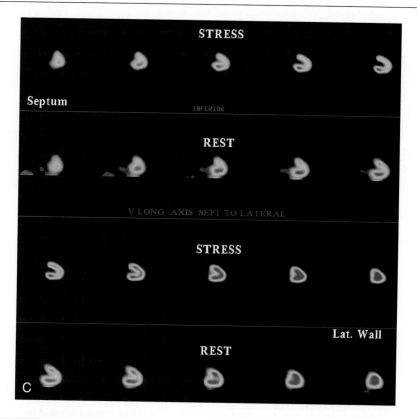

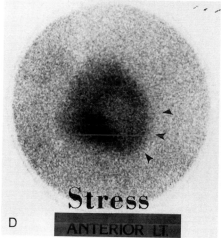

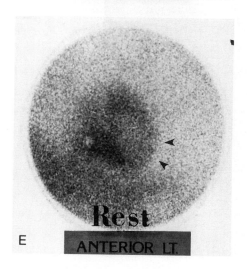

Patient 2: Nontransmural Anteroseptal and Apical Infarct

FIGURE 53–1   D and E.

Stress and Rest Anterior Planar Scans: The distal anterior wall and the apex have diminished thallium *(arrowheads)*.

FIGURE 53–1   F and G.

Stress and Rest 60 Degree LAO Scans: The septum has a fixed perfusion deficit, appearing thinner than the other walls. There is greater thallium accumulation in the posteroinferior wall than normal.

NOTE 1. If there is persistent thallium activity within a myocardial infarct, we define this as nontransmural. There appears to be no relationship between a nontransmural infarct on thallium scanning and the presence of Q waves on EKG.

NOTE 2. Increased activity in the posterior walls on planar scanning suggests an abnormality in the more anterior walls.

Illustration continued on following page

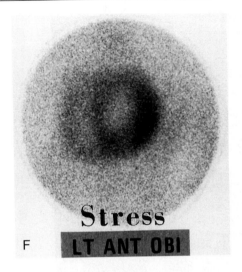

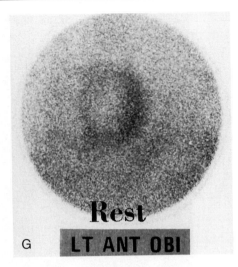

TRANSMURAL MYOCARDIAL INFARCTS ON STRESS/REST THALLIUM SCANS

Patient 1: Transmural Inferolateral Infarct Extending from Apex to Base

FIGURE 53–2   A.

Stress/Rest Short Axis SPECT Scans: There is no appreciable thallium in the inferolateral wall. The defect is present at both stress and rest.

FIGURE 53–2   B.

Stress/Rest Vertical Long Axis SPECT Scans.

FIGURE 53–2   C.

Stress/Rest Horizontal Long Axis SPECT Scans.

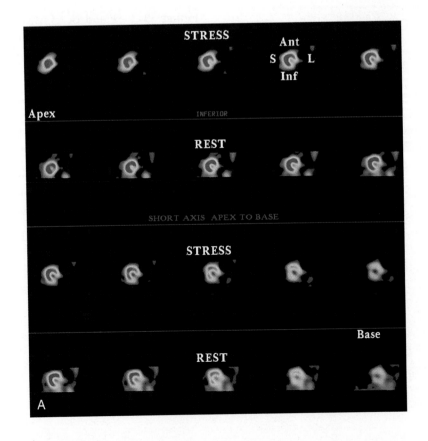

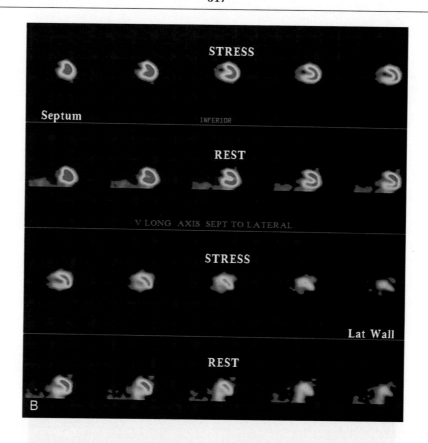

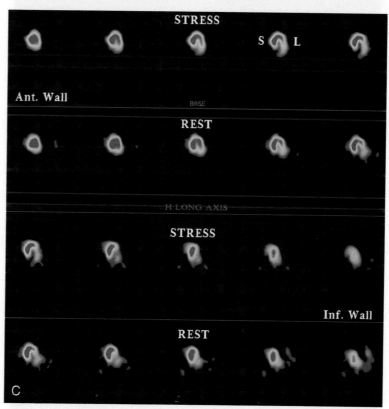

Illustration continued on following page

Patient 2: Multiple Infarcts

FIGURE 53–2   D and E.

Short Axis and Horizontal Long Axis Thallium SPECT Scan: There are fixed abnormalities involving the apex and inferior walls. The anterior wall has some viable, but ischemic, myocardium.

Patient 3: Inferior Infarct

FIGURE 53–2   F and G.

Stress and Rest Anterior Planar Scans: The entire inferior wall is infarcted (st = stress; r = rest).

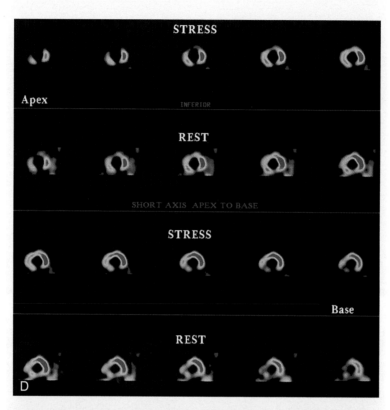

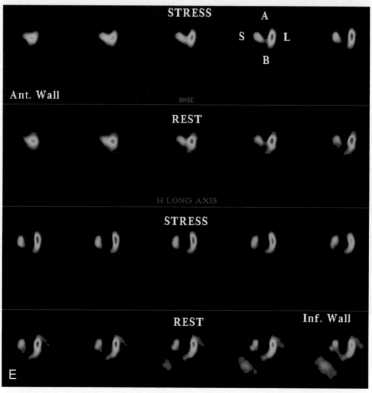

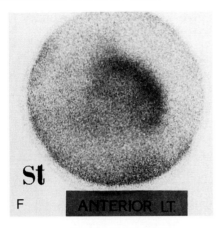

F ANTERIOR LT.

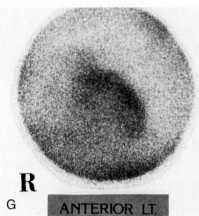

G ANTERIOR LT.

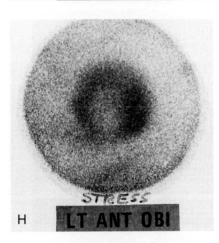

STRESS
H LT ANT OBI

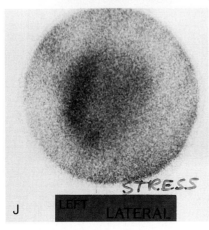

STRESS
J LEFT LATERAL

FIGURE 53–2 H and I.
Stress and Rest 45 Degree LAO Planar Scans: The inferior wall infarct is not as well seen, since this view sees the inferior wall "head-on."

FIGURE 53–2 J and K.
Stress and Rest Lateral Planar Scans: The inferior wall infarct extends up to the inferoapical junction.

NOTE. Transmural infarcts almost always have Q waves on EKGs.

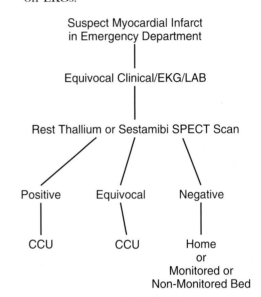

Suspect Myocardial Infarct
in Emergency Department

|

Equivocal Clinical/EKG/LAB

|

Rest Thallium or Sestamibi SPECT Scan

Positive   Equivocal   Negative

CCU   CCU   Home
                                 or
                                 Monitored or
                                 Non-Monitored Bed

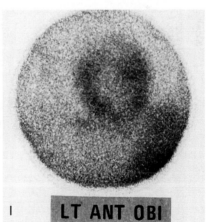

I LT ANT OBI

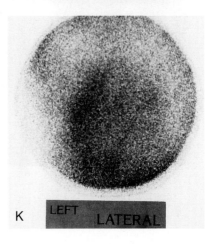

K LEFT LATERAL

REST THALLIUM MYOCARDIAL INFARCTION (MI) SCANS

Patient 1: Multiple Infarcts

FIGURE 53–3   A.

Short Axis SPECT Scan: The transmural inferior infarct extends from the base to just proximal to the apex. No residual viable myocardium is evident. There is also a smaller nontransmural anteroapical infarct.

Patient 2: Anteroseptal and Inferior Infarcts

FIGURE 53–3   B.

Short Axis SPECT Scan: The only "normal" myocardium is in the lateral wall. There is a small amount of viable myocardium in the septum.

Patient 3: Apical, Inferior, and Septal Infarcts

FIGURE 53–3   C.

Anterior Planar Scan: The infarct is well defined, involving the distal inferior wall and the apex.

FIGURE 53–3   D.

Forty-five Degree LAO Planar Scan: The infarct extends into the apex and septum *(arrowheads)*.

Patient 4: Five Year Old with Coronary Fistula and Anteroapical Infarct

FIGURE 53–3   E and F.

Anterior and 45 Degree LAO Planar Scan: The anteroapical myocardium has diminished thallium, indicating a nontransmural infarct with viable myocardium.

NOTE 1. Indications for resting myocardial imaging include (1) detection of an acute myocardial infarct; (2) detection of viable myocardium after MI; (3) detection of "hibernating" myocardium; and (4) detection of rest ischemia.

NOTE 2. A rest thallium or ^{99m}Tc-sestamibi scan can detect an acute MI immediately upon occurrence in virtually all cases, partly owing to the infarct and partly to the surrounding stunned myocardium and ischemic myocardium. A repeat resting scan in 3+ weeks will demonstrate a smaller infarct zone, since the stunned myocardium will have returned to normal.

NOTE 3. A rest thallium or sestamibi MI scan cannot distinguish a new infarct from an old one. ^{99m}Tc-pyrophosphate can distinguish acute infarcts from older ones within 10 days of their occurrence.

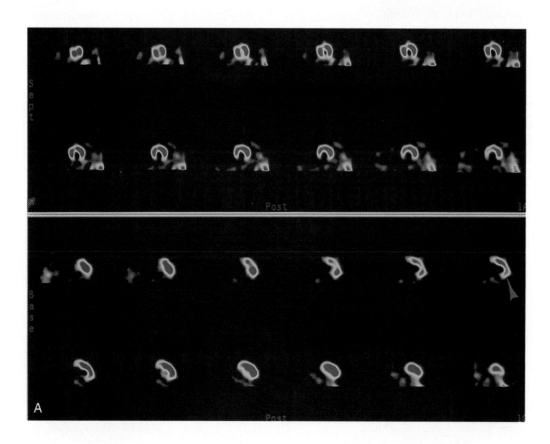

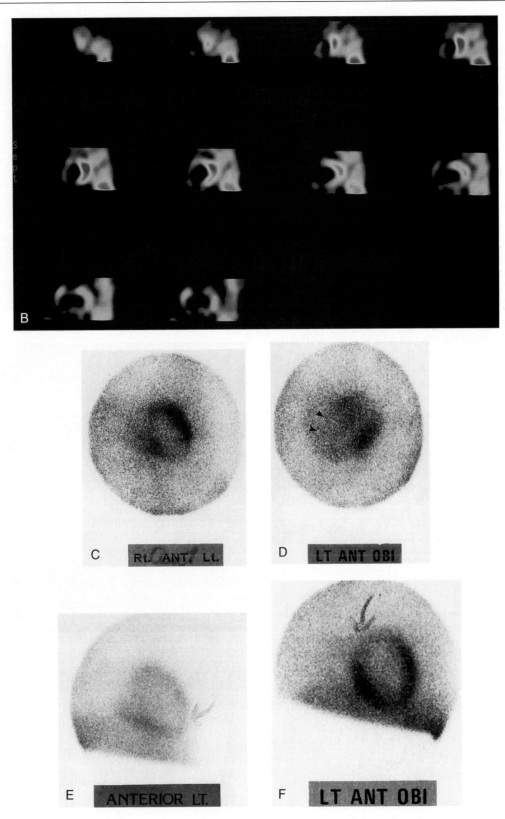

NOTE 4. Viable myocardium in an infarct zone can be better detected with thallium than with ^{99m}Tc-sestamibi.

NOTE 5. The SPECT scan, with its greater contrast, may better detect viable myocardium than planar imaging.

ACUTE MYOCARDITIS

Patient: Twenty-one Year Old with Acute Onset of Chest Pain

FIGURE 53–4   A.
Immediate Vertical Long Axis Thallium-201 Resting Myocardial Infarct SPECT Scan: The scan was performed 8 hours after admission and 10 hours after the onset of symptoms. The scan is normal.

FIGURE 53–4   B.
Eight Hour Delayed Vertical Long Axis Thallium SPECT Scan: The anterior wall now has markedly reduced blood flow.

FIGURE 53–4   C.
Eighteen Hour Coronal ^{99m}Tc-PYP SPECT Scan: This was performed immediately after the thallium examination. There are three areas of abnormal pyrophosphate accumulation: the anterior wall and the inferoapical and posteroinferior myocardium.

NOTE 1. This patient had elevated CPK values and anterior hypokinesia at the time of the scans. A coronary angiogram demonstrated perfectly normal coronary arteries. An endocardial biopsy demonstrated inflammatory cells and myocardial vacuoles.

NOTE 2. It is distinctly unusual for thallium to be normal in the face of myocardial infarction due to coronary artery disease. In acute myocarditis, with patent coronary arteries, the result may be dependent upon the stage of the disease.

NOTE 3. The abnormality seen on the delayed rest thallium scan is probably due to reduction in blood flow from myocardial necrosis and edema. The early scan may have reflected more normal flow and viable myocardium at that time.

NOTE 4. Separate areas of myocardial uptake of ^{99m}Tc-pyrophosphate is indicative of myocarditis and unlikely to represent a coronary artery process.

Cross References

Chapter 53: Myocardial Infarction—Rest Thallium MI Scans

Chapter 57: Infections—Viral Myocarditis

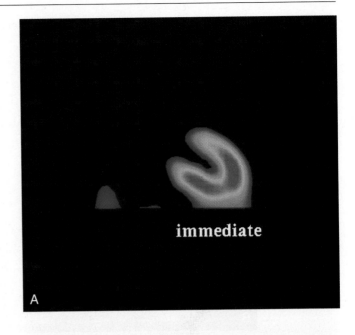

A

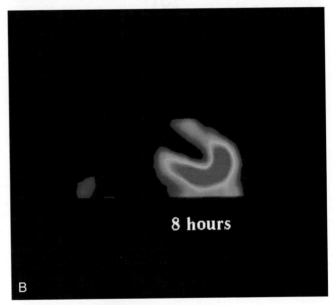

B

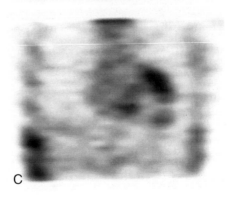

C

Chapter 54

^{99m}Tc-Pyrophosphate Scanning

NORMAL ^{99m}Tc-PYROPHOSPHATE (PYP) MYOCARDIAL INFARCT (MI) SCANS

FIGURE 54–1 A to D.

Planar ^{99m}Tc-PYP MI Scans: There is no accumulation of the radiopharmaceutical in the myocardium. The heart is just to the left of the xyphoid.

NOTE 1. ^{99m}Tc-PYP is best used if there is a history of previous MI and if a question of a new one exists.

NOTE 2. A ^{99m}Tc-PYP scan is most accurate 48 hours to 10 days after the event.

NOTE 3. Cardiac enzymes, if high enough, are usually sufficient for the diagnosis of acute MI. However, if the peaks were missed or the values nondiagnostic, ^{99m}Tc-PYP, especially with SPECT, can be useful.

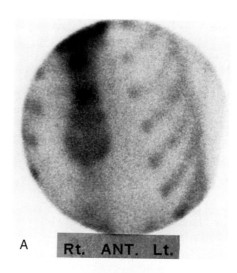

A   Rt. ANT. Lt.

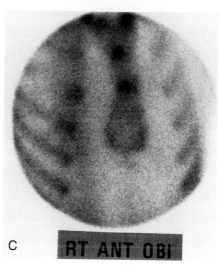

C   RT ANT OBl

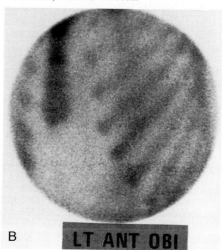

B   LT ANT OBl

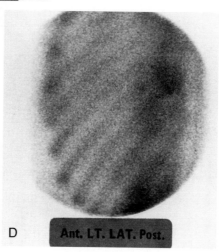

D   Ant. LT. LAT. Post.

ACUTE MYOCARDIAL INFARCT ON
^{99m}Tc-PYROPHOSPHATE SCANS

Patient 1: Apical Infarct

FIGURE 54–2 A to D.
Planar Scans: There is a small focus of activity between the ribs *(arrow)*, best seen on the anterior and RAO views.

Patient 2: Lateral Wall Infarct

FIGURE 54–2 E to H.
Planar Scans: The uptake in the lateral wall extends into the inferior and anterior walls, possibly representing areas of partial infarction or ischemia.

Patient 3: Subendocardial Infarct

FIGURE 54–2 I.
Planar Scans: The LAO view demonstrates a cavity surrounded by radiolabeled muscle.

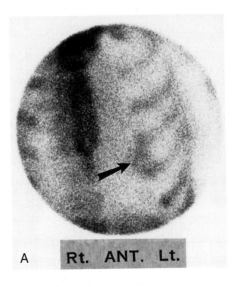

A   Rt. ANT. Lt.

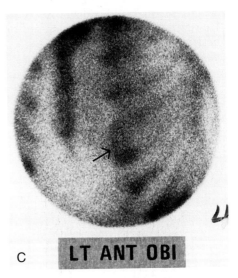

C   LT ANT OBI

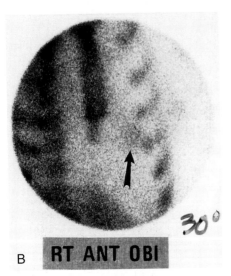

B   RT ANT OBI

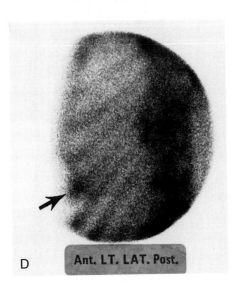

D   Ant. LT. LAT. Post.

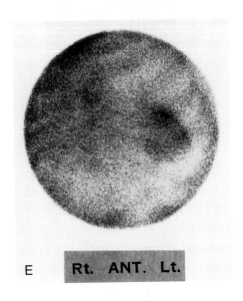

E   Rt. ANT. Lt.

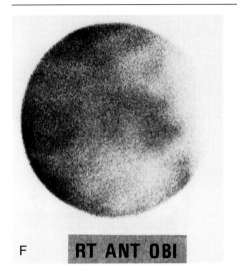

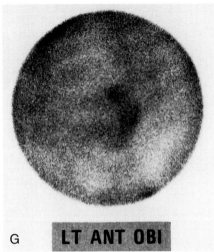

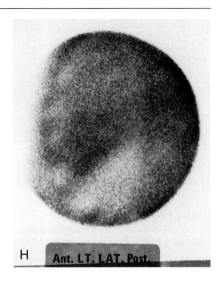

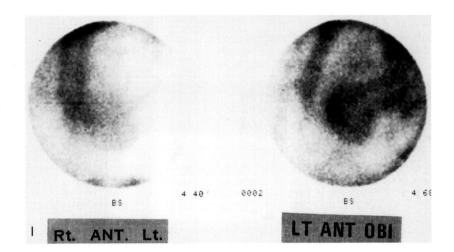

Patient 4: Right Ventricular Infarct

FIGURE 54–2 J.

Planar Scan: The inferior wall of the right ventricle *(arrow)* is abnormal, along with a subendocardial infarct of the left ventricle.

Illustration continued on following page

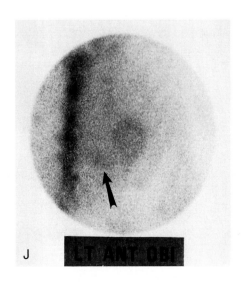

FIGURE 54–2 K.

Computer-Enhanced Scan: The right ventricular abnormality is more obvious.

Patient 5: Apical Infarct

FIGURE 54–2 L.

Anterior Planar Scan: The rib and costal cartilage activity obscures the myocardial activity.

FIGURE 54–2 M and N.

SPECT Scan: The apical activity extends along the septum.

Patient 6: Rib Fractures

FIGURE 54–2 O.

Anterior Planar Scan: There are three rib fractures, presumably the cause of the patient's left-sided chest pain.

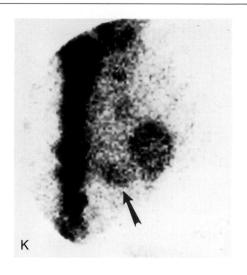

K

NOTE 1. A SPECT scan is more sensitive than planar imaging in detecting abnormal activity as well as in delineating muscle vs. blood pool.

NOTE 2. At least 3 to 5 hours should pass between injection of the medium and scanning in order to clear the blood pool. In almost all cases, ^{99m}Tc-PYP injected in the afternoon with the scan performed the following morning will eliminate the persistent blood pool that could confuse the issue.

NOTE 3. Right ventricular infarcts are difficult to evaluate with ^{99m}Tc-PYP, although SPECT, especially with multihead detectors, may improve sensitivity.

NOTE 4. A subendocardial infarct is suggested by diffuse uptake in all walls of the left ventricle.

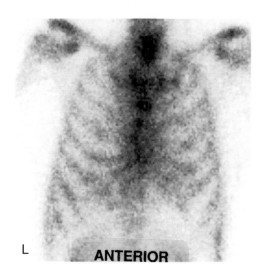

L **ANTERIOR**

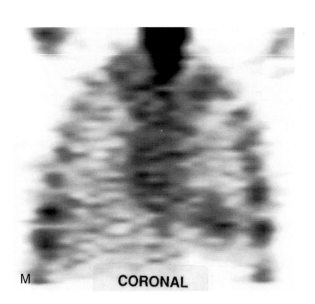

M **CORONAL**

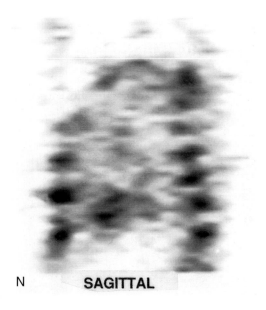

N **SAGITTAL**

PROCESSES THAT CAUSE MYOCARDIAL NECROSIS RESULTING IN POSITIVE MYOCARDIAL ^{99m}Tc-PYP SCANS

Acute myocardial infarction	Irradiation
Extension of previous infarct	Malignant or infected pericardial effusions
Severe angina pectoris	Cardiotoxic drugs
Pericarditis/myocarditis, including Chagas' disease	Cardiomyopathies
	Heart transplant rejection
Amyloidosis	Trauma with severe myocardial contusion
Hyperparathyroidism	Hyperphosphatemia
Electrical shock, including direct current cardioversion	Anoxic myocardial damage

Cross Reference

Chapter 11: Soft Tissue Abnormalities—Myocardial Infarction with MDP

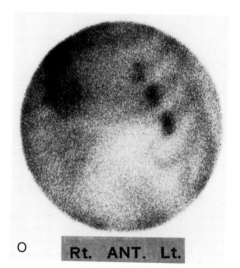

ANOXIC CARDIOMYOPATHY

Patient 1: Severe Congestive Heart Failure (CHF) Following Hypotensive Episode

FIGURE 54–3   A and B.

Twenty-four Hour Coronal and Sagittal SPECT Tc-PYP Scans: The massive heart has diffusely increased activity, indicating ongoing necrosis.

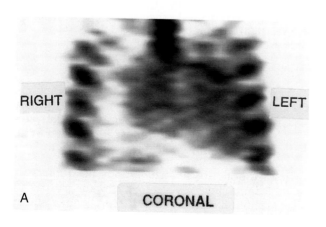

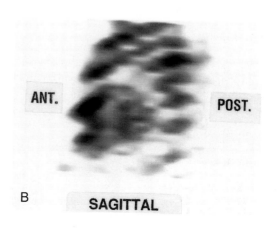

CARDIAC AMYLOIDOSIS

FIGURE 54–4   A.
Coronal SPECT ^{99m}Tc-Pyrophosphate Scan: The interventricular septum *(arrow)* has marked radiopharmaceutical accumulation, as does the liver.

FIGURE 54–4   B.
Transverse SPECT ^{99m}Tc-Pyrophosphate Scan: The lateral wall *(arrowheads)* is also abnormal.

NOTE. Cardiac amyloidosis is most often seen on bone scan as an asymptomatic process and is believed to be "senile amyloidosis."

Cross References

Chapter 11: Soft Tissue Abnormalities—Senile Amyloid of the Heart on Bone Scan; Diffuse Liver Activity

Chapter 14: Amyloid Liver Disease

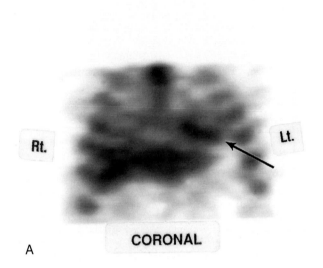

A   CORONAL

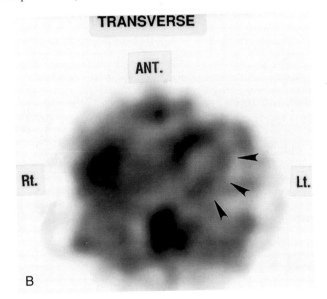

TRANSVERSE

ANT.

Rt.   Lt.

B

Chapter 55

Radionuclide Ventriculography

NORMAL MULTIPLE GATED ACQUISITION (MUGA)

Radionuclide Ventriculography

FIGURE 55–1   A.
Forty-five Degree LAO MUGA: All walls of both ventricles can be seen contracting synchronously (L = left ventricle; R = right ventricle).

FIGURE 55–1   B.
Wall Motion Histogram: The apex and all walls contract toward the isocenter.

FIGURE 55–1   C and D.
Three-Dimensional Surface Reconstruction of Radionuclide Ventriculogram (Gated SPECT RBC Scan): The view is from the right looking at the septum. The white color of the septum indicates normal contractility. The yellow-green represents reduced motion, normal for the membranous septum. The inferior, apical, and anterior contract toward the isocenter. ED = End diastole; ES = end systole.

NOTE 1. A complete MUGA study includes 15 degree RAO, anterior, 45 degree LAO, and left lateral acquisitions. Three-dimensional gated SPECT scans are now available.

NOTE 2. Although echocardiography has replaced radionuclide ventriculography for cardiac wall motion studies, the MCCGA scan is still the most accurate measure of ejection fractions.

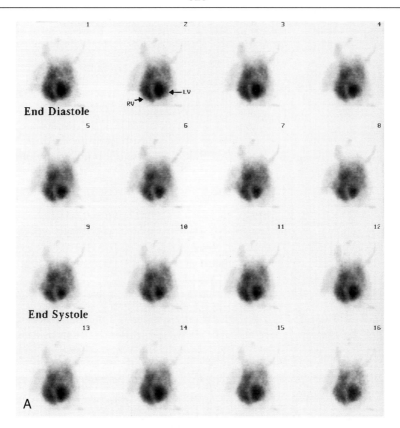

End Diastole

End Systole

A

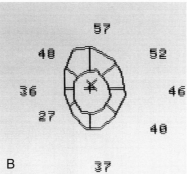

B

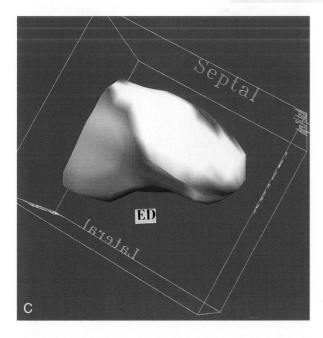

ED

C

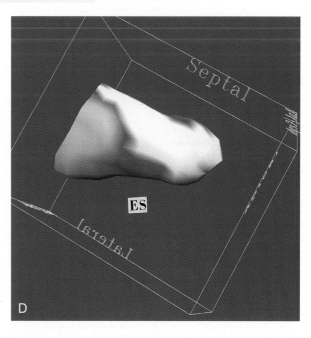

ES

D

VENTRICULAR ANEURYSM

FIGURE 55–2   A.
End-diastole MUGA in 30 Degree RAO View.

FIGURE 55–2   B.
End-systole MUGA: The apex gets larger with systole.

FIGURE 55–2   C.
Wall Motion Histogram: The dyskinetic motion of the apex, measured at 45 degree LAO, can be seen.

FIGURE 55–2   D.
PA Chest X-ray: The boot-shaped heart should raise the question of a ventricular aneurysm.

NOTE. Dyskinesia is the classic finding for aneurysm, although immediately after an infarct the stunned myocardium and infarcted muscle may be temporarily dyskinetic.

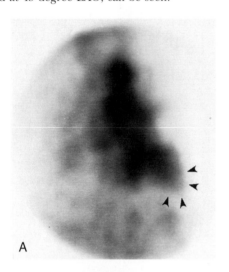

A

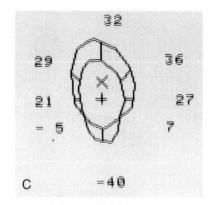

C

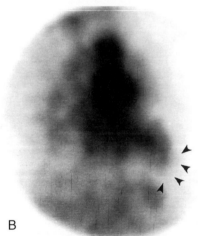

B

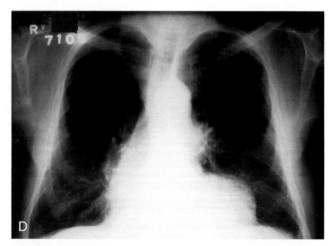

D

GLOBAL HYPOKINESIA

Patient 1: Idiopathic Cardiomyopathy (Early)

FIGURE 55–3   A.
MUGA: There is poor contractility of all walls except the base. The LVEF = 42% (normal = ≥ 53 +/–3%).

FIGURE 55–3   B.
Wall Motion Histogram: The motion of the base is better appreciated on the histogram.

NOTE. The last myocardium to lose contractility in virtually all forms of cardiomyopathy is at the base of the left ventricle.

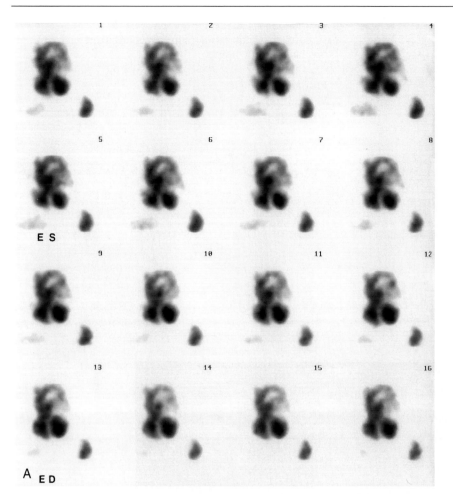

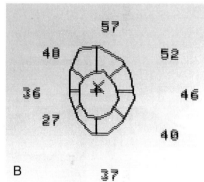

APICAL AKINESIA FROM INFARCTION

FIGURE 55–4   A and B.

Resting MUGA: The left ventricular apex contracts to the same
extent as the right apex. LVEF = 47%.

Illustration continued on following page

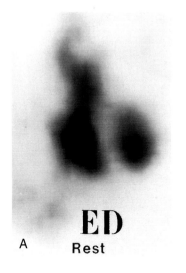

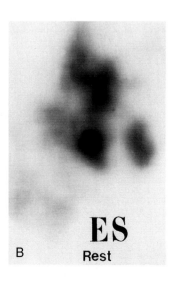

FIGURE 55–4   C and D.

Stress MUGA: The overall contractility is improved except for the LV apex, which does not reach the same level as the RV apex. LVEF = 51%.

FIGURE 55–4   E.

Stress Wall Motion Histogram: The apical akinesia is easily appreciated on the graph.

FIGURE 55–4   F.

Vertical Long Axis Stress/Rest Thallium SPECT Scan: The transmural apical infarct is evident. B = Base; Ap = apex.

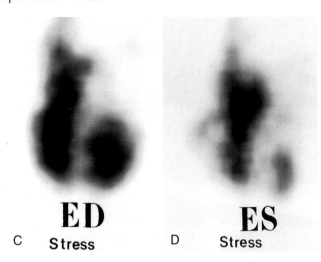

C   Stress

D   Stress

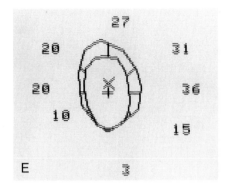

E

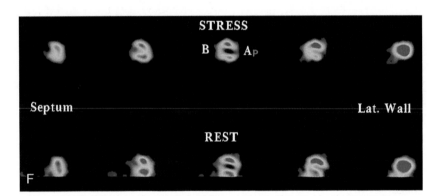

RIGHT VENTRICULAR CONTUSION

Patient 1: Steering Wheel Injury

FIGURE 55–5   A.

End-diastole MUGA: The right ventricle is moderately dilated.

FIGURE 55–5   B.

End-systole MUGA: The right ventricle does not contract normally, especially the apex. The RV ejection fraction was 35% (normal is >40%).

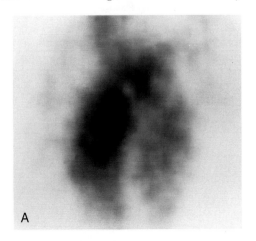

A

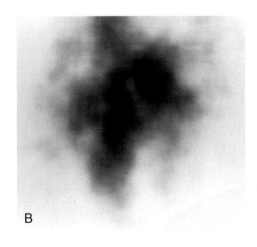

B

Patient 2: 11 Year Old Boy who Flipped an All-Terrain Vehicle

FIGURE 55–5 C.

Colloid Liver/Spleen Scan: The persistent blood pool after 1 hour can be seen with a halo of decreased activity due to hemopericardium and cardiac tamponade.

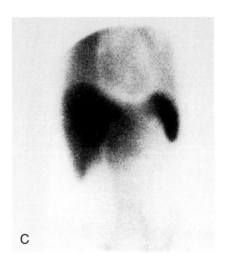

C

NOTE 1. The thorax gets more rigid with age, transmitting a blow to the precordium directly to the right ventricle, the anterior ventricle chamber. In the younger age groups, the pliable thoracic cage may allow the heart to be pushed against the vertebral column, damaging the left ventricle.

NOTE 2. EKG changes are not reliable in the diagnosis of ventricular contusion, nor are ^{99m}Tc-pyrophosphate or thallium scans, especially when the right ventricle is involved.

Chapter 56
Miscellaneous

ASYMMETRIC SEPTAL HYPERTROPHY

FIGURE 56–1.

45 Degree LAO Planar Thallium Scan: The septum has increased thickness compared with the rest of the myocardium.

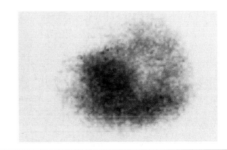

COR PULMONALE WITH SEVERE RIGHT VENTRICULAR HYPERTROPHY

FIGURE 56–2.

Planar Rest Thallium Scan: The right ventricle is well seen *(arrowheads)*, with myocardial hypertrophy and dilatation. There is an inferior wall myocardial infarct involving both ventricles.

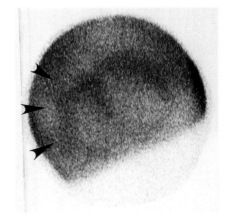

NOTE. If the right ventricle is well seen, it probably is hypertrophic.

Cross Reference

Chapter 52: Cardiac Ischemia—Infarct with Ischemia

RIGHT HEART FAILURE

Patient 1

FIGURE 56–3   A.

Anterior Technetium Blood Flow Study: During the pass of the radiopharmaceutical bolus through the right atrium, there is reflux down the inferior vena cava (I = IVC; A = aorta).

Patient 2

FIGURE 56–3   B.

Posterior ^{99m}Tc-DTPA Renal Blood Flow Scan: The right heart reflux is so severe that both the azygos and the hemiazygos veins fill retrograde for a long distance. The aorta is not well seen. The structure on the left empties in a cephalic direction.

Patient 3

FIGURE 56–3   C.

Posterior ^{99m}Tc-DTPA Renal Blood Flow Scan: The reflux into the inferior vena cava and hepatic veins occurs with each atrial systole (as).

Cross Reference

Chapter 13: Hepatomegaly—Right Atrial Reflux and Congestive Hepatomegaly

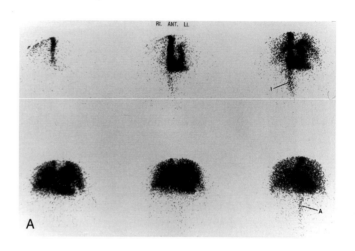

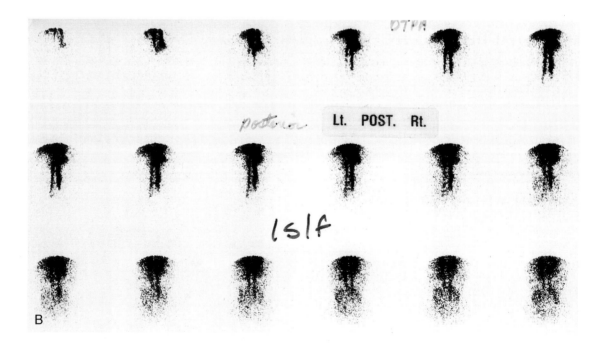

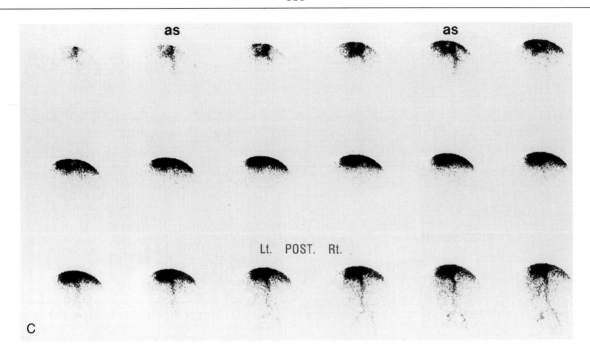

as   as

Lt. POST. Rt.

C

RIGHT-TO-LEFT SHUNTS

FIGURE 56–4   A to E.

^{99m}Tc Macroaggregate Albumin Lung Perfusion Scan; Multiple Views of the Entire Body: There is an abnormal distribution of the macroaggregated particles in the brain, kidneys, stomach, bowel, and even the extremities.

NOTE. Less than 10 percent of the injected particles can be outside the lungs in the normal situation.

Cross Reference

Chapter 44: Right-to-Left-Shunt with Pulmonary Embolism

Illustration continued on following page

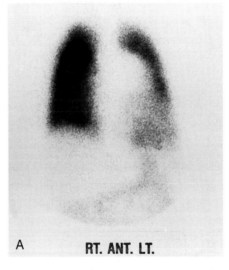

A   RT. ANT. LT.

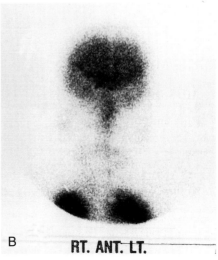

B   RT. ANT. LT.

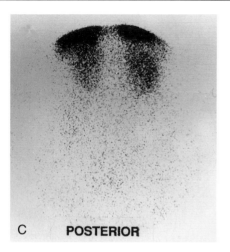

C   **POSTERIOR**

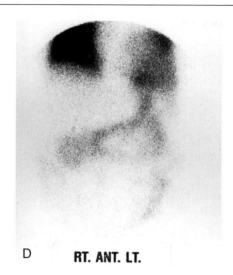

D   **RT. ANT. LT.**

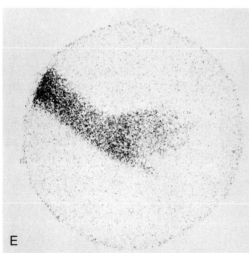

E

RIGHT-TO-LEFT SHUNTS
1. Cyanotic congenital heart disease
2. Eisenmenger's reaction: reversal of left-to-right shunt
3. Pulmonary hypertension with patent foramen ovale (including pulmonary embolism)
4. Pulmonary vascular dysplasia

Chapter 57
Cardiac Inflammation

PERICARDITIS/MYOCARDITIS

Patient 1: AIDS Myocarditis

FIGURE 57–1   A and B.
Gallium Scan: There is intense gallium activity in the pericardium/myocardium.

Patient 2: Active Idiopathic Cardiomyopathy

FIGURE 57–1   C.
Seventy-two Hour Gallium Scan: The massive heart has persistent gallium activity, indicating an active process.

Patient 3: Active Dilated Cardiomyopathy

FIGURE 57–1   D and E.
Gallium SPECT Coronal and Sagittal Scans: The massive heart has abnormal gallium accumulation in the muscle and/or pericardium.

Patient 4: Cocaine Myocarditis

FIGURE 57–1   F.
Twenty-four Hour ^{111}In-WBC Scan: The myocardial uptake *(arrow)* indicates an area of inflammation or infarction.

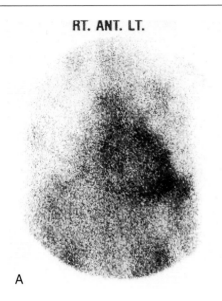

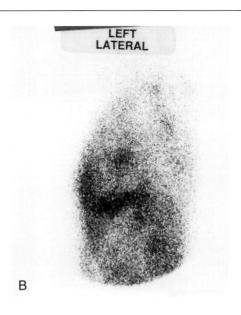

A

B

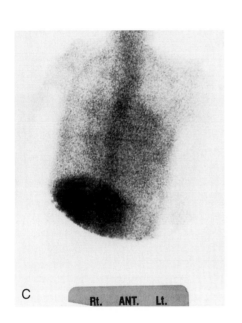

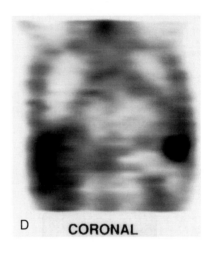

C

D   **CORONAL**

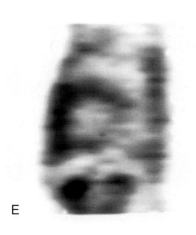

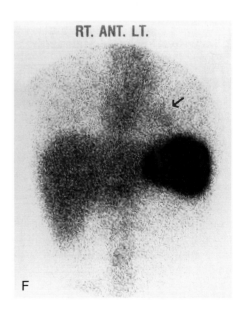

E

F

Illustration continued on following page

Patient 5: Viral Myocarditis

Figure 57–1   G.

Forty-eight Hour ^{111}In-WBC Scan: The diffuse myocardial uptake indicates active inflammation.

NOTE 1. Myocarditis cannot be distinguished from pericarditis.

NOTE 2. Delayed imaging with WBC scanning can avoid mistaking persistent blood pool for myocarditis.

NOTE 3. WBCs can accumulate in myocardial infarcts as well as in inflammatory lesions.

Cross References

Chapter 53: Myocardial Infarction—Acute Myocarditis

Chapter 71: Infectious Diseases—Mediastinitis; Bacterial Aortitis and Valvular Infections

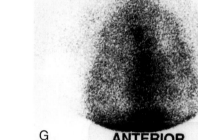

G   **ANTERIOR**

BACTERIAL ENDOCARDITIS

Patient 1: Thirty-nine Year Old Female with Aortic Valvular Infection

Figure 57–2   A and B.

Anterior and Left Lateral Planar ^{111}In-WBC Scans: There is a focal accumulation of WBCs in the left chest that cannot be localized on the lateral view

Figure 57–2   C to E.

Coronal, Transverse, and Sagittal ^{111}In-WBC SPECT Scans: The abnormal white cell accumulation can be localized within the chest, to the region of the aortic valve.

Patient 2: Sixty-five Year Old Male with Aortic Valvular Prosthetic Infection

Figure 57–2   F.

Anterior Planar ^{111}In-WBC Scan: There is a barely perceptible focus of white cells overlying the aortic valvular region.

Figure 57–2   G.

Coronal ^{111}In-WBC SPECT Scan: The infected valvular prosthesis can be identified with much greater assurance.

NOTE. There are significant numbers of false negative scans, but SPECT scanning certainly increases the sensitivity. Echocardiography can detect smaller vegetations.

Cross Reference

Chapter 71: Infectious Diseases—Bacterial Aortitis

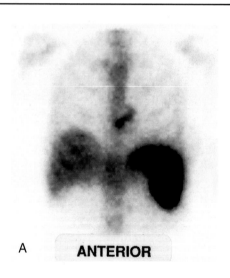

A   **ANTERIOR**

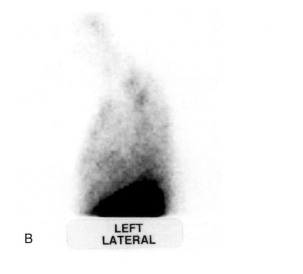

B LEFT
LATERAL

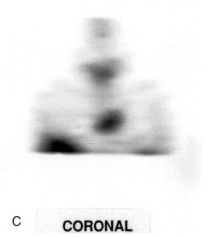

C CORONAL

TRANSVERSE

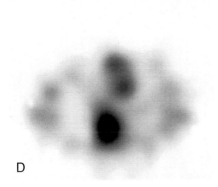

D

E SAGITTAL

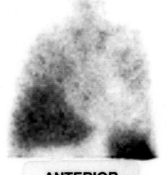

F ANTERIOR

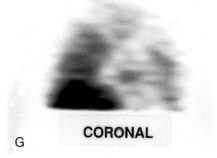

G CORONAL

SEPTIC THROMBUS

FIGURE 57–3   A and B.

Three Hour ⁹⁹ᵐTc-HMPAO WBC Scan: There is a focus of increased WBC aggregation in the apex of the left ventricle.

FIGURE 57–3   C.

Eighteen Hour ⁹⁹ᵐTc-HMPAO WBC Scan: The blood pool has cleared, leaving the WBC focus in the cardiac apex.

FIGURE 57–3   D.

Lower Extremities WBC Scan: Septic emboli have lodged in each thigh.

Cross Reference

Chapter 48—Lung Abscesses due to Infected Central Venous Catheter

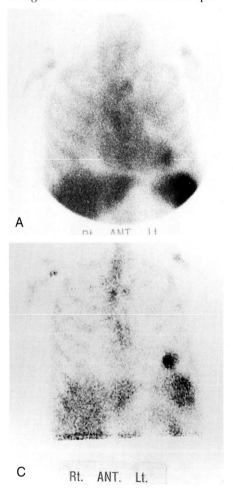

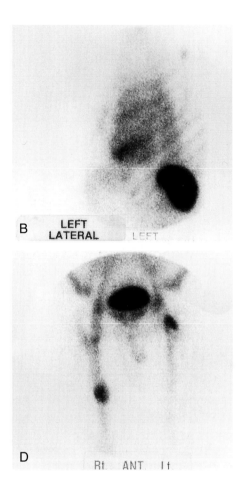

INFECTED PACEMAKER

FIGURE 57–4.

Forty-eight Hour Gallium Scan: The gallium along the periphery of the pacemaker *(arrow)* in the right upper thorax indicates an infection.

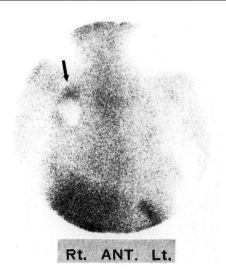

Chapter 58

Normal/Normal Variants

VALUE OF NUCLEAR VENOGRAM

1. Twenty-five gauge butterfly needles will cannulate almost any vein.

2. No pain on injection as opposed to contrast venography.

3. No side effects, no renal toxicity.

4. Can obtain V/Q scan if MAA is used to look for silent pulmonary emboli.

5. If done as routine part of V/Q scan, nuclear venogram can change probability of indeterminate V/Q; i.e., a positive venogram would upgrade an indeterminate V/Q scan to high probability. (Silent DVT occurs with PE 70+% of time.)

6. Silent pulmonary emboli will occur in 15 to 35% of acute thrombophlebitis.

7. MAA is diluted in normal saline; therefore, it is isotonic and provides a physiologic image of venous blood flow.

8. Nuclear venography is highly accurate in the pelvis and better than Doppler in the calves.

CRITERIA FOR POSITIVE NUCLEAR VENOGRAM

1. Obstruction of venous channels

2. Collaterals

3. Filling defects

4. Poorly filled deep veins

PREDISPOSING FACTORS FOR DEEP VENOUS THROMBOSIS

1. Malignancy

2. Venous stasis: bed rest, varicosity, long air or land travel

3. Recent blood transfusion

4. Recent surgery

5. Congestive heart failure

6. Infection

7. Pregnancy, especially immediately post partum

8. Hypercoagulability

NOTE 1. Clinical examination for deep venous thrombosis (DVT) is accurate about 30 percent of the time.

NOTE 2. A high percentage of patients with DVT will develop postphlebitic syndrome: pain, swelling, and erythema but no recurrent thrombosis.

NOTE 3. Chronic changes may be difficult to distinguish from acute changes unless a new pattern is seen on repeat venography.

NORMAL RADIONUCLIDE VENOGRAM

FIGURE 58–1   A.
Calf ⁹⁹ᵐTc-MAA Venogram: The deep veins appear as straight channels separate from the knee marker (k). The saphenous veins would be adjacent to the marker (T = ankle and knee tourniquets).

FIGURE 58–1   B.
Thigh ⁹⁹ᵐTc-MAA Venogram: The femoral vein (superficial femoral vein), the main deep vein of the thigh, has a curvilinear course, mirror-imaged on the opposite side.

FIGURE 58–1   C.
Pelvic ⁹⁹ᵐTc-MAA Venogram: The inferior vena cava and the iliofemoral veins can be well seen with or without ankle and knee tourniquets. The common iliac veins are less intense owing to inflow from the internal iliac veins and increased attenuation as the veins course posteriorly to form the inferior vena cava.

NOTE. The popliteal veins often have gaps in them that are not due to attenuation by bone or stretching with legs extended.

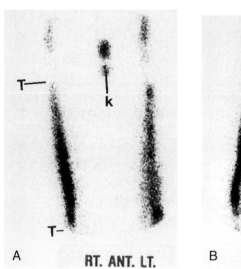

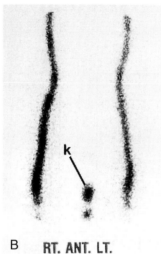

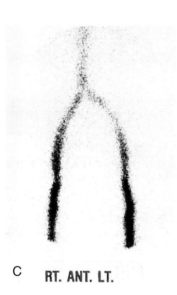

DOUBLE INFERIOR VENA CAVA (IVC)

Patient 1

FIGURE 58–2   A.
⁹⁹ᵐTc-MAA Venogram: There are two IVCs, a normal variant. The left one crosses at the renal level. No collaterals are seen.

Patient 2

FIGURE 58–2   B.
⁹⁹ᵐTc-MAA Venogram: There are two IVCs, the one on the left crossing at or above the diaphragm.

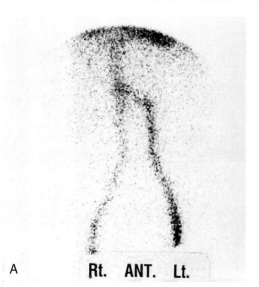

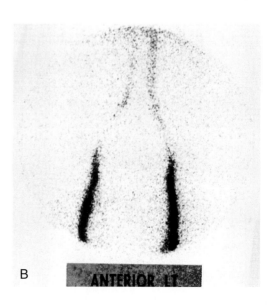

NORMAL SUPERIOR VENA CAVA

FIGURE 58–3.

Venogram: The injection was made in both arms simultaneously, demonstrating patent subclavian veins, innominate veins, and normal superior vena cava *(arrowheads)* (a = right atrium; v = right ventricle; p = main pulmonary trunk).

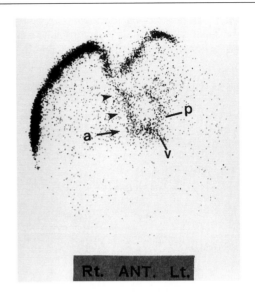

ANOMALOUS "DOUBLE" SUPERIOR VENA CAVA (SVC)

FIGURE 58–4   A.

SVC Venogram: The normal SVC drains the right side *(open arrow)*. The left side flows into an anomalous vein *(black arrow)*, which may cross over at the azygos level or fill the epidural venous plexus (midline vertical activity between the arrows).

Illustration continued on following page

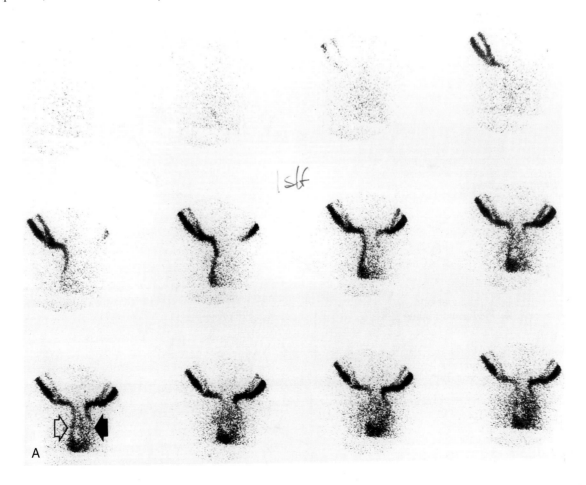

A

FIGURE 58–4   **B.**
Chest X-ray Detail: There is a soft tissue structure to the left of
the trachea *(arrow)* that represents the anomalous left SVC.

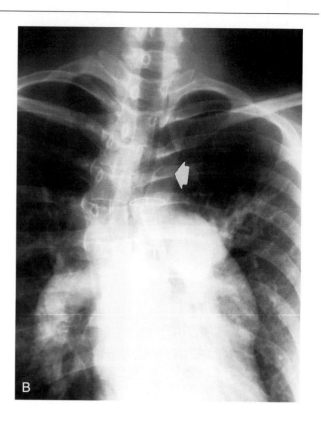

Chapter 59

Venous Thrombosis

CALF DEEP VENOUS THROMBOSIS

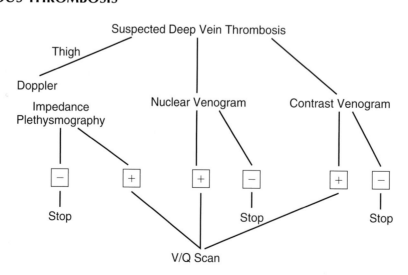

Patient 1

FIGURE 59–1   A.

Calf ^{99m}Tc-MAA Venogram: The left proximal calf demonstrates collateral bridging of some obstructed deep veins.

FIGURE 59–1   B.

Anteroposterior Contrast Venogram: The posterior tibial veins have filling defects from thrombi *(ink marks)*. Superficial collaterals are present.

Patient 2: "Fuzzy" Veins (Incomplete Filling of Collaterals or Normal Veins)

FIGURE 59–1   C.

Calf ^{99m}Tc-MAA Venogram of Left Leg: There are small, "fuzzy" veins seen adjacent to the patent veins. Right Leg: Although the ascending deep veins appear patent, there is a collateral *(arrowheads)* seen laterally, a finding only seen with DVT.

FIGURE 59–1   D.

Contrast Venogram: There are filling defects and poor filling of the peroneal and posterior tibial veins. The anterior tibial veins *(arrow)* are normal. The DVT was present in both calves.

Illustration continued on following page

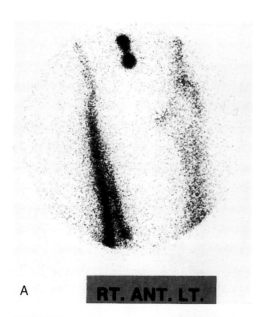

A

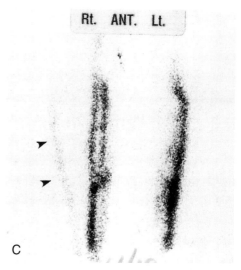

C

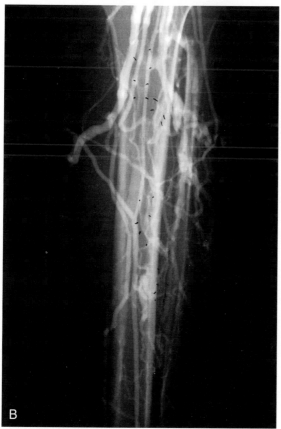

B

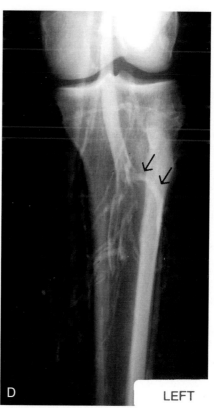

D

FIGURE 59–1   E.

^{99m}Tc-MAA Venogram 3 Weeks Later: There are now collaterals and incompetent perforators in the left calf and incomplete recanalization. The right calf deep veins are now patent.

NOTE 1. "Fuzzy" veins are probably small collateral veins or reflux into contributing veins adjacent to partially filled normal or collateral veins. When this is seen, it suggests nonocclusive thrombosis, late DVT with recanalization, or old scarred deep veins with valvular incompetence.

NOTE 2. The collaterals seen on a radionuclide venogram may not match those seen on a contrast venogram owing to the difference in densities and viscosities of the injected materials.

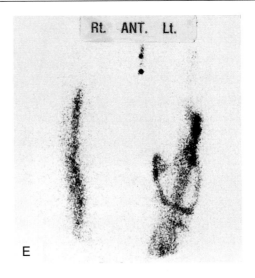

POPLITEAL DEEP VENOUS THROMBOSIS

Patient 1

FIGURE 59–2   A.

Calf ^{99m}Tc-MAA Venogram: The flow in the left calf deep veins abruptly terminates in a threadlike popliteal vein with multiple collaterals. A valve collects some MAA on the right *(arrow)*, next to the origin of a duplicate vein.

FIGURE 59–2   B.

Thigh Venogram: The superficial femoral vein is patent, but there are gaps *(arrows)* and collaterals, indicating extension of the clotting process proximally.

Patient 2: Bilateral Popliteal Thrombosis and Silent Pulmonary Embolism

FIGURE 59–2   C.

Calf ^{99m}Tc-MAA Venogram: The columns of deep venous flow end abruptly at the knees, with shunting into the saphenous veins.

FIGURE 59–2   D.

Thigh ^{99m}Tc-MAA Venogram: Multiple collaterals can be seen in both thighs, reconstituting the femoral veins proximally. The right saphenous vein overlies the knee marker *(arrow)*.

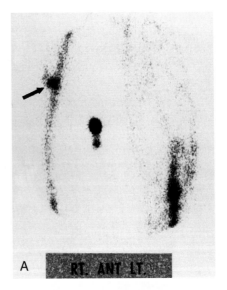

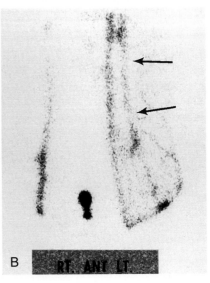

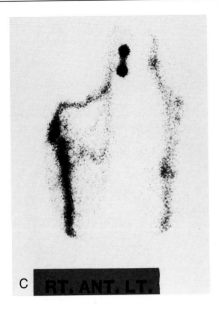

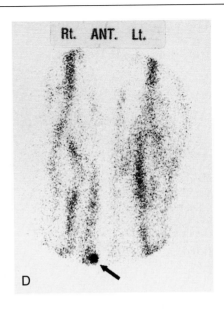

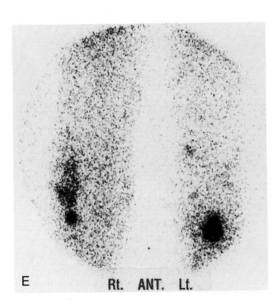

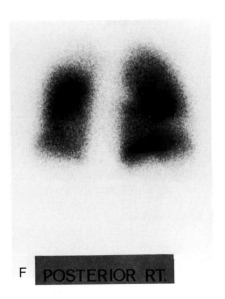

FIGURE 59–2   E.

Postvenography Scan: There is adherence of the ^{99m}Tc-MAA on clots in the popliteal region.

FIGURE 59–2   F and G.

Perfusion and Ventilation Lung Scans: There are several mismatched abnormalities, indicating a high probability for silent pulmonary emboli.

NOTE. Focal accumulation of the macroaggregated particles at the site of the clots is not always present in DVT; they may even be seen collecting under normal valves.

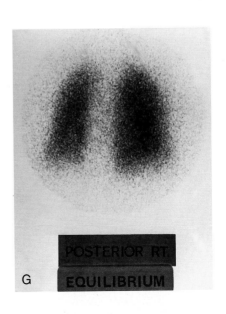

PELVIC DEEP VENOUS THROMBOSIS

Patient 1: Left Iliofemoral Thrombosis

FIGURE 59–3 A.

Pelvic ^{99m}Tc-MAA Venogram: The venous flow crosses from left to right through pudendal veins owing to obstruction of the left common iliac, external iliac, and common femoral veins.

Patient 2: Left Common Iliac Thrombosis

FIGURE 59–3 B.

Pelvic ^{99m}Tc-MAA Venogram: The left common iliac occlusion is bypassed by pudendal, transpelvic, and presacral collateral flow.

Patient 3: Phlegmasia Cerulea Dolens with Childbirth

FIGURE 59–3 C.

Pelvic ^{99m}Tc-MAA Venogram: The left iliofemoral veins are obstructed. There are numerous abdominal wall collaterals. The inferior vena cava is patent *(arrowhead)*.

Patient 4: Partial or Nonocclusive DVT, Acute vs. Chronic

FIGURE 59–3 D.

Pelvic ^{99m}Tc-MAA Venogram: The left femoral vein is "fuzzy" *(arrows)*, owing to reflux into contributing veins.

NOTE. Phlegmasia cerulea dolens is an old term for rapid, massive occlusion of the deep veins of an extremity, with pain, swelling, and skin mottling, and without an arterial abnormality. It may progress to gangrene ("venous gangrene"), with an attendant 45 percent mortality rate. The left leg is more commonly affected than the right. The condition is associated with malignant neoplasms, childbirth, recent surgery, trauma, ulcerative colitis, and congestive heart failure.

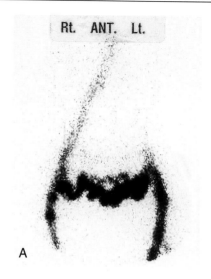

A

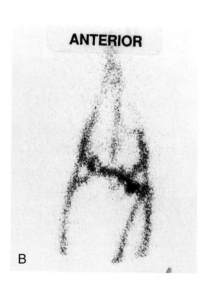

B

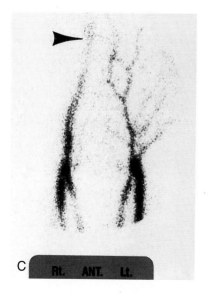

C

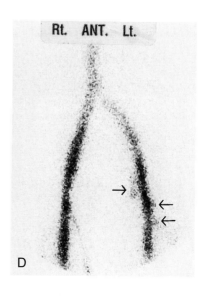

D

LIVER VISUALIZATION WITH IVC OBSTRUCTION

Patient 1

FIGURE 59–4   A.

Pelvic ^{99m}Tc-MAA Venogram: The iliofemoral veins and the IVC are not visualized, but numerous collaterals can be seen, including the inferior mesenteric vein *(arrow)*.

FIGURE 59–4   B.

Anterior Lung Scan: The liver has accumulated the labeled MAA diffusely. The spleen is not seen.

Patient 2

FIGURE 59–4   C.

Pelvic ^{99m}Tc-MAA Venogram: The inferior vena cava and common iliac veins are obstructed. There are no deep pelvic collaterals, only abdominal wall veins. The umbilical vein *(arrow)* drains into the liver *(curved arrow)*.

FIGURE 59–4   D and E.

Anterior and Right Lateral Lung Scan: A liver ''hot'' spot is evident.

Illustration continued on following page

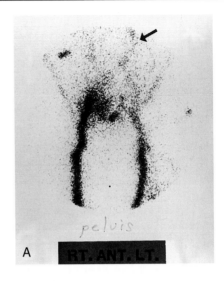

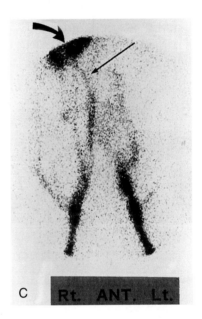

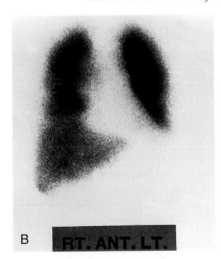

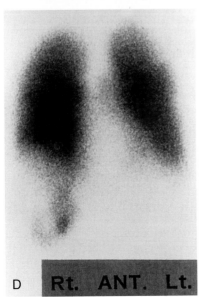

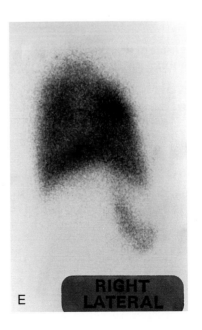

Patient 3

FIGURE 59–4 F.

Whole Body Lower Extremity Nuclear Venogram: The extensive abdominal collaterals shunt blood around pelvic venous and inferior vena caval thrombosis.

FIGURE 59–4 G.

Lung/Abdomen Scan: The liver is faintly seen owing to pelvic collaterals into the mesenteric and portal veins.

NOTE 1. Pelvic collaterals may include reverse flow in the internal iliac to hemorrhoidal veins, then to the inferior mesenteric vein, the splenic vein, and finally the portal vein into the liver.

NOTE 2. The umbilical vein drains into a small portion of the anterior right lobe of the liver.

NOTE 3. The inferior epigastric veins communicate with the internal mammary veins. The lateral abdominal wall veins drain into lateral thoracic veins. Both return blood via the superior vena cava. The paravertebral venous plexus can also be used as a collateral pathway.

Cross References

Chapter 18: "Hot" Spot in Liver

Chapter 59: Venous Thrombosis—Superior Vena Caval Obstruction

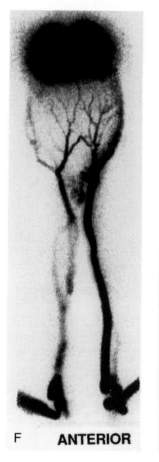

F ANTERIOR

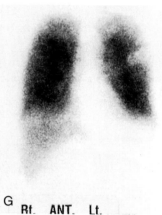

G Rt. ANT. Lt.

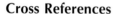

COMPRESSED VEIN VS. INTRALUMINAL CLOT

Patient 1: Thigh Hematoma with Vein Compression

FIGURE 59–5 A and B.

Anterior Nuclear Venogram: The left femoral vein is barely visible, although the veins are well filled above the inguinal ligament and in the distal thigh.

Patient 2: Seventy-one Year Old Male with Sudden Drop in Hematocrit Sent for GI Bleeding Scan

FIGURE 59–5 C and D.

Anterior Thigh Tagged RBC Scan: The femoral veins are draped over a photon-deficient mass that narrows the veins in segments. Veins not usually seen are present, including the deep femoral vein *(arrow)*.

Patient 3: Intraluminal Femoral Vein Clot in a Patient with Pulmonary Infarction

FIGURE 59–5 E.

Anterior Nuclear Venogram: There is decreased activity in the left femoral vein without collaterals. The right side has evidence of old venous disease with the presence of collaterals in the distal thigh.

FIGURE 59–5 F.

Contrast Venogram: There is intraluminal clot in the distal vein, with collaterals not seen on the radionuclide venogram.

NOTE 1. One should suspect DVT in a distal vein when it has less radioactivity than the proximal vein that it drains into.

NOTE 2. If the veins are displaced, a mass lesion should be suspected. Other clues include segmental or diffuse narrowing of the vein and visualization of normal veins that are not usually filled, e.g., deep femoral vein.

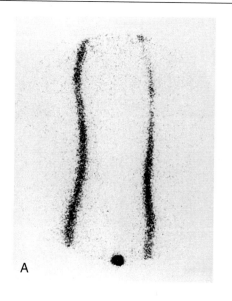

A

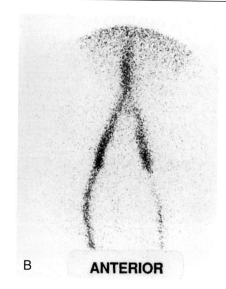

B   **ANTERIOR**

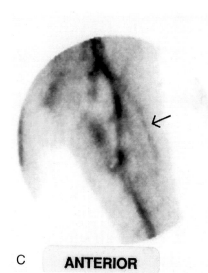

C   **ANTERIOR**

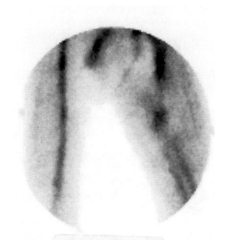

D   **Rt. ANT. Lt.**

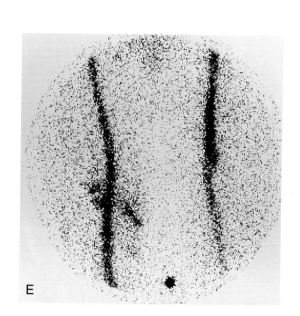

E

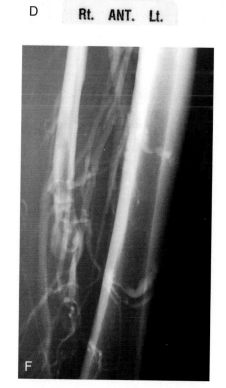

F

PELVIC VENOUS COMPRESSION

Patient 1: Neurogenic Bladder

FIGURE 59–6   A.

Pelvic ⁹⁹ᵐTc-MAA Venogram: The marked reduction in activity at the inguinal level raises the question of venous compression or attenuation by a pelvic mass.

Patient 2: Surgical Hematoma

FIGURE 59–6   B.

Pelvic ⁹⁹ᵐTc-MAA Venogram: The right iliofemoral veins are poorly seen, yet there are no collaterals.

NOTE. Prolonged compression by pelvic masses, including a neurogenic bladder, can cause venous thrombosis.

Cross Reference

Chapter 40: Bladder Abnormalities—Neurogenic Bladder with Secondary Hydronephrosis

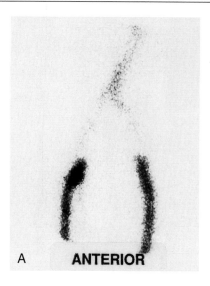

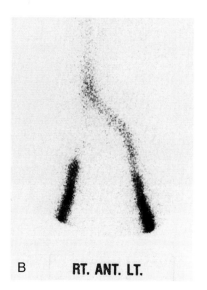

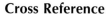

COMPRESSED INFERIOR VENA CAVA (IVC) BY ENLARGED LIVER

FIGURE 59–7   A.

Sagittal SPECT Tagged RBC Scan: The IVC is bowed backward and compressed *(between arrows).*

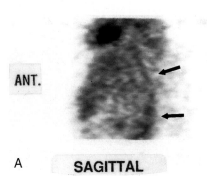

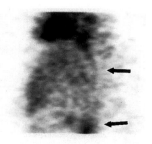

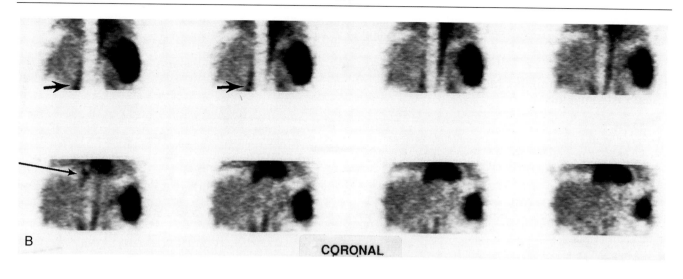

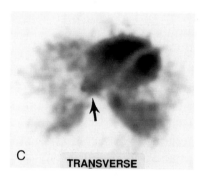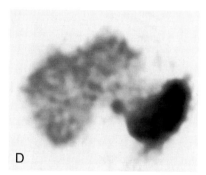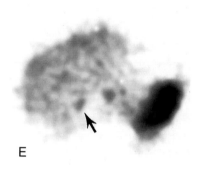

FIGURE 59–7   B.

Coronal SPECT Tagged-RBC Scan: The IVC *(arrows)* is seen well above and below the liver but poorly in between. The aorta can be seen in its entirety.

FIGURE 59–7   C to E.

Axial Cephalic to Caudal SPECT Tagged-RBC Scan: The IVC *(arrows)* virtually disappears at the midliver level (arrows = IVC).

WHITE BLOOD CELLS (WBCs) IN DEEP VENOUS THROMBOSIS

Patient 1: Thrombophlebitis

FIGURE 59–8   A.

^{111}In-WBC Scan: There is intense WBC accumulation in the left femoral vein.

Illustration continued on following page

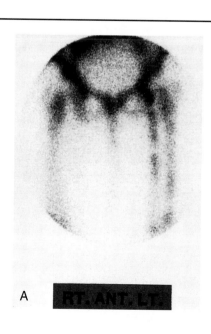

FIGURE 59–8   B.

Thigh Venogram: The left femoral vein is absent, indicating obstruction (arrow = saphenous vein).

Patient 2: Septic Thrombophlebitis and Spinal Osteomyelitis

FIGURE 59–8   C.

WBC Scan of the Pelvis: There is marked WBC accumulation over L5 and the overlying pelvic soft tissues. There is a subtle line of WBC activity *(arrowheads)* medial to the left femoral bone marrow activity *(arrow)*.

FIGURE 59–8   D.

^{99m}Tc-MAA Venogram: There is obstruction of the left iliofemoral veins extending distally into the thigh. Multiple collaterals in the pelvis can be seen.

FIGURE 59–8   E.

Posterior Delayed Bone Scan: There is increased osteogenesis of L5.

FIGURE 59–8   F.

CT of Abdomen: There is a soft tissue mass eroding the anterior L5 vertebral body.

NOTE. WBCs can accumulate in septic or "aseptic" thrombophlebitis and may help differentiate acute disease in patients with postphlebitic syndrome.

Cross Reference

Chapter 3: Spinal Abnormalities—Spinal Osteomyelitis Associated with Hydronephrosis

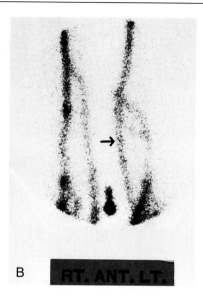

B

RT. ANT. LT.

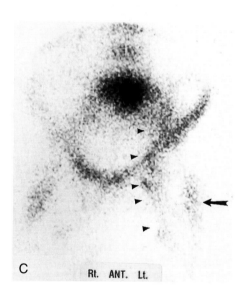

C

Rt.   ANT.   Lt.

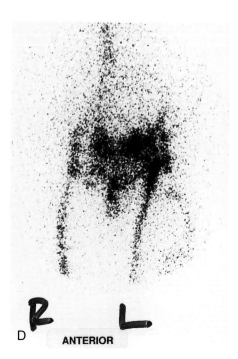

D   ANTERIOR

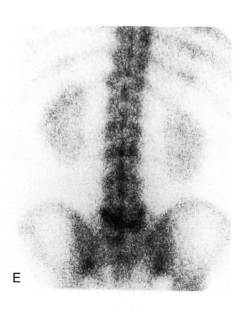

E

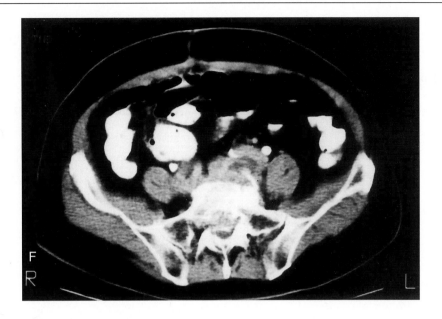

VARICOSE VEINS

FIGURE 59–9.

Calf ⁹⁹ᵐTc-MAA Venogram: The major ascending deep veins appear normal in the left calf. Multiple tortuous channels are seen, especially laterally. There are also incompetent perforating veins shunting blood from the deep system to the saphenous vein.

NOTE. Varicose veins and incompetent perforating veins are probably due to previous thrombophlebitis, usually silent, destroying valves.

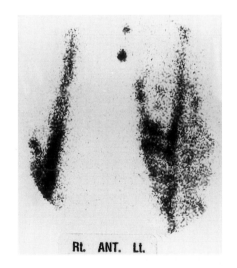

LEG HEMANGIOMA ON TAGGED RED BLOOD CELL (RBC) SCAN

Patient: Thirteen Year Old Female with Chronically Enlarged Left Leg

FIGURE 59–10 A to C.

Anterior, Medial, and Lateral ⁹⁹ᵐTc-RBC Scan of Both Lower Legs: There are dilated veins draining the left calf hemangioma *(arrowheads)*. Normal deep veins are present.

Illustration continued on following page

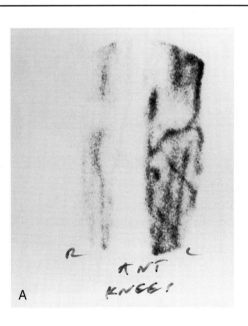

NOTE 1. The presence of deep veins rules out congenital absence of the deep veins, as seen with Osler-Weber-Trenauney syndrome.

NOTE 2. Hemangiomas are a common cause of hemihypertrophy and should be looked for when a child has enlargement of a single limb.

Cross References

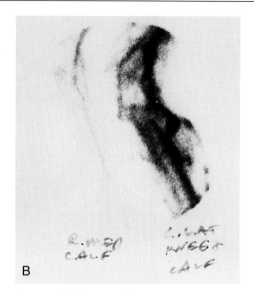

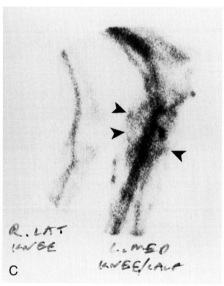

SUPERIOR VENA CAVAL (SVC) OBSTRUCTION

Patient 1

FIGURE 59–11   A.

SVC ⁹⁹ᵐTc-Albumin Colloid Venogram: The right subclavian vein and the left innominate veins are obstructed. Collaterals include internal mammary and lateral thoracic veins.

Patient 2

FIGURE 59–11   B.

SVC ⁹⁹ᵐTc-Albumin Colloid Venogram: The right arm injection demonstrates multiple intercostal and thoracic wall collaterals with some blood flow into the umbilical vein, forming a "hot" spot in the liver *(arrow).*

FIGURE 59–11   C.

Lateral Liver Scan: The "hot" spot from collateral flow through the umbilical vein can be seen in the anterior liver *(arrow).*

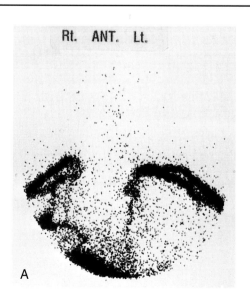

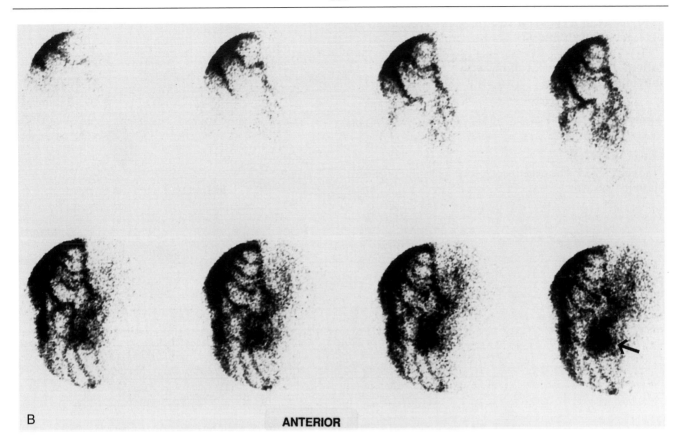

B   **ANTERIOR**

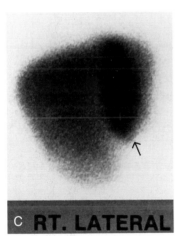

C **RT. LATERAL**

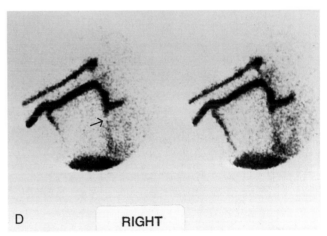

D   **RIGHT**

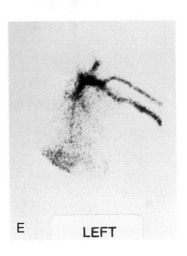

E   **LEFT**

Patient 3

FIGURE 59–11   D.

SVC ^{99m}Tc-Albumin Colloid Venogram: There is retrograde flow into the left innominate vein from the right arm injection as a result of a high-grade partial obstruction of the superior vena cava *(arrow)* and left subclavian obstruction.

FIGURE 59–11   E.

SVC Venogram: The left arm injection demonstrates left subclavian obstruction. The left arm was clinically normal.

Cross Reference

Chapter 59: Venous Thrombosis—Liver Visualization with IVC Obstruction

¹¹¹INDIUM-PLATELET SCAN IN SUBCLAVIAN VENOUS THROMBOSIS

Patient 1: Left Arm Swelling with Subclavian Catheter

FIGURE 59–12   A.

Left Arm Venogram: The left subclavian vein is obstructed *(arrow)*. Chest wall collaterals are present *(arrowheads)*.

FIGURE 59–12   B.

¹¹¹In-Platelet Scan: The platelets aggregate along the proximal left subclavian vein.

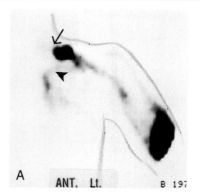

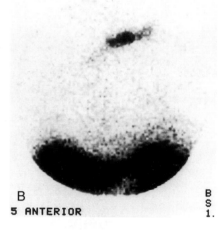

Chapter 60

Arterial Disease

ATHEROSCLEROTIC ILIOFEMORAL ARTERIES

FIGURE 60–1.

Technetium Flow Scan: The iliofemoral arteries are patent but tortuous owing to advanced atherosclerosis.

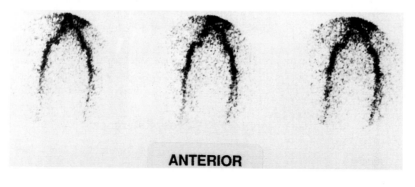

KINKED AORTA

Patient 1

FIGURE 60–2 A.

Technetium Flow Study: The abdominal aorta is kinked to the right at the level of the renal arteries.

Patient 2

FIGURE 60–2 B.

Tagged RBC Scan: The aorta is dilated and kinked to the left.

NOTE 1. The abdominal aorta frequently develops a kink or becomes tortuous with advanced atherosclerosis.

NOTE 2. Any technetium compound can be used for first-pass flow studies.

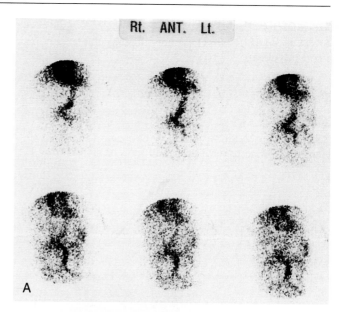

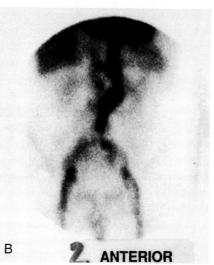

ABDOMINAL AORTIC ANEURYSMS

Patient 1

FIGURE 60–3 A.

Anterior Tagged RBC Scan: There is a fusiform aneurysm at the bifurcation of the aorta that does not extend into the common iliac arteries.

Illustration continued on following page

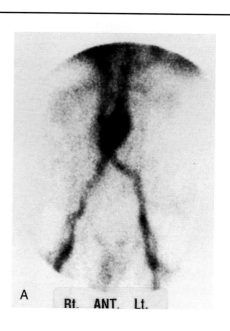

FIGURE 60–3   B.

LAO Tagged RBC Scan: The aneurysm projects anteriorly, making it palpable.

Patient 2

FIGURE 60–3   C.

Technetium Flow Study: The aortic bifurcation aneurysm empties slowly owing to turbulence and stasis of blood within it.

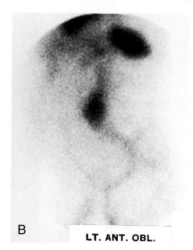

B   **LT. ANT. OBL.**

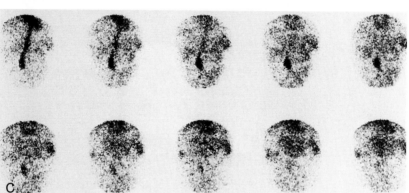

DISSECTING ANEURYSM

FIGURE 60–4.

Posterior ^{99m}Tc-DTPA Scan: The aortic true lumen is patent and persists along the right side of the aorta. The false lumen fills slowly and ends above the renal arteries and is along the left side of the aorta. In this case, both kidneys are perfused through the true lumen.

NOTE 1. The false lumen virtually always descends along the left side and may compromise the left renal and left iliac arteries.

NOTE 2. Renal artery patency, especially that of the left kidney, can be determined with a nuclear scan.

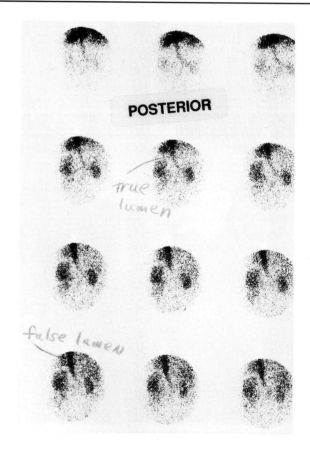

MYCOTIC ANEURYSM

FIGURE 60–5   A.

Posterior Technetium Blood Flow Study: There is a round collection of blood *(arrow)* outside the normal course of the aorta.

FIGURE 60–5   B and C.

Posterior and Anterior ^{111}In-WBC Scan: The marked WBC accumulation *(arrow)* indicates an active infection.

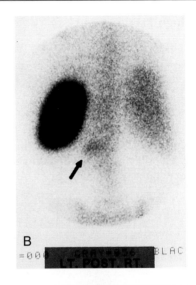

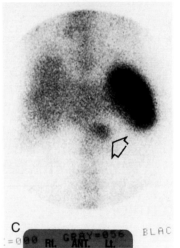

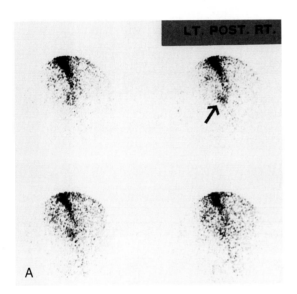

PSEUDOANEURYSM AFTER TRAUMA

Patient 1: Calf Pseudoaneurysm

FIGURE 60–6   A.

Tagged RBC Scan: The localized intense RBC collection *(arrow)* in the proximal right lower leg is cephalad to a photon-deficient area representing a hematoma. (Courtesy of Dr. Amiel Z. Rudavsky, New York, NY.)

Illustration continued on following page

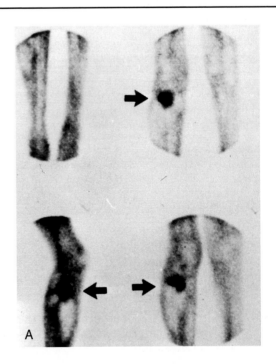

Patient 2: Thigh Pseudoaneurysm

FIGURE 60-6   B.

Tagged RBC Scan: The pseudoaneurysm is surrounded by a large hematoma. (Courtesy of Dr. Amiel Z. Rudavsky, New York, NY.)

NOTE. A pseudoaneurysm, or even a transection of an artery, can occur with preservation of distal pulses and may be asymptomatic.

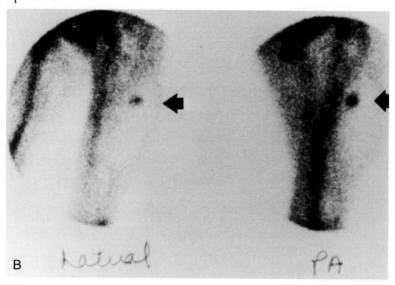

B

AORTIC OCCLUSION

FIGURE 60-7   A.

Composite Film of Renal Blood Flow: The aorta comes to an abrupt halt at the level of the renal arteries. The left kidney has no appreciable blood flow.

FIGURE 60-7   B.

DTPA Renal Scan: The kidneys are functional, although the left kidney demonstrates defects due to infarcts. The left kidney, therefore, must have a collateral blood supply.

FIGURE 60-7   C.

Subtraction Angiogram: The right renal artery is patent *(arrows)*, whereas the left renal artery is occluded *(arrowhead)*.

FIGURE 60-7   D and E.

Renal Function Curves: The left kidney's glomerular filtration and tubular excretion are poor but are preserved owing to collateral blood flow.

NOTE 1. Thrombosis of the aorta usually occurs below the renal arteries because of atherosclerosis and sluggish flow. High flow in the renal arteries usually prevents thrombotic occlusion of the aorta at this level.

NOTE 2. Collaterals to the kidneys can come from lumbar, intercostal, adrenal, ureteric, capsular, and phrenic arteries.

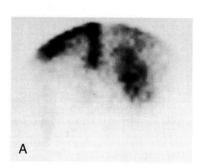

A

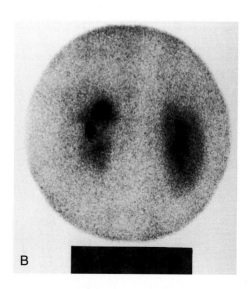

B

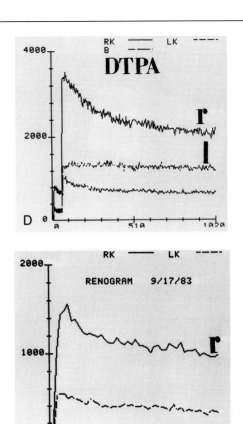

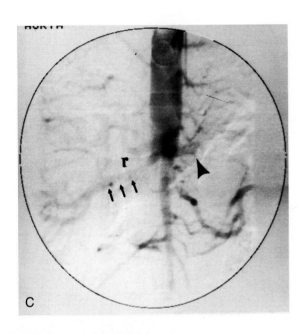

HYPEREMIA FOLLOWING ARTERIAL EMBOLISM

Patient: Painful Right Lower Leg with Normal Distal Pulses

FIGURE 60–8   A.

[99mTc]-MDP Flow Scan: The right popliteal artery is not seen, yet flow is faster and greater on the right.

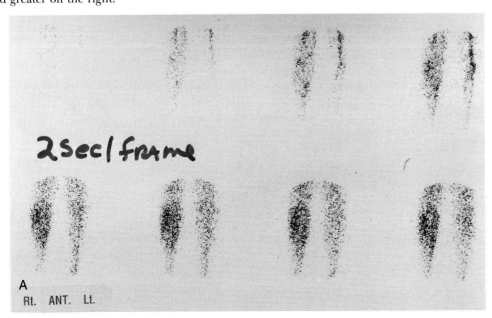

Illustration continued on following page

FIGURE 60–8 B.
Contrast Arteriogram: The intra-arterial clot can be seen occluding the right popliteal artery.

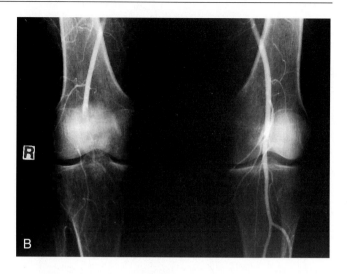

NOTE. Hyperemia can be explained by distal vasodilatation from ischemia, collateralization, and partial occlusion of the arterial lumen.

THALLIUM PERFUSION SCANNING IN CLAUDICATION

FIGURE 60–9.
Posterior Calf Thallium Planar Scans: The right lower leg has less thallium than the left.

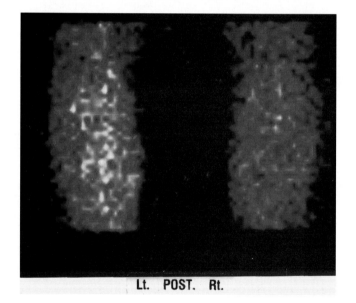

Lt. POST. Rt.

NOTE. Thallium accumulates in skeletal muscle as it does in cardiac muscle. It can be used to determine the hemodynamic significance of an arterial stenosis in the legs or arms.

Cross Reference

Chapter 8: Hyperemia—Claudication Simulating Hyperemia in the Opposite Leg

BLOOD FLOW STUDY IN GANGRENE

FIGURE 60–10 A.
Intra-Arterial ^{99m}Tc-MAA: The arterial blood supply stops in the distal forearm.

FIGURE 60–10 B.
Intra-Arterial ^{99m}Tc-MAA: The blood flow stops at the ankle.

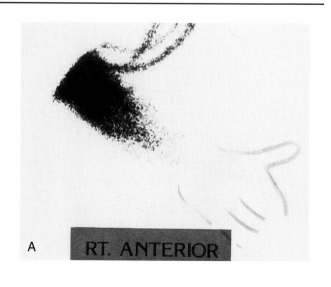

RT. ANTERIOR

NOTE 1. Intra-arterial macroaggregated albumin particles will follow the arterial distribution and may help in deciding the level of amputation.

NOTE 2. A tagged RBC scan is an alternative technique to intra-arterial MAA.

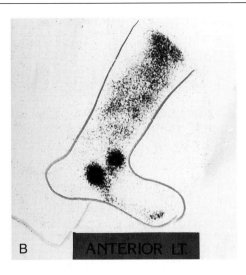

GRAFT OCCLUSION

FIGURE 60–11.

Technetium Flow Study: The left iliac limb of the aortoiliac graft is occluded. The native aorta is faintly filled *(arrow)*.

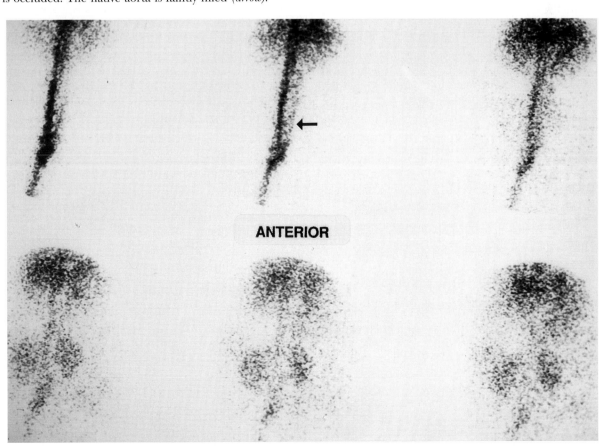

ARTERIAL GRAFT INFECTION

FIGURE 60–12.

^{111}In-WBC Scan: There is intense accumulation of the WBCs along the left femoropopliteal graft. (Courtesy of Dr. Arnold Jacobson, Seattle, WA.)

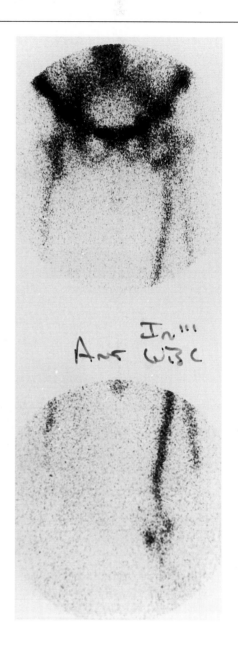

DIALYSIS FISTULA INFECTION

FIGURE 60–13.

Four Hour Forearm ^{99m}Tc-HMPAO WBC Scan: There is a focal abnormality at the apex of the shunt loop. Blood pool is seen in the rest of the graft.

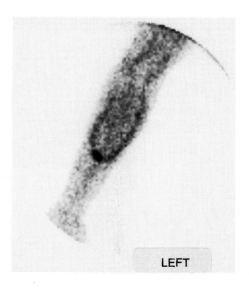

INTERNAL MAMMARY LYMPHOSCINTIGRAPHY

Patient 1: Breast Cancer

FIGURE 61–1 A.

Anterior Chest ^{99m}Tc-Antimony Colloid Lymphoscintigraphy: The lymph nodes on both sides are seen, with no skip areas.

Patient 2: Breast Cancer

FIGURE 61–1 B and C.

Anterior and Lateral Chest ^{99m}Tc-Antimony Colloid Lymphoscintigraphy: There are lymph nodes filling in the inferior and superior internal mammary chain but a substantial gap in between.

Patient 3: Breast Cancer

FIGURE 61–1 D.

Anterior Abdominal ^{99m}Tc-Antimony Colloid Lymphoscintigraphy: The initial injection was intraperitoneal rather than between the rectus abdominis muscle and the peritoneum. Markers = Costal margin.

NOTE 1. Poor filling of lymph nodes is presumed to represent tumor involvement.

NOTE 2. Internal mammary lymphoscintigraphy can be used to set the radiation ports accurately.

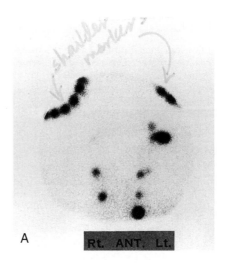

A   Rt. ANT. Lt.

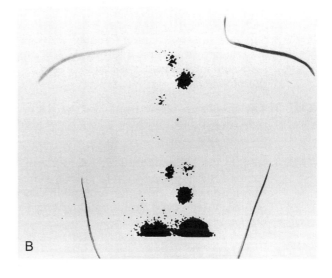

B

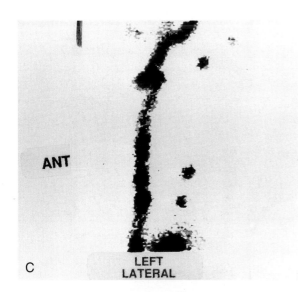

C   LEFT LATERAL

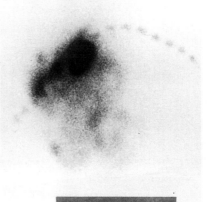

D   Rt. ANT. Lt.

LYMPHOSCINTIGRAPHY FOR SENTINEL NODE IDENTIFICATION

Patient 1: Anterior Chest Wall Melanoma

FIGURE 61–2 A.

Thirty Minute ⁹⁹ᵐTc-Human Serum Albumin Lymphoscintigraphy: The right inferior axillary lymph node was first to fill and thus is the "sentinel" node.

FIGURE 61–2 B.

Three Hour ⁹⁹ᵐTc-Human Serum Albumin Lymphoscintigraphy: The lymphatic channels are well seen along with the more superior axillary lymph nodes.

Patient 2: Right Upper Quadrant Abdominal Wall Melanoma

FIGURE 61–2 C and D.

Three Hour Anterior Chest and Upper Abdomen ⁹⁹ᵐTc-Antimony Colloid Lymphoscintigraphy: The melanoma injection site, near the midline and just below the liver, drains into both axillary and inguinal lymph node groups (b = bladder).

NOTE 1. Resection and histopathology of sentinel lymph nodes are used to determine the need for greater nodal resection.

NOTE 2. Sappey's line is a circumferential watershed area demarcating truncal lymphatic flow superiorly and inferiorly. It is at a variable level near the umbilicus.

NOTE 3. The lymphatics of the trunk also drain left or right, depending on which side of the midline they are on.

NOTE 4. Despite the generalization of Notes 2 and 3, cutaneous lesions can drain to other quadrant lymph nodes; therefore, if lymph node dissection is contemplated, lymphoscintigraphy can be helpful.

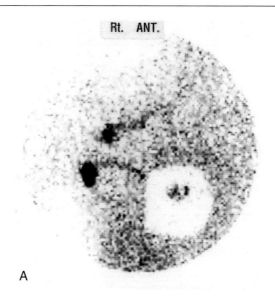

A

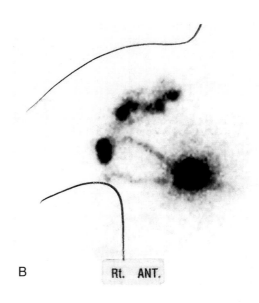

B

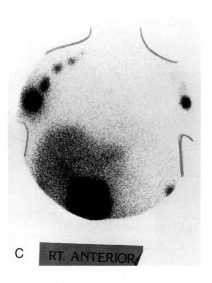

C

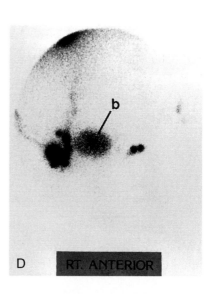

D

LYMPHATIC OBSTRUCTION

Patient 1: Idiopathic Right Leg Lymphedema

FIGURE 61–3   A to C.

Bilateral Leg and Pelvic Lymphoscintigraphy: There is obstruction of the right popliteal lymphatic channels, although some collaterals exist. The left side is normal.

Patient 2: Filariasis Affecting Both Legs

FIGURE 61–3   D to F.

Bilateral Leg ⁹⁹ᵐTc-Antimony Colloid Lymphoscintigraphy: There is a single dilated lymphatic channel in the right leg that ends at the inguinal region. In the right thigh and calf there is dispersion of the colloid. The left leg does not have demonstrable lymphatic flow.

Illustration continued on following page

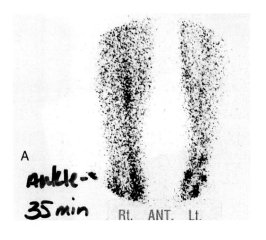

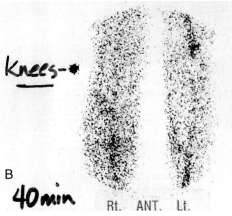

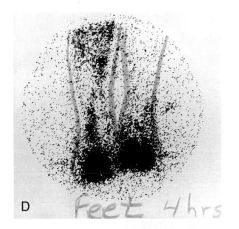

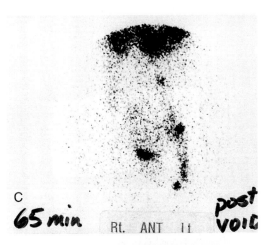

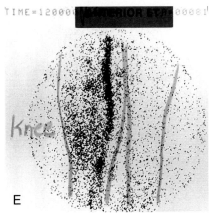

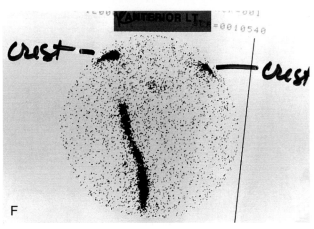

Patient 3: Right Arm Swelling Following Surgery

FIGURE 61–3 G and H.

99mTc-HSA Lymphoscintigraphy: The left arm lymphatics can be seen *(arrowheads)*, but the right arm has no flow.

FIGURE 61–3 I.

Two Hour Delayed Lymphoscintigraphy: The radiopharmaceutical is in the subcutaneous tissue (dermal backflow), indicative of lymphatic obstruction.

FIGURE 61–3 J.

Two Hour Delayed Lymphoscintigraphy: Eventually the axillary lymph nodes fill.

NOTE. Lymph normally flows from the dermis to the deep lymphatics. In lymphatic obstruction, the dermal lymphatics act as collateral channels (dermal backflow).

Cross Reference

Chapter 11: Soft Tissue Abnormalites—Lymphedema on Bone Scan

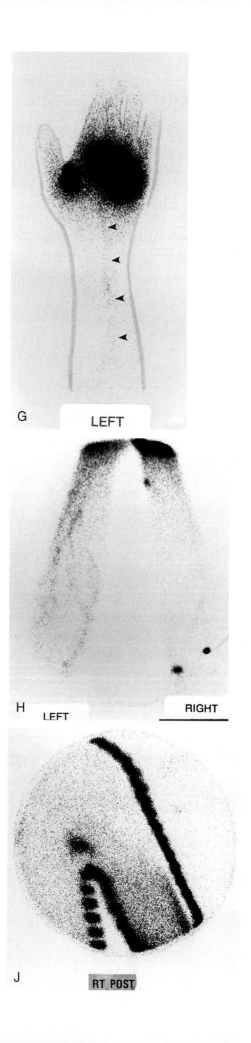

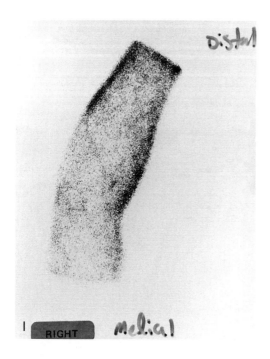

CONGENITAL ABSENCE OF LYMPHATICS

Patient 1: Milroy's Disease

FIGURE 61–4   A.
Leg Thigh Stump Bone Scan: There is a sac of lymphatic fluid hanging off the left leg.

FIGURE 61–4   B.
^{99m}Tc-Antimony Colloid Lymphoscintigraphy: There is no uptake of the intradermal colloid into lymphatics.

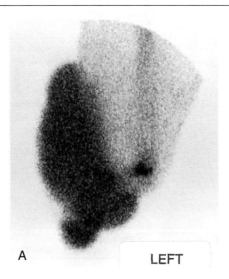

A   LEFT

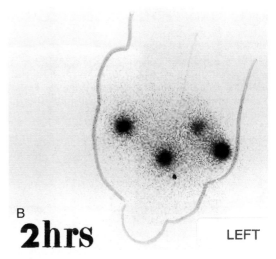

B   **2hrs**   LEFT

Chapter 62

Perfusion Scanning

NORMAL BRAIN PERFUSION SPECT SCAN

FIGURE 62–1   A to C.

Transverse, Sagittal, and Coronal ^{99m}Tc-HMPAO SPECT Scan: There is even distribution of perfusion throughout the supratentorial gray matter, including the basal ganglia. The cerebellum has the greatest blood flow. (Red is normal flow.)

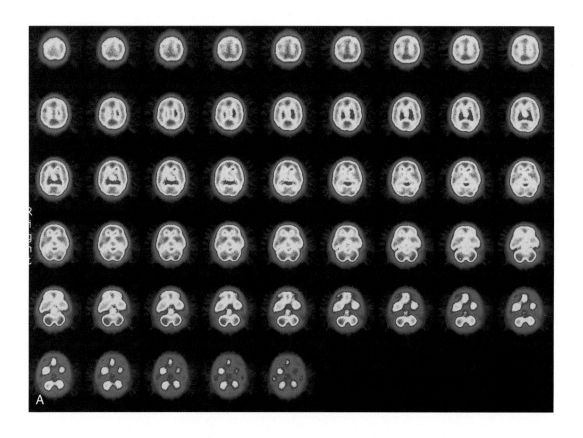

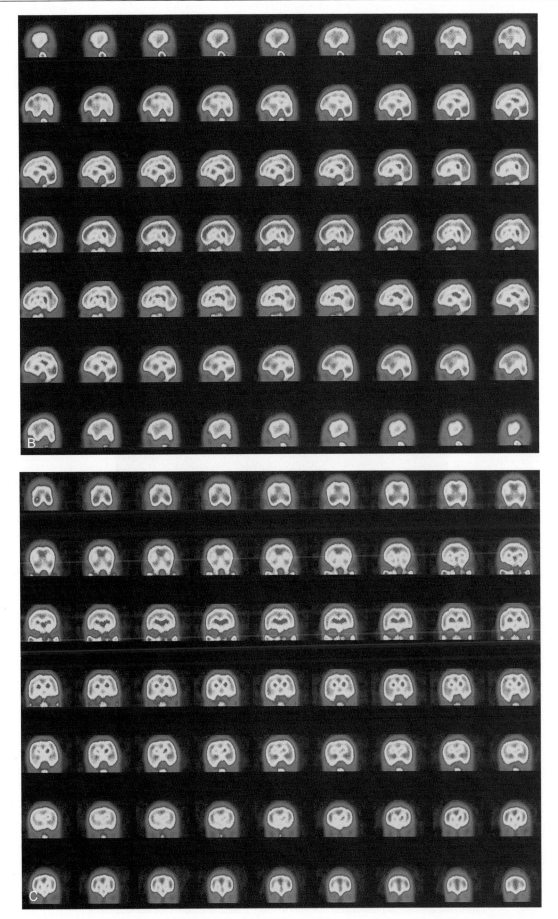

Illustration continued on following page

FIGURE 62–1 D.

Lateral View of 3-D Surface Reconstruction of Cerebral Perfusion.

FIGURE 62–1 E.

Vertex View of 3-D Surface Reconstruction of Cerebral Perfusion.

NOTE. Attenuation correction is important in order to properly evaluate the basal ganglia.

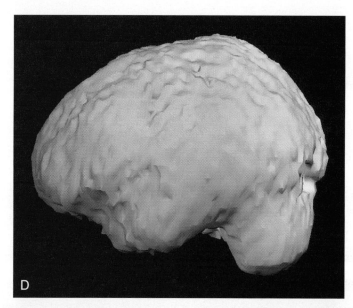

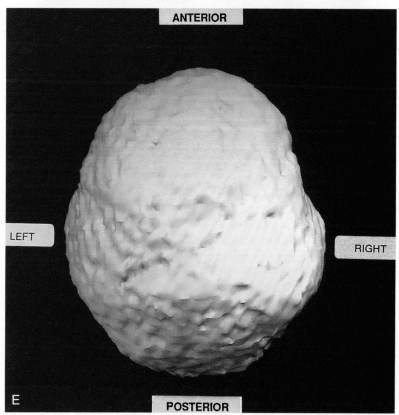

HERPES ENCEPHALITIS

FIGURE 62–2 A.

Transverse ^{99m}Tc-HMPAO SPECT Scan: There is hyperperfusion of the left mesial temporal lobe and the midlateral right temporal lobe (white areas).

FIGURE 62–2 B to D.

Left and Right Sagittal and Coronal ^{99m}Tc-HMPAO SPECT Scans 2 Weeks Later: The temporal lobe hyperemia is so great that the remaining brain perfusion is poorly visualized.

NOTE 1. In the late stages of herpes encephalitis there is necrosis of brain tissue and subsequent hypoperfusion of the affected areas.

NOTE 2. Increased regional cerebral blood flow is not specific. It can be seen with other viral encephalitides, with seizure disorders, and in luxury perfusion after stroke or trauma.

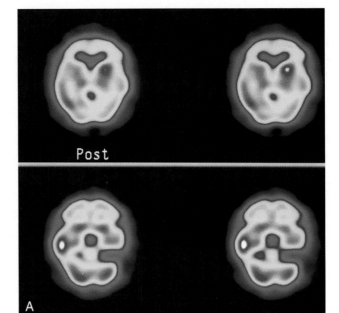

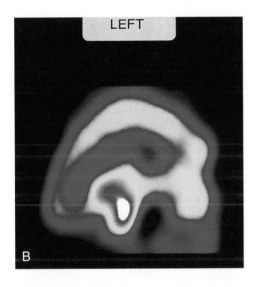

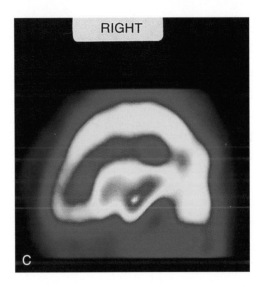

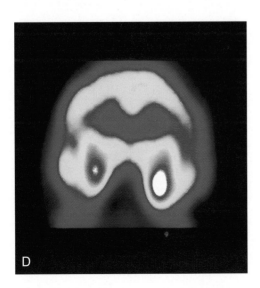

MENINGITIS

FIGURE 62–3   A and B.

Anterior and Left Lateral WBC Scan: There are multiple focal areas of WBC accumulation along the periphery of the brain as well as in the upper cervical spine *(arrowhead)*.

NOTE. These findings suggest that meningitis may have focal areas of infection as well as diffuse inflammation.

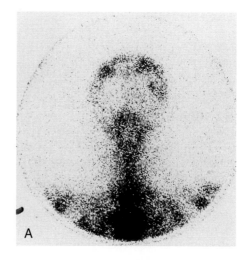

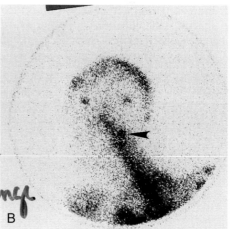

BRAIN ABSCESS

Patient 1: Fifty-three Year Old Male with Fever, Headache, and Pneumonia

FIGURE 62–4   A.

Lateral Head ^{111}In-WBC Scan: There is a focus of WBC aggregation in the right frontal lobe (frontal view confirmed localization) from *Staphylococcus*.

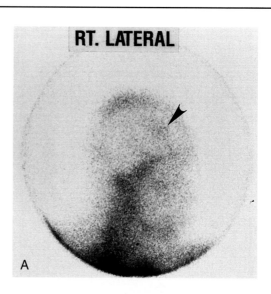

Patient 2: Sixty-six Year Old Male with AIDS

FIGURE 62–4 B and C.

Lateral and Anterior Gallium Scan: There are multiple foci of gallium accumulation in the brain.

FIGURE 62–4 D.

Contrast-Enhanced CT Scan: The multiple contrast-enhancing abnormalities proved to be cysticercosis.

NOTE. Although rarely used for brain abnormalities, WBC scans may help separate infection from tumor. Sestamibi or thallium SPECT scans could also be used.

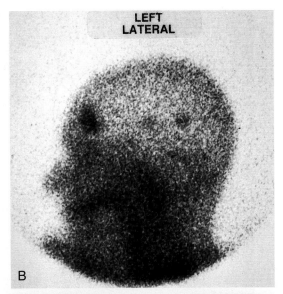

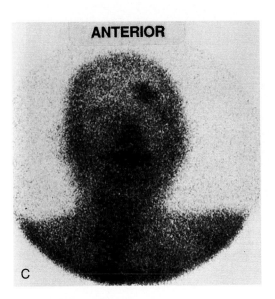

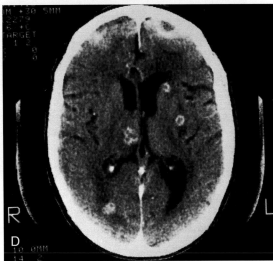

SEVERE COGNITIVE AND MOTOR DEFICITS AFTER TRAUMA

Patient: Twenty Year Old Female 2 Years After Jumping Out of a Moving Car

FIGURE 62–5 A.

Transverse ^{99m}Tc-HMPAO SPECT Scan: There is a perfusion defect in the left vertex.

FIGURE 62–5 B.

Transverse ^{99m}Tc-HMPAO SPECT Scan: The inferior right frontal, temporal, and occipital lobes and the right cerebellar hemisphere have markedly reduced perfusion.

NOTE. Although anatomic abnormalities may be demonstrated by CT or MRI, perfusion abnormalities are thought to more accurately represent functional deficits. Perfusion abnormalities are often seen in areas that are normal on CT and MRI.

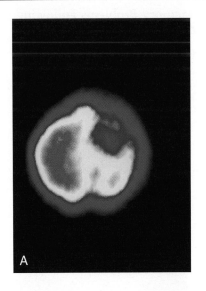

Illustration continued on following page

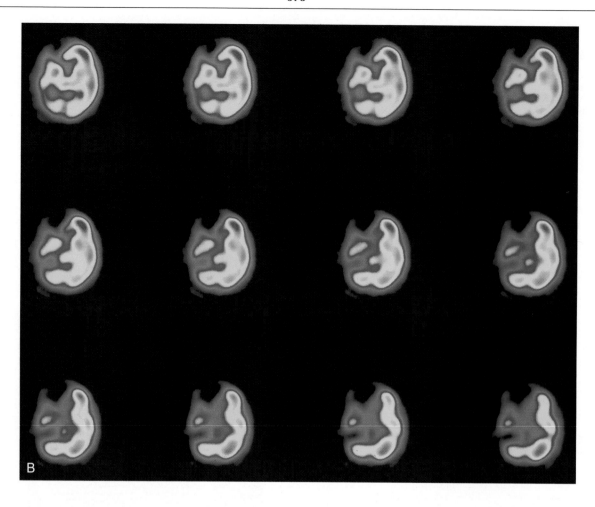

MEMORY AND PERSONALITY DEFICITS FOLLOWING TRAUMA

Patient 1: Memory Problems Following an Auto Accident

FIGURE 62–6   A and B.

Transverse and Sagittal ^{99m}Tc-HMPAO SPECT Scan: There is a focal perfusion deficit in the left frontal lobe (*arrows*). CT scan of the head was normal.

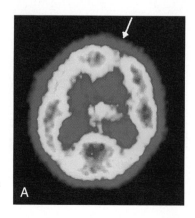

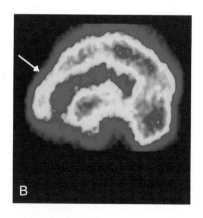

FIGURE 62–6   C and D.

Vertex and Anterior Views of 3-D Reconstruction of Cerebral Perfusion: The left frontal deficit is easily appreciated.

Patient 2: Thirty-nine Year Old Male with Personality Disorder and Memory Deficit Following Removal of a Frontal Meningioma

FIGURE 62–6   E to G.

Transverse, Sagittal, and Coronal ^{99m}Tc-HMPAO SPECT Scan: There is a well-defined defect in the posterior frontal lobe.

Illustration continued on following page

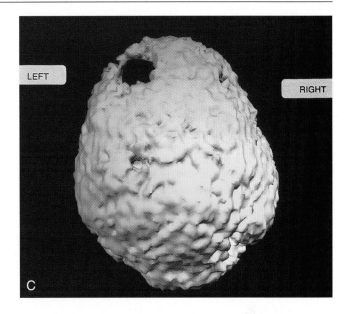

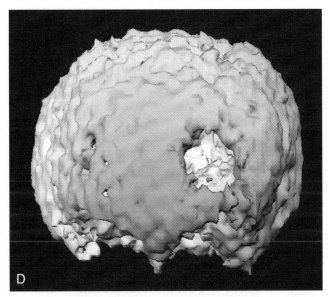

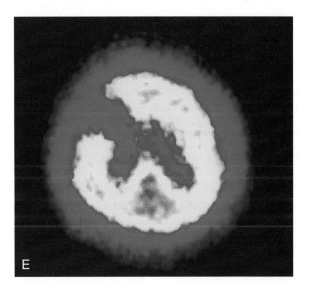

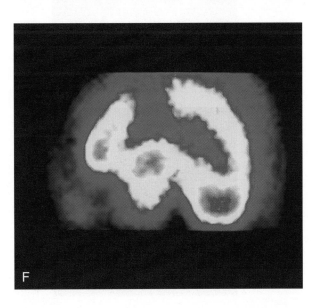

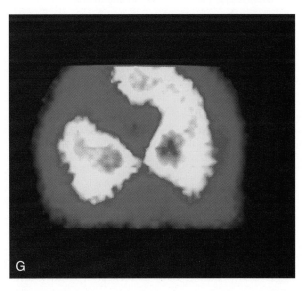

FIGURE 62–6 H.

Right Lateral View of 3-D Surface Reconstruction of Cerebral Perfusion: The distribution of the perfusion defect is better appreciated with surface reconstruction.

NOTE 1. A craniotomy by itself should not produce extensive brain changes on perfusion scanning.

NOTE 2. Even though a meningioma is an extra-axial mass, there are extensive effects on the brain, probably beyond simple pressure effects.

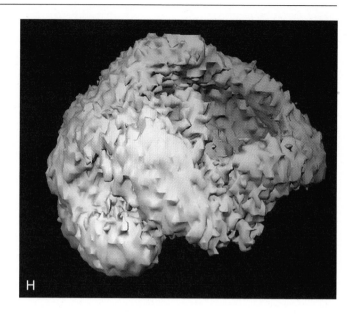

MIDDLE CEREBRAL ARTERY INFARCT

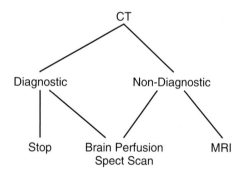

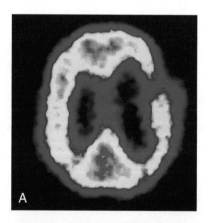

FIGURE 62–7 A and B.

Transverse ⁹⁹ᵐTc-HMPAO Perfusion SPECT Scans: There is a broad area of perfusion deficit involving the left frontoparietal lobes.

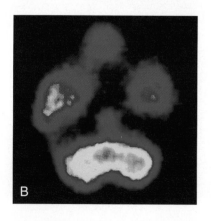

FIGURE 62–7   C and D.

Vertex and Left Lateral Views of 3-D Surface Reconstruction of Cerebral Perfusion: The large perfusion deficit in the left middle cerebral artery distribution spares some of the temporal lobe.

FIGURE 62–7   E.

Follow-Up of CT Scan: The infarct can be seen as low density within the left hemisphere.

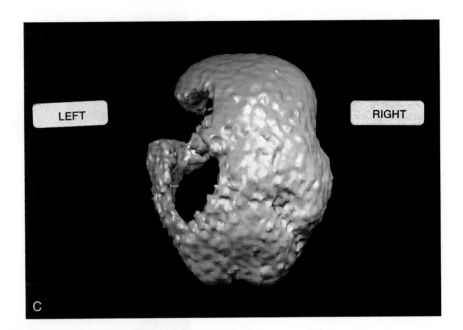

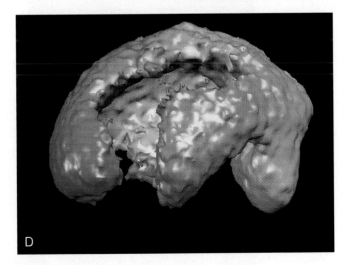

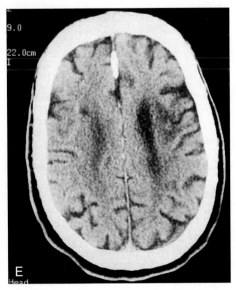

TRAUMA FOLLOWING STROKE

Patient: Brain Death Study in Patient Found Unresponsive and Requiring Life Support

FIGURE 62–8   A and B.

Transverse ^{99m}Tc-HMPAO Brain Death SPECT Scan: There is no perfusion to the right thalamic region (black), whereas the left hemisphere has diffusely decreased perfusion (yellow). The right caudate and other basal ganglia are not as well perfused as those of the left.

FIGURE 62–8   C.

CT Scan: A hemorrhagic infarct of the right thalamus is present, with bleeding into the lateral ventricle. The soft tissues overlying the left calvarium are swollen.

NOTE 1. It would be quite unusual for trauma to cause intracerebral hemorrhage in the thalamus while sparing the overlying brain. Thus, the CVA occurred first.

NOTE 2. The brain perfusion demonstrates that there is considerable viable brain and that life support should not be withdrawn. Clinical recovery was made, albeit with deficits.

Cross Reference

Chapter 62: Perfusion Scanning—Brain Death Studies

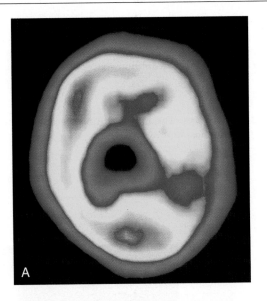

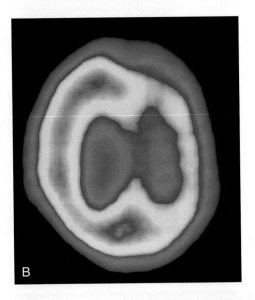

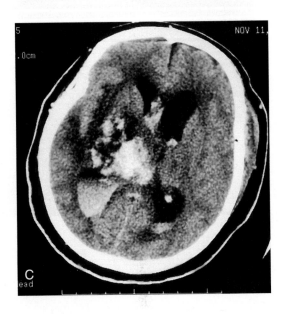

CROSSED CEREBELLAR DIASCHISIS

FIGURE 62–9   A and B.

Transverse ^{99m}Tc-HMPAO Perfusion SPECT Scans: The perfusion deficit involves the right frontal, parietal, and temporal lobes as well as the right basal ganglia. The left cerebellar hemisphere has reduced perfusion.

NOTE. Although the cause of crossed cerebellar diaschisis is unknown, it probably represents disruption of the corticopontocerebellar pathway. This can occur with strokes, vascular malformations, or supratentorial tumors causing a reduction in blood flow and metabolism in the contralateral cerebellar hemisphere. Atrophy of the cerebellar hemisphere can occur.

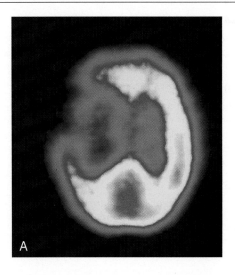

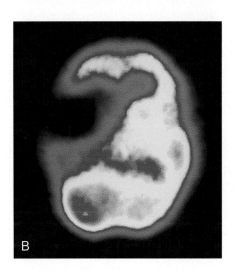

NEW AND OLD CVAs

Patient: Sixty-six Year Old Female, with Known Infarct of Right Frontal Lobe, Presented with Mild Right-Sided Weakness

FIGURE 62–10   A.

Transverse ^{99m}Tc-HMPAO Perfusion Scan: There is a mild reduction in perfusion to the left frontoparietal cortex *(arrow)*. There is a more severe and focal defect of the right frontal lobe with hypoperfusion of the adjacent brain.

Illustration continued on following page

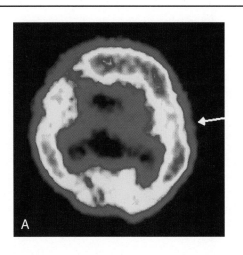

FIGURE 62–10   B.

Transverse ⁹⁹ᵐTc-HMPAO Perfusion Scan: The right cerebellar hemisphere has reduced perfusion, indicative of crossed cerebellar diaschisis.

FIGURE 62–10   C.

Vertex View of 3-D Surface Reconstruction of Cerebral Perfusion: The old right middle cerebral artery infarct and the new smaller left frontoparietal infarct are seen. The right cerebellar hemisphere appears smaller than the left owing to the reduced perfusion.

FIGURE 62–10   D.

CT Scan: The old right infarct *(arrow)* on CT is smaller than the HMPAO perfusion abnormality. The left infarct is too acute to be seen.

NOTE 1. An acute infarct usually is missed on CT for the first few days unless there is hemorrhage. It will be evident on a ⁹⁹ᵐTc-HMPAO SPECT scan immediately.

NOTE 2. The SPECT perfusion abnormality is usually larger as compared with the CT or MRI abnormalities, partly owing to a reflection of cerebral function.

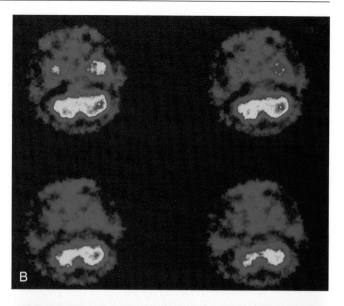

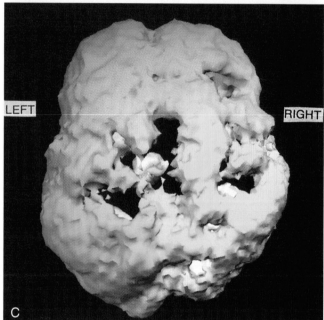

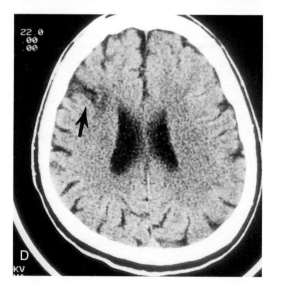

POST CENTRAL GYRAL STROKE

Patient: Fifty Year Old Female with Numbness of the Right Leg and Trunk

FIGURE 62–11   A and B.

Transverse and Coronal ^{99m}Tc-HMPAO SPECT Scan: There is diminished perfusion in the region of the left sensory cortex.

FIGURE 62–11   C.

Left Lateral View of 3-D Surface Reconstruction of Cerebral Perfusion: There is a patchy perfusion deficit in the lower left parietal lobe in the region of the sensory cortex.

NOTE. A brain perfusion SPECT scan often demonstrates areas of abnormality when symptoms or signs are quite mild or difficult to otherwise objectively measure.

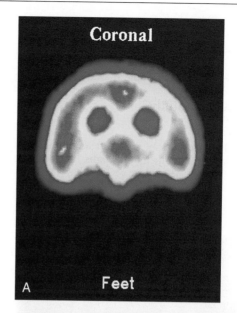

A Coronal Feet

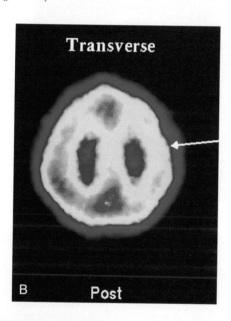

B Transverse Post

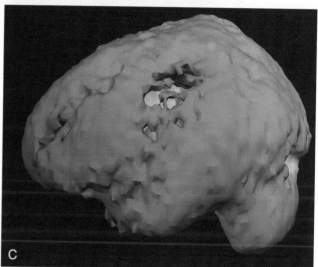

C

SEIZURE FOCI

INTRACTABLE SEIZURE DISORDERS

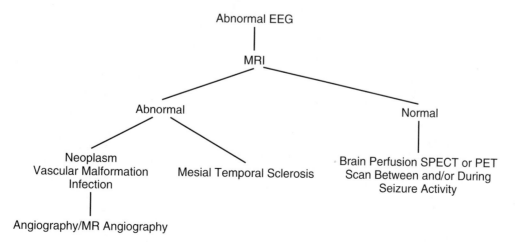

Illustration continued on following page

Patient 1: Active Seizure Focus

FIGURE 62–12   A and B.

Transverse and Sagittal ^{99m}Tc-HMPAO SPECT Scan: There is increased blood flow in the right temporal lobe *(arrows)*.

Patient 2: Ictal Seizure Study

FIGURE 62–12   C.

Transverse ^{18}F-FDG PET Brain Scan: The left temporal lobe, especially the hippocampus and the left thalamus, have marked increased metabolic activity. (Courtesy of Dr. Shay Lee, Los Angeles, CA.)

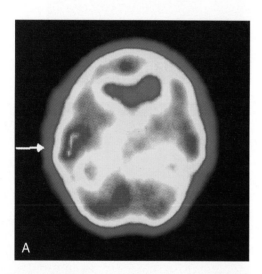

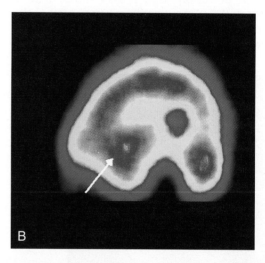

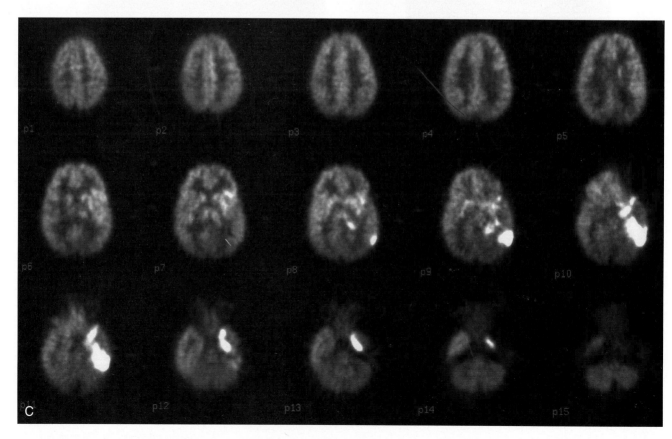

Patient 3: Interictal Seizure Focus

FIGURE 62–12 D and E.

Transverse and Coronal ⁹⁹ᵐTc-HMPAO SPECT Scan: The left temporal lobe has diminished perfusion.

Patient 4: Interictal Temporal Lobe Seizure Disorder

FIGURE 62–12 F.

Transverse ¹⁸F-FDG PET Brain Scan: The right temporal lobe has less activity than the remaining cortex and basal ganglia. (Courtesy of Dr. Shay Lee, Los Angeles, CA.)

Patient 5: Normal FDG PET Scan

FIGURE 62–12 G.

Transverse ¹⁸F-FDG PET Brain Scan: There is homogeneous activity throughout the gray matter. (Courtesy of Dr. Shay Lee, Los Angeles, CA.)

NOTE. ⁹⁹ᵐTc-HMPAO and other brain perfusion agents produce SPECT scans that are relatively insensitive in detecting interictal seizure foci. If the injection is made when seizure activity is present clinically or on EEG, the sensitivity of these agents is excellent.

Illustration continued on following page

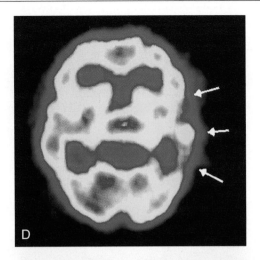

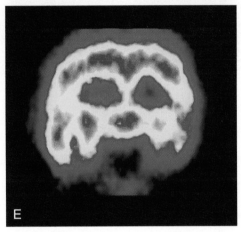

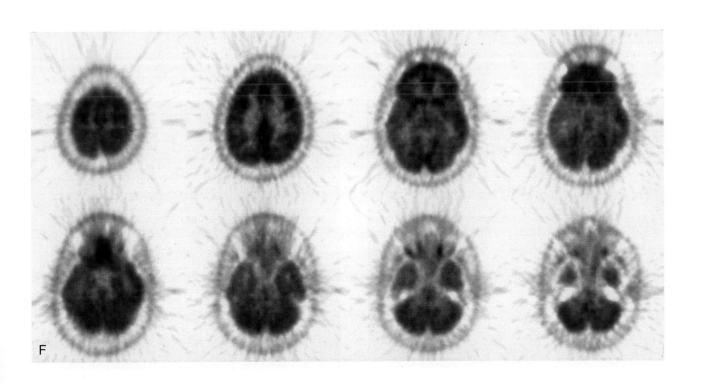

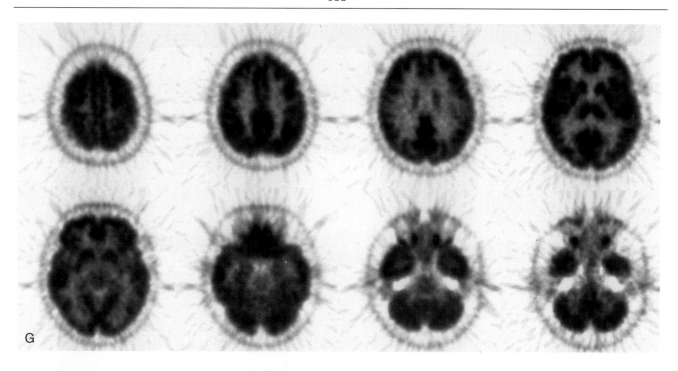

DIFFUSE WHITE MATTER INFARCTS

Patient: Sixty-six Year Old with Dementia

FIGURE 62–13   A and B.

Transverse and Coronal ⁹⁹ᵐTc-HMPAO Perfusion SPECT Scans: There is diffusely reduced perfusion to virtually the entire cerebrum. The vertex is relatively spared.

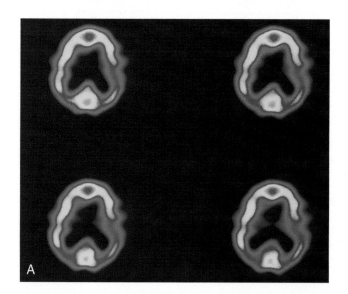

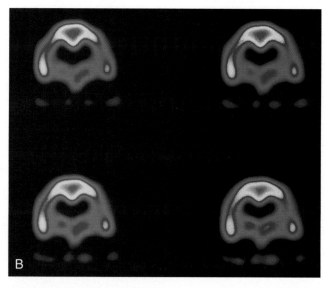

FIGURE 62–13   C and D.

Lateral Views of 3-D Surface Reconstructions of Cerebral Perfusion: There is marked reduction of perfusion throughout both hemispheres. The superiormost brain is better perfused.

FIGURE 62–13   E.

Transverse T2 MRI: The white matter has foci of abnormally high signal, most indicative of infarcts, along with sulcal enlargement due to cortical atrophy.

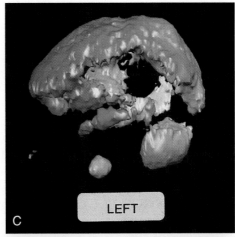

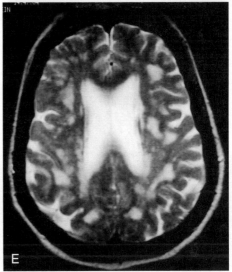

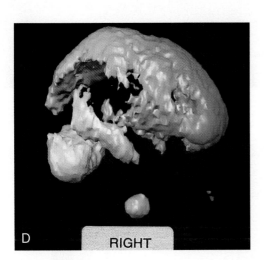

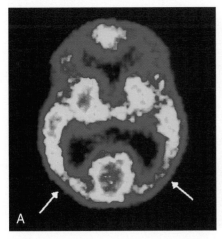

ALZHEIMER'S TYPE DEMENTIA

Patient 1

FIGURE 62–14   A and B.

Transverse ^{99m}Tc-HMPAO SPECT Scan: There is decreased perfusion *(arrows)* to both parietal lobes and the posterior temporal lobes. There is also mild frontal lobe hypoperfusion.

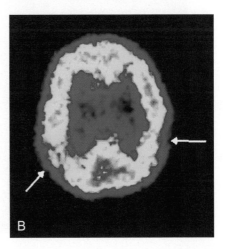

Illustration continued on following page

FIGURE 62–14   C and D.

Lateral and Vertex Views of 3-D Surface Reconstructions: The reduction in perfusion is in the classic distribution.

Patient 2

FIGURE 62–14   E and F.

Transverse and Left Sagittal ^{99m}Tc-HMPAO SPECT Scan: The hypoperfusion is asymmetric, affecting the left temporal lobe to a greater extent. The frontal lobes are spared in this patient.

FIGURE 62–14   G.

Left Lateral View of 3-D Surface Reconstruction: There is reduction of posterior temporal lobe perfusion extending into the left posterior parietal lobe.

NOTE 1. The posterior temporoparietal perfusion deficits may be symmetric or asymmetric.

NOTE 2. Alzheimer's type dementia may also have frontal lobe perfusion abnormalities.

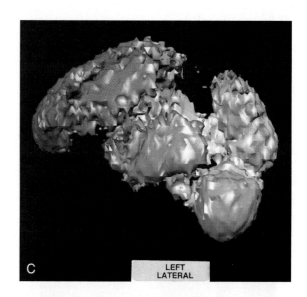

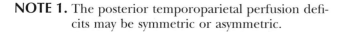

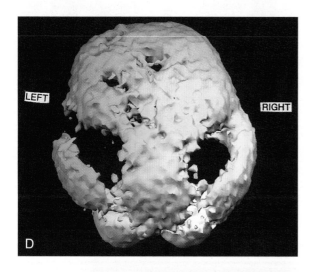

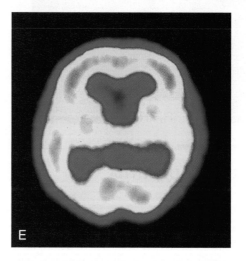

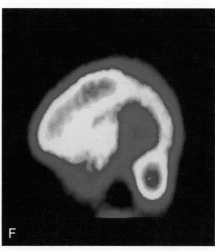

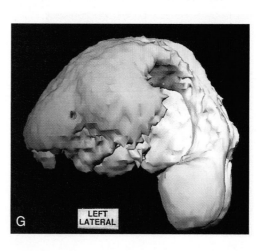

PICK'S DISEASE

Patient 1: Dementia Clinically of Alzheimer's Type

FIGURE 62–15   A and B.
Transverse and Sagittal ^{99m}Tc-HMPAO SPECT Scans: The frontal lobes have diminished perfusion, whereas the parietal and posterior temporal lobes have relatively normal perfusion.

FIGURE 62–15   C.
Right Lateral View of 3-D Surface Reconstruction: The perfusion of the posterior temporal and parietal lobes are normal, but the frontal lobes have reduced perfusion.

Patient 2: Dementia of Alzheimer's Type

FIGURE 62–15   D.
Vertex View of 3-D Surface Reconstruction: There is reduced perfusion of the frontal lobes bilaterally, with sparing of the temporoparietal area.

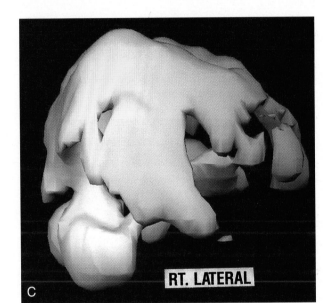

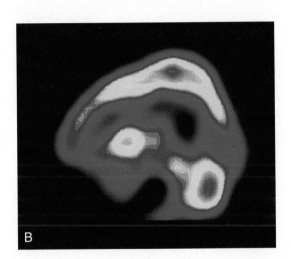

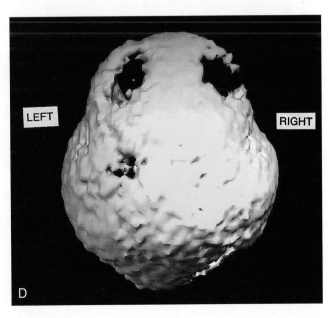

NOTE. Pick's disease should be suspected in patients with Alzheimer's type dementia who have normal temporoparietal perfusion but decreased frontal lobe perfusion.

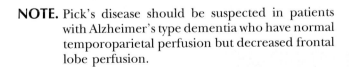

DEPRESSION

Patient 1: Severe Depression

FIGURE 62–16 A and B.

Transverse and Sagittal ⁹⁹ᵐTc-HMPAO SPECT Scan: The entire cerebral cortex has markedly reduced perfusion. The basal ganglia and the cerebellum are normal.

FIGURE 62–16 C.

Left Lateral View of 3-D Surface Reconstruction: The severe perfusion deficits of the frontal, parietal, and anterior temporal lobes can be well appreciated.

Patient 2: Moderate Depression

FIGURE 62–16 D.

Sagittal ⁹⁹ᵐTc-HMPAO SPECT Scan: The left frontal lobe has reduced perfusion. The right side is also involved but to a lesser degree.

NOTE 1. The left hemisphere usually is more profoundly affected in depression.

NOTE 2. This pattern will improve or revert to normal after successful therapy.

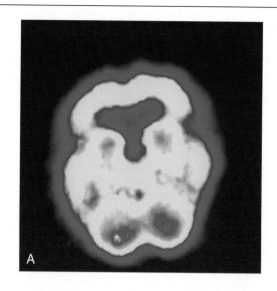

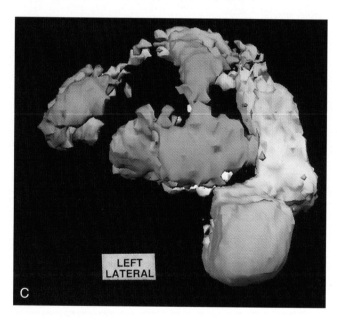

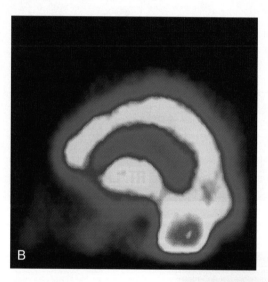

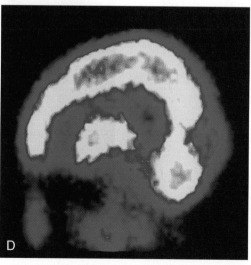

"YOUR BRAIN ON DRUGS"

Patient History: Recent Cocaine Use

FIGURE 62–17   A and B.
Transverse ⁹⁹ᵐTc-HMPAO SPECT Scans: There are multiple small areas of decreased perfusion (yellow) separated by more normal areas of blood flow (red).

FIGURE 62–17   C and D.
Vertex and Left Lateral Views of 3-D Surface Reconstruction: There are multiple small areas of perfusion deficit scattered throughout the frontal and, to a lesser extent, the parietal lobes.

Patient 2: Chronic Methamphetamine Abuse

FIGURE 62–17   E.
Vertex View of ⁹⁹ᵐTc-HMPAO 3-D Surface Reconstruction: The perfusion has diffused focal abnormalities throughout the entire cortex.

NOTE 1. This pattern can be seen with polydrug or single drug abuse.

NOTE 2. These changes *may* be transitory if the patient becomes drug-free.

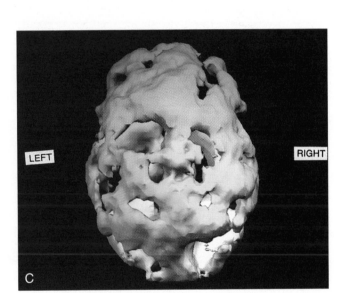

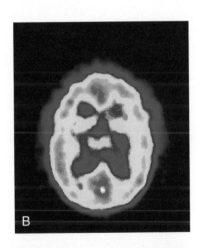

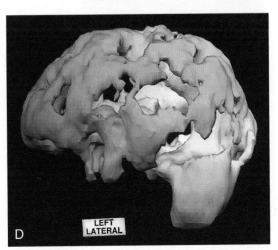

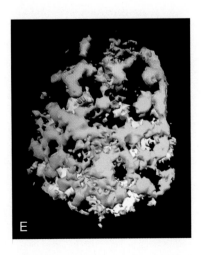

BRAIN DEATH STUDIES

Patient 1: Normal Cerebral Blood Flow

FIGURE 62–18   A.

^{99m}Tc-HMPAO Cerebral Blood Flow: The blood flow through the middle and anterior cerebral arteries is symmetric.

FIGURE 62–18   B and C.

Anterior and Lateral ^{99m}Tc-HMPAO Planar Brain Scans: The diffuse brain activity reflects blood flow through intracerebral blood vessels.

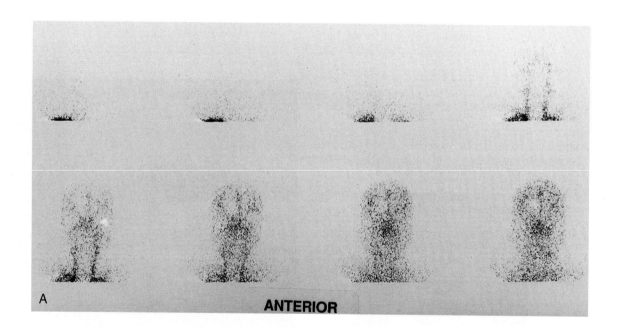

A   ANTERIOR

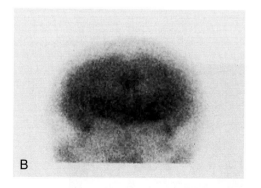

B

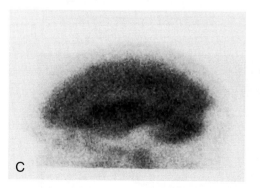

C

Patient 2: Brain Death

FIGURE 62–18   D.

^{99m}Tc-HMPAO Cerebral Blood Flow: The internal carotid blood flow stops at the base of the skull. The external carotid blood flow can be seen surrounding the brain and in the scalp.

FIGURE 62–18   E and F.

Anterior and Lateral ^{99m}Tc-HMPAO Planar Brain Scans: There is no supratentorial or infratentorial brain perfusion. All activity is in the surrounding scalp.

Illustration continued on following page

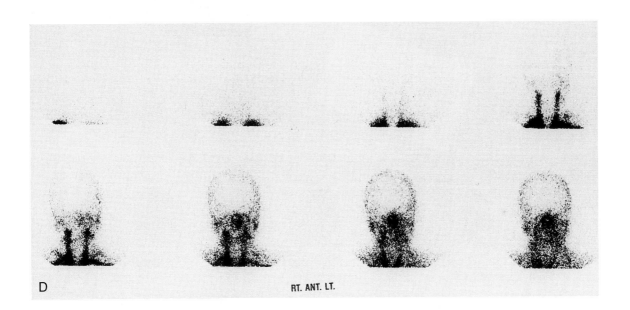

D   RT. ANT. LT.

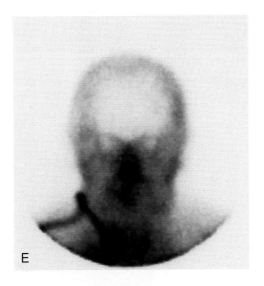

E

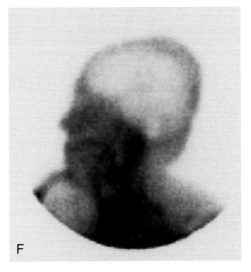

F

FIGURE 62–18   G.

Lateral Brain Arteriogram: The injection was made in the right common carotid artery. Internal carotid blood flow stops at the carotid siphon. Meningeal branches from the external carotid artery are filled. Vertebral blood flow stopped at the skull base.

Patient 3: Head Trauma

FIGURE 62–18   H.

⁹⁹ᵐTc-Glucoheptonate Cerebral Blood Flow: There is good perfusion of the right hemisphere but poor blood flow to the left.

Patient 4: Coma After Head Trauma

FIGURE 62–18   I.

⁹⁹ᵐTc-Glucoheptonate Cerebral Blood Flow Delayed Planar Scan: There is minimal residual blood flow beneath a left epidural hematoma *(arrow)*. This may be meningeal blood flow or compressed brain. There is also sagittal sinus visualization. This activity is not enough to sustain life.

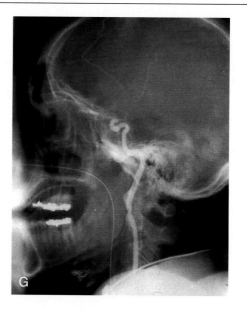

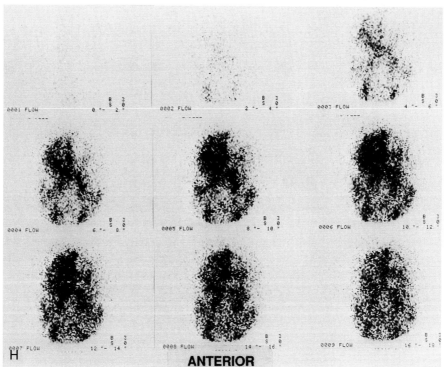

NOTE 1. Significant residual cerebral blood flow is a reliable sign for some degree of recovery, although by no means is it capable of predicting residual disabilities.

NOTE 2. The advantage of using a brain perfusion agent, such as ⁹⁹ᵐTc-HMPAO, is the availability of delayed scans, which can give greater information as to the amount of brain being perfused. It can also act as a backup if the cerebral blood flow study is lost or improperly acquired.

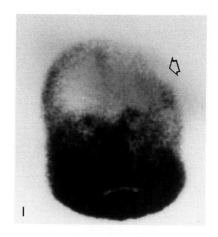

Cross Reference

Chapter 62: Perfusion Scanning—Trauma Following Stroke

Chapter 63
Cerebrospinal Fluid Flow Studies

NORMAL CEREBROSPINAL FLUID FLOW

Patient 1

FIGURE 63–1   A and B.

Five Hour ¹⁶⁹Yb-DTPA Cisternogram: The radiolabeled cerebrospinal fluid (CSF) can be seen in the basal cisterns but not in the cerebral ventricles.

FIGURE 63–1   C and D.

Twenty-four Hour Cisternogram: The CSF flow is over the frontal, temporal, and parietal lobes.

FIGURE 63–1   E and F.

Forty-eight Hour Cisternogram: Resorption in the midline, through the pacchionian (arachnoid) granulations, has occurred.

Illustration continued on following page

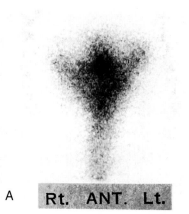

A   Rt. ANT. Lt.

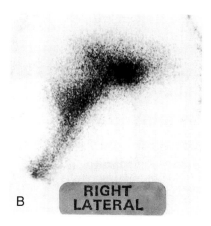

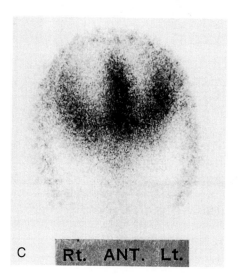

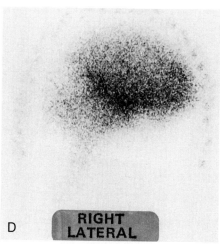

B   RIGHT LATERAL

C   Rt. ANT. Lt.

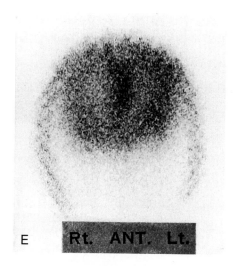

D   RIGHT LATERAL

E   Rt. ANT. Lt.

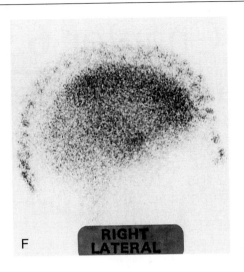

F   **RIGHT LATERAL**

Patient 2: Cortical Atrophy

FIGURE 63–1   G and H.

Right and Left Lateral 72-Hour Cisternogram: There are focal collections of CSF overlying the parietal lobes.

FIGURE 63–1   I and J.

Anterior and Posterior Cisternogram: The peripheral CSF collections can be seen.

NOTE 1. To be normal, the cisternogram must demonstrate flow over the parietal lobes, without ventricular penetration of the labeled CSF, and resorption at the vertex by 48 hours.

NOTE 2. CSF flow must be seen over the parietal and occipital lobes and not just over the frontal lobes.

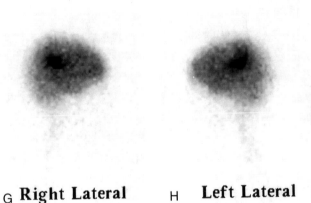

G **Right Lateral**   H **Left Lateral**   I **Anterior 72 hours**   J **Posterior 72 hours**

COMMUNICATING HYDROCEPHALUS

Patient 1: Normal Pressure Hydrocephalus (NPH)

FIGURE 63–2   A.

Twenty-four Hour ^{169}Yb-DTPA Cisternogram: There is ventricular penetration.

FIGURE 63–2   B.

Forty-eight Hour Cisternogram: The ventricular activity remains, and CSF flow over the vertex is absent. Flow over the frontal lobes can be seen with NPH.

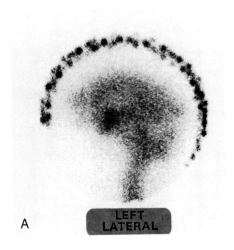

A   **LEFT LATERAL**

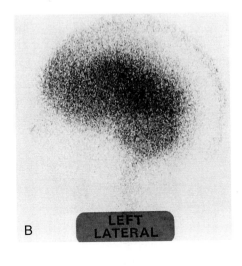

B   **LEFT LATERAL**

Patient 2: Slow Ventricular CSF Clearance

FIGURE 63–2   C and D.

Four Hour [169]Yb-DTPA Cisternogram: There is early CSF flow into the ventricles.

FIGURE 63–2   E and F.

Twenty-four and 48 Hour Cisternogram: The ventricles retain some radioactivity, but there is some flow around the brain.

FIGURE 63–2   G and H.

Seventy-two Hour Cisternogram: There is CSF flow around the brain and the ventricles have cleared, but there is no concentration in the midline arachnoid villi.

NOTE 1. NPH can be seen after subarachnoid hemorrhage, e.g., ruptured aneurysms or trauma, but most often it is idiopathic.

NOTE 2. Communicating hydrocephalus includes NPH, central atrophy (e.g., cerebrovascular disease), arrested hydrocephalus, and overproduction of CSF (i.e., choroid plexus papilloma).

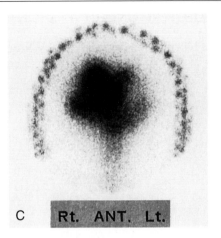

C   Rt. ANT. Lt.

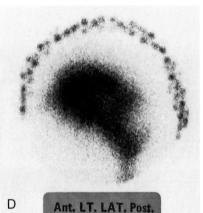

D   Ant. LT. LAT. Post.

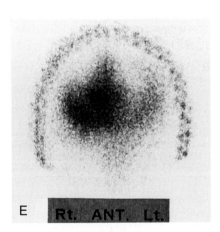

E   Rt. ANT. Lt.

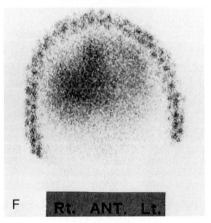

F   Rt. ANT. Lt.

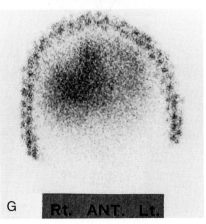

G   Rt. ANT. Lt.

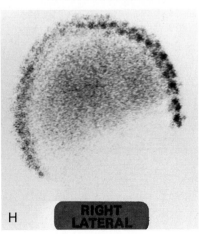

H   RIGHT LATERAL

VENTRICULOPERITONEAL (VP) SHUNTS

Patient 1: Normal VP Shunt Patency Study

FIGURE 63–3   A to C.

⁹⁹ᵐTc-DTPA VP Shunt Scan: The flow is continuous from the shunt reservoir down into the abdomen, with intraperitoneal dispersion.

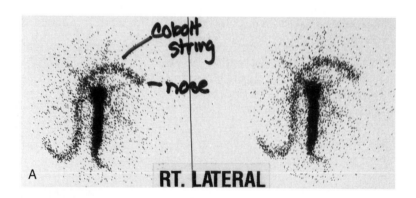

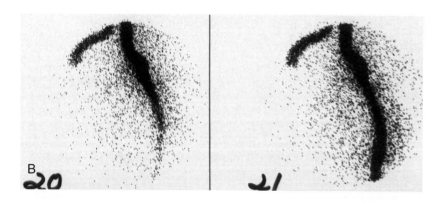

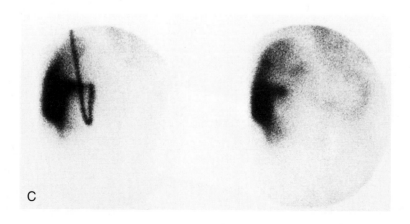

Patients 2 and 3: Intraperitoneal Pseudocyst

Figure 63–3   D and E.
⁹⁹ᵐTc-DTPA VP Shunt Scan: There is a loculated collection of the radiopharmaceutical at the distal tip of the shunt tubing.

Patient 4: Bowel Perforation by VP Shunt

Figure 63–3   F to H.
⁹⁹ᵐTc-DTPA VP Shunt Scan: There is visualization of small bowel lumen over 30 minutes.

Illustration continued on following page

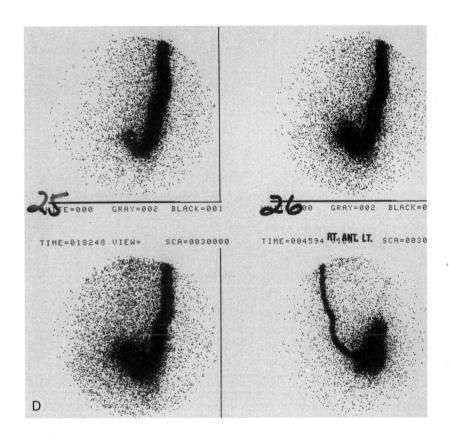

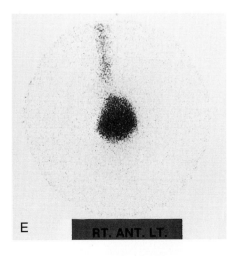

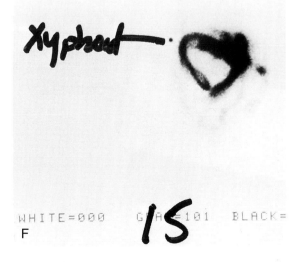

Patient 5: Reflux into the Cerebral Ventricles

FIGURE 63–3 I.

^{99m}Tc-DTPA VP Shunt Scan: After injection into the shunt reservoir, there is reflux into the cerebral ventricles due to an incompetent one-way valve.

Patient 6: Obstructed VP Shunt Reservoir

FIGURE 63–3 J.

^{99m}Tc-DTPA VP Shunt Scan: There is reflux into the ventricles and down the spine but no antegrade flow from the reservoir into the shunt tubing.

NOTE 1. Reservoir injections should be made with extremely small radiopharmaceutical volumes with high specific activity and as little force as possible.

NOTE 2. The pseudocyst is formed by fibrinous material and can sometimes be removed through a laparoscopic approach, without removing the shunt tubing.

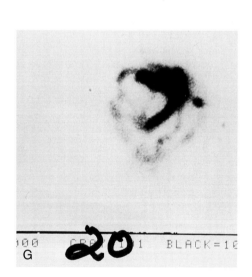

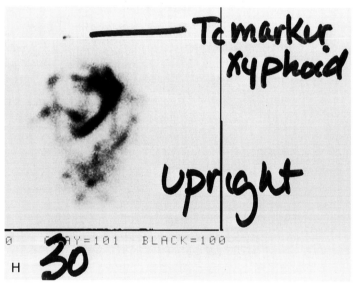

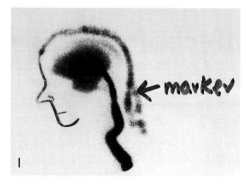

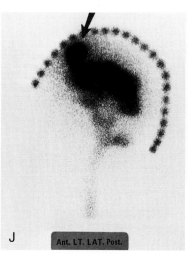

SPINAL BLOCK

Patient: Spinal Block from Metastatic Breast Carcinoma

FIGURE 63–4.

Posterior ⁹⁹ᵐTc-DTPA Nuclear Myelogram: The T3 CSF block is well delineated *(small arrows)*. The activity in the right cerebellopontine angle *(wavy arrow)* is due to the patient's lying on her right side most of the time.

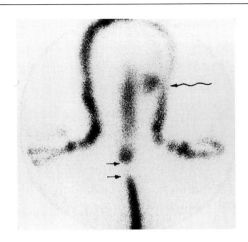

CSF LEAKS

Patient 1: Sphenoid Sinus Fracture

FIGURE 63–5   A.

One Hour ⁹⁹ᵐTc-DTPA Hyperbaric Cisternogram: There is good CSF flow into the basal cisterns, under the frontal lobes, and into the sylvian fissures.

FIGURE 63–5   B and C.

Three Hour ⁹⁹ᵐTc-DTPA Hyperbaric Cisternogram: There is an accumulation of the labeled CSF in the region of the sphenoid sinus *(curved arrow)*.

Illustration continued on following page

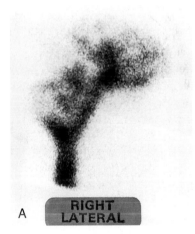

A   **RIGHT LATERAL**

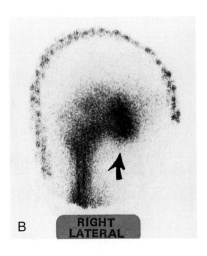

B   **RIGHT LATERAL**

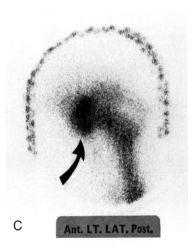

C   **Ant. LT. LAT. Post.**

Patient 2: Petrous Ridge Fracture

FIGURE 63–5   D.

Two Hour ^{99m}Tc-DTPA Hyperbaric Cisternogram: Radioactivity can be seen in the nose.

FIGURE 63–5   E.

Two Hour ^{99m}Tc-DTPA Hyperbaric Cisternogram: The leak in the right petrous ridge *(arrow)* flows into the eustachian canal and nose.

Patient 3: Craniotomy CSF Leak Only When the Patient Lies Down

FIGURE 63–5   F and G.

Twenty-four Hour Lateral ^{99m}Tc-DTPA Hyperbaric Cisternogram: The CSF flows around the frontal lobes in the interhemispheric fissure and flows out the craniotomy site into the subgaleal soft tissues.

NOTE 1. Cotton pledgets can be placed in the external auditory orifices, eustachian canals, and sphenoid orifices. They are pulled out after 2 to 4 hours of the cisternogram and counted. The highest counts indicate the site of the leak. The test can also be done with the pledgets in place overnight.

NOTE 2. Hyperbaric cisternography is accomplished by using 10 percent glucose/saline to dilute the radiopharmaceutical. With the patient in a Trendelenburg position, this moves the radioactivity away from the lumbar puncture site as a bolus.

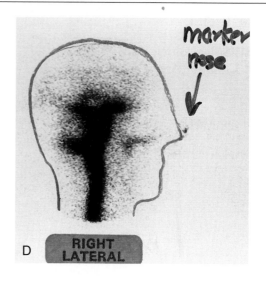

D RIGHT LATERAL

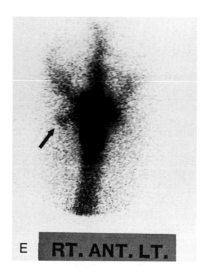

E RT. ANT. LT.

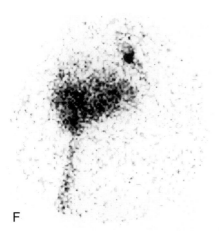

F

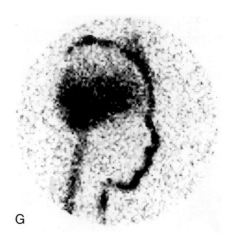

G

ARACHNOID CYST

Patient 1

FIGURE 63–6   A and B.

Immediate Anterior and Vertex ^{99m}Tc-DTPA Shunt Reservoir Injection: There is a large collection of radiolabeled CSF overlying the brain. The cyst was injected directly.

FIGURE 63–6   C and D.

Five Minute and 1 Hour ^{99m}Tc-DTPA Scans: The shunt is patent, but flow is slow.

FIGURE 63–6   E.

CT Scan: The large CSF collection and shunt can be seen. The shift of the midline was due to recent surgery and intracerebral hemorrhage.

Illustration continued on following page

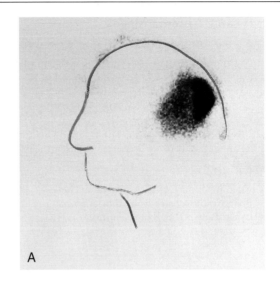

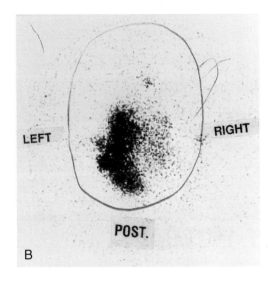

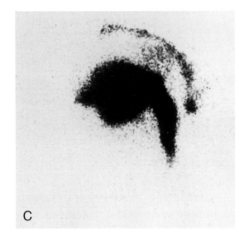

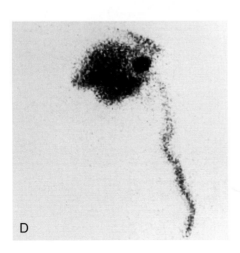

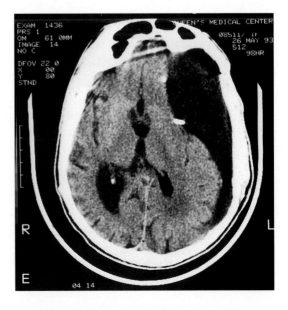

Patient 2: Large Cisterna Magna

FIGURE 63–6   F.

Sagittal T1 MRI Scan: The large CSF fluid collection in the posterior fossa represents a large cisterna magna or arachnoid cyst.

FIGURE 63–6   G.

Six Hour ^{111}In-DTPA Cisternogram: The radiolabeled CSF fills a large cisterna magna (EAM = external auditory meatus).

FIGURE 63–6   H.

Twenty-four Hour ^{111}In-DTPA Cisternogram: There is complete clearance of the radioactivity from the large cisterna magna. (Courtesy of Dr. Calvin Dela Plane, Honolulu, HI.)

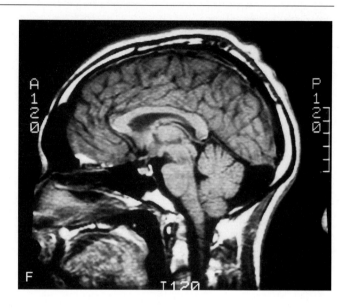

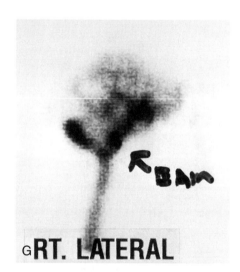

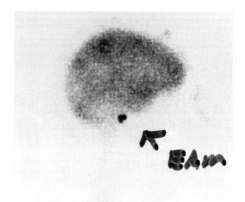

Chapter 64

Normal/Normal Variants

NORMAL THYROID SCANS

Patient 1

FIGURE 64–1   A to C.
Thirty Minute ^{99m}Tc-Pertechnetate Scan: Three views of the thyroid reveal homogeneous activity, reflecting the trapping mechanism activity.

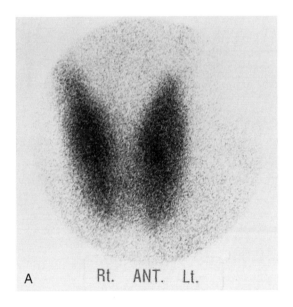

A   Rt.   ANT.   Lt.

Illustration continued on following page

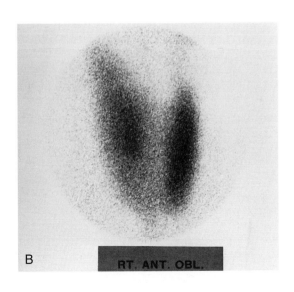

B   RT. ANT. OBL.

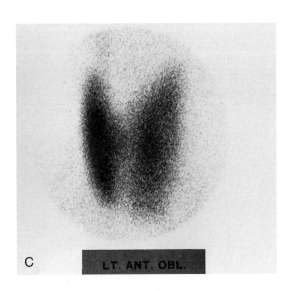

C   LT. ANT. OBL.

Patient 2

FIGURE 64–1   D to F.

Six Hour ¹²³I Scan: There is homogeneous activity, indicative of organification and storage. (Courtesy of Dr. Michael Kipper, Vista, CA.)

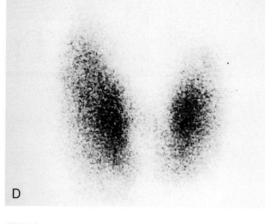

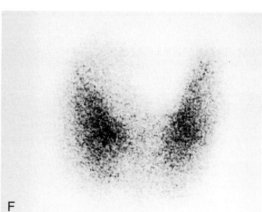

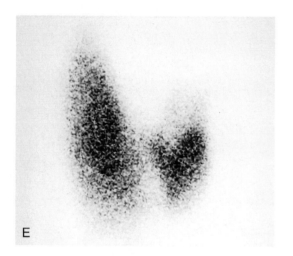

ASYMMETRIC THYROID LOBES

Patient 1

FIGURE 64–2   A and B.

Anterior and RAO ⁹⁹ᵐTc-Pertechnetate Thyroid Scan: The right lobe extends inferiorly below the right clavicular head.

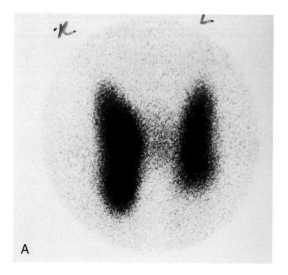

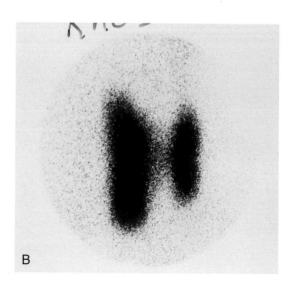

Patient 2: Solitary Hypertrophic Lobe

FIGURE 64–2 C.

⁹⁹ᵐTc-Pertechnetate Thyroid Scan: The left lobe is normal while the right lobe is large. The patient was euthyroid.

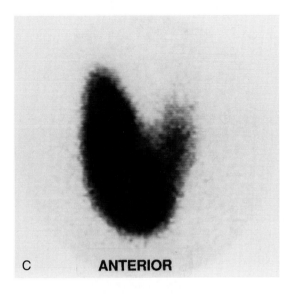

Patient 3: Small Left Lobe

FIGURE 64–2 D.

⁹⁹ᵐTc-Pertechnetate Thyroid Scan: The left lobe measured small, 2 cm in length.

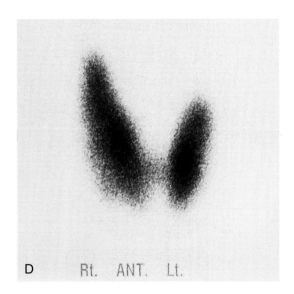

FREE TECHNETIUM PERTECHNETATE DISTRIBUTION

FIGURE 64–3.

Total Body Scan: There is only soft tissue accumulation of technetium pertechnetate. Activity is seen in the parotids, submandibular glands, oropharynx, thyroid, stomach, kidneys, and urinary bladder. Minimal blood pool can be seen in the heart.

NOTE 1. Technetium pertechnetate will accumulate and be secreted or excreted by those organs that take up, secrete, or excrete inorganic iodine.

NOTE 2. If any of the glandular organs is seen on a bone scan, free technetium pertechnetate should be suspected. A check of the thyroid, salivary glands, and stomach should detect free technetium pertechnetate.

NOTE 3. If a woman being scanned for thyroid disease is breast feeding, she should milk her breasts and not breast feed for 24 hours.

Cross References

Chapter 11: Soft Tissue Abnormalities—Differential Diagnosis of Soft Tissue Uptake of Bone Scanning Agents

Chapter 73: Breast Diseases—Normal Breast Activity with Various Radiopharmaceuticals

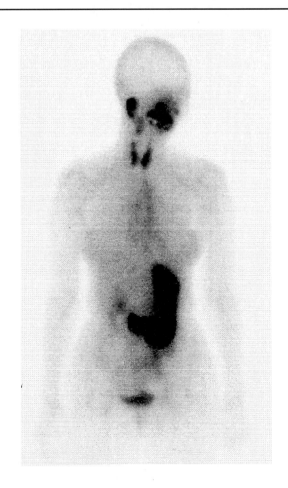

LINGUAL THYROID

FIGURE 64–4   A.
Anterior Neck Thyroid Scan: There is no normal thyroid activity.

FIGURE 64–4   B.
Anterior Face Scan: There is a focus of activity in the midline *(arrow)* that corresponded to a lingual mass (the patient's head is slightly tilted).

FIGURE 64–4   C.
Right Lateral Face Scan: The activity *(arrow)* is seen at the back of the oral cavity.

Cross Reference

Chapter 65: Diffuse Disease—Subacute Thyroiditis

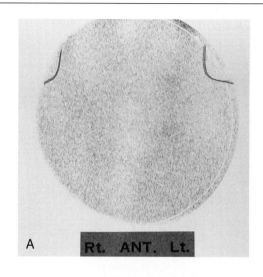

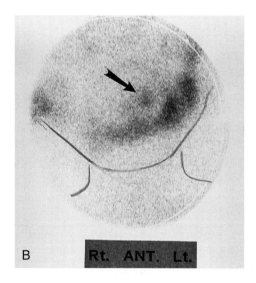

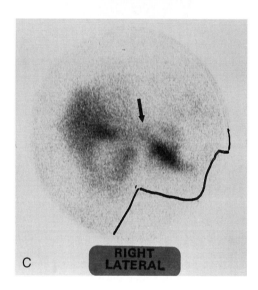

THYROGLOSSAL DUCT CYST

Patient 1: Thirty-six Year Old Woman with a Midline Neck Mass

FIGURE 64–5   A.
Anterior Scan of the Neck: There is no appreciable activity in the midline mass, outlined by four technetium markers *(arrowheads)* above the normal thyroid.

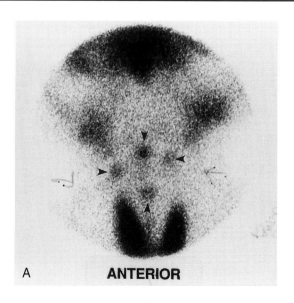

Patient 2: Forty-six Year Old Woman with a Nodular Thyroid

FIGURE 64–5 B to E.

Anterior, LAO, and RAO Pinhole Views of the Neck and Thyroid: The activity in the midline above the thyroid was not palpable, nor was it diminished or washed away with repeated drinks of water. No mass was palpable.

NOTE 1. Ectopic functioning thyroid, as well as thyroid carcinomas, may occur in thyroglossal duct cysts.

NOTE 2. These scans are done preoperatively to make sure that there is functioning thyroid tissue in the normal location and that the thyroglossal duct cyst does not contain the only functioning thyroid.

NOTE 3. Thyroid tissue rests may occur along the migrational tract of embryologic tissue, from the back of the tongue to beneath the sternum.

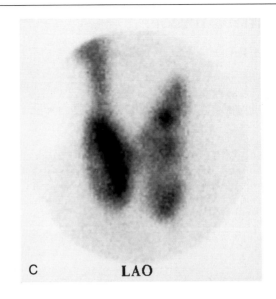

C   LAO

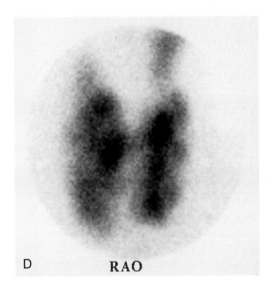

D   RAO

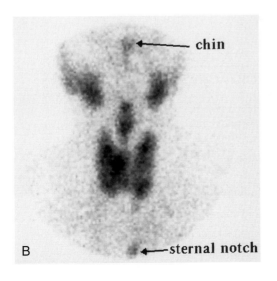

B

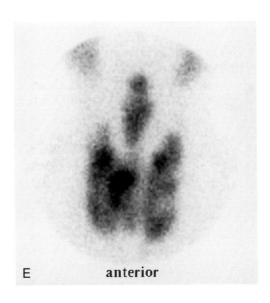

E   anterior

SUBSTERNAL THYROID

Patient 1

FIGURE 64–6   A.

^{99m}Tc-Pertechnetate Scan of Neck: There is a large mass of functioning thyroid tissue within the superior mediastinum.

Patient 2

FIGURE 64–6   B.

^{99m}Tc-Pertechnetate Thyroid Scan: There is a sliver of functioning thyroid extending into the superior mediastinum. (The patient swallowed water prior to the scan.)

NOTE 1. Retained activity in the esophagus from swallowed saliva can simulate substernal thyroid tissue. Swallowing water prior to scanning can clear the esophagus.

NOTE 2. A mediastinal thyroid may be the only thyroid tissue.

NOTE 3. Substernal goiters may present as dyspnea, dysphasia, or venous engorgement of the neck ("superior vena cava syndrome").

NOTE 4. Superior mediastinal masses include thyroid, thymus, and metastatic disease as well as lymphoma and teratoma.

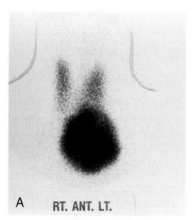

A   RT. ANT. LT.

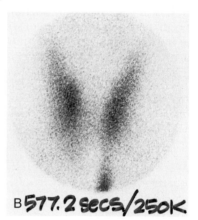

B 577.2 secs/250K

Chapter 65
Diffuse Disease

DECREASED OR ABSENT THYROID ACTIVITY IN THE NECK

DECREASED OR ABSENT THYROID ACTIVITY IN THE NECK	
1. Hypothyroidism	6. Thyroidectomy, ^{131}I Ablation
2. Ectopic thyroid	7. High-iodine diet (e.g., seaweed)
3. Subacute thyroiditis, lymphocytic or granulomatous	8. Lithium therapy
4. Thyroid suppression, e.g., PTU, methimazole, T3, T4	9. Radiation therapy
	10. Amiodarone therapy
5. Contrast media	11. Cretinism

SUBACUTE THYROIDITIS

FIGURE 65–1.

Technetium Thyroid Scan: There is no thyroid seen in this patient with subacute thyroiditis.

NOTE 1. Patients are usually referred for scanning because of their elevated T4 and suppressed TSH serum levels, caused by release of stored hormone by the inflamed thyroid.

NOTE 2. If the gland is tender, it is usually due to granulomatous (de Quervain's) thyroiditis. If it is painless, it is usually due to lymphocytic thyroiditis.

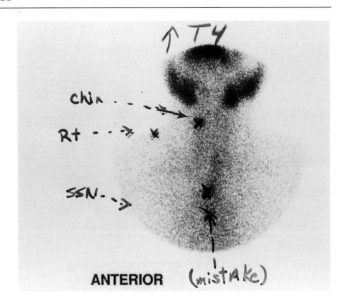

DIFFUSE TOXIC GOITER (GRAVES' DISEASE)

FIGURE 65–2 A to C.

Technetium Thyroid Scan: Both thyroid lobes have convex margins. There is also activity in the pyramidal lobe.

NOTE 1. A shortened time of acquisition of each scan is also indicative of the hyperthyroid state.

NOTE 2. Graves' disease and Hashimoto's thyrotoxicosis may not be associated with an enlarged thyroid gland.

NOTE 3. Thyroid carcinoma can arise in a Graves' disease gland, and a "cold" nodule should be biopsied.

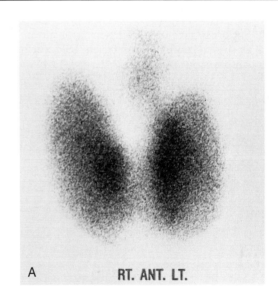

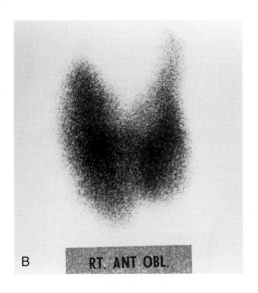

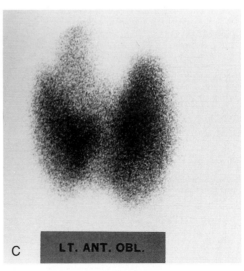

SUPPRESSIBLE HOT NODULE

FIGURE 66–1 A.

Technetium Thyroid Scan: There is a functioning nodule in the inferior pole of the right lobe.

FIGURE 66–1 B.

Thyroid Scan During T3 Suppression Test: There is suppression of the normal thyroid gland as well as the hot nodule.

FIGURE 66–1 C.

Thyroid Scan After ¹³¹Iodine Therapy: The hot nodule is no longer evident.

NOTE. Suppressible hot nodules are not autonomous, as they respond to decreased TSH during a T3 suppression test.

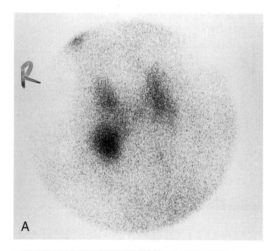

A

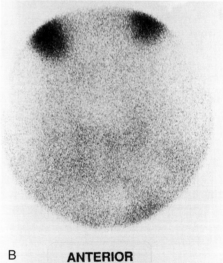

B **ANTERIOR**

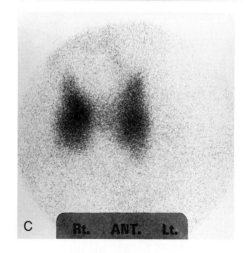

C Rt. ANT. Lt.

SUSPECT THYROID NODULE

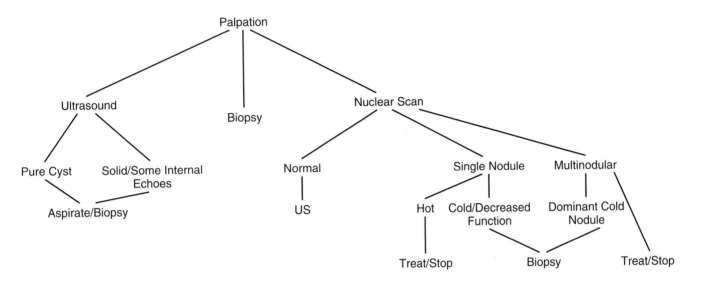

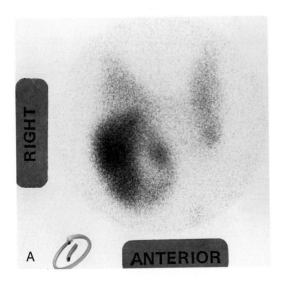

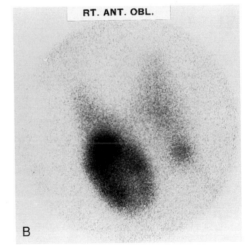

THYROID ADENOMA

Patient 1

FIGURE 66–2   A to C.

^{99m}Tc-Pertechnetate Thyroid Scan: There is a hot nodule containing areas of decreased function. The remaining thyroid gland is suppressed.

Illustration continued on following page

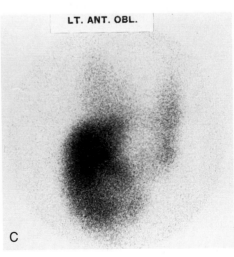

Patient 2

FIGURE 66–2 D.

⁹⁹ᵐTc-Pertechnetate Thyroid Scan: The entire left lobe is "hot," with decreased function centrally and suppression of the right lobe.

Patient 3

FIGURE 66–2 E and F.

Anterior and RAO ⁹⁹ᵐTc-Pertechnetate Thyroid Scan: The hot nodule has homogeneous activity, without complete suppression of the normal thyroid tissue.

Patient 4

FIGURE 66–2 G.

⁹⁹ᵐTc-Pertechnetate Thyroid Scan: There is a solitary hot nodule in the right lobe, which has homogeneous activity.

FIGURE 66–2 H.

¹³¹Iodine Thyroid Scan: The nodule remains hot on this scan, indicating its ability to organify iodine.

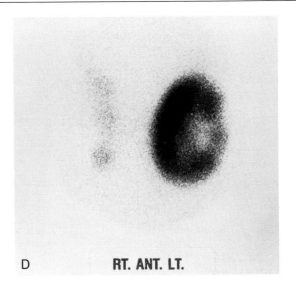

D   RT. ANT. LT.

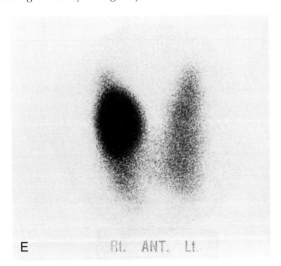

E   Rt. ANT. Lt.

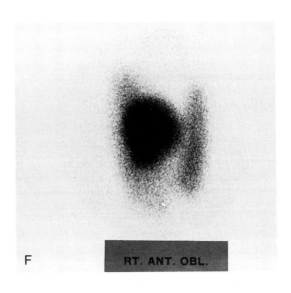

F   RT. ANT. OBL.

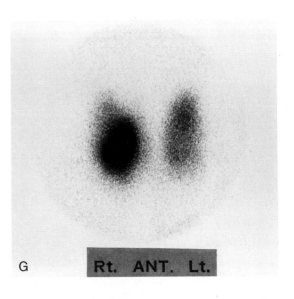

G   Rt. ANT. Lt.

NOTE 1. Thyroid adenomas often hemorrhage within themselves, creating sudden focal swelling of the thyroid gland, pain, and tenderness.

NOTE 2. Adenomas that hemorrhage may present with small areas of photopenia or as cold nodules.

NOTE 3. A warm nodule that does not completely suppress the remaining thyoid tissue has approximately a 1 percent chance of being a well-differentiated thyroid carcinoma. Activity on a 24 hour ^{131}I scan for organification properties is usually sufficient to allow conservative therapy. Lack of activity on the 24 hour ^{131}I scan is an indication for biopsy or removal.

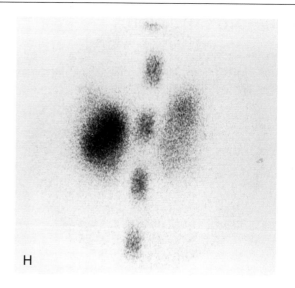

H

PLUMMER'S NODULE

FIGURE 66–3   A.

Technetium Thyroid Scan: There is only a solitary hot nodule visible, with complete suppression of the remaining normal thyroid.

FIGURE 66–3   B.

[131]Iodine Scan During Therapy: Virtually all the ^{131}I goes to the nodule, effectively treating it and sparing the normal gland.

NOTE. A Plummer nodule is a toxic adenoma that is nonsuppressible (autonomous) and usually presents as hyperthyroidism.

Cross Reference

Chapter 67: Multiple Nodules—Toxic Multinodular Goiter

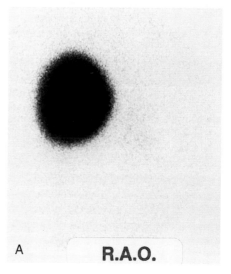

A   **R.A.O.**

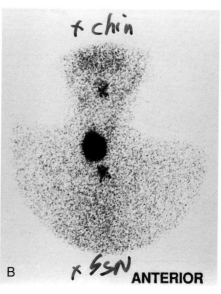

B   **ANTERIOR**

HASHIMOTO'S THYROIDITIS

FIGURE 66–4.

Anterior Thyroid Scan: There is a large right lobe mass with irregular areas of functioning tissue.

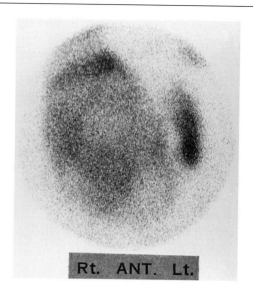

COLD NODULE–COLLOID CYST

FIGURE 66–5   A to C.

Thyroid Scan: There is a large nonfunctioning nodule within the right lobe.

NOTE. All solitary cold or poorly functioning nodules >1 cm should be biopsied.

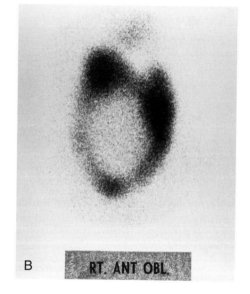

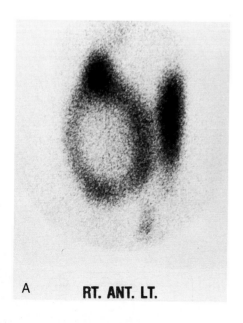

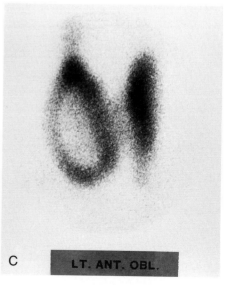

ISTHMUS COLD NODULE

Patient 1: Colloid Cyst

FIGURE 66-6 A.
Thyroid Scan: The isthmus is wider and more convex than normal owing to a nodule with little function.

Patient 2: Epithelioid Thymoma

FIGURE 66-6 B.
Thyroid Scan: The isthmus is more prominent than usual. By palpation there was a mass.

NOTE 1. Isthmus nodules may be difficult to detect on scanning. Correlation with palpation is mandatory.

NOTE 2. Prominent thyroid cartilage as well as a mass can be separating the lobes.

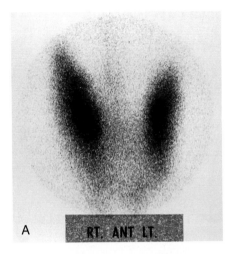

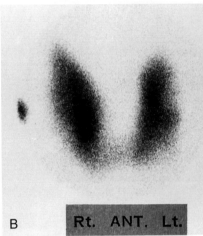

DISCORDANT NODULE

Patient: Papillary Carcinoma

FIGURE 66-7 A.
Technetium Thyroid Scan: There are several warm nodules, including a palpable one in the left upper pole *(arrow)*.

FIGURE 66-7 B.
^{131}Iodine Thyroid Scan: The upper pole nodule is not apparent on this scan.

NOTE 1. Technetium pertechnetate scans reflect the trapping mechanism, whereas radioiodine scanning reflects organification.

NOTE 2. Some well-differentiated thyroid carcinomas have the ability to trap iodine and technetium but do not organify the iodine. They appear as discordant, i.e., "hot," nodules, with ^{99m}Tc-pertechnetate but as "cold" nodules on delayed radioiodine scan.

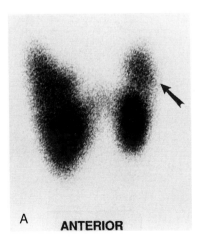

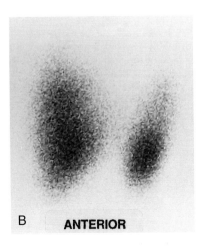

FOLLICULAR CARCINOMA

FIGURE 66–8   A and B.

Technetium Thyroid Scan: The nodule in the inferior pole of the left lobe has some functioning tissue and is not absolutely "cold."

NOTE 1. As with cold nodules, those with some function can be benign or malignant and should be biopsied.

NOTE 2. Follicular carcinoma is difficult to distinguish from follicular adenoma by fine needle biopsy. Vascular or capsular invasion is a helpful criterion used to diagnose follicular carcinoma.

Cross Reference

Chapter 68: Cancer—Papillofollicular Carcinoma

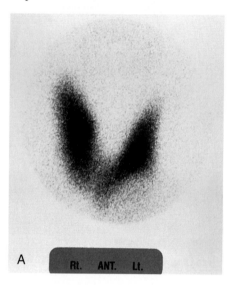

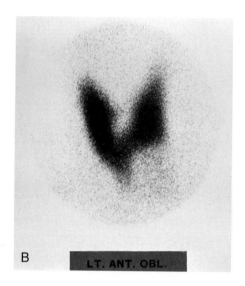

Chapter 67
Multiple Nodules

THYROID NODULES: ONE HOT, ONE COLD

FIGURE 67–1   A.

Anterior Technetium Thyroid Scan: There is a warm nodule in the inferior pole of the right lobe and a poorly functioning nodule in the inferior pole of the left lobe.

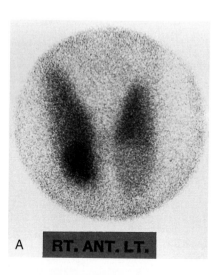

FIGURE 67–1   B.

[131]Iodine Thyroid Scan: There is organification in the right lower pole but decreased function on the left.

NOTE. Radioiodine should be used when there is a warm nodule without suppression of the remaining thyroid tissue. If there is organification, no biopsy is necessary.

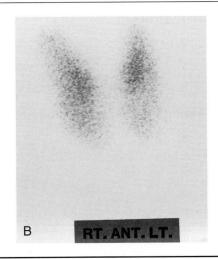

TOXIC MULTINODULAR GOITERS

Patient 1: Toxic Multinodular Goiter

FIGURE 67–2   A to D.

Technetium Pertechnetate Thyroid Scan: This huge thyroid consists mainly of cold nodules. Despite a long acquisition time (354 seconds) the uptakes were unusually high for a multinodular gland: 17 percent at 6 hours and 28 percent at 24 hours. (Normal in our laboratory is under 15 percent and under 30 percent, respectively.) The serum values were also at the upper limits of normal.

Illustration continued on following page

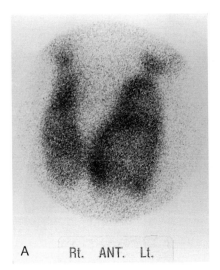

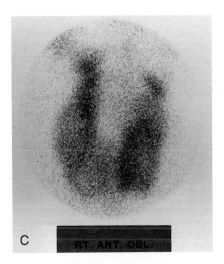

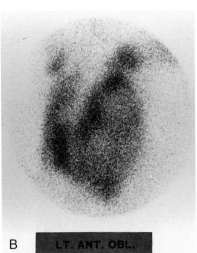

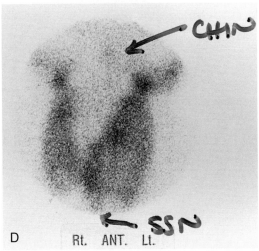

Patient 2: Hashitoxicosis

FIGURE 67–2   E to G.

Anterior, RAO, and LAO Scans: There are numerous nonpalpable nodules associated with increased activity.

Patient 3: Multiple Autonomous Nodules

FIGURE 67–2   H.

Presuppression Anterior Thyroid Scan: There are six hyperfunctioning nodules.

FIGURE 67–2   I.

Post-T3 Suppression Thyroid Scan: Although the more normal gland has further decreased its uptake of the technetium pertechnetate, the nodules are still hyperfunctioning.

Cross Reference

Chapter 66: Solitary Nodules—Plummer's Nodule

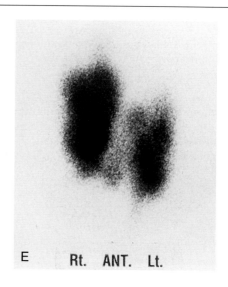

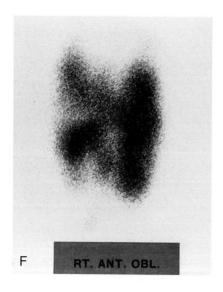

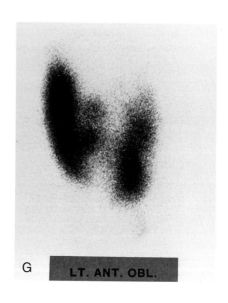

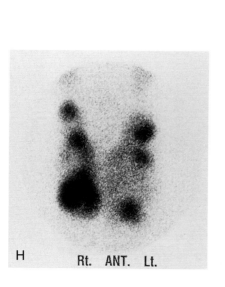

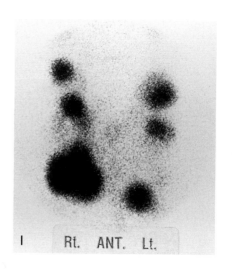

UNILATERAL MULTINODULAR THYROID DISEASE

Patient: Lymphocytic Thyroiditis

FIGURE 67–3   A and B.

Anterior and LAO Thyroid Scan: The left lobe is enlarged, with areas of increased, normal, and decreased function. The right lobe is mildly suppressed.

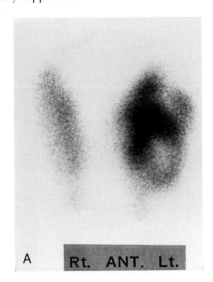

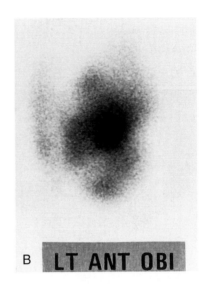

MULTINODULAR DISEASE

Patient 1: Multinodular Thyroid

FIGURE 67–4   A to C.

^{99m}Tc-Pertechnetate Thyroid Scan: There are multiple nonfunctioning nodules bilaterally but neither distinct hot nodules nor a dominant cold nodule are present.

Illustration continued on following page

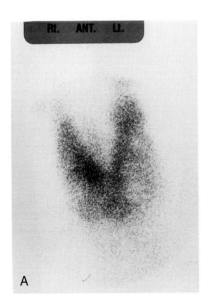

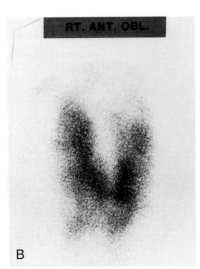

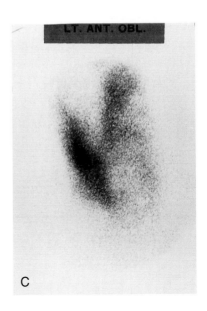

Patient 2: Organification Demonstrated by ¹³¹I in Multinodular Thyroid

FIGURE 67–4   D to F.

Twenty-four Hour Anterior, RAO, and LAO ¹³¹I Thyroid Scan: There are several small functioning nodules as well as nonfunctioning portions of the gland. (Courtesy of Dr. Michael Kipper, Vista, CA.)

Patient 3: Bilateral Papillary Carcinoma in Multinodular Goiter

FIGURE 67–4   G to I.

⁹⁹ᵐTc-Pertechnetate Thyroid Scan: There is a large cold nodule arising from the right lobe (dominant "cold" nodule) along with other "cold" nodules in both lobes.

NOTE 1. Multinodular thyroid glands may have nodules that have increased, normal, or decreased trapping and organification.

NOTE 2. It is often difficult to palpate more than one nodule or, occasionally, any nodule.

NOTE 3. Bilateral thyroid carcinoma occurs in <5 percent of thyroid cancer cases.

NOTE 4. Multinodular goiter has the same incidence of thyroid carcinoma as do normal glands. Biopsy of the dominant "cold" nodule is a practical compromise.

Cross Reference

Chapter 68: Cancer—Bilateral Synchronous Papillary Carcinoma

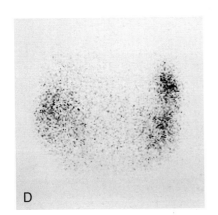

D

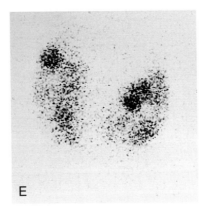

E

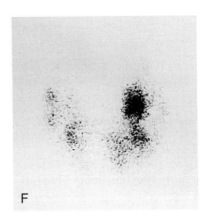

F

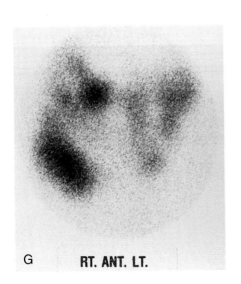

G   RT. ANT. LT.

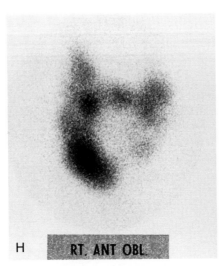

H   RT. ANT OBL

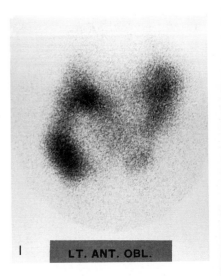

I   LT. ANT. OBL.

HUGE HASHIMOTO'S THYROIDITIS NODULES

FIGURE 67–5   A.

⁹⁹ᵐTc-Pertechnetate Scan of the Neck: The markers outline two huge masses extending beneath both sternocleidomastoid muscles.

FIGURE 67–5   B.

Pinhole View of the Thyroid: There is irregular uptake within both thyroid lobes, with only a small (<1 cm) "cold" nodule evident in the lower pole of the right lobe.

NOTE. Nonfunctioning nodules that do not appear to arise from the thyroid may still represent thyroid disease. They presumably arise from the periphery of the gland and grow outward and do not indent or displace the normal thyroid tissue.

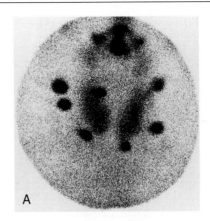

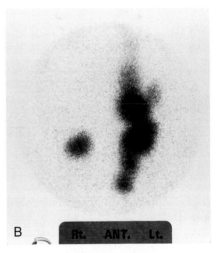

POST-THYROIDECTOMY "NODULES"

Patient 1

FIGURE 67–6   A.

Anterior Preoperative ⁹⁹ᵐTc-Pertechnetate Thyroid Scan: The cold nodule in the right lobe proved to be a papillary carcinoma.

FIGURE 67–6   B and C.

Postoperative Anterior and LAO Thyroid Scan: There are small "nodules" of residual thyroid.

Illustration continued on following page

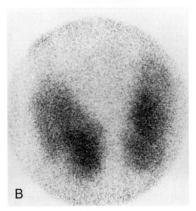

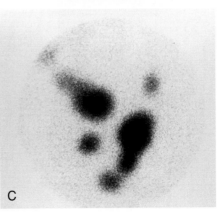

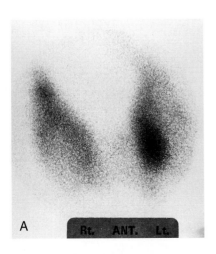

Patient 2: Postoperative Hypertrophic Nodule

FIGURE 67–6   D and E.

Anterior and LAO ^{99m}Tc-Pertechnetate Thyroid Scan: The left upper pole nodule was palpable 2 years after surgery.

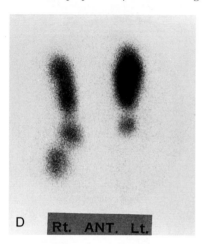

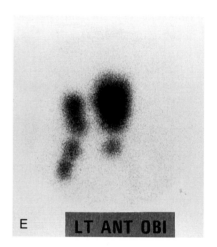

Chapter 68
Thyroid Cancer

PAPILLOFOLLICULAR CARCINOMA

FIGURE 68–1   A and B.

Thyroid Scan: There is a large "cold" mass in the left upper pole (outlined by four markers on Fig. 68–1B).

NOTE 1. Cold nodules >1 cm in diameter should be biopsied.

NOTE 2. Most malignant thyroid neoplasms have papillary and follicular elements, usually with one cell type dominating.

Cross Reference

Chapter 68: Cancer—Follicular Carcinoma

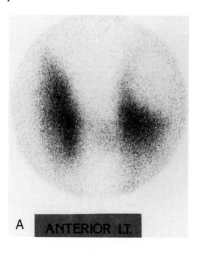

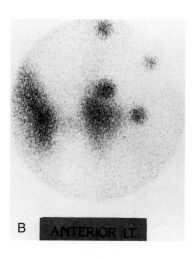

BILATERAL SYNCHRONOUS PAPILLARY CARCINOMA

FIGURE 68–2.

Thyroid Scan: There are cold nodules of the right lower pole and the left upper pole.

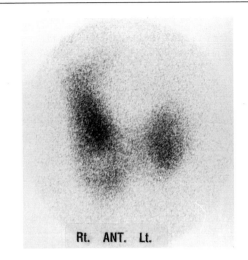

NOTE. Bilateral malignancies occur in <5 percent cases and can be synchronous, as in this case, or metachronous (at different times). There may be separate tumor foci in the same lobe as well.

Cross Reference

Chapter 67: Multiple Nodules—Multinodular Thyroid Disease

NORMAL ¹³¹IODINE WHOLE BODY DISTRIBUTION POST THYROIDECTOMY

FIGURE 68–3 A.

Anterior and Posterior ¹³¹Iodine Whole Body Scan: The iodine will be seen in the mouth and salivary glands, the stomach, the bowel (especially the colon), the urinary bladder, and, often, the liver. Residual thyroid tissue will also be seen.

Illustration continued on following page

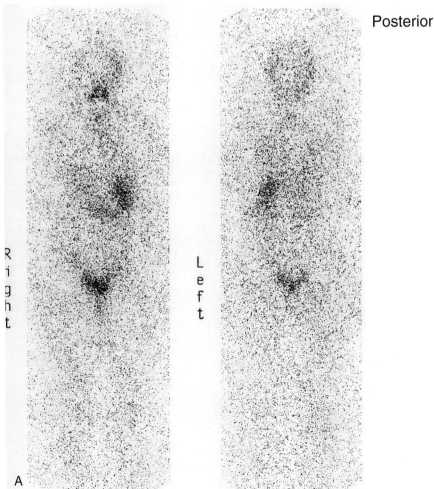

FIGURE 68–3   B.

Pinhole View of Neck: There is no appreciable residual thyroid activity after total thyroidectomy and radioiodine ablation.

NOTE 1. A pinhole view of the neck is essential to pick up metastatic lymph nodes, especially when there is residual normal thyroid tissue.

NOTE 2. A TSH of >40 is optimal for effective screening for functioning metastases.

NOTE 3. The whole body scan should be done 5 to 7 days after an ablative dose, or 48 to 72 hours after a diagnostic (5mCi ^{131}I) dose.

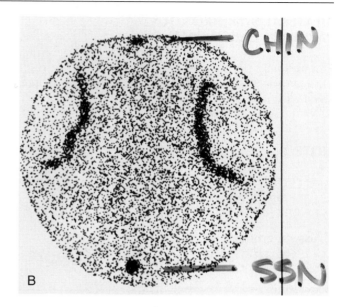

FUNCTIONING THYROID METASTASES

Patient 1: Sixty-three Year Old Female with Follicular Carcinoma

FIGURE 68–4   A.

Thyroid Scan: The dominant cold nodule in the left lower pole was follicular carcinoma. There are several additional "cold" nodules *(arrowheads)*.

FIGURE 68–4   B.

^{131}Iodine Scan of the Lungs 6 Weeks Later: The lungs have diffuse, multiple metastases in a macronodular pattern.

FIGURE 68–4   C.

CT Scan: There are numerous nodules throughout both lungs.

FIGURE 68–4   D.

Right Lateral ^{131}Iodine Scan of the Head 3 Years Later: There is intense ^{131}I accumulation in the posterior parietal region.

FIGURE 68–4   E.

Bone Scan: There is a "doughnut" lesion in the posterior right parietal bone.

FIGURE 68–4   F.

Plain Film X-ray of the Skull: There is a lytic lesion in the posterior right parietal bone.

FIGURE 68–4   G.

CT Scan: The lytic lesion of the skull is seen. Soft tissue windows did not demonstrate brain involvement.

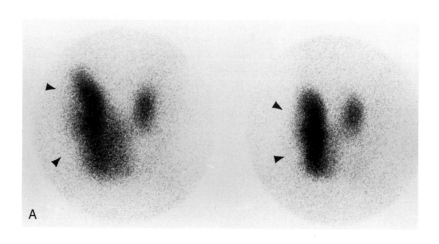

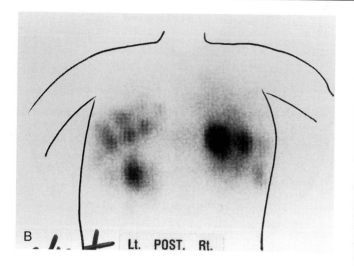

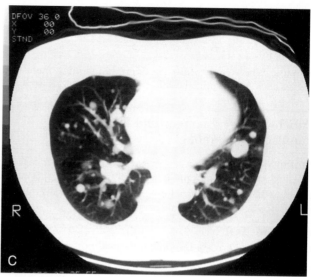

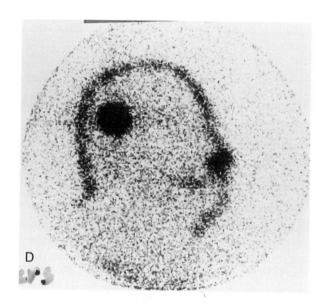

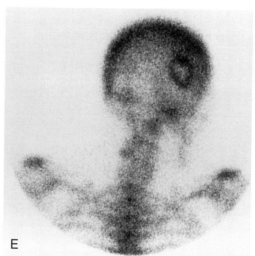

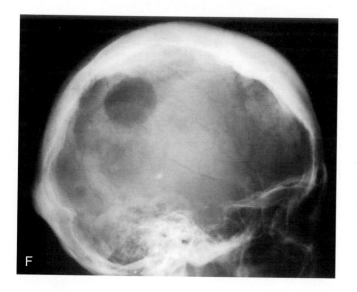

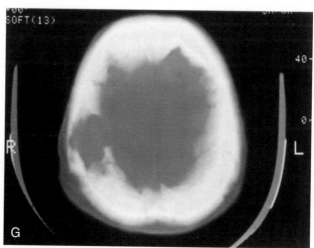

Illustration continued on following page

Patient 2: Fifty Year Old Male with Papillary Carcinoma

FIGURE 68–4   H.

[131]Iodine Whole Body Scan: There are functioning metastases in the neck, right supraclavicular fossa, and mediastinum.

Patient 3: Forty-six Year Old Female with Papillary Carcinoma

FIGURE 68–4   I.

[131]Iodine Scan: There is diffuse radioactive accumulation in the lungs, without a nodular pattern. Other metastases are present in the neck, liver, and abdomen.

FIGURE 68–4   J.

Chest X-ray: There are innumerable small nodules.

NOTE 1. Pulmonary metastases can be tolerated for long periods, particularly in young patients.

NOTE 2. Although older patients have a worse prognosis, they may still survive many years.

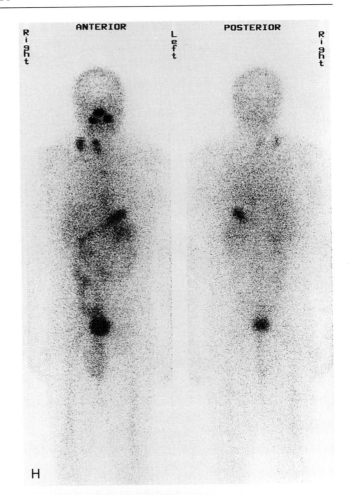

H

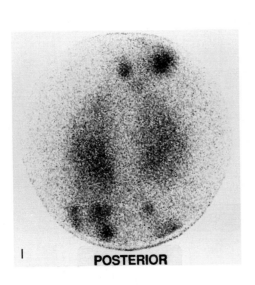

I   POSTERIOR

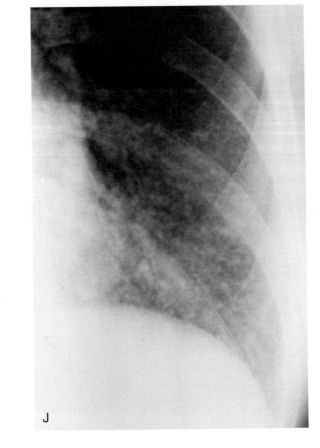

J

¹³¹IODINE DOSE–DEPENDENT METASTASES

Patient 1

FIGURE 68–5 A.
Five mCi ¹³¹Iodine Pinhole Neck Scintigram: There are three subtle foci of radioactivity representing metastases from papillary thyroid carcinoma in the right neck *(short arrows)*.

FIGURE 68–5 B.
Ten Days Later, 150 mCi ¹³¹Iodine Pinhole Neck Scintigram: The metastases are more apparent with the higher dose.

Patient 2

FIGURE 68–5 C.
Ten mCi ¹³¹Iodine Scan: The preablative dose demonstrated only residual thyroid tissue.

FIGURE 68–5 D.
One Week After Ablation, 150 mCi ¹³¹Iodine Scan: The postablation scan demonstrates a right cervical lymph node *(arrowhead)*.

Patient 3

FIGURE 68–5 E.
Ten mCi ¹³¹Iodine Chest Scan: There are no appreciable foci of abnormal ¹³¹I activity. Markers are at the manubrium and xiphoid.

FIGURE 68–5 F.
Eight Days Post 146 mCi ¹³¹Iodine Therapy Chest Scan: The lungs demonstrate diffuse pulmonary activity as well as foci of intense ¹³¹I accumulation.

Illustration continued on following page

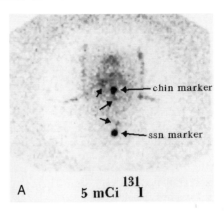

A   5 mCi ¹³¹I

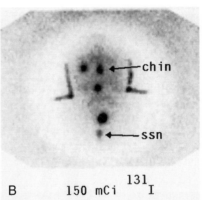

B   150 mCi ¹³¹I

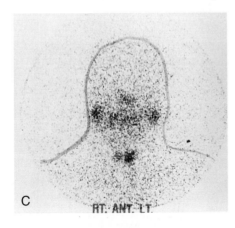

C   RT. ANT. LT.

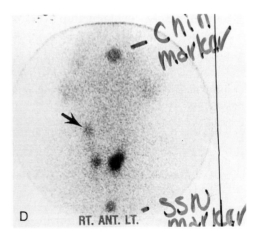

D   RT. ANT. LT.

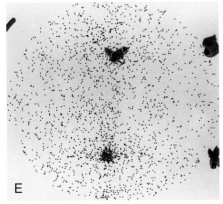

E

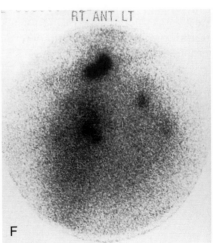

F

Patient 4

FIGURE 68–5   G.

5 mCi [131]Iodine Pinhole Neck Scintigram: There is faint visualization of right neck nodal uptake of the radioiodine (hot spot in midline is a sternal notch marker).

FIGURE 68–5   H.

Anterior 5 mCi [131]Iodine Chest Planar Scan: There is an ill-defined radioiodine accumulation in the mediastinum.

FIGURE 68–5   I.

[99m]Technetium Sestamibi Pinhole Neck Scan: There is a solitary right lower neck focal abnormality.

FIGURE 68–5   J.

[99m]Technetium Sestamibi Planar Anterior Chest Scan: There is no abnormal sestamibi accumulation within the lungs or mediastinum.

FIGURE 68–5   K.

144 Hour, 150 mCi [131]Iodine Pinhole Neck Scan: There are multiple functioning metastases within the neck.

FIGURE 68–5   L.

144 Hour, 150 mCi [131]Iodine Whole Body Scan: The functioning metastasis is evident in the mid-mediastinum.

NOTE 1. Postablation therapy scans may demonstrate more metastases in about 15 percent of cases, presumably from the larger dose given.

NOTE 2. [131]Iodine scans may not demonstrate all metastases whether 1 mCi or 10 mCi is used. Thallium or sestamibi may show some metastases but miss others.

NOTE 3. The 10 mCi [131]Iodine used for scanning may stun some tumor foci as well as normal tissue, possibly interfering with the ability to ablate metastases. We now use 2 to 5 mCi ^{131}I for whole body scanning, except in those patients with elevated serum thyroglobulin levels or other clinical evidence for metastatic disease.

NOTE 4. In those patients who are to receive radioiodine ablative therapy, preablation scans are often unnecessary except to help determine the therapeutic dose.

NOTE 5. In low-risk patients, 29 mCi [131]Iodine may be enough to ablate residual normal tissue. Low risk is defined as a small (<1 cm) primary tumor, no microvascular or capsular invasion, and no cervical lymph node involvement.

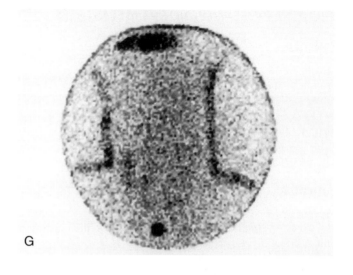

G

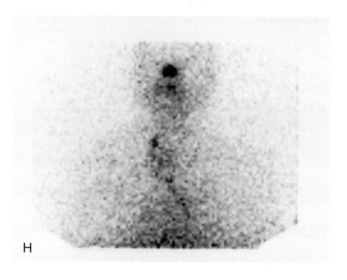

H

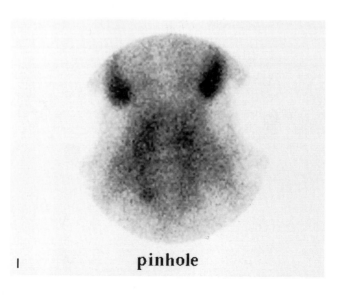

I   **pinhole**

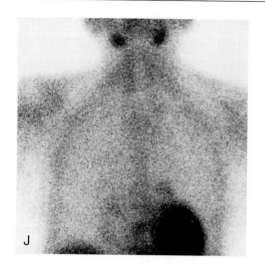

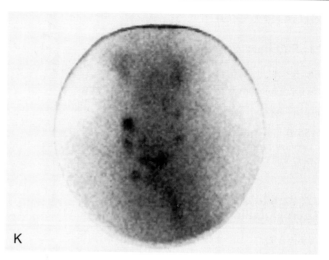

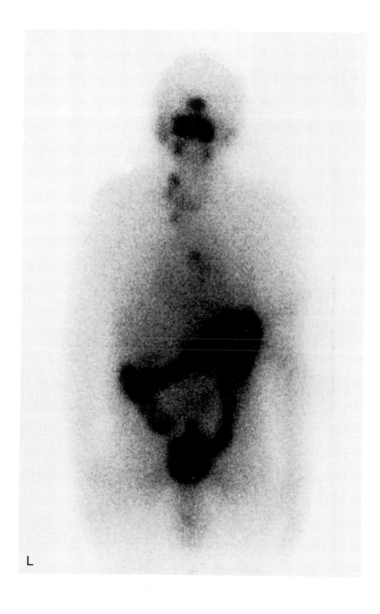

FALSE NEGATIVE ¹³¹IODINE SCAN

Patient 1: Papillary Carcinoma

FIGURE 68–6   A.

¹³¹Iodine Scan: The scan is negative in the chest and neck.

FIGURE 68–6   B and C.

Thallium Scan: There are metastases in the left lung, right posterior cervical lymph node, and skull. (Courtesy of Dr. Michael Kipper, Vista, CA.)

Patient 2: Papillofollicular Carcinoma with Rising Thyroglobulin

FIGURE 68–6   D.

Anterior ⁹⁹ᵐTc-Sestamibi Scan: There is a focus in the lower neck that could not be seen with a 5 mCi ¹³¹I scan.

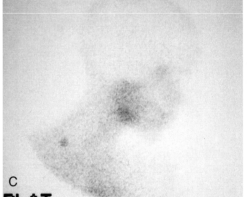

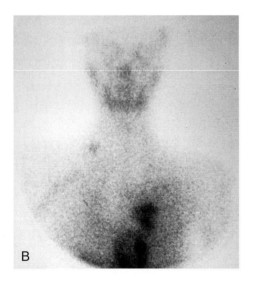

Patient 3

FIGURE 68–6   E.

Five mCi ¹³¹I Pinhole Neck Scan: There is no appreciable radioiodine accumulation in the neck. Markers are at the chin and sternal notch.

FIGURE 68–6   F.

Coronal ⁹⁹ᵐTc-Sestamibi SPECT Scan: There is diffuse accumulation in both sides of the neck and the superior mediastinum.

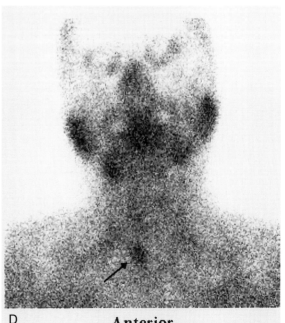

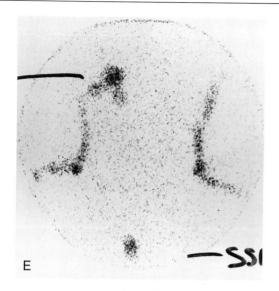

E

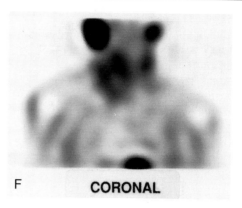

F   **CORONAL**

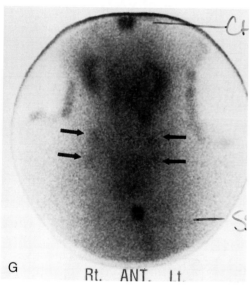

G   Rt. ANT. Lt.

FIGURE 68–6   G.

Postablation Scan 5 Days After 125 mCi [131]I Scan: Several metastatic foci in both sides of the neck and upper mediastinum are barely discernible *(arrows)*. The diffuse activity is due to scatter from the radioiodine in the infiltrative tumor.

NOTE. An elevated serum thyroglobulin with a negative ^{131}I scan is an indicator for a sestamibi or thallium scan.

FALSE NEGATIVE THALLIUM TUMOR SCAN

FIGURE 68–7   A.

Bone Scan: There is a "cold" metastasis to the manubrium and proximal clavicles.

FIGURE 68–7   B and C.

Anterior [201]Thallium Scan: The left clavicular metastasis is evident as well as some lung lesions *(arrows)*.

Illustration continued on following page

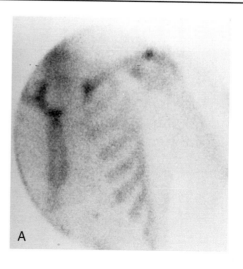

A

FIGURE 68–7   D and E.

Anterior ¹³¹Iodine Scan: There is a large mediastinal mass *(arrowhead)* not seen on the thallium scan.

FIGURE 68–7   F and G.

¹³¹Iodine and ²⁰¹Thallium Scans 6 Months Later: There are numerous pulmonary metastases not evident on the thallium scan (arrow = xyphoid marker). (Courtesy of Dr. Michael Kipper, Vista, CA.)

NOTE. Well-differentiated papillary or follicular carcinoma of the thyroid may be negative on thallium owing to its slow growth rate and relatively low blood flow.

Cross Reference

Chapter 72: Tumors—Soft Tissue Metastases

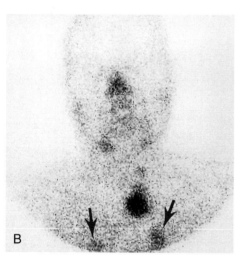

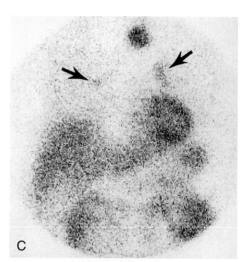

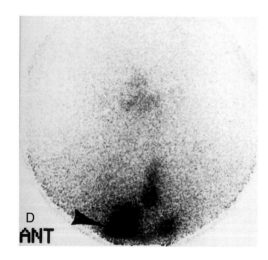

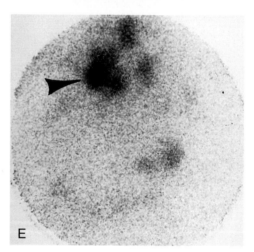

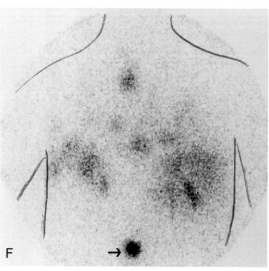

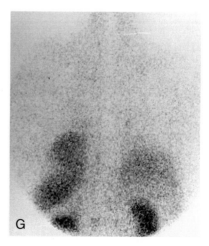

FALSE POSITIVE ¹³¹IODINE SCAN

Patient: Papillary Carcinoma

FIGURE 68–8   A.
¹³¹I-Whole Body Scan: There is intense iodine accumulation in the region of the lower pole of the left kidney. This persisted over 6 days.

FIGURE 68–8   B.
Contrast-Enhanced CT Scan: The left lower pole hydronephrosis and cortical scarring from chronic pyelonephritis are evident.

NOTE 1. It is unusual to have thyroid metastases below the diaphragm, or even in the chest, before neck nodal involvement.

NOTE 2. Other causes of "false-positive" ¹³¹I scans include sialadenitis, Warthin's tumor, sinusitis, tracheostomy, lung cancer, inflammatory lung disease, uptake in normal organs (breast, gallbladder, liver), renal cyst, gastroesophageal reflux, hiatal hernia, ectopic gastric mucosa (Barrett's esophagus and Meckel's diverticulum), Zenker's diverticulum, gastric adenocarcinoma, cystadenoma of ovary, and scrotal hydrocoele. (From McDougall IR: Whole-body scintigraphy with radioiodine-131. Clin Nucl Med 20:869, 1995.)

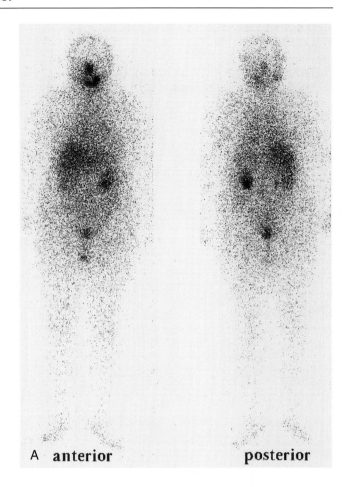

A   **anterior**   **posterior**

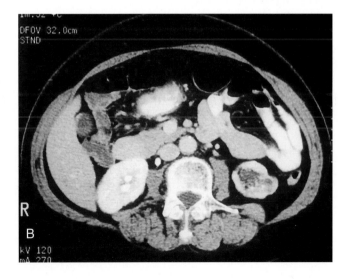

SESTAMIBI IN MEDULLARY CARCINOMA OF THE THYROID

Patient: Rising Serum Calcitonin and Negative CT of the Neck and Chest

FIGURE 68–9.

Anterior Planar ^{99m}Tc-Sestamibi Scan: There are several foci of radiopharmaceutical accumulation in the left neck and one behind the right clavicle *(arrow)* that represent lymph node metastases. (The asymmetry of the salivary glands is unexplained.)

NOTE. Imaging of medullary carcinoma metastases can be performed with radiolabeled octreotide, ^{99m}Tc-sestamibi, ^{131}I, or ^{123}I-MIBG.

Cross Reference

Chapter 72: Tumors—Octreotide: Multiple Endocrine Neoplasia Syndrome IIb

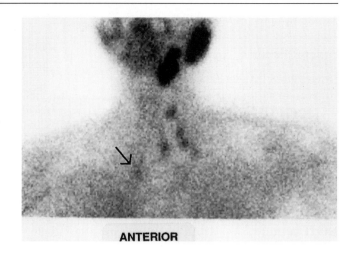

ANTERIOR

THYROID LYMPHOMA

FIGURE 68–10.

Gallium Scan: There is marked gallium accumulation in the thyroid. (Courtesy of Dr. Michael Kipper, Vista, CA.)

NOTE 1. Gallium uptake can be seen in Graves' disease, thyroid carcinoma (especially anaplastic carcinoma), lymphoma, thyroiditis, and some metastases.

NOTE 2. On rare occasions, Hodgkin's disease may first manifest itself as a cold nodule within the thyroid.

Cross Reference

Chapter 72: Tumors—Gallium Avid Lymphomas

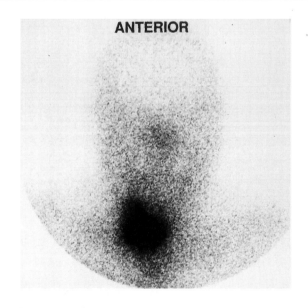

ANTERIOR

Chapter 69

Parathyroid Diseases

NORMAL DUAL ISOTOPE PARATHYROID SCAN

FIGURE 69–1 A and B.

Pinhole Thallium Scan and Pinhole Technetium Pertechnetate Scan: There is homogeneous activity within the thyroid bed.

FIGURE 69–1 C.

Computer Subtraction Scan: The technetium and thallium scans match, subtracting completely.

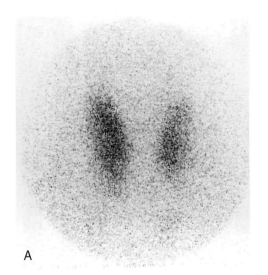

A

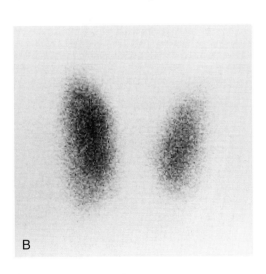

B

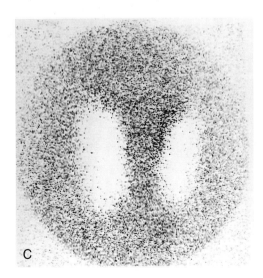

C

NORMAL SESTAMIBI PARATHYROID SCAN

FIGURE 69–2 A.

⁹⁹ᵐTc-Sestamibi Scan 20 Minutes Post Injection: The thyroid gland picks up the sestamibi, as do the salivary glands.

FIGURE 69–2 B.

Three Hour Delayed Sestamibi Scan: There is no residual radio-pharmaceutical in the thyroid or thyroid bed.

FIGURE 69–2 C and D.

Twenty Minute and 3 Hour Mediastinal Scans: The mediastinum does not accumulate sestamibi.

NOTE. Thallium–technetium pertechnetate subtraction scan requires more time, greater patient immobility, and greater computer interaction than the sestamibi technique.

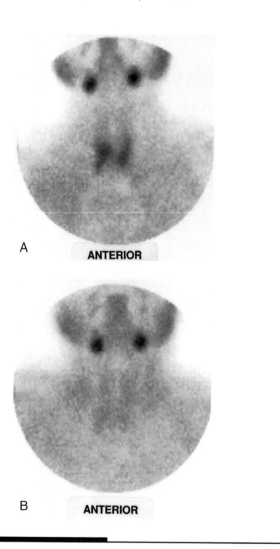

A   **ANTERIOR**

B   **ANTERIOR**

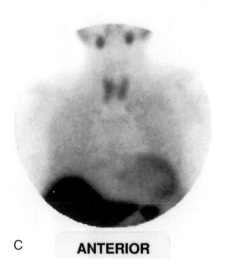

C   **ANTERIOR**

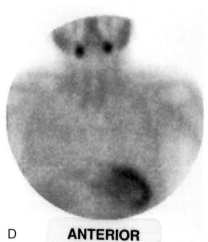

D   **ANTERIOR**

PARATHYROID ADENOMA ON ²⁰¹T1-⁹⁹ᵐTC SCAN

FIGURE 69–3 A and B.

Pinhole Thallium and ⁹⁹ᵐTc-Pertechnetate Scans: There is thallium activity in the right lower pole defect seen on the technetium scan.

FIGURE 69–3 C.

Computer Subtraction of Technetium from Thallium: The residual activity is the thallium in the adenoma. (Courtesy of Dr. Michael Kipper, Vista, CA.)

NOTE. In most cases visual inspection achieves the same result as computer subtraction.

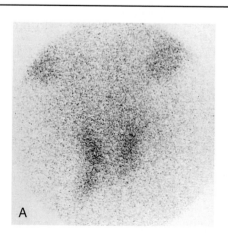

A

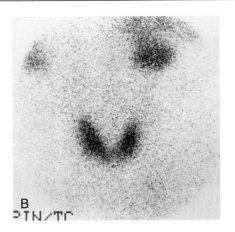
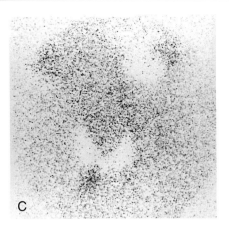

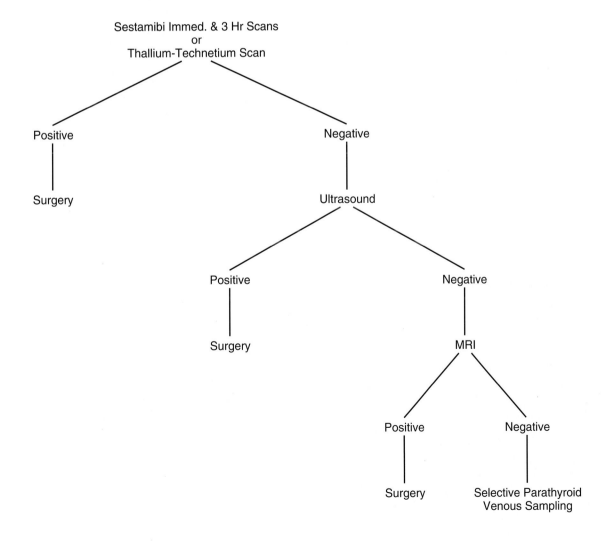

SUSPECTED HYPERTHYROIDISM

Sestamibi Immed. & 3 Hr Scans
or
Thallium-Technetium Scan

Positive — Negative

Surgery

Ultrasound

Positive — Negative

Surgery

MRI

Positive — Negative

Surgery — Selective Parathyroid
Venous Sampling

PARATHYROID ADENOMAS ON SESTAMIBI SCAN

Patient 1: Solitary Parathyroid Adenoma

FIGURE 69–4   A and B.

Immediate and Delayed ^{99m}Tc-Sestamibi Scans: There is increased activity in the region of the left lower pole of the thyroid, which persists over 3 hours.

FIGURE 69–4   C.

Ultrasound Scan: A 2.2 cm solid mass is present beneath the left lower pole of the thyroid.

Patient 2: Multiple Adenomas

FIGURE 69–4   D.

Three Hour Delayed ^{99m}Tc-Sestamibi Scan: The three foci of retained radioactivity were reproducible over 6 months and proved to be adenomas (s = sternal notch marker; arrows = adenomas).

Patient 3: Bilateral Adenomas

FIGURE 69–4   E and F.

Immediate and 3 Hour Delayed ^{99m}Tc-Sestamibi Scans: The right lower pole nodule, evident on both scans, was palpable, although the left lower pole nodule was detected only on the delayed scan.

Patient 4: Mediastinal Adenoma

FIGURE 69–4   G and H.

Immediate and 3 Hour Delayed ^{99m}Tc-Sestamibi Scans: The focus of activity in right mediastinum persisted over time.

NOTE. Ectopic mediastinal parathyroids may be buried within a thymic remnant or isolated. The thymic remnant may need to be serially sectioned in order to locate the ectopic parathyroid.

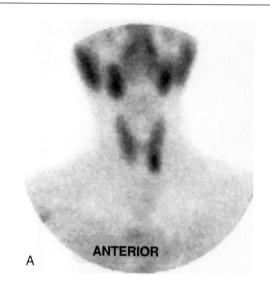

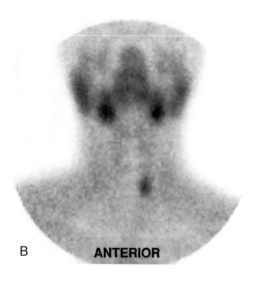

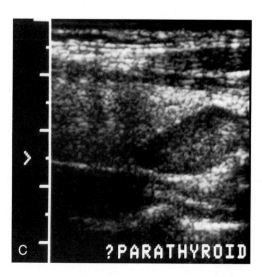

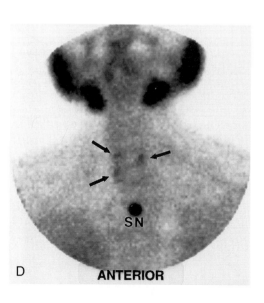

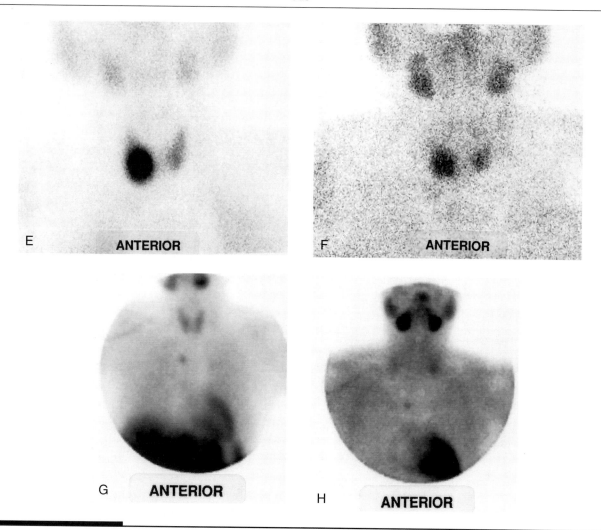

E   **ANTERIOR**

F   **ANTERIOR**

G   **ANTERIOR**

H   **ANTERIOR**

VALUE OF PINHOLE IMAGING FOR PARATHYROID ADENOMA

FIGURE 69–5   A and B.

Anterior Immediate and Digitally Magnified Delayed ^{99m}Tc-Sestamibi Scans: Both the immediate and the delayed scans are normal.

Illustration continued on following page

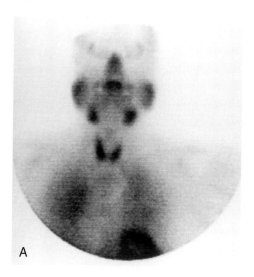

A

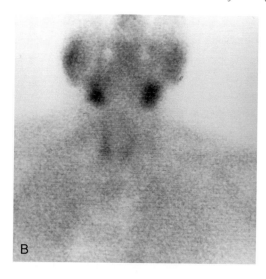

B

FIGURE 69-5 C.

Pinhole Delayed Scan: The right lower pole parathyroid adenoma is now obvious. (Courtesy of Dr. Michael Kipper, Vista, CA.)

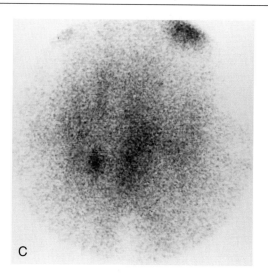

NOTE. Pinhole imaging has proved invaluable in the detection of small parathyroid adenomas when the planar and digitally magnified scans are negative.

CONCURRENT THYROID AND PARATHYROID ADENOMAS

FIGURE 69-6 A.

Pinhole Thallium Scan: There is some increased activity in the right lower pole of the thyroid.

FIGURE 69-6 B.

Pinhole Technetium Pertechnetate Scan: There is a "cold" nodule along the lateral margin of the left lobe.

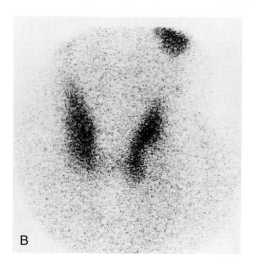

FIGURE 69-6 C.

Computer Subtraction Scan: There is residual thallium in the right lower pole (parathyroid adenoma) and the left lateral margin (thyroid adenoma).

NOTE. Thallium or sestamibi can accumulate in thyroid carcinomas and adenomas as well as in parathyroid adenomas.

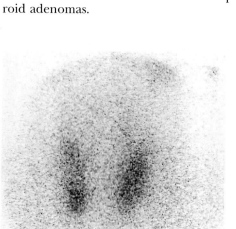

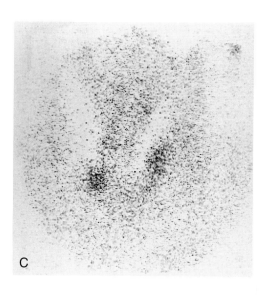

FUNCTIONING PARATHYROID CARCINOMA

FIGURE 69–7   A.

Thallium/Technetium Pertechnetate Subtraction Scan: There is a large thallium collection in the lower half of the right thyroid bed.

FIGURE 69–7   B.

Ultrasound Scan: The large retrothyroid mass is solid.

FIGURE 69–7   C and D.

Anterior and RAO Bone Scans: The mass has intense radiopharmaceutical retention, along with the remaining thyroid and the lungs. The patient was only mildly hypercalcemic.

Cross Reference

Chapter 11: Soft Tissue Abnormalities—Metastatic Calcification from Functioning Parathyroid Carcinoma

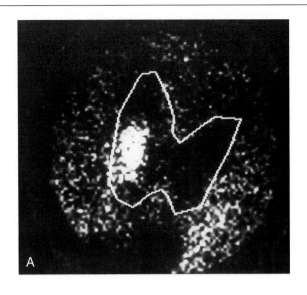

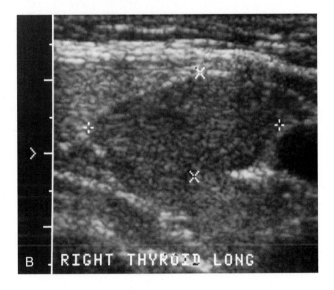

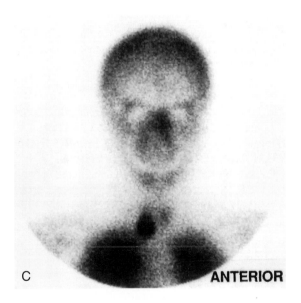

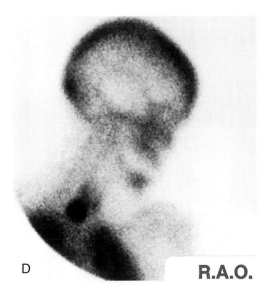

PHEOCHROMOCYTOMA

FIGURE 70–1.

Posterior ^{123}I MIBG Image of Abdomen: There is a focus of activity in the region of the right adrenal gland, indicating a right adrenal pheochromocytoma. No other foci of uptake were seen. (Courtesy of Dr. James Sisson, Ann Arbor, MI.)

NOTE 1. MIBG is most valuable in locating extra-adrenal pheochromocytomas.

NOTE 2. Octreotide imaging can also detect pheochromocytomas. Both agents may be necessary to detect some tumors.

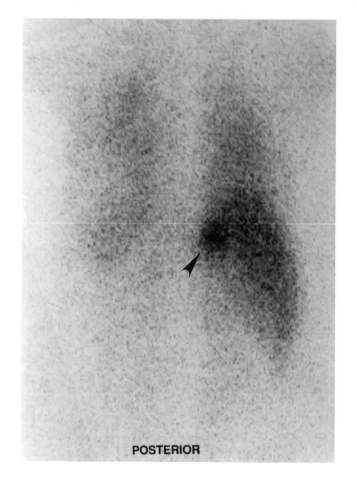

POSTERIOR

MINIMUM LABORATORY DATA FOR INTERPRETING ^{131}I-IODOCHOLESTEROL STUDIES (NUCLEAR MEDICINE DIVISION, UNIVERSITY OF MICHIGAN, 1993)

1. CUSHING'S SYNDROME

   a. Urinary free cortisol and/or

   b. Suppression test (at least serum cortisol in A.M. after 1 mg dexamethasone in evening)

   c. ACTH (serum)

2. ALDOSTERONISM (PRIMARY)

   a. Serum K and

   b. Plasma renin (upright more than 1 h) and

   c. Plasma aldosterone (upright more than 1 h)

3. HYPERANDROGENISM

   a. Serum testosterone and

   b. Serum dehydroepiandrosterone sulfate

4. EUADRENAL TUMORS

   a. If BP normal and K normal: None

   b. If BP elevated and/or K reduced
      As for Cushing's syndrome *and* aldosteronism

   Also helpful: Urinary catecholamines and metabolites.

Courtesy of Dr. James Sisson, University of Michigan, Ann Arbor, MI.

PRIMARY ALDOSTERONISM

Patient 1: Hypertension and Hypokalemia

FIGURE 70–2 A.

CT Scan: There is a subtle hypodense mass *(arrowhead)* in the inferior limb of the right adrenal gland.

FIGURE 70–2 B.

[131]I-Iodocholesterol Scan: The increased activity in the right adrenal gland *(white arrow)* indicates an aldosteronoma (surgically proven). (Courtesy of Dr. James Sisson, Ann Arbor, MI.)

Patient 2: Fifty-five Year Old Male with Elevated Aldosterone Levels

FIGURE 70–2 C.

[131]I-Iodocholesterol Scan: The focal accumulation of the radiopharmaceutical did not move despite laxatives. The CT scan did show a slightly enlarged left adrenal above a low left kidney.

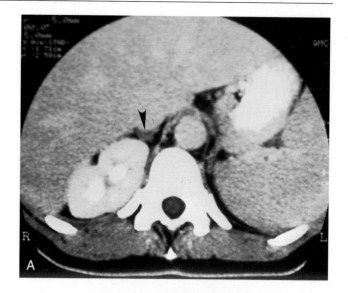

A

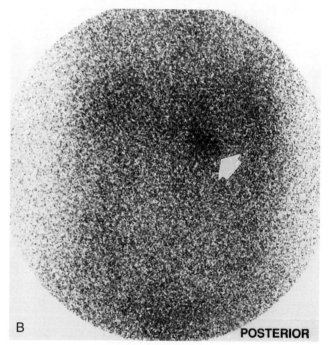

B   POSTERIOR

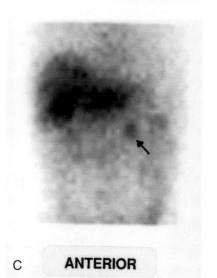

C   ANTERIOR

"INCIDENTALOMA" VS. METASTASIS

Patient 1: Sixty-two Year Old Male with Malignant Fibrous Histiocytoma

FIGURE 70–3   A.

Abdominal CT: The left adrenal is large, measuring 2 cm.

FIGURE 70–3   B.

Posterior Abdominal ^{131}I-Iodocholesterol Scan 8 Days After Injection: Radioactivity is seen in each adrenal gland. The greater activity on the left side indicates that the mass apparent on CT is a functioning left adrenal adenoma rather than a metastasis. (Courtesy of Dr. James Sisson, Ann Arbor, MI.)

Patient 2: Seventy-seven Year Old Female with Breast Cancer with No Known Metastases

FIGURE 70–3   C.

Posterior ^{131}I-Iodocholesterol Scan: The large right adrenal found at CT can be seen to be functioning and to be larger than the left.

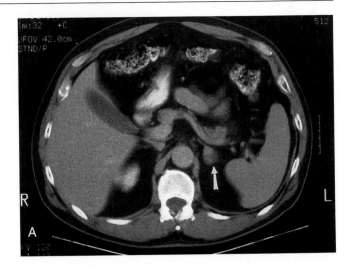

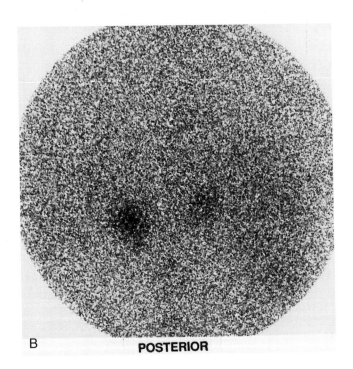

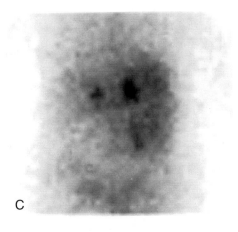

SECTION XV

INFECTION

Chapter 71

Infectious Diseases

WBC SCANNING

Best for

- Acute infections, soft tissue or bone, and abdominal processes, especially bowel, i.e., Crohn's disease and ulcerative colitis.

    Cross Reference

    Chapter 33: Gastrointestinal and Abdominal Infections—GI Infections

- Orthopedic prosthetic infections (along with radiocolloid)

    Cross Reference

    Chapter 10: Prostheses—WBC/Colloid Subtraction in Prosthetic Infection

- Tumor patients with fever
- Vascular infections, i.e., graft infections or mycotic aneurysm

    Cross Reference

    Chapter 60: Mycotic Aneurysm

    Chapter 60: Arterial Graft Infection

- Renal infections

    Cross Reference

    Chapter 36: Acute Pyelonephritis

- Active arthritis

    Cross Reference

    Chapter 2: Multiple Bony Abnormalities—Rheumatoid Arthritis on WBC Scan

    Chapter 3: Spinal Abnormalities—Abnormal WBC Accumulation in Bone

Possible False Positive Findings

- Atelectasis and ARDS

    Cross Reference

    Chapter 49: Adult Respiratory Distress Syndrome

- Occasional neoplasms, especially necrotic masses; lymphoma

    Cross Reference

    Chapter 71: Infectious Diseases—WBCs in Tumor

- Swallowed WBCs from pneumonia or sinusitis

    Cross Reference

    Chapter 33: Gastrointestinal and Abdominal Infections—Swallowed WBCs

- Acute fractures

    Cross Reference

    Chapter 1: Solitary Bony Abnormalities—WBC Accumulation in Fracture Fragment

- Orthopedic prostheses (packed marrow)

    Cross Reference

    Chapter 11: Prostheses—Marrow Compression with Normal Hip Prosthesis

- Active GI bleeding

    Cross Reference

    Chapter 33: Gastrointestinal and Abdominal Infections—GI Hemorrhage on WBC Scan

- Hematomas
- Heterotopic ossification
- Large osteophytes or sesamoid bones with marrow
- Paget's disease
- Ostomies, e.g., tracheostomies, ileostomies
- Nares from indwelling tubes
- Intramuscular injection sites

Possible False Negative Findings

- Spinal osteomyelitis/diskitis ("cold")

Cross Reference

Chapter 3: Spinal Abnormalities—Decreased WBCs, Increased Gallium in Spinal Osteomyelitis

- Parasitic and fungal infections, including TB
- Chronic infections, e.g., chronic osteomyelitis
- Splenic or perisplenic abscess

Cross Reference

Chapter 20: Disorders of the Spleen—Subphrenic Abscess Simulating Spleen

- Poor preparation

(WBC scans *may* be positive with diskitis, parasitic and fungal infections, and chronic infections, but overall accuracy may be less than that of gallium in these entities.)

GALLIUM SCANNING

Best for

- Spinal osteomyelitis/diskitis

Cross Reference

Chapter 3: Spinal Abnormalities—Value of SPECT in Gallium Scanning for Spinal Osteomyelitis and Diskitis

- Infections that do not elicit a strong WBC response
- Chronic infections
- Pulmonary infection in immunosuppressed patients

Cross Reference

Chapter 49: Pneumocystis Pneumonia

- Leukopenic patients
- Splenic abscess
- Parasitic and fungal infections of the chest and head

Cross References

Chapter 48: Aspergillosis

Chapter 72: Lung Nodules—Aspergillosis

Possible False Positive Finding

- Neoplasms
- Fractures
- Kidney disease
- Inactive chronic osteomyelitis
- Normal colon activity vs. colitis
- Ostomies
- Nares and paranasal sinuses, e.g., from nasogastric tubes
- Intramuscular injection sites
- Granulation tissue

Cross Reference

Chapter 10: Prostheses—Granulation Tissue with Prosthetic Hip

Possible False Negative Findings

- Iron overload (including hemolytic anemias and multiple
- blood transfusions)
- High ascorbic acid intake
- Chronic osteomyelitis

NORMAL GALLIUM SCAN

Patient 1

FIGURE 71–1 A.
Forty-eight Hour Anterior and Posterior Whole Body Gallium Scans: Normal accumulation can be seen in the liver, lacrimal glands, bone marrow, and, to a variable degree, spleen and kidneys.

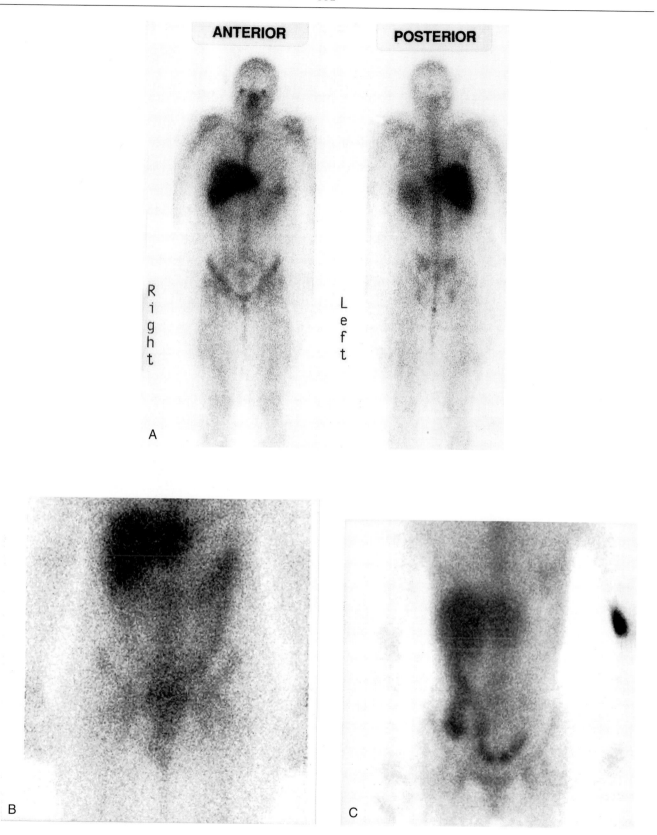

Patients 2 and 3

FIGURE 71–1   B and C.

Forty-eight Hour Anterior Abdominal Gallium Scans: The normal colon may have varying degrees of gallium accumulation.

NORMAL WHITE CELL SCAN

FIGURE 71–2   A.
Anterior Head ¹¹¹In-WBC Scan: The activity is only within the bone marrow, none within the paranasal sinuses.

FIGURE 71–2   B and C.
Anterior and Posterior Chest ¹¹¹In-WBC Scan: The lungs do not have any appreciable white cell accumulation. The splenic activity should be greater than the liver activity.

FIGURE 71–2   D and E.
Anterior and Posterior Abdomen and Pelvis ¹¹¹In-WBC Scan: There is no bowel or kidney activity normally.

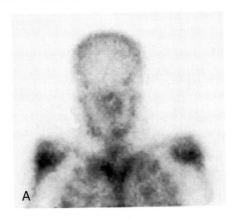
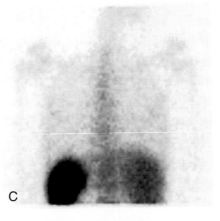
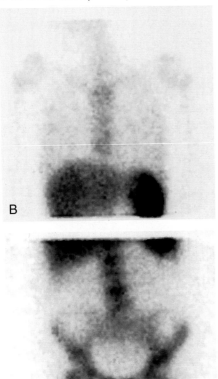
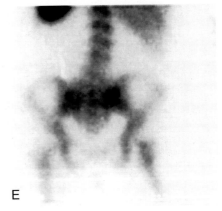

NORMAL WBCs IN RECENT SURGICAL INCISION

FIGURE 71–3.
Anterior Abdominal ¹¹¹In-WBC Scan: The linear vertical activity is in the recent surgical wound. The radiolabeled autologous white blood cells were infused back into the patient 2 hours prior to exploratory laparotomy. The scan was performed 18 hours after the reinjection, 12 hours after surgery.

NOTE. White blood cell or gallium activity in the surgical wound decreases rapidly after surgery, and hardly any activity should be present by 3 days.

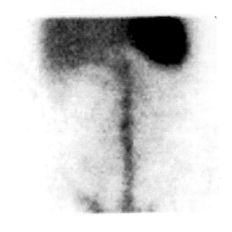

NORMAL TRACHEOSTOMY ON WBC SCANS

FIGURE 71–4.

WBC Scan: The tracheostomy has moderate WBC accumulation, which is normal.

NOTE. Colostomy and ileostomy sites also attract increased WBCs.

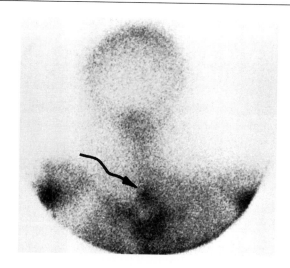

MAXILLARY ANTRUM WBC ACTIVITY DUE TO NASOGASTRIC TUBING

FIGURE 71–5.

WBC Scan: The left naris has increased WBCs from a nasogastric tube.

NOTE. Paranasal sinus WBC activity can be the cause of an FUO, although it is a common finding with indwelling nasal tubes, regressing with the removal of obstructing tube.

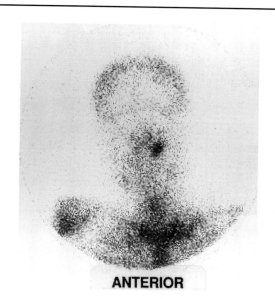

GALLIUM UPTAKE IN BENIGN FRACTURES

FIGURE 71–6.

Gallium Scan: There is uptake of gallium in benign, postoperative rib fractures.

NOTE. Gallium can accumulate in recent benign post-traumatic fractures as well as in pathologic fractures and bony metastases.

Cross Reference

Chapter 1: Solitary Bony Abnormalities—WBC Accumulation in a Fracture Fragment

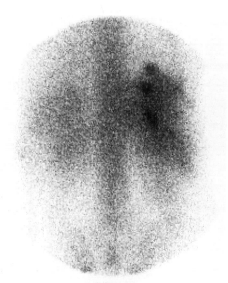

SYMMETRIC THORACIC INLET INFECTION

Patient: Left Sternoclavicular Joint Pain and a 100°F Fever

FIGURE 71–7   A.

Anterior ¹¹¹In-WBC Scan: There is symmetric abnormal white cell activity in what was thought to be both clavicular heads, without a manubrial abnormality.

FIGURE 71–7   B.

CT Scan: The left clavicular head and the right first rib are substantially destroyed. There is minimal soft tissue swelling on the left.

NOTE. Knowledge of normal patterns will help separate symmetric disease from normal variants.

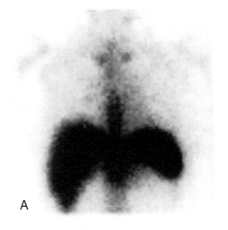

A

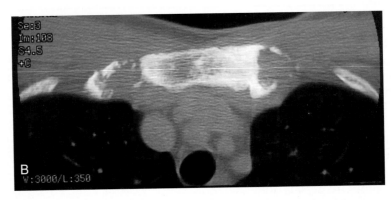

B

INFLAMMATORY LYMPH NODES

Patient 1: *Mycobacterium avium-intracellulare* Infection

FIGURE 71–8   A.

Gallium Scan: There is abnormal accumulation in the superior mediastinal and supraclavicular lymph nodes.

FIGURE 71–8   B.

Gallium Scan: The central abdominal gallium activity represents mesenteric/para-aortic lymph nodes.

Patient 2: Diffuse Interstitial Pneumonitis in Rheumatoid Arthritis

FIGURE 71–8   C.

Planar Chest Gallium Scan: It is difficult to appreciate the focal areas of more intense gallium uptake because of the diffuse gallium activity.

FIGURE 71–8   D to F.

Coronal and Sagittal Gallium SPECT Scans: The rheumatoid nodules are better delineated using SPECT.

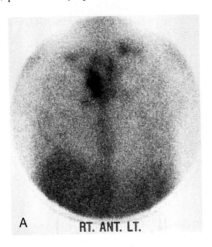

A   RT. ANT. LT.

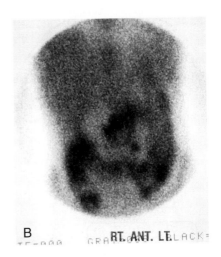

B   RT. ANT. LT.

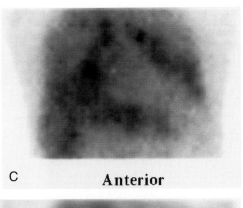

C   **Anterior**

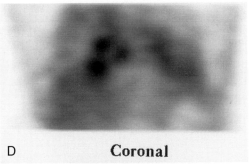

D   **Coronal**

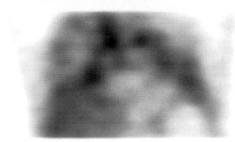

E   **Coronal**

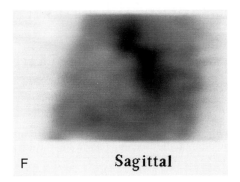

F   **Sagittal**

NOTE 1. Lymph node activity does not always require lymph node enlargement.

NOTE 2. Rheumatoid arthritis involves the lungs with diffuse interstitial pneumonitis, pleuritis, and intrapulmonary rheumatoid nodules.

NOTE 3. Caplan's syndrome is a combination of rheumatoid arthritis and a dust-related pneumoconiosis associated with coal dust, silicosis, and asbestosis.

NOTE 4. False positive WBC and gallium scans for infection can be seen with nodes involved with tumors, especially lymphomas and leukemias.

Cross References

Chapter 48: Active Interstitial Pneumonitis

Chapter 71: WBCs in Tumor

MEDIASTINITIS

FIGURE 71–9.

Anterior Gallium Scan: There is considerable gallium accumulation in the mediastinum.

DIFFERENTIAL DIAGNOSIS OF MEDIASTINITIS	
Perforated esophagus	Tuberculosis
Infected penetrating wounds or surgery	Methysergide therapy
Histoplasmosis	

NOTE. Mediastinal activity may also be due to inflammatory and neoplastic nodes.

Cross Reference

Chapter 57: Pericarditis/Myocarditis

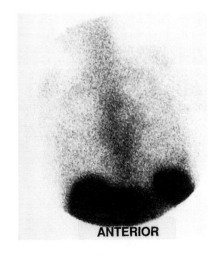

ANTERIOR

BACTERIAL AORTITIS AND PULMONARY ARTERY INFECTION

Patient: Sixty-five Year Old Male with Fever, Aortic Regurgitation, and *Staphylococcus aureus* Septicemia

FIGURE 71–10   A and B.

Anterior and LAO Chest ^{111}In-WBC Scans: There is intense white cell accumulation in the ascending aorta and the left pulmonary artery *(arrow)*.

NOTE 1. The infection spreads to the pulmonary artery through the ductus arteriosus.

NOTE 2. The most common cause of mycotic aneurysm in the thoracic aorta is dental disease.

Cross References

Chapter 57: Pericarditis/Myocarditis

Chapter 57: Bacterial Endocarditis

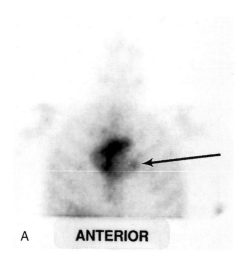

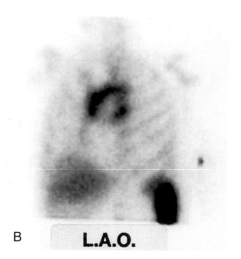

UNSUSPECTED ABSCESSES

Patient 1: Forty-five Year Old Diabetic Man with Painful, Swollen Left Proximal Thigh

FIGURE 71–11   A and B.

Anterior and Posterior ^{111}In-WBC Scans: There is marked white cell accumulation in the left greater trochanteric bursa and along myofascial planes.

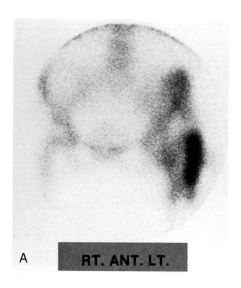

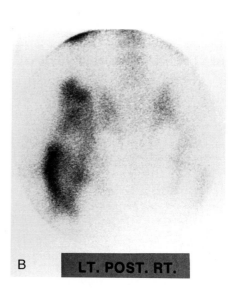

FIGURE 71–11   C.

Posterior Chest ¹¹¹In-WBC Scan: The posterior pleural abscess was unsuspected and asymptomatic.

Patient 2: Eighty-three Year Old Male with a Right Hip Prosthesis Complaining of Hip and Thigh Pain

FIGURE 71–11   D and E.

Anterior Hip and Pelvic ¹¹¹In-WBC Scans: The right hip activity on the WBC scan matched that seen on a ⁹⁹ᵐTc-albumin colloid scan. The unsuspected appendiceal abscess was the cause of the referred pain.

NOTE 1. With gallium or WBC scanning, anterior and posterior chest, abdomen and pelvis, and anterior face (for occult paranasal sinusitis) scans should be obtained for asymptomatic sites of infection.

NOTE 2. Other views in addition to the symptomatic site are necessary because of the possibility of referred pain.

Cross Reference

Chapter 33: Diverticulitis and Appendiceal Abcess

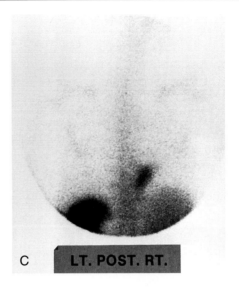

C   LT. POST. RT.

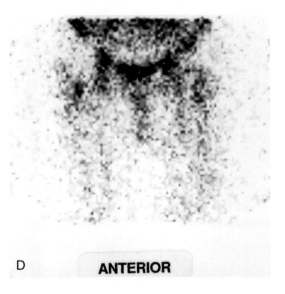

D   ANTERIOR

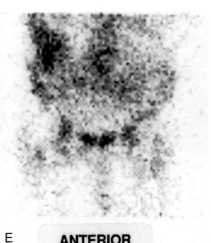

E   ANTERIOR

INFECTED SUBCLAVIAN AND JUGULAR VEINS

FIGURE 71–12   A.
Anterior ¹¹¹In-WBC Scan: There is intense white cell accumulation in the left subclavian and jugular veins.

FIGURE 71–12   B.
Left Subclavian ⁹⁹ᵐTc-Albumin Colloid Venogram: The left subclavian and innominate veins are patent.

NOTE 1. White cell accumulation in veins can be due to infection or thrombosis.

NOTE 2. The site of injection of the white cells should be recorded, since a "hot spot" often occurs at the injection site.

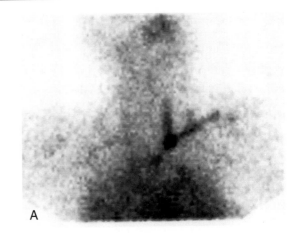

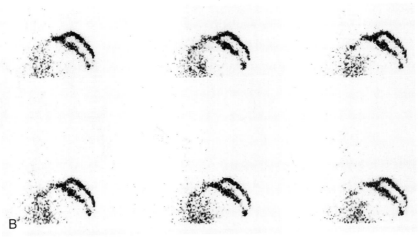

EXTREMITY SOFT TISSUE INFECTIONS

Patient 1: Disseminated Streptococcal Soft Tissue Infection

FIGURE 71–13   A.
Posterior ¹¹¹In-WBC Scan: The lungs are diffusely abnormal.

FIGURE 71–13   B and C.
¹¹¹In-WBC Scans: The right arm has focal areas of WBC accumulation in the soft tissues and axillary nodes. The left arm has a massive infection of the muscle.

FIGURE 71–13   D.
¹¹¹In-WBC Scan: The left cheek, salivary gland, neck and nose are all infected.

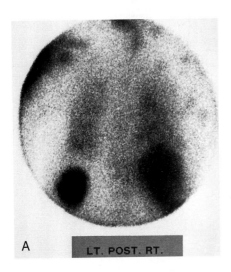

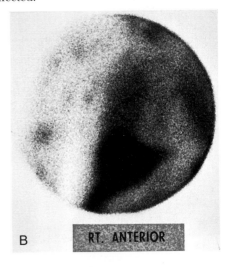

Patients 2 to 4: Necrotizing Fasciitis in Diabetes (Various Patients)

FIGURE 71–13   E.

^{111}In-WBC Scan of Thighs: The elongated activity suggests infection of the muscles and/or fascia.

FIGURE 71–13   F and G.

Gallium Scan: The lateral muscle/fascial soft tissues are abnormal.

Illustration continued on following page

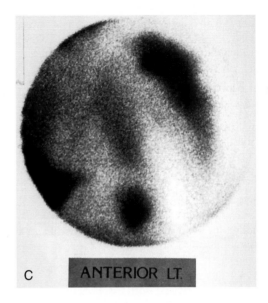

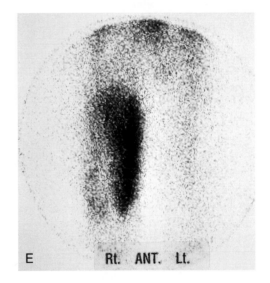

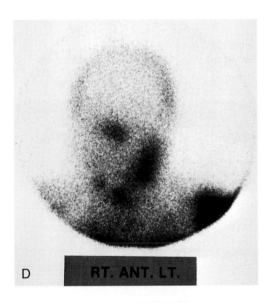

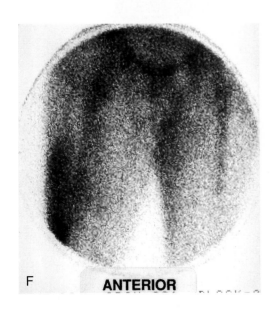

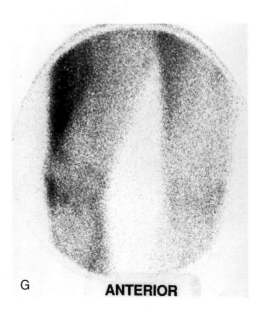

FIGURE 71–13   H.

Posterior Lumbar Region ^{111}In-WBC Scan: The muscle planes can be seen in this patient with massive fasciitis. Note the liver tumor, which did not accumulate white cells *(arrow)*.

Patient 5: Tuberculous Myofasciitis

FIGURE 71–13   I and J.

Gallium Scan: There is a focal abscess *(arrow)* as well as more diffuse soft tissue infection in the right elbow and forearm.

Patient 6: Chronic Coccidioidomycosis

FIGURE 71–13   K and L.

Gallium Scan: There is a soft tissue abscess in the lateral right knee, along with left distal femoral metaphyseal and left tibial metaphyseal infections.

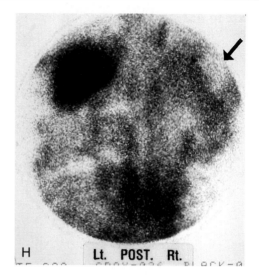

NOTE 1. Any increased soft tissue activity on WBC or gallium scanning should represent an active inflammatory site.

NOTE 2. Elongated soft tissue activity, especially in diabetes, suggests a fasciitis.

NOTE 3. Fungal and tuberculous infections will be positive with labeled WBCs despite predominance of mononuclear cells.

Cross Reference

Chapter 2: Multiple Bony Abnormalities—Multiple Septic Joints

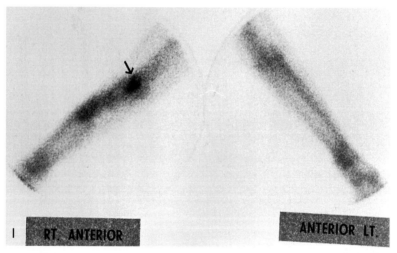

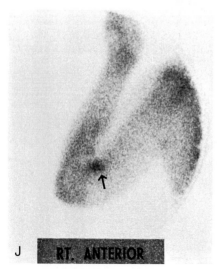

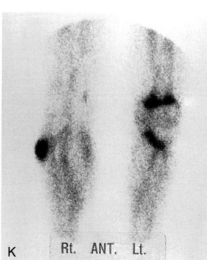

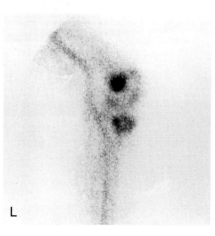

PARASPINAL ABSCESS

Patient: Low Back and Abdominal Pain

FIGURE 71–14   A.

Posterior Lumbar Bone Scan: The scan is normal.

FIGURE 71–14   B.

Planar Gallium Scan: There is intense and localized gallium accumulation at the left thoracolumbar junction.

FIGURE 71–14   C.

Coronal Gallium SPECT Scan: The abnormality extends both lateral to the margin of the vertebral column *(arrow)* and medially *(arrowhead)* toward the spinal canal.

FIGURE 71–14   D.

Detail of Plain Film of Thoracic Spine: There is widening of the left paraspinal stripe.

FIGURE 71–14   E.

Coronal MRI: The T2 weighted tomogram demonstrates a left paravertebral mass displacing the crus of the diaphragm laterally. The high signal of two thoracic vertebrae indicates marrow edema, but surgery and follow-up did not demonstrate osteomyelitis.

Illustration continued on following page

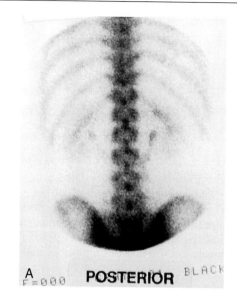

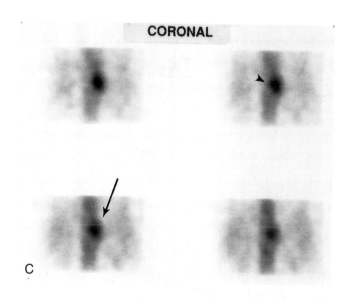

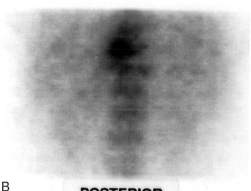

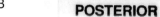

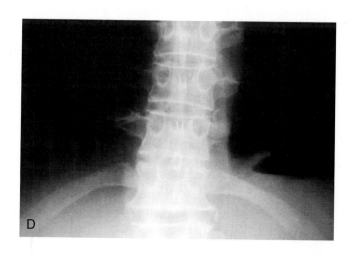

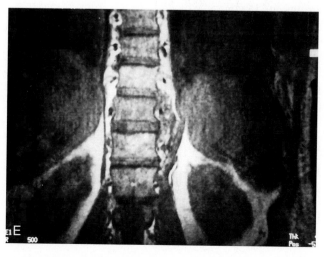

FIGURE 71–14 F.

Transverse MRI Scan: The abscess invades the left neuroforamen, obliterating the normal bright fat signal, to become an epidural abscess.

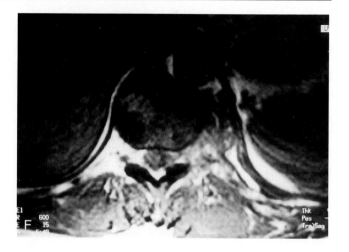

NOTE 1. Epidural or neuroforaminal extension of infection without osteomyelitis should be suspected when the gallium scan is abnormal overlying the spine but the bone scan is normal.

NOTE 2. Epidural abscesses may have presenting symptoms below their level of involvement and may not have fever or leukocytosis. The symptoms may simulate those of herniated disk, pyelonephritis, cholecystitis, aortic dissection, pulmonary embolism, myocardial infarction, or progressive paralysis.

Cross Reference

Chapter 3: Spinal Abnormalities—Value of SPECT in Gallium Scanning for Spinal Osteomyelitis and Diskitis

PSOAS ABSCESS

Patient 1

FIGURE 71–15 A.

Anterior Abdomen ^{111}In-WBC Scan: There is abnormal WBC accumulation over the left sacral ala and left ilium. The L3 vertebra has decreased WBCs and is also infected.

FIGURE 71–15 B.

WBC SPECT Scan: The abscess can be seen anterior and to the left of the spine *(arrow)*.

FIGURE 71–15 C.

CT Scan: The soft tissue mass in the left pelvis corresponds to the area of abnormality on the WBC scan.

FIGURE 71–15 D.

Higher Level CT Scan: The gas-filled abscess is eroding the left side of L3, but the vertebral body is not diffusely abnormal.

FIGURE 71–15 E.

Bone Scan: The left kidney upper pole collecting system is obstructed. The left side of the L3 vertebra has decreased bone radiopharmaceutical, while the right side has increased osteogenesis.

FIGURE 71–15 F.

Plain Film X-ray: The collapse of L3 is greatest on the left side.

Patient 2

FIGURE 71–15 G and H.

Anterior and Posterior Planar Gallium Scan: The oblique course of the gallium accumulation *(arrowheads)* suggests a psoas infection.

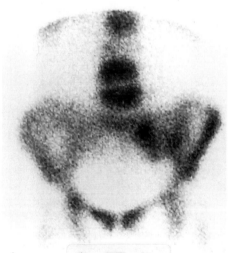

A   Rt. ANT. Lt.

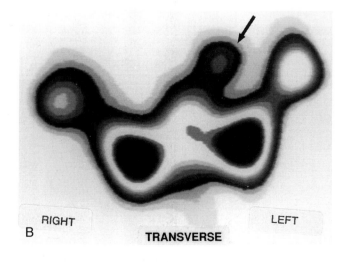

B   RIGHT   LEFT
       TRANSVERSE

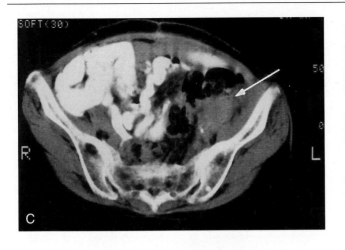

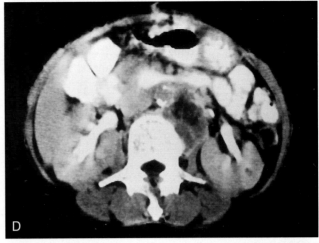

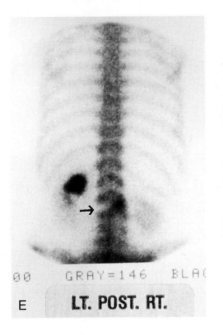

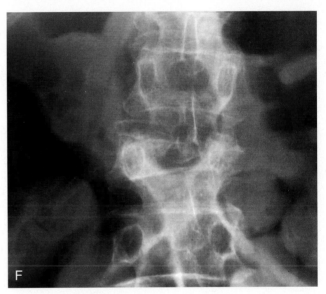

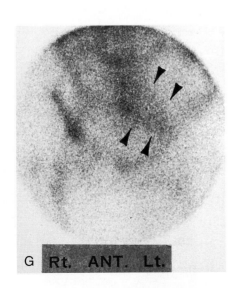

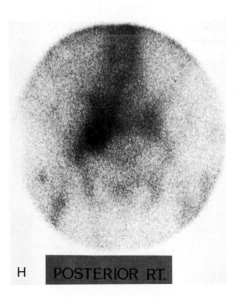

Illustration continued on following page

Patient 3

FIGURE 71–15 I and J.

Anterior and Posterior WBC Scan: There are bilateral psoas infections, L3 osteomyelitis, and dissection of the infections into the hips.

NOTE 1. Worldwide, tuberculosis is the most common cause of psoas abscesses, but suppurative organisms can also be responsible.

NOTE 2. Intraspinal involvement should be checked for, as extension into the epidural space is not uncommon.

NOTE 3. Spinal and psoas abscesses may be a consequence of an infected hydronephrosis.

Cross References

Chapter 3: Spinal Abnormalities—Spinal Osteomyelitis Associated with Hydronephrosis

Chapter 9: "Cold" Abnormalities—"Cold" Osteomyelitis of the Spine

Chapter 36: Urinary Obstruction with "Flip-Flop" Function

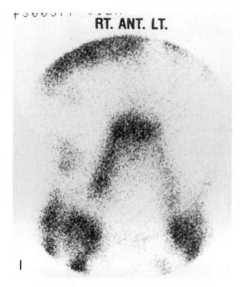

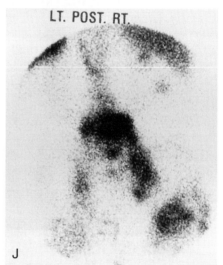

DECREASED WBCS WITH OSTEOMYELITIS

FIGURE 71–16 A.

Pelvic Bone Scan: The left ischium, including the inferior acetabulum, is abnormal.

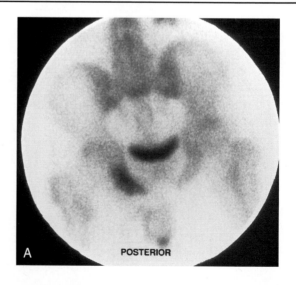

FIGURE 71–16 B.

Pelvic WBC Scan: The ischial tuberosity *(arrowheads)* is devoid of WBCs, although the acetabular component of the ischium has increased WBC accumulation.

NOTE. Decreased marrow activity could be due to fibrosis secondary to chronic osteomyelitis. The bone scan would remain abnormal.

Cross Reference

Chapter 3: Spinal Abnormalities—Decreased WBCs, Increased Gallium in Spinal Osteomyelitis

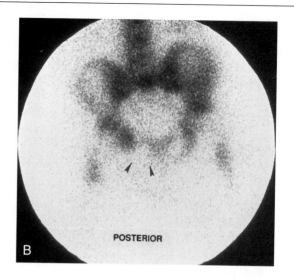

ACUTE CHOLECYSTITIS ON WBC SCAN

FIGURE 71–17.

^{111}In-WBC Scan: The gallbladder has intense WBC accumulation. The small bowel activity is presumed to be due to infected bile released into the gut.

Cross Reference

Chapter 22: Incomplete Gallbladder Distention

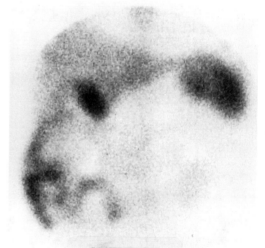

PELVIC ABSCESSES

Patient 1: Postpartum Tubo-ovarian Abscess

FIGURE 71–18 A.

Anterior ^{111}In-WBC Scan: The horizontal WBC activity in the pelvis represents the tubo-ovarian abscess, which spread to form a retrocecal abscess.

Illustration continued on following page

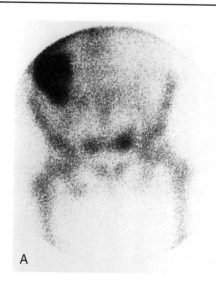

Patient 2: Tubo-ovarian Abscess

FIGURE 71–18   B and C.

Planar and SPECT Gallium Scans: There is a midline circular mass with activity in the periphery.

Patient 3: Massive Diverticular Abscess

FIGURE 71–18   D.

WBC Scan: There is a multiloculated WBC accumulation in the pelvis.

FIGURE 71–18   E.

CT Scan: The pelvic abscess has necrotic material that accumulated WBCs, an unusual finding.

Cross Reference

Chapter 33: Gastrointestinal and Abdominal Infections—Diverticular and Appendical Abscesses; Inflammatory Bowel Disease

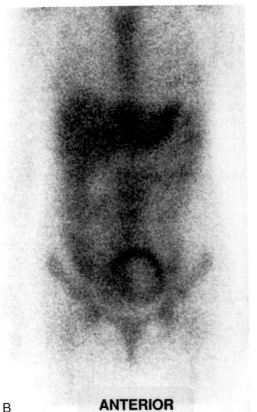

B   **ANTERIOR**

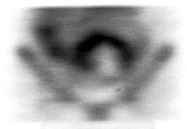

C   **CORONAL**

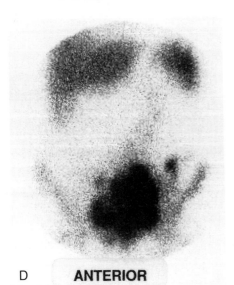

D   **ANTERIOR**

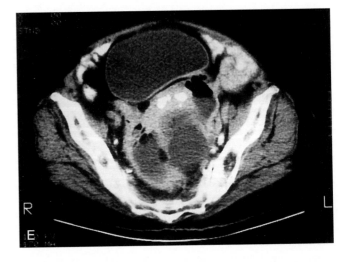

URETHRAL INFECTION

FIGURE 71–19   A.

WBC Scan: There is abnormal WBC accumulation in the penis.

FIGURE 71–19   B.

^{99m}Tc-Colloid Scan: This was done in evaluation of a bony abnormality. It shows hyperemia of the penis. (Courtesy of Dr. Thomas Owens, Honolulu, HI.)

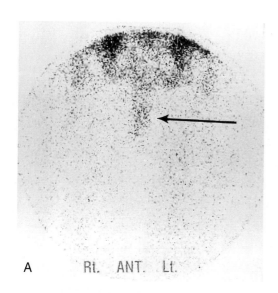

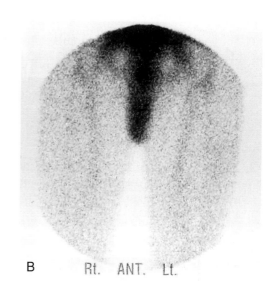

WBCs IN TUMOR

Patient 1: Lymphoma

FIGURE 71–20   A.

WBC Scan: There are foci of WBC accumulation in the midabdomen, probably in the periphery of the lymphomatous mass seen on CT.

FIGURE 71–20   B.

CT Scan: There is a mass just anterior to the aorta.

Illustration continued on following page

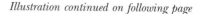

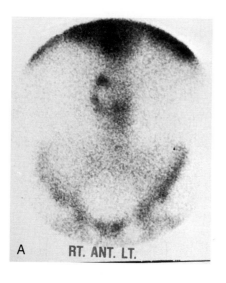

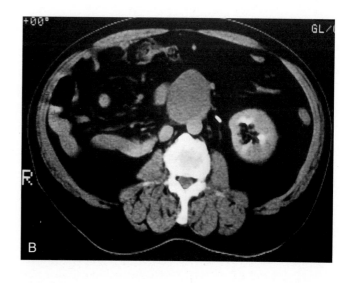

Patient 2: Schwannoma

FIGURE 71–20 C.

Posterior WBC Scan: The WBCs accumulate in an oblique fashion in the right pelvis, suggesting a psoas infection or active thrombophlebitis.

FIGURE 71–20 D.

CT Scan: The mass in the right paraspinal area elevates the psoas muscle. Other CT sections demonstrated its course along the psoas muscle.

NOTE 1. The incidence of WBC accumulation in neoplasms is 2 to 3 percent.

NOTE 2. Although unusual, WBCs will accumulate in a wide variety of neoplasms, both malignant and benign as well as solid and necrotic. Primary and secondary tumors and malignant lymph nodes may have increased WBCs.

NOTE 3. Tumors accumulating WBCs include lymphomas, leukemias, osteosarcomas, eosinophilic granuloma, pigmented villonodular synovitis, and schwannomas.

Cross References

Chapter 50: Tumors—WBC Uptake in Lung Tumor

Chapter 71: Infectious Diseases—Inflammatory Lymph Nodes

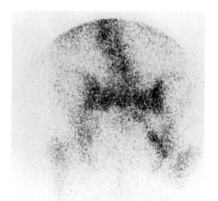

C   Lt. POST. Rt.

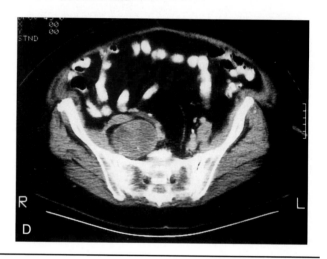

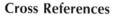

METASTASES TO THE LIVER ON WBC SCAN

FIGURE 71–21 A and B.

Anterior and Posterior Abdomen ^{111}In-WBC Scan: The liver has multiple photon-deficient defects due to metastatic involvement.

Cross Reference

Chapter 15: Subhepatic Abscess

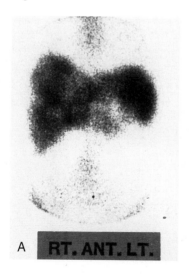

A RT. ANT. LT.

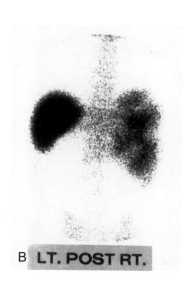

B LT. POST RT.

Chapter 72
Tumors

TUMOR SCANNING AGENTS

TUMOR SCANNING AGENTS
1. Gallium
2. Thallium
3. ^{99m}Tc-sestamibi
4. ^{99m}Tc-glucoheptonate
5. ^{99m}Tc-HMPAO
6. Monoclonal antibodies
7. ^{18}F-FDG
8. Labeled peptides

NOTE. Occasionally, labeled WBCs or ^{99m}Tc-MDP can be seen in neoplasms or neoplastic nodes.

Cross References

Chapter 11: Soft Tissue Abnormalities—Multiple Soft Tissue Metastases with Mucin-Secreting Colon Cancer on Bone Scan

Chapter 71: Infectious Diseases—WBCs in Tumor

GALLIUM-AVID LYMPHOMAS

Patient 1: Lymphoma in Salivary Glands

FIGURE 72–1   A and B.

Gallium Scans: The disease is present only in the left parotid and submandibular glands.

Illustration continued on following page

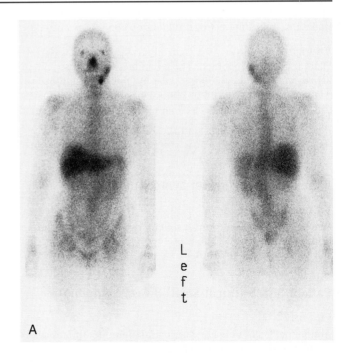

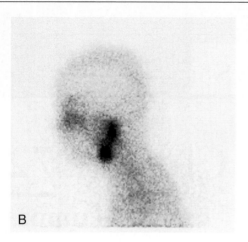

B

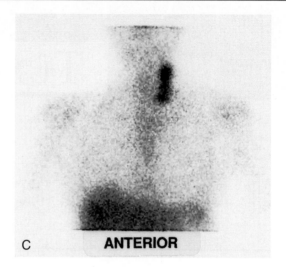

C **ANTERIOR**

Patient 2: Disease Limited to the Neck

FIGURE 72–1 C.

Gallium Scan: The left neck lymph nodes are markedly abnormal.

Patient 3: Mediastinal and Renal Lymphocytic Lymphoma

FIGURE 72–1 D and E.

Chest X-rays 6 Months Apart: The mediastinal mass is smaller on the later examination, but the right paratracheal nodes have not changed their size over the 6 months.

FIGURE 72–1 F and G.

CT Scans of Mediastinum 6 Months Apart: The subcarinal nodes are unchanged or slightly smaller.

FIGURE 72–1 H.

Gallium Scan at Time of 6 Month Follow-up: The right paratracheal and mediastinal lymph nodes have intense gallium accumulation, indicating active residual disease.

FIGURE 72–1 I.

Gallium Scan of Abdomen: The left kidney has intense gallium activity in the upper and lower poles but not in the midportion. The right kidney is diffusely abnormal.

FIGURE 72–1 J.

CT Scans of Kidneys: The kidneys are enlarged without discernible masses.

Patient 4: Small Bowel Lymphoma

FIGURE 72–1 K.

Whole Body Gallium Scan: A solitary right lower quadrant abdominal gallium-avid mass is present in this AIDs patient. The spleen may also be abnormal.

Patient 5: Multifocal Small Bowel Lymphoma

FIGURE 72–1 L.

Abdominal Gallium Scan: The jejunum and ileum (*arrow*) are involved with active lymphoma.

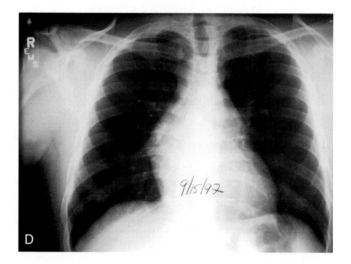

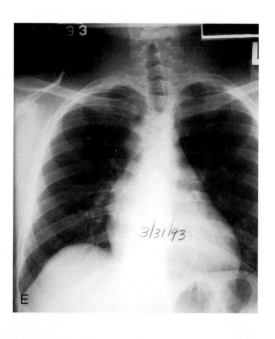

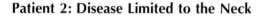

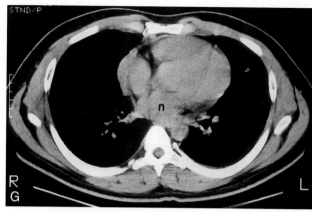

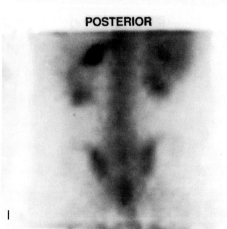

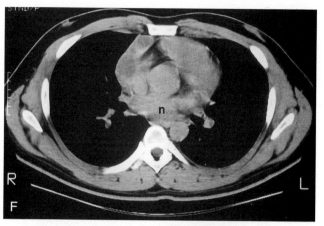

ANTERIOR

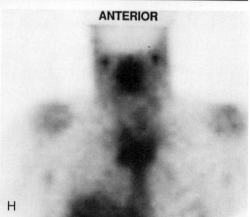

POSTERIOR

H

I

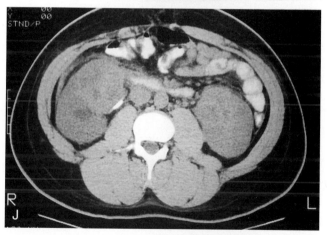

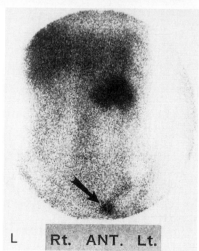

ANTERIOR   POSTERIOR

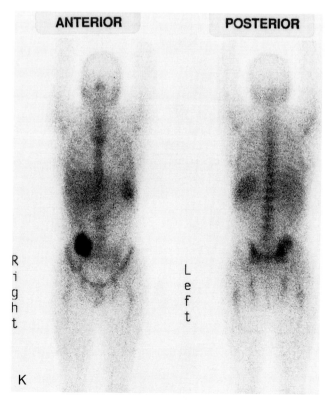

L   Rt. ANT. Lt.

K

Illustration continued on following page

Patient 6: Disseminated Lymphoma

FIGURE 72–1   M.

Whole Body Gallium Scan: There are numerous foci of gallium accumulation, indicating lymphomatous involvement of the neck, axillae, lung, spine, and abdomen.

Patient 7: Non-Hodgkin's Lymphoma

FIGURE 72–1   N and O.

Pre-Chemotherapy Anterior and Lateral Head and Neck Gallium Scans: There is intense gallium accumulation in the right forehead mass as well as in right neck lymph nodes.

FIGURE 72–1   P and Q.

Anterior and Lateral Head and Neck Gallium Scans 6 Months Post Chemotherapy: The forehead mass and the neck lymph nodes have been successfully treated, as evidenced by the absence of gallium activity. (Courtesy of Dr. Michael Kipper, Vista, CA.)

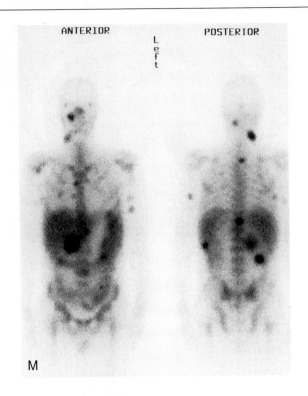

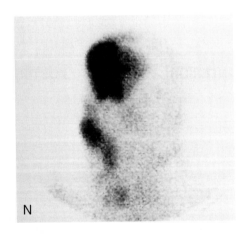

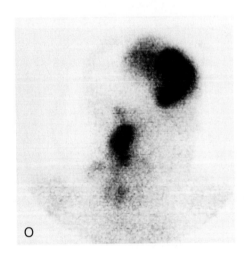

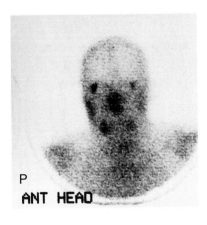

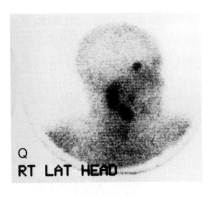

Patient 8: Partially Treated Non-Hodgkin's Lymphoma, Negative on Sestamibi Scan

FIGURE 72–1 R and S.

Anterior Planar and Coronal SPECT Gallium Scans: The huge retroperitoneal lymph nodes that were seen on CT have viable tumor, as evidenced by the gallium accumulation (biopsy proven).

Illustration continued on following page

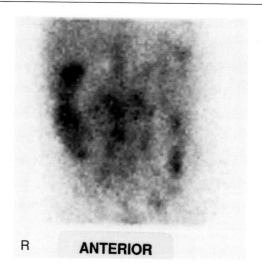

R ANTERIOR

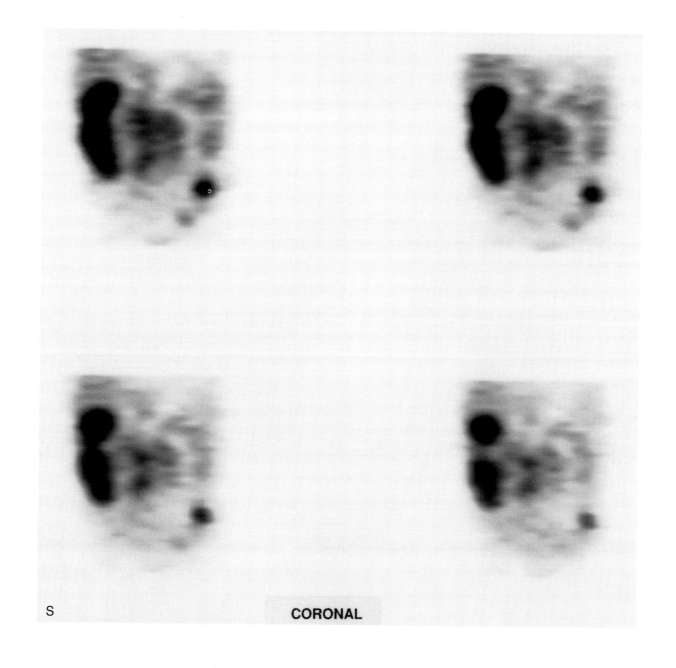

S CORONAL

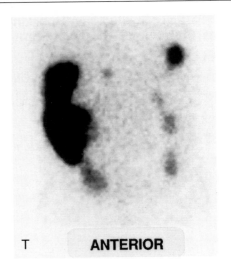

FIGURE 72–1 T.

Anterior Planar ^{99m}Tc-Sestamibi Scan: Neither the planar nor the SPECT scans demonstrated any activity within the lymph nodes. This scan was performed simultaneously with the gallium scan.

NOTE 1. If a lymphoma is gallium-avid initially, gallium scanning can be used to monitor the patient's therapy for residual or recurrent disease.

NOTE 2. Thallium SPECT scans of the chest combined with gallium SPECT scans of the abdomen and pelvis may be the best combination to follow lymphoma. Thallium is very sensitive, but there is too much bowel activity to allow abdominal scanning. A gallium scan at 7 to 10 days post injection usually has little bowel or renal activity.

NOTE 3. Gallium activity in the salivary glands is variable. Physical examination or MRI/CT examinations may help assure salivary gland involvement with disease.

NOTE 4. SPECT scanning has improved the detection of gallium avidity of tumors, especially non-Hodgkin's lymphomas.

NOTE 5. A negative sestamibi scan suggests multidrug resistance.

Cross References

Chapter 50: Tumor Extent on Gallium Scan vs. Chest X-ray

Chapter 68: Thyroid Cancer—Thyroid Lymphoma

Chapter 72: Tumors—Octreotide: Lymphomas; PET: Metastatic Disease

Chapter 73: Breast Diseases—Gallium Scanning of Breast Cancer

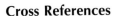

PERICARDIAL MESOTHELIOMA

FIGURE 72–2.

Anterior Gallium Scan: The intense gallium accumulation in the mediastinum extends over the great vessels and heart.

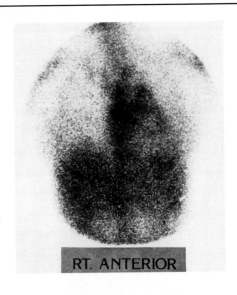

AGGRESSIVE RETROPERITONEAL FIBROMATOSIS (DESMOID)

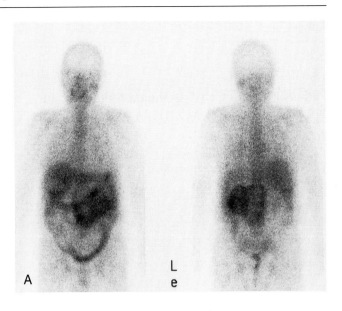

FIGURE 72–3 A.
Anterior and Posterior Gallium Whole Body Scan: There is a lobulated mass in the left posterior abdomen.

FIGURE 72–3 B.
Coronal Gallium SPECT Scan: The medial mass has an inactive center, and the lateral lobulation is more uniformly gallium-avid.

FIGURE 72–3 C.
Transverse Gallium SPECT Scan: The mass is posterior.

NOTE 1. The sestamibi SPECT scan was negative, suggesting that this was not a malignant process.

NOTE 2. Gallium may go to benign or malignant neoplasms as well as to inflammatory conditions. In this case, it may be the ''inflammatory'' component that causes the gallium accumulation.

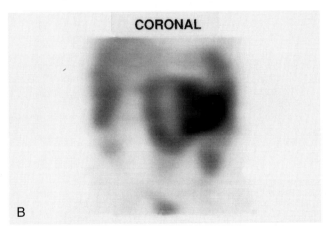

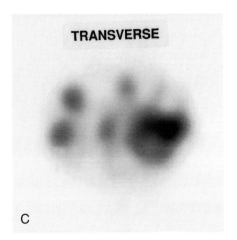

SOFT TISSUE METASTASES

Patient 1: Lung Metastases to Neck Lymph Nodes

FIGURE 72–4 A.
Anterior Thallium Scan: The neck mass accumulates greater thallium than the submandibular or parotid glands.

Illustration continued on following page

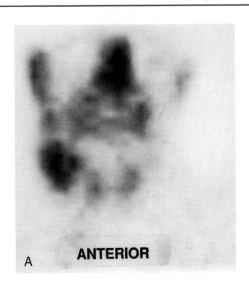

FIGURE 72–4   B.

CT Scan: The enlarged lymph nodes are evident on the right side.

Patient 2: Small Cell Carcinoma Metastatic to the Paraspinal Muscles

FIGURE 72–4   C to E.

Coronal, Transverse, and Sagittal ⁹⁹ᵐTc-Sestamibi SPECT Scan: There is abnormal sestamibi along the left side of the paraspinous muscles *(arrowhead)*.

FIGURE 72–4   F.

Transverse STIR MR Scan: The left paraspinal tumor mass is invading the left lamina and pedicle while replacing the normal muscle.

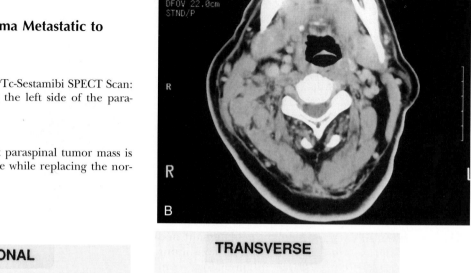

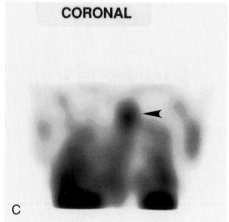

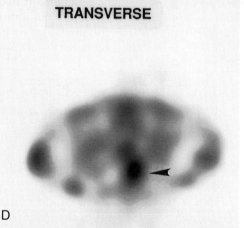

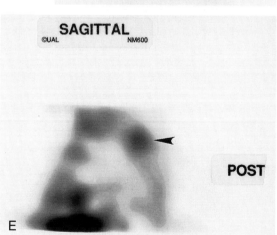

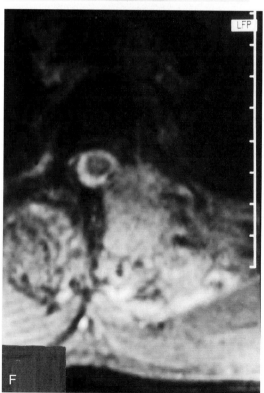

Patient 3: Soft Tissue Sarcoma

FIGURE 72–4   G.

Transverse Thallium SPECT Scan of Upper Neck: The tumor *(arrowheads)* crosses the midline just below the mandible. A metastatic lymph node(s) *(arrow)* in the right anterior cervical chain is present.

FIGURE 72–4   H.

Sagittal Thallium SPECT Scan: The right cervical lymph node and the palpable right tumor are seen (arrowhead = thyroid).

Patient 4: Leiomyosarcoma Metastatic to an Inguinal Lymph Node

FIGURE 72–4   I and J.

Planar and Coronal SPECT Thallium Scans: A metastatic lymph node is present just proximal to the tumor mass.

Illustration continued on following page

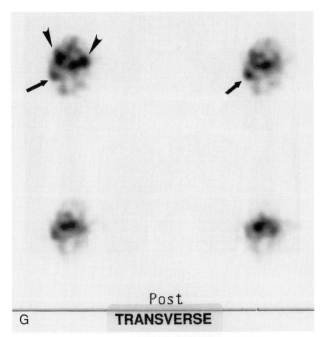

G   TRANSVERSE

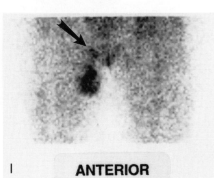

I   ANTERIOR

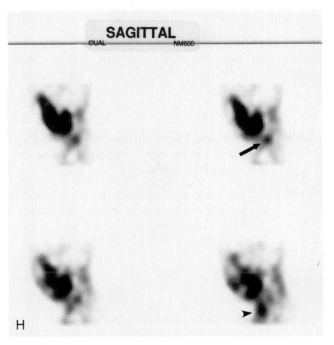

SAGITTAL

H

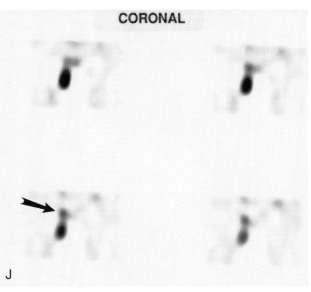

CORONAL

J

Figure 72–4   K and L.

Coronal T2 Weighted MRI Scans: The mass *(black arrow)* and lymph node *(white arrow)* have smooth, well-marginated borders.

Patient 5: Breast Cancer Metastatic to Pleura

Figure 72–4   M.

Coronal Thallium SPECT Scan: There is thallium accumulation in the left apex, in what was thought to be radiation-induced pleural scarring on chest x-ray.

Patient 6: Lung Carcinoma Metastatic to Bone, Axilla, and Mediastinum (Value of SPECT)

Figure 72–4   N.

Coronal Gallium SPECT Scan of Chest: There are gallium-avid metastases in the right scapula, the right axilla, the left humeral head, both hila, and the right paratracheal nodes.

Figure 72–4   O.

Planar Gallium Scan: The right axillary lymph nodes seen on the SPECT scan are not visible on the planar scan. The hilar nodes are barely discernible.

NOTE 1. An MRI may suggest malignancy only if there are irregular margins and invasion of surrounding fat or muscle.

NOTE 2. SPECT scanning improves the confidence of the scan interpretation of subtle abnormalities as well as detecting additional tumor sites, when compared with planar imaging.

Cross Reference

Chapter 68: Thyroid Cancer—Sestamibi in Medullary Carcinoid of the Thyroid; False Negative Thallium Tumor Scan

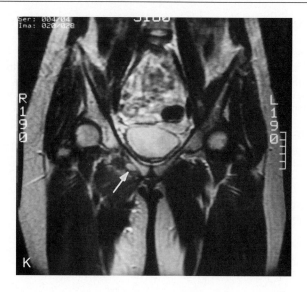

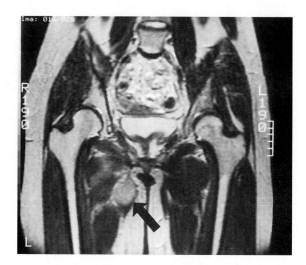

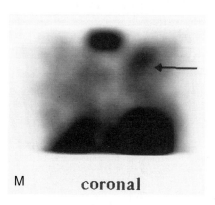

M   coronal

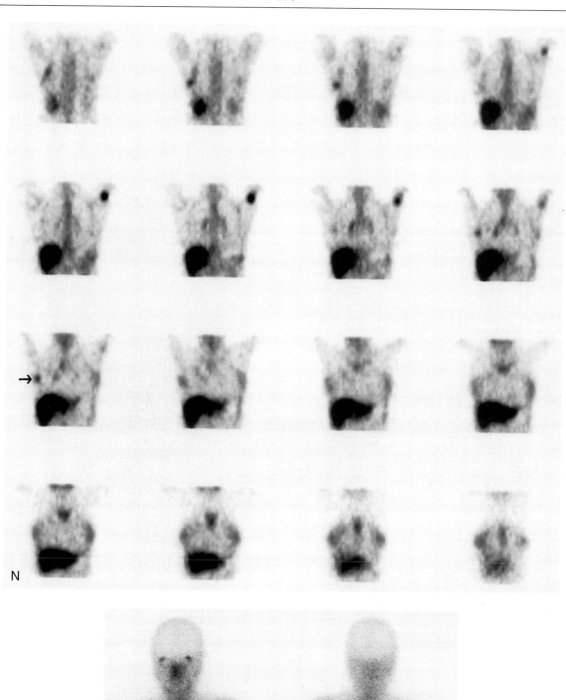

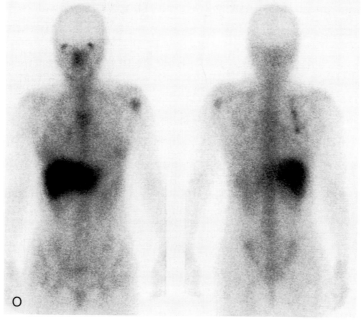

BONE AND SOFT TISSUE METASTASES WITH SESTAMIBI

Patient: Fifty-nine Year Old Female with Gastric Carcinoma

FIGURE 72–5   A.

Anterior and Posterior Planar Chest ^{99m}Tc-Sestamibi Scans: There are several abnormal areas of sestamibi, including the right superior mediastinum, right axilla *(short arrow)*, and right humerus *(long arrow)*.

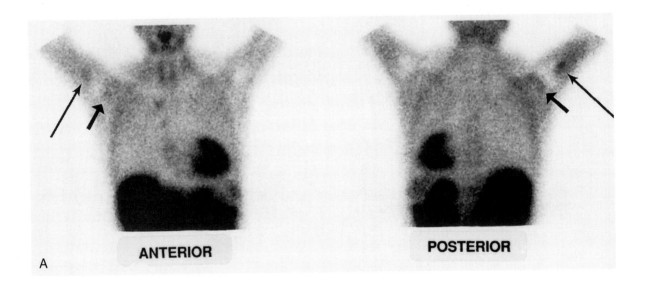

A   **ANTERIOR**   **POSTERIOR**

FIGURE 72–5   B and C.

Sagittal and Coronal Sestamibi SPECT Scans: A midthoracic vertebra is abnormal, although not evident on the planar scan.

NOTE 1. This study was done originally as a scintimammography examination in an asymptomatic patient.

NOTE 2. It appears that most tumor scanning agents are effective for both soft tissue and bony metastases.

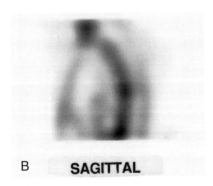

B   **SAGITTAL**

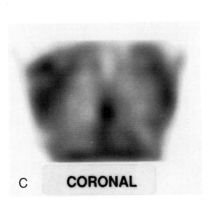

C   **CORONAL**

RECURRENT BRAIN TUMOR

Patient 1: Astrocytoma Grade II–III, S/P Radiation Therapy

FIGURE 72–6   A.

Transverse T2 MRI: There is diffuse white matter high signal and medial mass effect in the left temporal lobe.

FIGURE 72–6   B and C.

Transverse and Coronal Thallium SPECT Scans: There is intense thallium accumulation in the left medial temporal lobe, indicative of viable neoplasm.

Illustration continued on following page

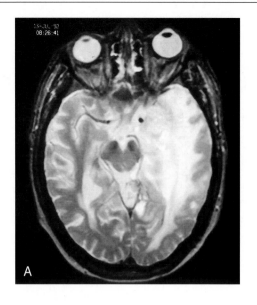

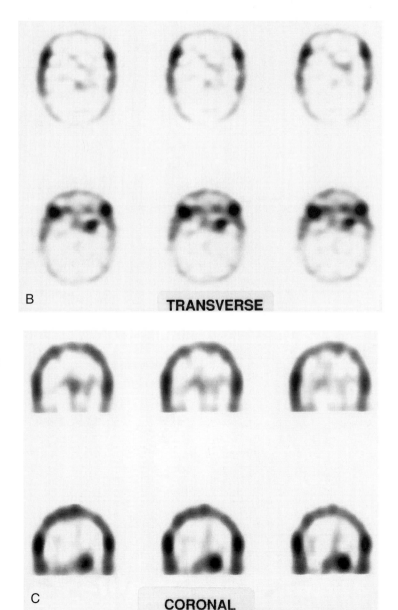

Patient 2: Oligodendroglioma

FIGURE 72–6   D and E.

Coronal and Sagittal Thallium SPECT Scans: Recurrent tumor can be seen in the midline and medial left temporal lobe.

Patient 3: Glioblastoma Multiforme

FIGURE 72–6   F and G.

Transverse and Coronal ^{18}F-FDG PET Brain Scans: The increased activity *(arrows)* in the left centrum semiovale (white matter in the vertex) and cortex of the vertex is indicative of metabolically active tumor. (Courtesy of Dr. Shay Lee, Los Angeles, CA.)

NOTE 1. Thallium or ^{99m}Tc-sestamibi can be helpful to differentiate radiation necrosis from recurrent, viable neoplasms.

NOTE 2. The more malignant the tumor, the greater the radiopharmaceutical accumulation, i.e., benign or low-grade neoplasms may have little or no uptake.

NOTE 3. PET scanning with ^{18}F-FDG or ^{11}C-methionine can also be used for recurrent tumor detection, but normal cortical activity may equal that of a cortical tumor, rendering it difficult to distinguish the two.

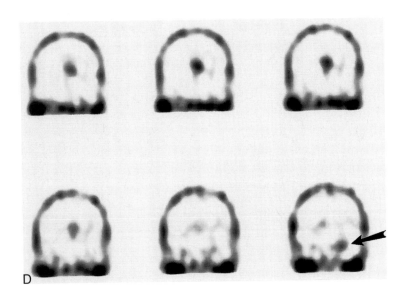

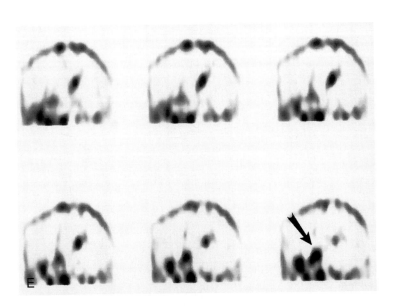

TRANSVERSE

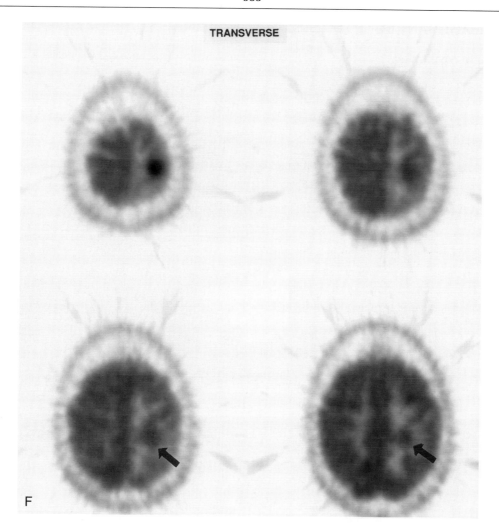

F

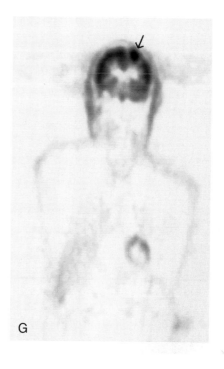

G

THALLIUM IN MALIGNANT BONE TUMORS

Patient 1: Multiple Myeloma

FIGURE 72–7   A.

Plain Film X-ray: The left femoral diaphysis has a motheaten appearance.

FIGURE 72–7   B.

Planar Thallium Scan: The region of the abnormality has intense thallium accumulation.

Patient 2: Osteosarcoma

FIGURE 72–7   C.

Plain Film X-ray: The classic bony production of an osteosarcoma can be seen.

FIGURE 72–7   D.

Planar Thallium Scan: The intense perifemoral activity makes the marrow involvement less evident.

FIGURE 72–7   E.

Sagittal T1 MRI Scan: The marrow involvement (loss of the normal fatty high signal) is evident along with the surrounding tumor mass.

Cross Reference

Chapter 1: Solitary Bony Abnormalities—Osteosarcoma

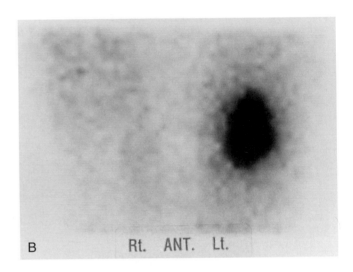

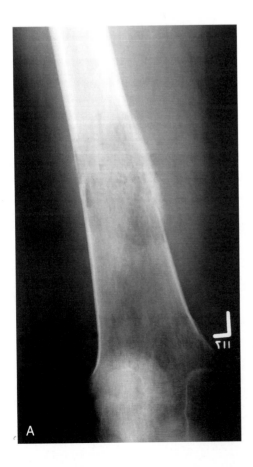

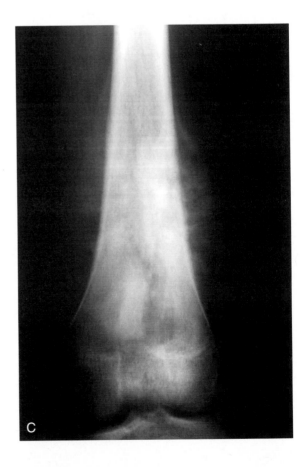

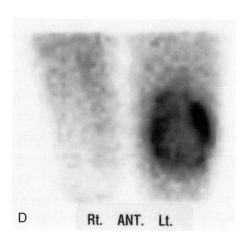

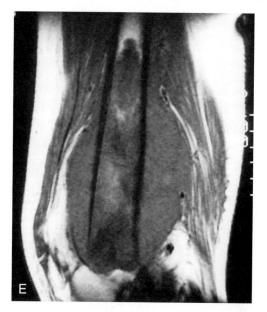

THALLIUM IN BENIGN BONE CONDITIONS

Patient 1: Benign Enchondroma

FIGURE 72–8 A.

Plain Film X-ray: There is an expansile lesion arising in the medullary canal of the fibula.

Illustration continued on following page

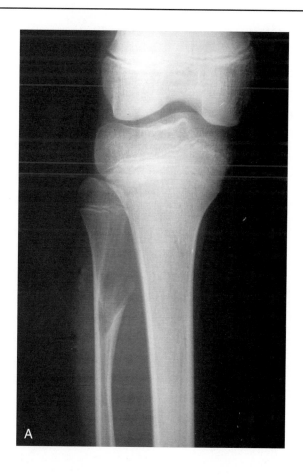

FIGURE 72–8   B.

CT Scan: There is a lobulated lesion without a calcified rim but with internal calcification *(white arrow)*.

FIGURE 72–8   C and D.

Blood Pool and Delayed Bone Scintigrams: There is hyperemia and mildly increased activity involving the fibula.

FIGURE 72–8   E and F.

Thallium Tumor SPECT Scan: There is normal accumulation of thallium in the region of the tumor.

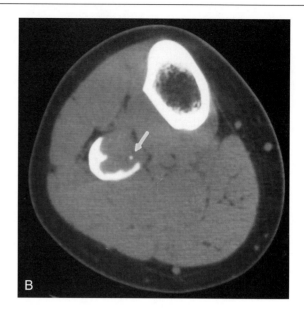

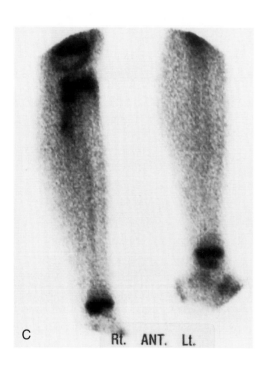

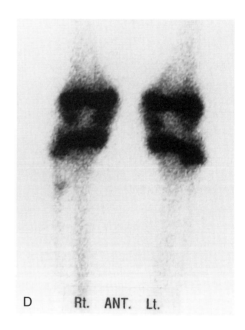

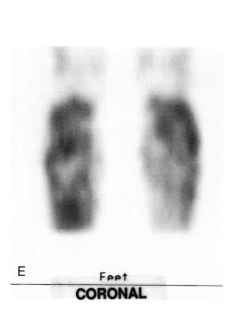

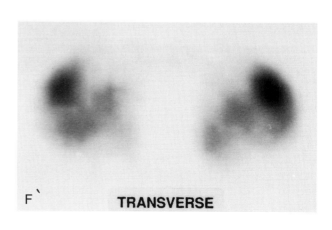

Patient 2: Paget's Disease

FIGURE 72–8 G.

Anterior Pelvic Bone Scan: The ilium and pubic bone as well as the lower lumbar vertebrae have such intense uptake that the normal bones barely show up.

FIGURE 72–8 H.

Coronal Thallium Scan: There is minimal thallium accumulation in the anterior left iliac wing *(arrow)*. The intense activity is bowel.

Patient 3: Fibrous Dysplasia

FIGURE 72–8 I and J.

Anterior and Posterior Pelvic Planar Bone Scan: There is increased activity along the right ilium, extending to the sacroiliac joint. There is also activity in the left-sided L5 hypertrophic spur.

Illustration continued on following page

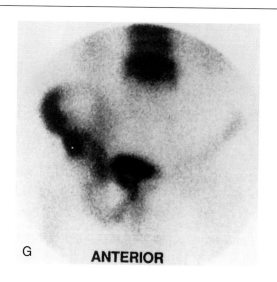

G **ANTERIOR**

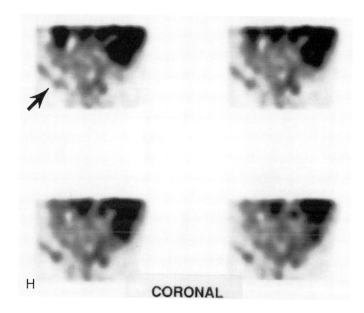

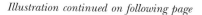

H **CORONAL**

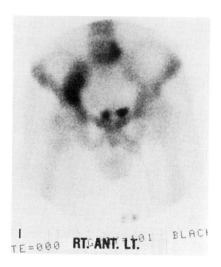

I TE=000 **RT. ANT. LT.** BLACK

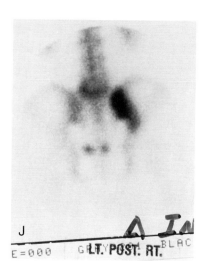

J E=000 **LT. POST. RT.** BLAC

FIGURE 72–8   K and L.

Axial and Coronal Bone SPECT Scans: The iliac lesion and the hypertrophic L5 spur *(arrow)* are well seen.

FIGURE 72–8   M and N.

Axial and Coronal Thallium SPECT Scans: The iliac abnormality has mild thallium accumulation *(arrows)*, whereas the hypertrophic spur has none (open arrow = bowel).

FIGURE 72–8   O.

CT Scan: The right ilium has a lytic expansile lesion.

NOTE. Most benign processes have little or no thallium or sestamibi accumulation.

Cross Reference

Chapter 1: Solitary Bony Abnormalities—Value of Negative [201]Thallium Tumor Scan

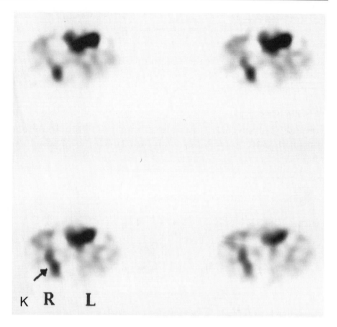

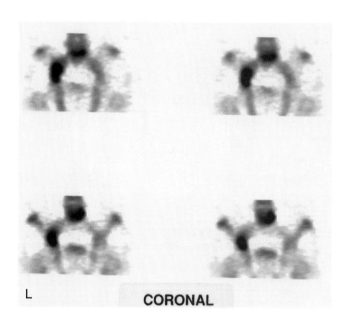

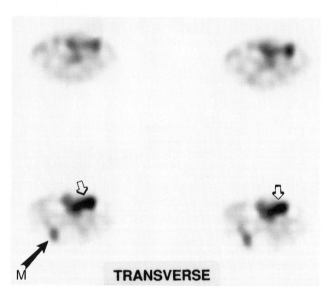

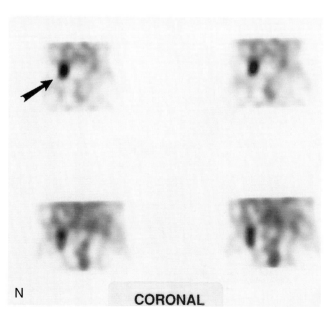

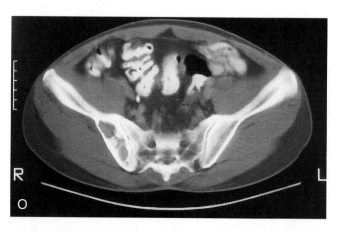

RETROPERITONEAL UNDIFFERENTIATED LIPOSARCOMA METASTATIC TO PLEURA

FIGURE 72–9   A.

Coronal Thallium SPECT Scan: There are two abnormal thallium accumulations: one over the left pararenal retroperitoneum, the primary site *(arrow)*, and the other over the dome of the liver.

FIGURE 72–9   B.

Right Sagittal Thallium SPECT Scan: The mass above the liver proved to be a metastatic focus.

NOTE. The purpose of tumor scanning in bone or soft tissue masses is to give a preoperative estimate of tumor grade and to look for involvement of proximal lymph nodes ("sentinel" nodes) and metastatic foci.

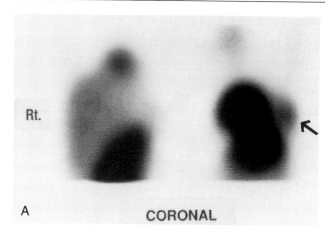

A   CORONAL

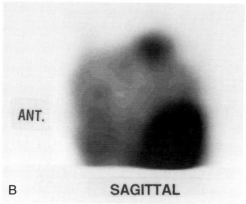

B   SAGITTAL

LUNG NODULES

Patient 1: Adenocarcinoma of the Lungs

FIGURE 72–10   A.

Posterior Planar Sestamibi Scan: The left upper lobe has a focal accumulation of the radiopharmaceutical.

FIGURE 72–10   B.

Transverse SPECT Scan: The focal activity on the planar scan actually is a summation of two nodules, as seen on SPECT *(arrows)*.

Illustration continued on following page

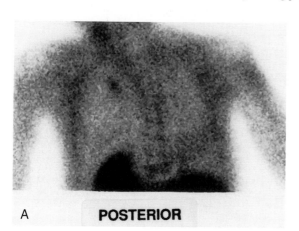

A   **POSTERIOR**

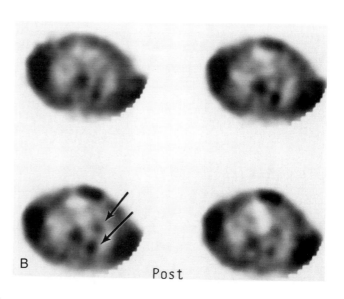

B   Post

Patient 2: Large Cell Carcinoma of the Lungs

FIGURE 72–10   C to E.

Transverse, Sagittal, and Coronal Sestamibi SPECT Scan: There is a large mass with a photopenic center and lymph node involvement *(arrow)*.

FIGURE 72–10   F.

Transverse CT Scan: The mass and abnormal right hilar lymph nodes can be seen.

Patient 3: Aspergillosis

FIGURE 72–10   G.

PA Chest X-ray: There is a density in the left upper lobe extending to the pleura.

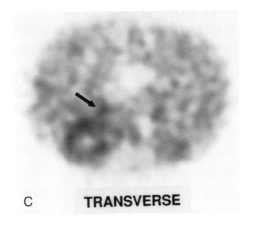

C   TRANSVERSE

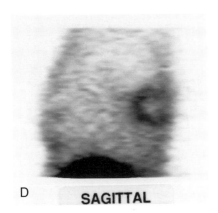

D   SAGITTAL

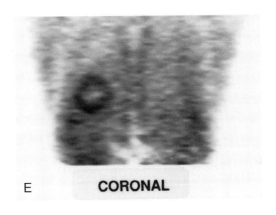

E   CORONAL

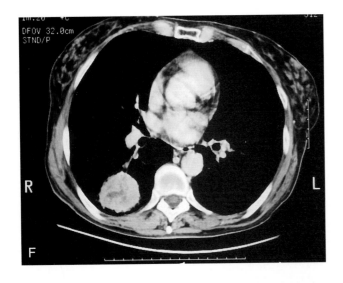

F

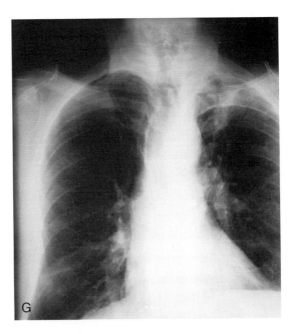

G

FIGURE 72–10 H and I.

Planar Anterior and Posterior Thallium Scan: There is only mild, diffuse thallium accumulation throughout the left upper lobe, without a focus of intense activity.

FIGURE 72–10 J.

Thallium Coronal SPECT Scan: The diffuse increased thallium accumulation in the left lung can be seen above the heart.

SOLITARY PULMONARY NODULE

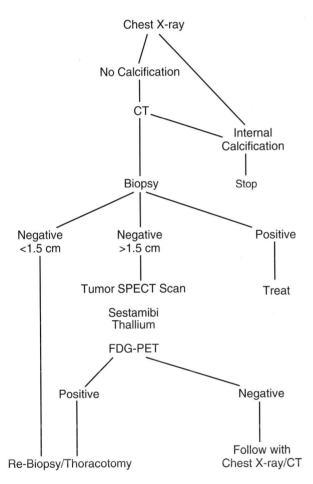

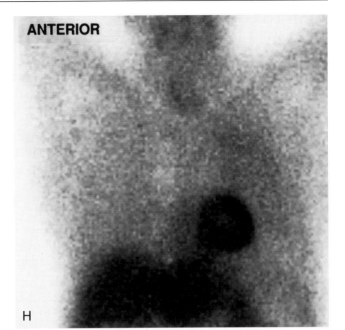

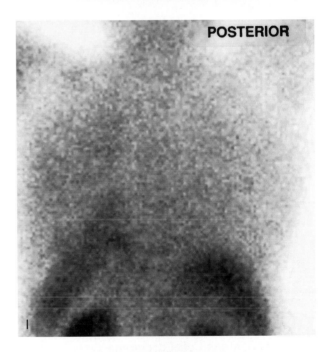

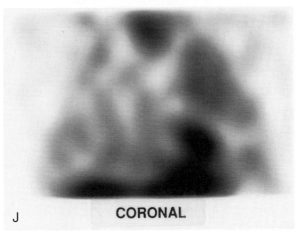

NOTE 1. Either thallium or sestamibi SPECT scans for "solitary" pulmonary nodules can be helpful to determine whether a "solitary" pulmonary nodule needs to be re-biopsied. If mediastinal nodes are visualized, then tumor involvement is likely.

NOTE 2. Nonlocalized activity, especially when mild, is less likely to represent malignancy, usually indicating an inflammatory process.

NOTE 3. The most common false positive tumor scan in the lung is tuberculosis

Cross Reference

Chapter 50: Tumors—Lung Tumor Scanning (Several Cases)

RECURRENT TUMOR WITH CHEST INFECTION

Patient: Seventy-seven Year Old Male with Fever 2 Years After Partial Pneumonectomy for Lung Carcinoma

FIGURE 72–11   A.

Anterior Chest ^{99m}Tc-Sestamibi Scan: There are two foci of sestamibi in the right chest. The remaining right thorax has minimal activity.

FIGURE 72–11   B.

Anterior Chest ^{111}In-WBC Scan: There is intense WBC accumulation in the peripheral right chest but not in the areas of tumor.

FIGURE 72–11   C.

AP Chest X-ray: The right hemithorax is partially opacified by fluid and fibrosis, with considerable loss of volume.

NOTE. Sestamibi generally does not accumulate avidly in areas of active infection, i.e., obstructive pneumonias.

Cross Reference

Chapter 48: Progression of Pneumonia

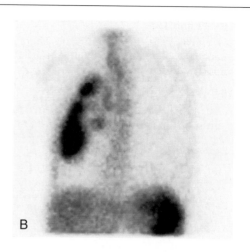

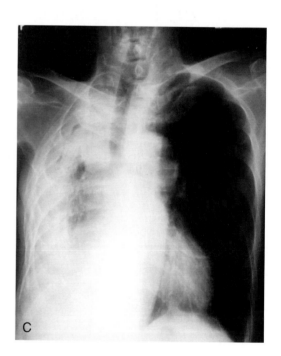

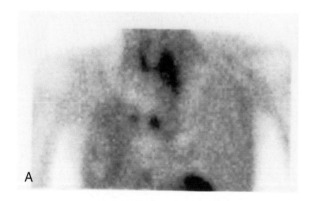

UTERINE TUMORS

Patient 1: Squamous Cell Carcinoma

FIGURE 72–12   A and B.

Anterior Pelvic Gallium Scan: The gallium-avid mass does not change with voiding.

Patient 2: Uterine Sarcoma

FIGURE 72–12   C.

Post-Void Anterior Pelvic Gallium Scan: There is a localized gallium collection in the central pelvis that did not change with voiding.

NOTE. There are no recent studies on the efficacy of gallium scanning, especially using SPECT, with uterine tumors.

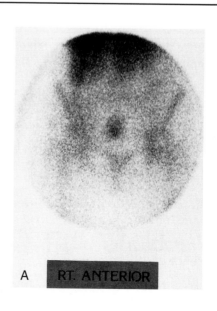

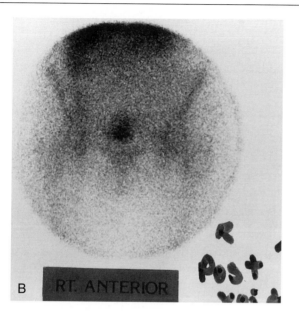

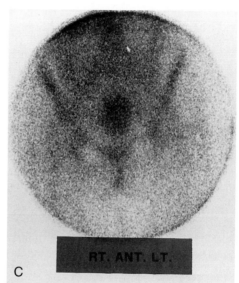

ANTIBODY SCANNING

Patient 1: Metastatic Colon Carcinoma

FIGURE 72–13   A.

Seven Day Planar Abdomen ^{111}In-Anti-TAG-72 (OncoScint CR/OV) Scan: The para-aortic nodes are diffusely abnormal.

Patient 2: Twenty-eight Year Old with Metastatic Colon Carcinoma

FIGURE 72–13   B.

Seven Day Planar Abdomen ^{111}In-Anti-TAG-72 (OncoScint CR/OV) Scan: Abnormal abdominal lymph nodes are evident.

Illustration continued on following page

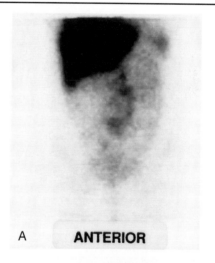

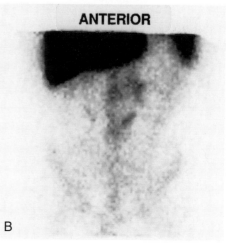

FIGURE 72–13 C and D.

Coronal and transverse Anti-TAG-72 (OncoScint CR/OV) Scans: The metastatic lymph nodes extend anterior from the aorta into the mesentery.

FIGURE 72–13 E.

CT with Contrast: This scan has no evident adenopathy.

Patient 3: Metastatic Ovarian Carcinoma

FIGURE 72–13 F.

Planar Anterior Pelvic ^{111}In-Anti-TAG-72 (OncoScint CR/OV) Scan: There is a faint increase in activity deep in the pelvis, which was not seen on the posterior planar views.

FIGURE 72–13 G to I.

Coronal, Transverse, and Sagittal SPECT Anti-TAG-72 (Onco-Scint CR/OV) Scan: There is intense activity between the urinary bladder and the rectum *(arrow)*.

FIGURE 72–13 J.

CT Scan of Pelvis: A mass *(asterisk)* can be seen anterior to the rectum.

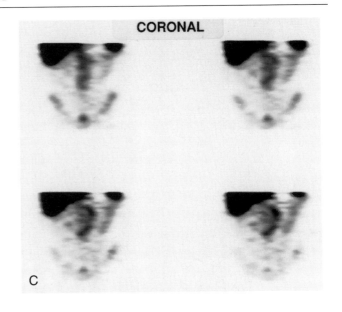

C

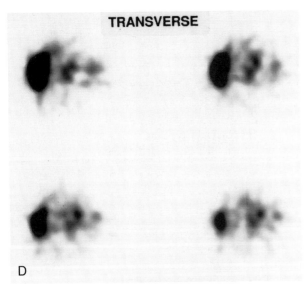

TRANSVERSE

D

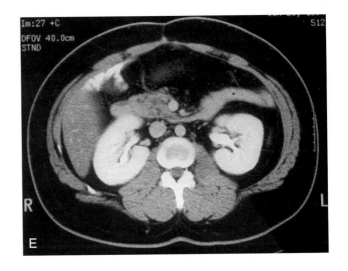

E

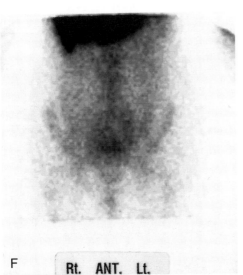

F   Rt. ANT. Lt.

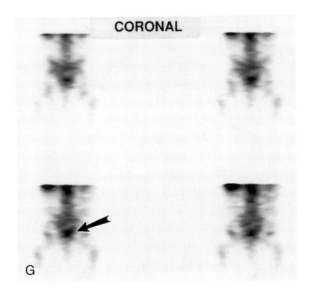

CORONAL

G

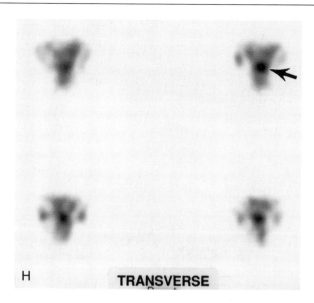

H **TRANSVERSE**

Patient 4: Normal Colostomy Activity Without Evidence of Recurrent Rectal Carcinoma

FIGURE 72–13 K.

Planar Anterior Abdomen ^{111}In-Anti-TAG-72 (OncoScint CR/OV) Scan: There is a focal "abnormality" in the left lower quadrant.

FIGURE 72–13 L to N.

Coronal, Sagittal, and Transverse Anti-TAG-72 (OncoScint CR/OV) SPECT Scans: The colostomy can be seen in the lower left abdominal wall *(arrow)*.

Illustration continued on following page

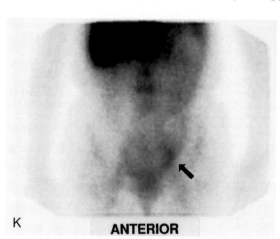

K **ANTERIOR**

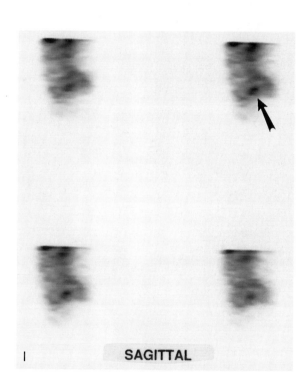

I **SAGITTAL**

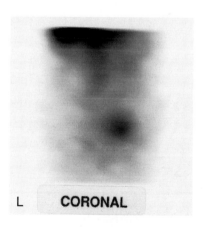

L **CORONAL**

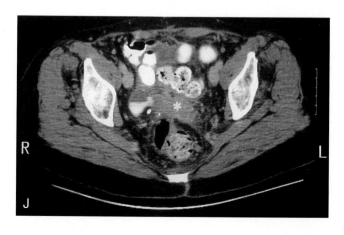

J

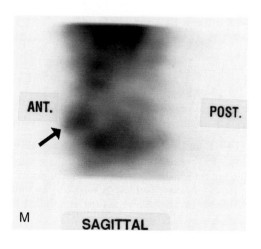

ANT. POST.

M **SAGITTAL**

Patient 5: Prostate Carcinoma Metastatic to Retroperitoneal Lymph Nodes

FIGURE 72–13 O.

Whole Body ¹¹¹In-Anti-CYT-356 (ProstaScint) and ¹⁸F-FDG PET Scans: The metastases are clearly visible in the midabdomen on the monoclonal antibody study but are not seen with the FDG PET scan. (Courtesy of Dr. Michael Haseman, Sacramento, CA.)

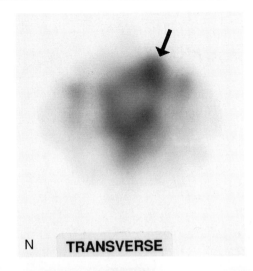

NOTE 1. Planar and SPECT scans should be done in all cases, to feel confident that all potentially detectable metastatic deposits are seen.

NOTE 2. Some metastatic deposits may not show up with radiolabeled antibody imaging, whereas other metastatic foci in the same patient may have intense accumulation.

NOTE 3. Inflammatory foci, such as abscesses and colostomy stoma, may accumulate radiolabeled antibodies.

NOTE 4. PET scanning with ¹⁸F-FDG for prostate carcinoma does not appear to be sensitive.

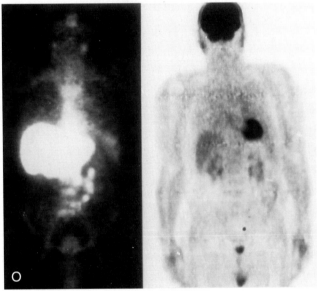

NORMAL OCTREOTIDE SCAN

FIGURE 72–14 A and B.

Twenty-four Hour Anterior and Lateral Head and Neck ¹¹¹In-Octreotide Scans: There is only mild octreotide accumulation in the thyroid and none in the choroid plexus.

FIGURE 72–14 C and D.

Twenty-four Hour Anterior Chest ¹¹¹In-Octreotide Scan: There is no activity in the lungs or the heart.

FIGURE 72–14 E and F.

Twenty-four Hour Anterior and Posterior Abdomen: The liver activity is mild, but the spleen has intense radiopeptide accumulation. The major excretory pathway is through the kidneys, making the kidneys intense. Bowel activity is reduced by cathartics.

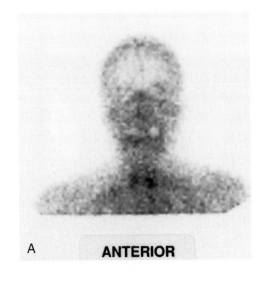

NOTE 1. Radiolabeled octreotide is a peptide that binds to the somatostatin receptor. It is useful in localizing neuroendocrine tumors, lymphomas, some pituitary tumors, meningiomas, and sarcoid.

NOTE 2. Neuroendocrine tumors include carcinoid, small cell carcinoma of the lung, endocrine tumors of the pancreas, gastrinomas, Merkel cell tumors, medullary carcinoma of the thyroid, neuroblastoma, pheochromocytoma, melanoma, mucocutaneous neuromas, VIPomas, and APUDomas.

NOTE 3. Radiolabeled octreotide peptides can accumulate in non-neuroendocrine tumors, such as adenocarcinomas of the breast and lung.

NOTE 4. Successful treatment with somatostatin can be predicted by accumulation of a radiolabeled somatostatin analog. A negative scan indicates dedifferentiation of a tumor and a predictable lack of response to somatostatin.

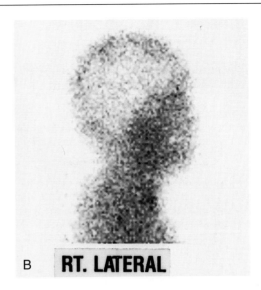

B **RT. LATERAL**

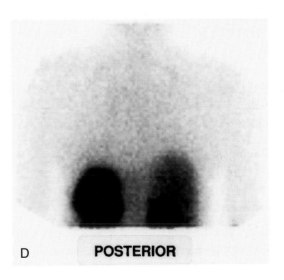

D **POSTERIOR**

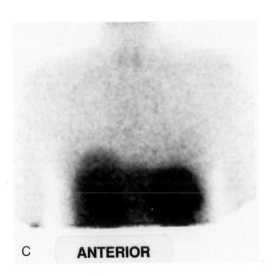

C **ANTERIOR**

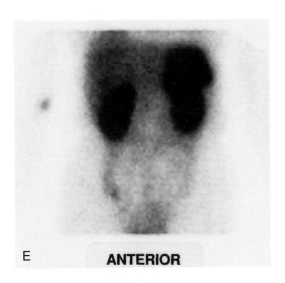

E **ANTERIOR**

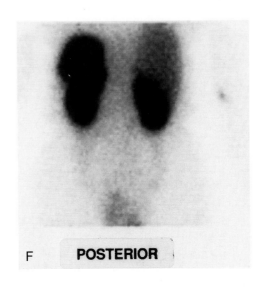

F **POSTERIOR**

OCTREOTIDE: MULTIPLE ENDOCRINE NEOPLASIA SYNDROME IIB

Patient 1: Medullary Carcinoma of the Thyroid with Mucocutaneous Neuromas

FIGURE 72–15 A.

Twenty-four Hour Anterior Neck ^{111}In-Octreotide Scan: Both lobes of the thyroid have intense uptake of the octreotide.

FIGURE 72–15 B.

Twenty-four Hour Anterior Abdomen ^{111}In-Octreotide Scan: The transverse and descending colon have intense uptake in the neuromas, while lesser uptake is present in the uninvolved small bowel and ascending colon. (Courtesy of Dr. Michael Kipper, Vista, CA.)

Patient 2: Paraganglioma and Pheochromocytoma

FIGURE 72–15 C and D.

Anterior and Left Lateral Planar ^{111}In-Octreotide Scans: The intense accumulation in the left neck is indicative of a neuroendocrine tumor.

FIGURE 72–15 E.

Posterior Planar Abdominal ^{111}In-Octreotide Scan: The left adrenal gland is barely visible *(arrow)*. The kidneys are small from chronic hypertension, causing arteriolar nephrosclerosis.

FIGURE 72–15 F to H.

Sagittal, Transverse, and Coronal Abdominal ^{111}In-Octreotide SPECT Scans: The SPECT scan confirms the abnormal accumulation of the octreotide.

Patient 3: Multiple Paragangliomas

FIGURE 72–15 I and J.

Anterior and Right Lateral ^{111}In-Octreotide Planar Scans: There is an intense accumulation in the upper right neck, a recurrent carotid body tumor.

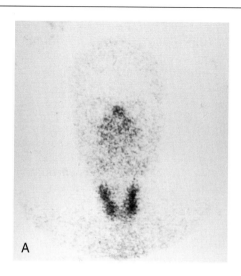

A

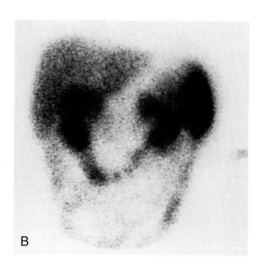

B

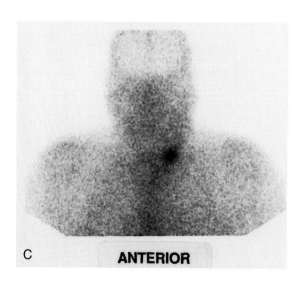

C **ANTERIOR**

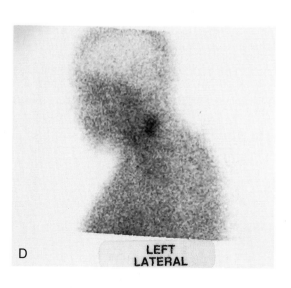

D **LEFT LATERAL**

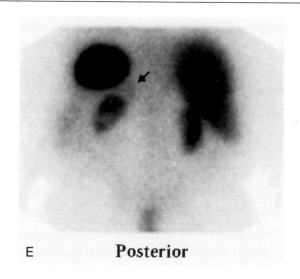

E **Posterior**

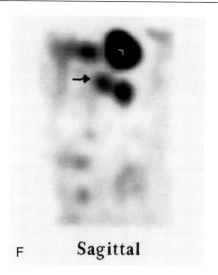

F **Sagittal**

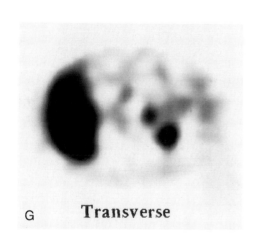

G **Transverse**

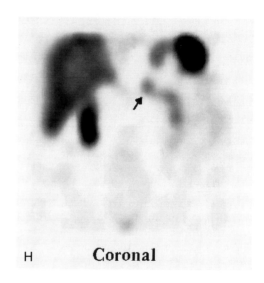

H **Coronal**

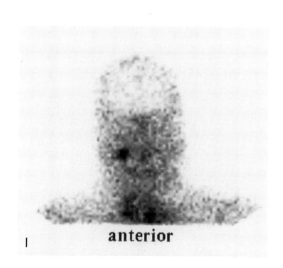

I **anterior**

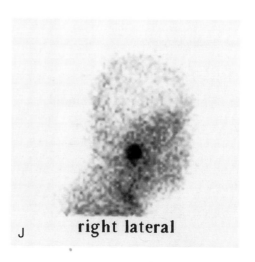

J **right lateral**

Illustration continued on following page

FIGURE 72–15 K.

Anterior Chest ¹¹¹In-Octreotide Scans: An additional tumor site is seen in the lower mediastinum. Normal activity is seen in the thyroid gland. The activity to the left of the thyroid is due to recent surgery in which a paraganglioma was removed.

FIGURE 72–15 L.

Anterior ¹¹¹In-Octreotide Scan: Activity can be seen in both adrenal glands from asymptomatic tumors *(arrows)*.

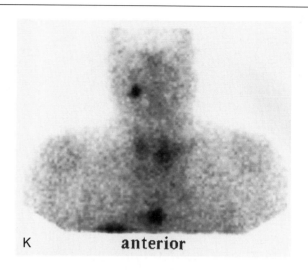

K   **anterior**

MULTIPLE ENDOCRINE NEOPLASIA SYNDROMES			
Lesions	MEN I	MEN IIA	MEN IIB or III
Pituitary	++++	0	0
Medullary carcinoma of thyroid	+	++++	++++
Parathyroid	++++	++	+
Adrenal cortex	++++	+	+
Pheochromocytoma	0	++++	++++
Pancreas	++++	0	0
Peptic ulcer	++++	0	0
Mucocutaneous neuromas	0	0	++++

From Cotran R, Kumar V, Robbins S: Pathologic Basis of Disease, 4th ed. Philadelphia, W.B. Saunders, 1989.

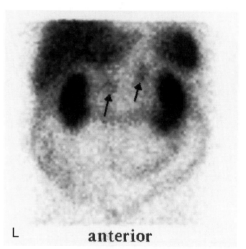

L   **anterior**

NOTE 1. SPECT scans of the neck, chest, abdomen and pelvis are necessary to detect and localize abnormalities.

NOTE 2. Multiple paragangliomas can be found in 20 percent of patients without MEN syndrome.

Cross Reference

Chapter 68: Cancer—Sestamibi in Medullary Carcinoma of the Thyroid

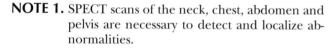

OCTREOTIDE: CARCINOID

Patient 1: Primary Bronchial Carcinoid

FIGURE 72–16 A.

Twenty-four Hour Posterior Chest ¹¹¹In-Octreotide Scan: There is an intense focus of radioactivity in the right lower lobe. The milder activity peripheral to the neoplasm is in an obstructive pneumonia.

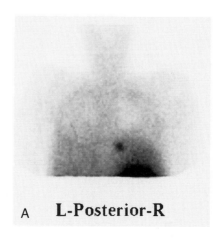

A   **L-Posterior-R**

Patient 2: Carcinoid in the Liver

FIGURE 72–16 B and C.

Twenty-four Hour Anterior and Posterior Abdomen ^{111}In-Octreotide Scans: The liver activity is normal.

FIGURE 72–16 D and E.

Twenty-four Hour Transverse and Coronal Liver ^{111}In-Octreotide SPECT Scans: There is focal increased octreotide accumulation in the lateral right lobe *(arrows)*.

FIGURE 72–16 F.

Transverse T2 MRI Scan: Two small high-signal nodules are seen along the lateral right lobe of the liver. (Courtesy of Dr. Michael Kipper, Vista, CA.)

Illustration continued on following page

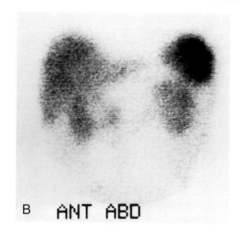

B   ANT ABD

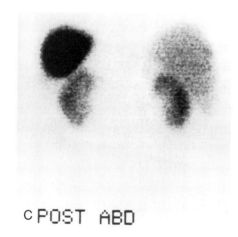

C POST ABD

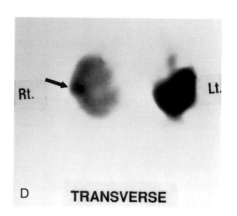

D   TRANSVERSE

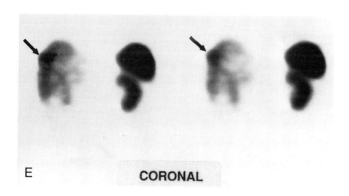

E   CORONAL

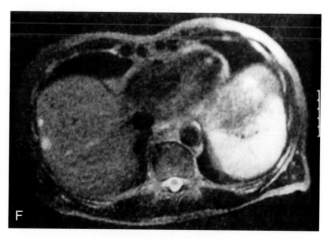

F

Patient 3: Recently Developed Liver Mass Diagnosed on CT, Ultimately Proven to be a Healed Abscess.

FIGURE 72–16   G.

Anterior ^{99m}Tc-Octreotide Scan: There is a subtle photon-deficient defect in the dome of the right lobe of the liver.

FIGURE 72–16   H.

Coronal SPECT Scan: The lack of octreotide indicates that the mass does not have somatostatin receptors.

FIGURE 72–16   I and J.

Anterior and Right Lateral 3 Hour Delayed Planar Liver ^{99m}Tc-Sestamibi Scans: After 3 hours the sestamibi has washed out of the liver. The mass does not have any retained radiopharmaceutical.

NOTE 1. The relatively low liver activity allows SPECT scans to evaluate the liver in cases of tumors known to accumulate octreotide.

NOTE 2. Virtually all extrahepatic carcinoid sites will be detected as long as the tumor has not dedifferentiated.

NOTE 3. A radio-octreotide scan should be performed preoperatively, since unexpected sites of involvement are frequent despite the use of CT.

Cross Reference

Chapter 50: Octreotide—A Non–Small Cell Carcinoma of the Lung

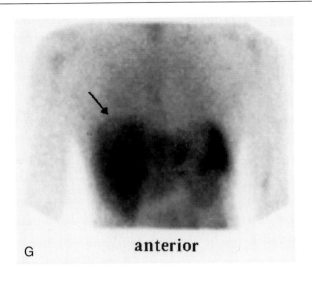

G   **anterior**

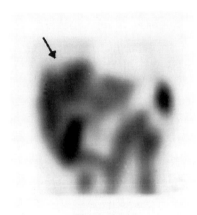
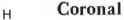

H   **Coronal**

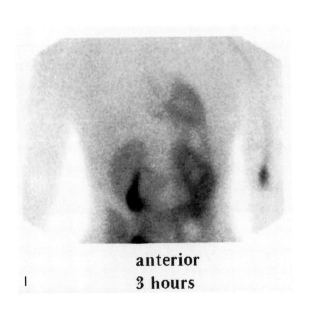

anterior

I   **3 hours**

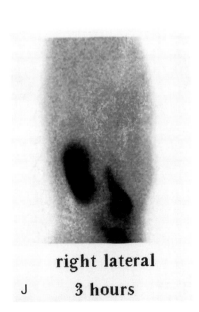

right lateral

J   **3 hours**

OCTREOTIDE: LYMPHOMAS

Patient 1: Nasopharyngeal and Neck Non-Hodgkin's Lymphoma

FIGURE 72–17   A to C.

Twenty-four Hour Anterior, Posterior, and Right Lateral ^{111}In-Octreotide Scans: There is abnormal accumulation of the octreotide within the nasopharynx and the right neck.

Patient 2: Viable Lymphomatous Lymph Nodes Following Chemotherapy and Radiation Therapy

FIGURE 72–17   D and E.

Anterior and Posterior 15 Minute Postinjection ^{99m}Tc-Octreotide Scans: Several abnormal tumor masses are present. The largest appears to have a necrotic center.

NOTE. Radiolabeled octreotide accumulation is thought to occur as a result of activated lymphocytes in lymphomas, and in somatostatin receptors on surrounding venules with non-small cell carcinomas of the lung.

Cross Reference

Chapter 72: Tumors—Gallium-Avid Lymphomas

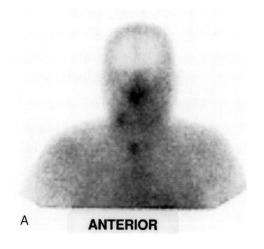

A   **ANTERIOR**

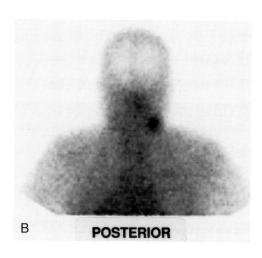

B   **POSTERIOR**

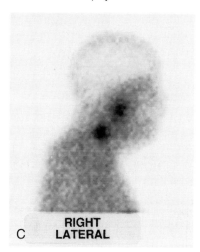

C   **RIGHT LATERAL**

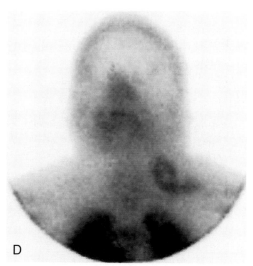

D

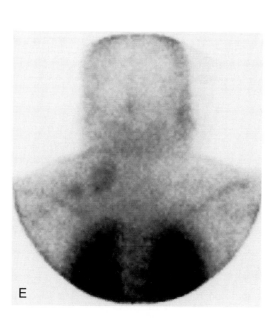

E

GIANT HEMANGIOMA (KASABACH-MERRITT SYNDROME)

Patient: Three Month Female with Severe Thrombocytopenia and Masses in the Right Shoulder and Left Flank

FIGURE 72–18   A and B.

Anterior and Posterior ^{111}In-Platelet Scans: There is abnormal accumulation of the platelets in the right chest and shoulder hemangioma but none in the left flank hemangioma.

NOTE. Kasabach-Merritt syndrome has thrombocytopenia due to thrombosis and platelet sequestration in one or more giant cavernous hemangiomas.

Cross References

Chapter 7: Hands and Feet—Bone and Soft Tissue Hemangioma of the Foot

Chapter 11: Soft Tissue Abnormalities—Hemangioma

Chapter 15: Hemangioma

Chapter 17: Multiple Hepatic Hemangiomata

Chapter 59: Leg Hemangioma on Tagged RBC Scan

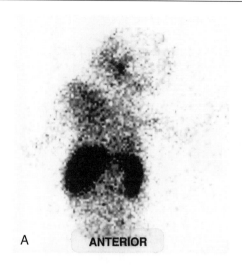

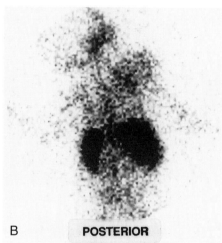

NORMAL WHOLE BODY TOMOGRAPHIC PET SCAN

FIGURE 72–19   A and B.

^{18}F-FDG Whole Body PET Scans: Normal high activity is present in the brain, heart, kidneys, bladder, and segments of colon. Minor activity can be seen in the lungs, liver, spleen, and bone marrow. (Courtesy of Dr. Shay Lee, Los Angeles, CA.)

PROPOSED METASTATIC WORK-UP

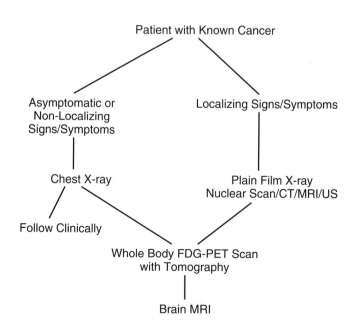

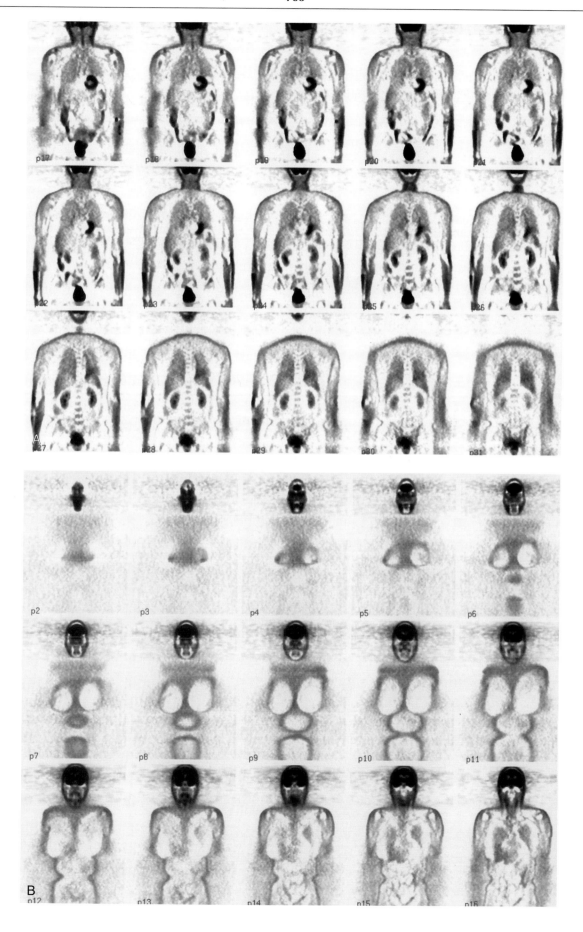

RECURRENCE AT MASTECTOMY SITE

FIGURE 72–20.

18F-FDG Whole Body Scan: The right mastectomy site has increased glucose metabolism, indicative of tumor recurrence. (Courtesy of Dr. Shay Lee, Los Angeles, CA.)

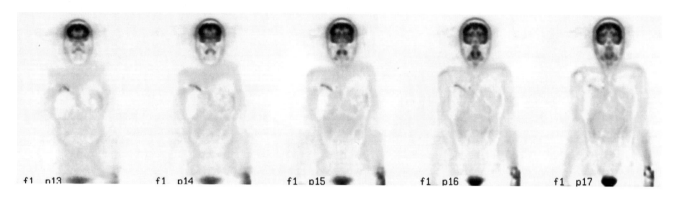

PET: METASTATIC DISEASE

Patient 1: Melanoma

FIGURE 72–21   A.

18F-FDG Whole Body Scan: A focus of increased metabolism is present in the right neck. (Courtesy of Dr. Shay Lee, Los Angeles, CA.)

Patient 2: Melanoma

FIGURE 72–21   B.

18F-FDG Whole Body Scan: Mediastinal, hilar, and possibly bone (*arrow*) metastases are seen. (Courtesy of Dr. Shay Lee, Los Angeles, CA.)

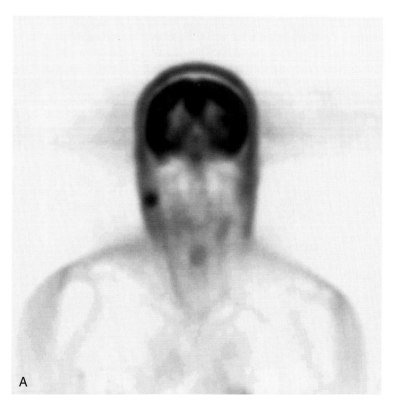

A

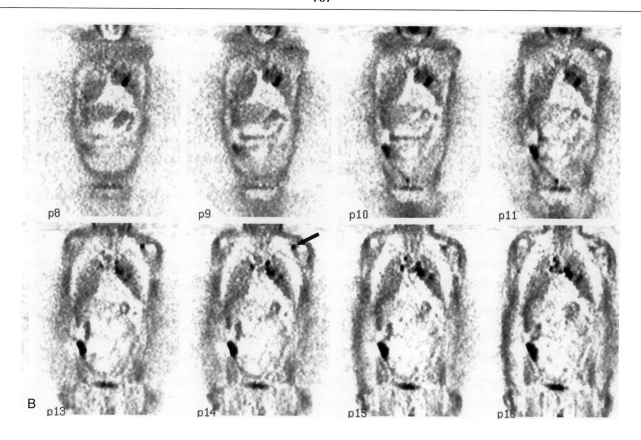

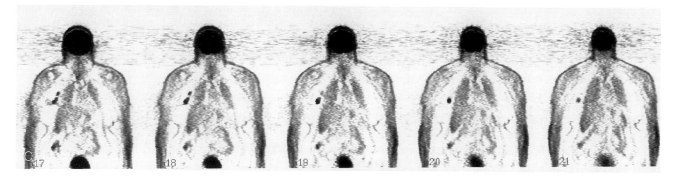

Patient 3: Metastatic Preoperative Breast Carcinoma

FIGURE 72–21 C.

^{18}F-FDG Whole Body Scan: There is intense activity in several right axillary lymph nodes. (Courtesy of Dr. Shay Lee, Los Angeles, CA.)

Patient 4: Breast Carcinoma

FIGURE 72–21 D.

Sagittal and Coronal ^{18}F-FDG Whole Body Scan: Three metastatic foci can be seen in the right superior mediastinum and hila. The smallest detectable lesion measured 5 mm on a concurrent CT scan. (Courtesy of Dr. David Lilien, Newport Beach, CA.)

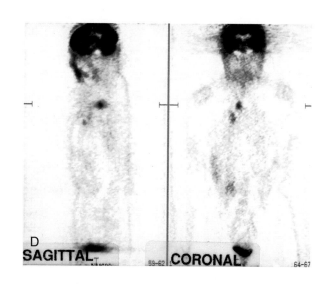

Illustration continued on following page

Patient 5: Colon Carcinoma

FIGURE 72–21   E and F.

Coronal and Transverse ^{18}F-FDG PET Scans: There are several foci of increased metabolic activity in the periphery of the right lobe of the liver. (Courtesy of Dr. Sushama Bharghava, Indianapolis, IN.)

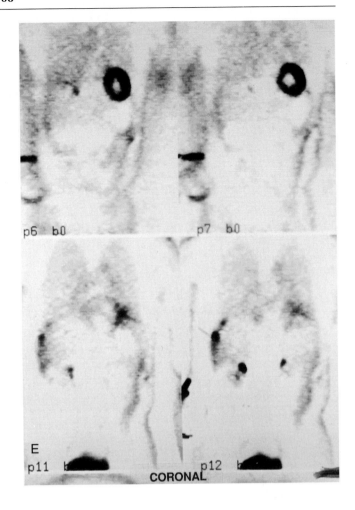

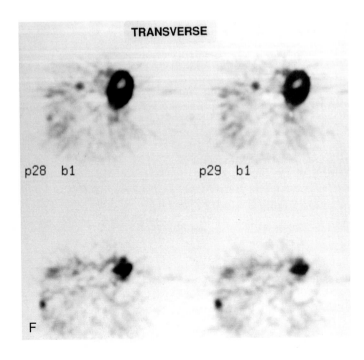

Chapter 73
Breast Diseases

NORMAL BREAST ACTIVITY WITH VARIOUS RADIOPHARMACEUTICALS

Patient 1: Postmenopausal Woman

FIGURE 73–1 A.
Bone Scintigraphy: The normal breast can be seen in both premenopausal and postmenopausal women.

Patient 2: Lactating Mother

FIGURE 73–1 B.
Anterior Bone Scan: The breasts have diffuse increased activity.

Illustration continued on following page

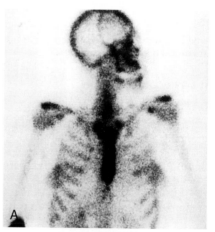

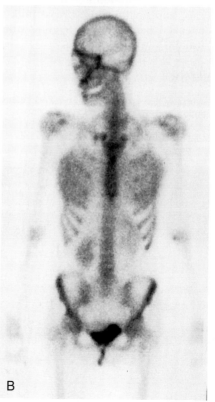

Patient 3: Normal Gallium Breast Activity

FIGURE 73–1   C and D.
Anterior and Left Lateral Gallium Scans: There is mild gallium accumulation in both breasts.

FIGURE 73–1   E.
Supine Coronal Gallium SPECT Scan: The symmetric activity overlies the inferior axillae and partially obscures the anterior lung fields.

Patient 4: Gallium Activity in Lactating Breast

FIGURE 73–1   F.
Anterior Gallium Scan: The breasts have considerable gallium accumulation.

Patient 5: Technetium Pertechnetate in the Lactating Breast

FIGURE 73–1   G.
Thyroid Scan: Technetium pertechnetate is excreted in lactating breast tissue, as is inorganic iodine.

Patient 6: Gynecomastia

FIGURE 73–1   H.
Bone Scan: The right breast activity is due, in this case, to prostate cancer therapy with diethylstilbestrol.

NOTE 1. With most technetium radiopharmaceuticals, 24 hours should elapse before breast feeding resumes, assuming normal renal functions.

NOTE 2. With ^{131}I compounds, ^{111}In radiopharmaceuticals, and gallium, the breast milk should be checked before breast feeding resumes. It is usually safe at 2 weeks.

Cross Reference

Chapter 64: Normal/Normal Variants—Free Technetium Pertechnetate Distribution

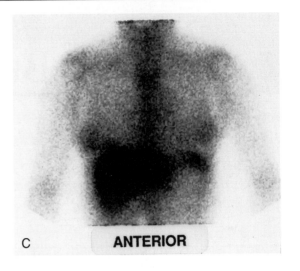

C   **ANTERIOR**

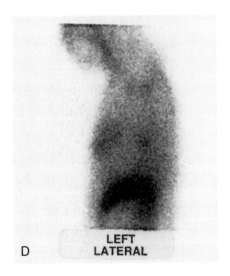

D   **LEFT LATERAL**

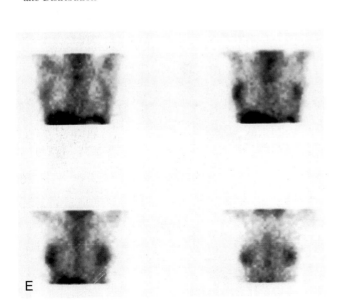

E

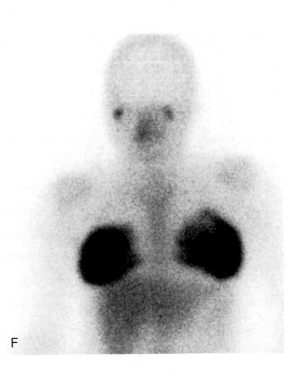

F

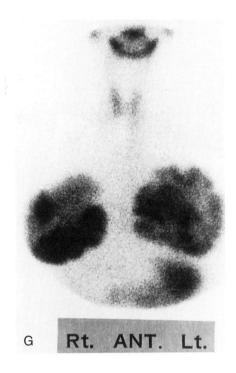

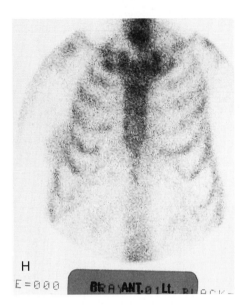

BREAST CANCER ON BONE SCAN

FIGURE 73–2.

Total Body Bone Scan: The left breast is markedly enlarged with increased accumulation of the ^{99m}Tc-MDP.

NOTE. There is no correlation between breast activity on bone scan and presence of breast carcinoma.

Illustration continued on following page

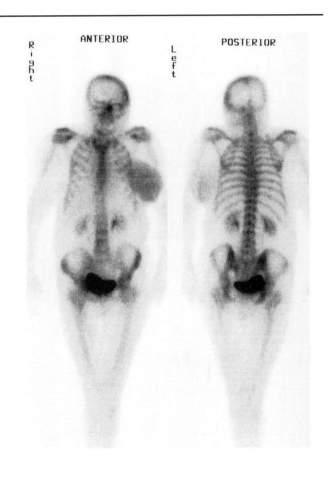

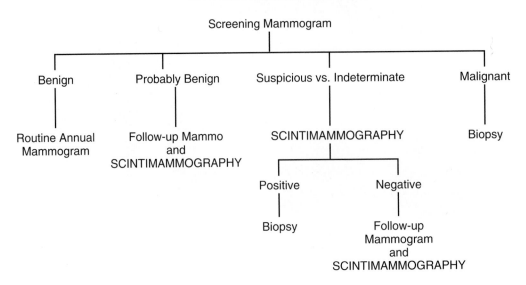

MANAGEMENT OF NONPALPABLE MASSES
WITH SCINTIMAMMOGRAPHY

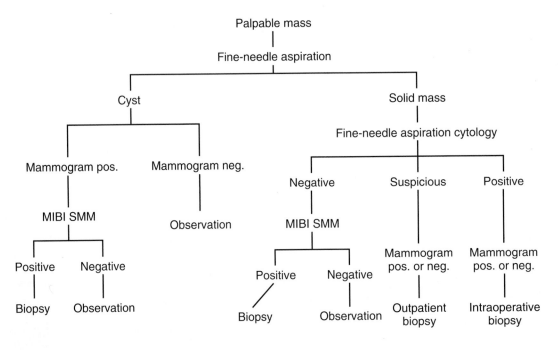

MANAGEMENT OF PALPABLE MASSES WITH SMM

SESTAMIBI SCINTIMAMMOGRAPHY

Patient 1: Normal Dense Breast

FIGURE 73–3   A.

Lateral and Posterior Oblique ^{99m}Tc-Sestamibi Breast Scans:
There is homogeneous radioactivity throughout the breasts.

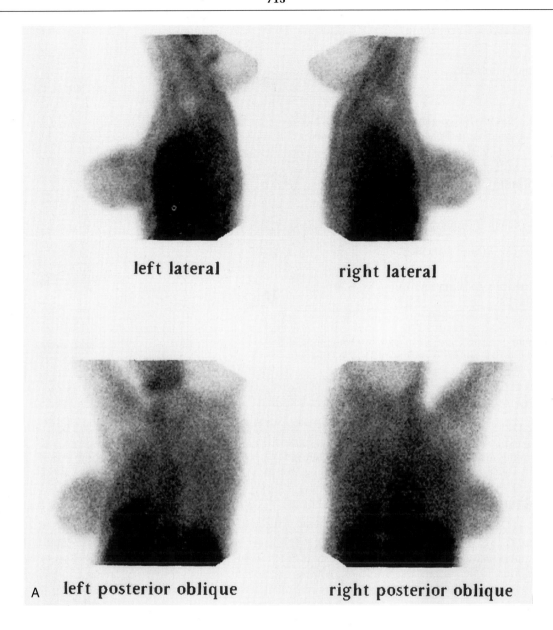

left lateral right lateral

left posterior oblique right posterior oblique

A

Patient 2: Fibroadenoma

FIGURE 73–3 B.

LPO ^{99m}Tc-Sestamibi Breast Scan: There is homogeneous activity within the breast. (Courtesy of Dr. Iraj Khalkhali, Torrance, CA.)

Illustration continued on following page

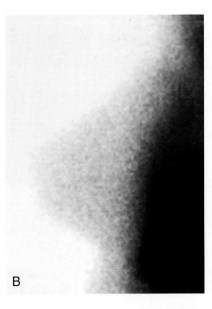

B

Patient 3: Medullary Carcinoma

FIGURE 73–3 C.

LPO [99mTc]-Sestamibi Breast Scan: An intense focus of radioactivity is present.

FIGURE 73–3 D.

Post-lumpectomy LPO [99mTc]-Sestamibi Breast Scan: The breast has no abnormal accumulation. (Courtesy of Dr. Iraj Khalkhali, Torrance, CA.)

Patient 4: Inflammatory Carcinoma

FIGURE 73–3 E.

Prone [99mTc]-Sestamibi Scintimammogram: The elongated breast cancer has metastasized to the axillary lymph nodes. (Courtesy of Dr. J.W. Birsner, Lancaster, CA.)

Patient 5: Multiple Axillary Lymph Node Metastases

FIGURE 73–3 F.

Prone [99mTc]-Sestamibi Scan: There are at least four lymph nodes involved with the breast cancer. (Courtesy of Dr. J.W. Birsner, Lancaster, CA.)

Patient 6: Five Millimeter Breast Cancer

FIGURE 73–3 G.

Prone [99mTc]-Sestamibi Scan: The tumor-to-background activity is very high, allowing small lesions to be detected. (Courtesy of Dr. J.W. Birsner, Lancaster, CA.)

Patients 7 and 8: Active Fibrocystic Disease

FIGURE 73–3 H and I.

Prone [99mTc]-Sestamibi Scans: There is an ill-defined area of abnormality in the upper outer quadrant that does not appear as intensely abnormal as the cancers. (Figure 73–3 I courtesy of Dr. J.W. Birsner, Lancaster, CA.)

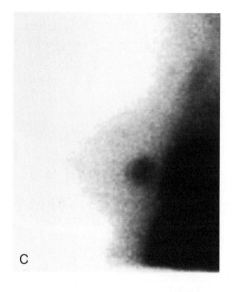

C

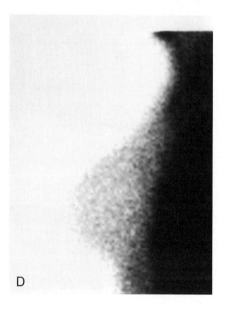

D

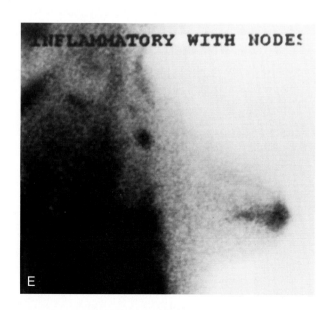

E

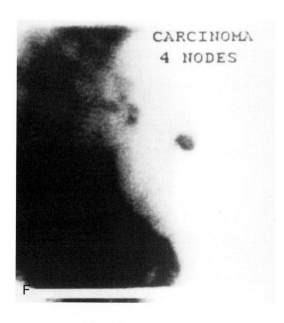

F

Patient 9: Breast Abscess

FIGURE 73–3 J.

Prone ⁹⁹ᵐTc-Sestamibi Scan: The abscess appears as a focal but ill-defined area of low-intensity uptake. (Courtesy of Dr. J.W. Birsner, Lancaster, CA.)

Patient 10: Infiltrating Ductal Carcinoma on SPECT but False Negative for Lymph Node Involvement

FIGURE 73–3 K and L.

Prone Anterior and RPO Planar ⁹⁹ᵐTc-Sestamibi Scans: There is an ill-defined linear area of sestamibi uptake in the right breast. There are no involved lymph nodes evident.

Illustration continued on following page

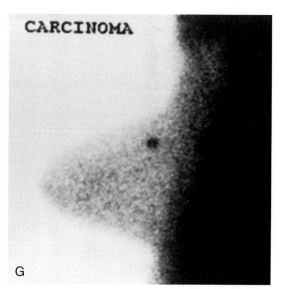

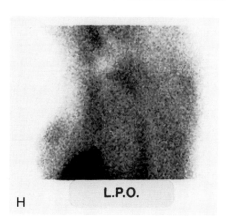

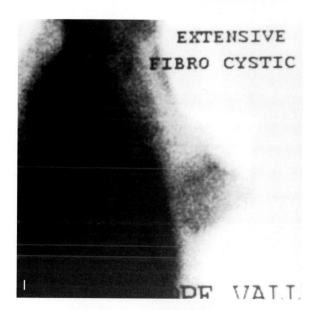

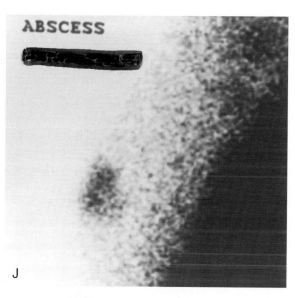

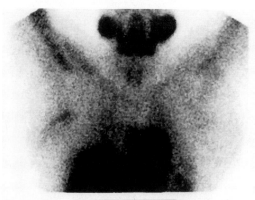

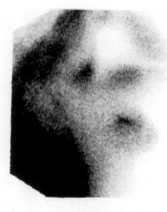

FIGURE 73–3   M to O.

Coronal, Sagittal, and Transverse Reconstructions of ^{99m}Tc-Sestamibi SPECT Scan: The breast tumor can be easily localized to the right mid-upper breast. Right axillary lymph nodes were later positive on biopsy.

Patient 11: Breast Carcinoma in Patient with Breast Implants

FIGURE 73–3   P.

Prone LPO Planar ^{99m}Tc-Sestamibi Scan: There is increased radiopharmaceutical accumulation in the superior breast above the photopenic breast implant.

FIGURE 73–3   Q.

Prone RPO Planar ^{99m}Tc-Sestamibi Scan: The right breast tissue has normal, homogeneous activity, although the breast implant is not as well visualized.

NOTE 1. SPECT scanning in scintimammography can enhance detection and localization of small tumors or metastatic lymph nodes. It may be most useful in determining the depth of the tumor.

NOTE 2. The sensitivity of sestamibi scintimammography for axillary lymph node metastases is not as high as its accuracy in detecting breast malignancies.

NOTE 3. Given the difficulty of imaging breasts with implants, as well as those that are dense on mammography, sestamibi scintimammography may be useful in high-risk patients and in those with suspicious clinical or mammographic findings.

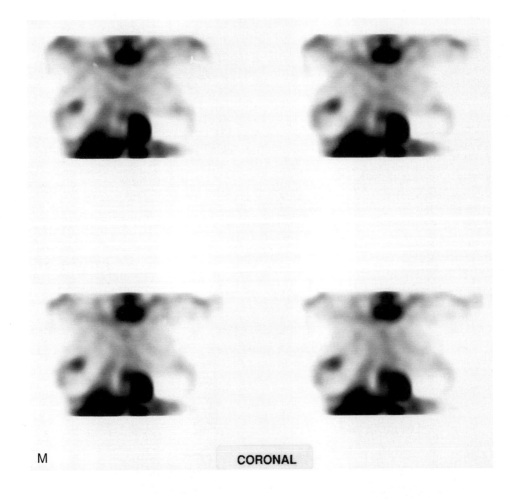

M   CORONAL

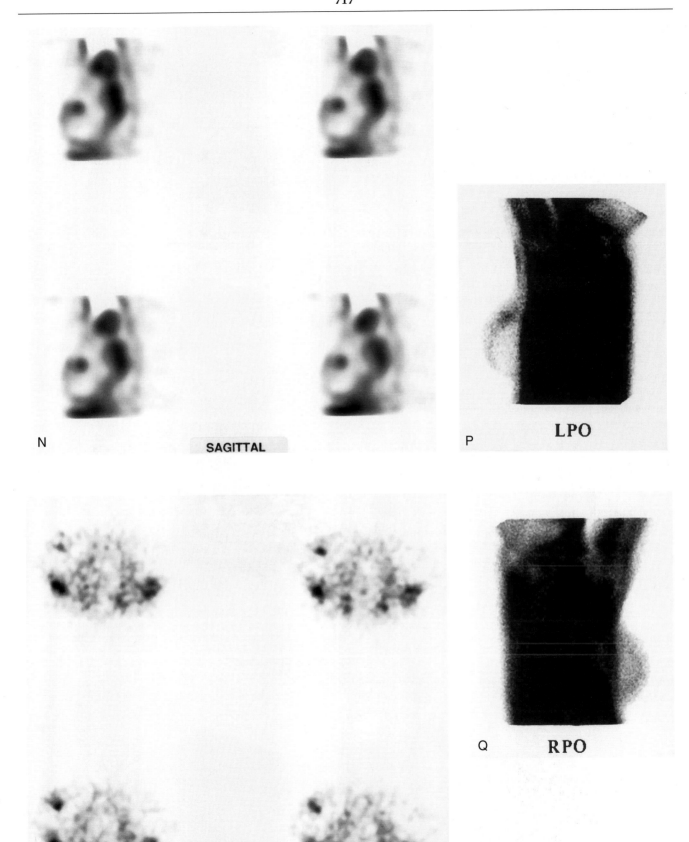

N   SAGITTAL   P   LPO

Q   RPO

O   TRANSVERSE

BILATERAL BREAST CANCER WITH BONY METASTASES WITH SESTAMIBI

FIGURE 73–4   A and B.

Right and Left Lateral Planar ^{99m}Tc-Sestamibi Breast Scan: There is a solitary abnormality in the left breast and two adjacent abnormalities in the right breast.

FIGURE 73–4   C.

Anterior, Planar, ^{99m}Tc-Sestamibi Breast Scan: The breast abnormalities can be faintly seen as well as a left axillary focus of activity.

FIGURE 73–4   D.

Posterior Planar ^{99m}Tc-Sestamibi Scan: The posterior ribs have a mottled appearance on the left, suggesting bony metastases.

FIGURE 73–4   E.

Coronal ^{99m}Tc-Sestamibi SPECT Scan: There are definite rib metastases accumulating the sestamibi.

FIGURE 73–4   F.

Coronal ^{99m}Tc-Sestamibi SPECT Scan: The left axillary lymph node(s) has marked sestamibi accumulation.

FIGURE 73–4   G and H.

Sagittal ^{99m}Tc-Sestamibi SPECT Scans: The two right breast and the solitary left breast abnormalities are clearly seen in the anterior breast.

NOTE 1. SPECT scans of the breast can be helpful in looking for bony, lung, and axillary metastases.

NOTE 2. Although it appears that there are two lesions in the right breast, the pathology demonstrated continuity between the two masses.

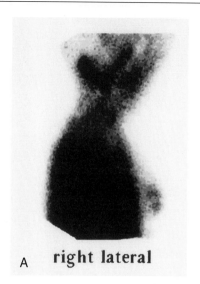

A   right lateral

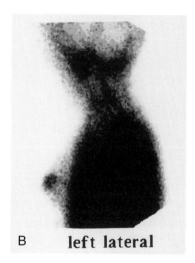

B   left lateral

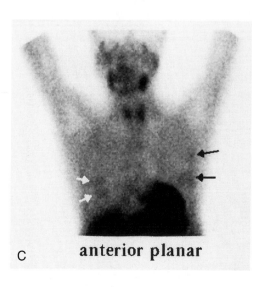

C   anterior planar

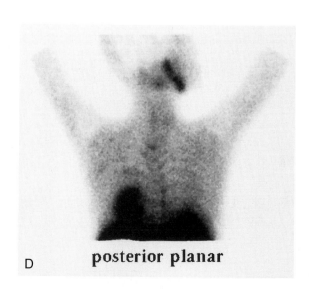

D   posterior planar

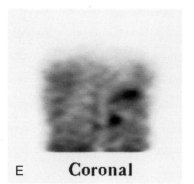

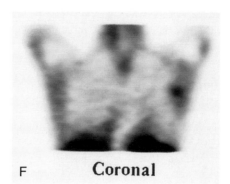

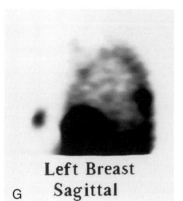

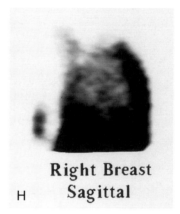

GALLIUM SCANNING IN BREAST CANCER

Patient 1: Bilateral Breast Implants with Adenocarcinoma of Breast

FIGURE 73–5 A.

Planar Anterior Chest Gallium Scan: The focus of abnormal gallium accumulation *(arrow)* is barely noticeable.

Illustration continued on following page

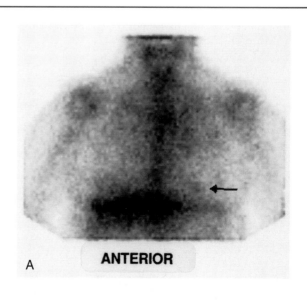

FIGURE 73–5   B and C.

Coronal and Sagittal Gallium SPECT Scans: The abnormality is clearly visible in the inferior left breast.

Patient 2: Lymphoma of Breast

FIGURE 73–5   D.

Anterior Planar Gallium Scan: There is irregular intense gallium activity in the left breast. Activity in a lymph node *(arrow)* is discernible in the left axilla.

Cross Reference

Chapter 72: Tumors—Gallium-Avid Lymphomas

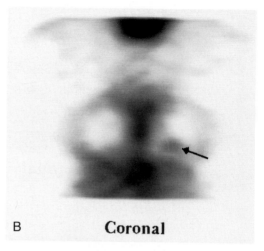

B   **Coronal**

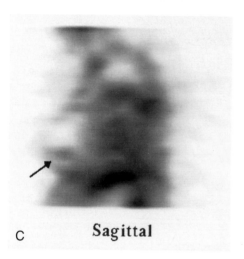

C   **Sagittal**

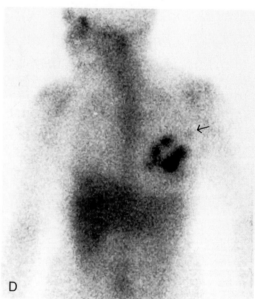

D

BREAST PROSTHESES ON BONE SCAN

FIGURE 73–6.

Anterior Bone Scan (film darkened): The prostheses attenuate the activity of the ribs.

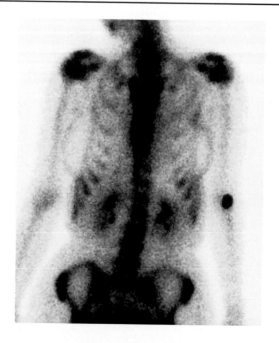

BREAST PROSTHESIS INFLAMMATION

FIGURE 73–7   A and B.

Anterior and Lateral Gallium Scan: There is abnormal gallium accumulation around the periphery of the left breast prosthesis. The right breast prosthesis is normal except for the mild attenuation *(arrowheads)*.

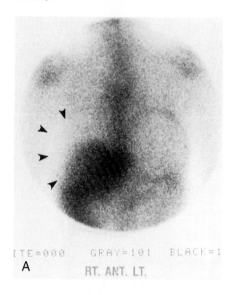

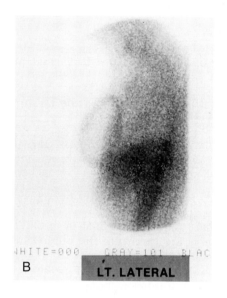

RADIONUCLIDE HYSTEROSALPINGOGRAPHY

Patient 1: Normal Fallopian Tube Function

FIGURE 73–8   A.

Contrast Hysterosalpingogram: There is bilateral spillage into the peritoneum.

Illustration continued on following page

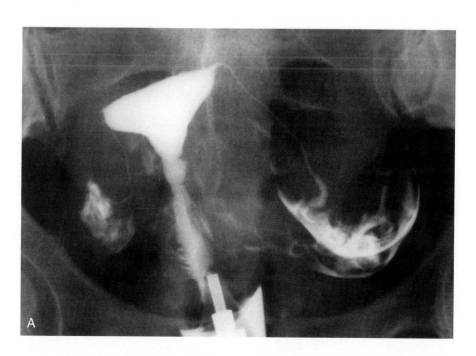

FIGURE 73–8   B.

⁹⁹ᵐTc-Macroaggregated Albumin Hysterosalpingogram: The fallopian tubes and the peritoneal spillage are evident bilaterally. (Courtesy of Drs. Thompson and M. Uszler, Santa Monica, CA.)

Patient 2: Unilateral Fallopian Tube Dysfunction

FIGURE 73–8   C.

⁹⁹ᵐTc-MAA Hysterosalpingogram: There is unilateral spillage. (Courtesy of Drs. Thompson and M. Uszler, Santa Monica, CA.)

Patient 3: Bilateral Fallopian Tube Dysfunction

FIGURE 73–8   D and E.

One Hour and 4 Hour ⁹⁹ᵐTc-MAA Hysterosalpingogram: The radioactivity remains in the uterus and never progresses out along the fallopian tubes.

NOTE. Ciliary action is essential in fertility because it carries the sperm up the uterus and fallopian tubes. Radionuclide hysterosalpingography is a technique that can directly measure ciliary function. Most other techniques determine patency but do not measure ciliary function.

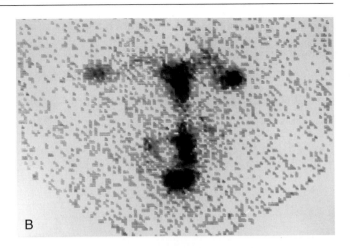

B

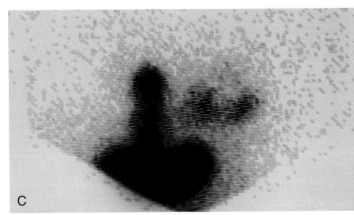

C

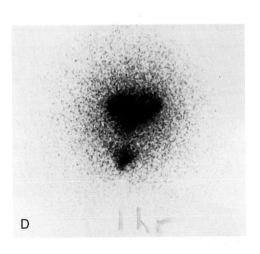

D

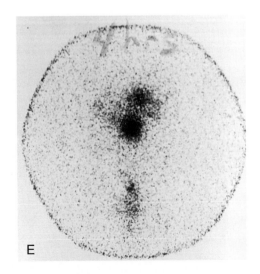

E

Index

Note: Page numbers in *italics* refer to illustrations;
page numbers followed by b refer to boxed material.

ISBN 0-7216-3578-4

90038